Contents

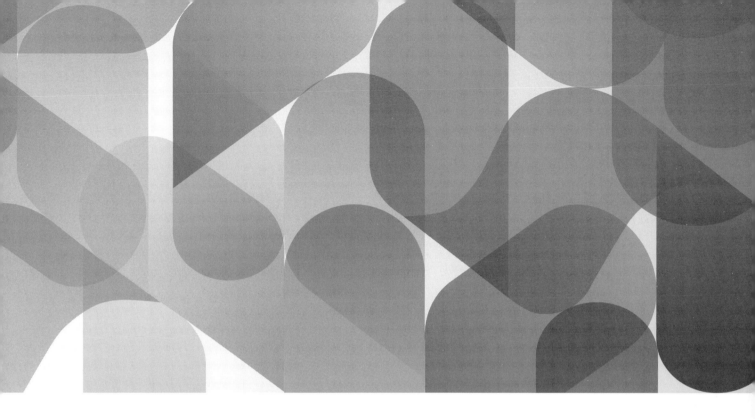

ADULT-GERONTOLOGY PRIMARY CARE NURSE PRACTITIONER

CERTIFICATION REVIEW

JoAnn Zerwekh, EdD, RN

President/CEO
Nursing Education Consultants, Inc.
Chandler, Arizona;
Director of Nursing Education
Picmonic, Inc
Tempe, Arizona;

Faculty
University of Phoenix Online
Phoenix, Arizona

ELSEVIER

ELSEVIER

3251 Riverport Lane
St. Louis, Missouri 63043

ADULT-GERONTOLOGY PRIMARY CARE NURSE
PRACTITIONER CERTIFICATION REVIEW   ISBN: 978-0-323-53198-6

Notices

Knowledge and best practice in this field are constantly changing. As new research and experience broaden our understanding, changes in research methods, professional practices, or medical treatment may become necessary.

Practitioners and researchers must always rely on their own experience and knowledge in evaluating and using any information, methods, compounds, or experiments described herein. In using such information or methods they should be mindful of their own safety and the safety of others, including parties for whom they have a professional responsibility.

With respect to any drug or pharmaceutical products identified, readers are advised to check the most current information provided (i) on procedures featured or (ii) by the manufacturer of each product to be administered, to verify the recommended dose or formula, the method and duration of administration, and contraindications. It is the responsibility of practitioners, relying on their own experience and knowledge of their patients, to make diagnoses, to determine dosages and the best treatment for each individual patient, and to take all appropriate safety precautions.

To the fullest extent of the law, neither the Publisher nor the authors, contributors, or editors, assume any liability for any injury and/or damage to persons or property as a matter of products liability, negligence or otherwise, or from any use or operation of any methods, products, instructions, or ideas contained in the material herein.

Library of Congress Cataloging-in-Publication Data

Names: Zerwekh, JoAnn Graham, author.
Title: Adult-gerontology primary care nurse practitioner certification review
    / JoAnn Zerwekh.
Description: St. Louis, Missouri : Elsevier, [2019] | Includes index.
Identifiers: LCCN 2017041739 | ISBN 9780323531986 (pbk. : alk. paper)
Subjects: | MESH: Nursing Care | Nurse Practitioners | Advanced Practice
    Nursing | Geriatric Nursing | Test Taking Skills | Certification |
    Examination Questions
Classification: LCC RC954 | NLM WY 18.2 | DDC 618.97/0231076--dc23 LC record
available at https://lccn.loc.gov/2017041739

Executive Content Strategist: Lee Henderson
Director, Content Development: Laurie Gower
Associate Content Development Specialist: Elizabeth Kilgore
Publishing Services Manager: Jeff Patterson
Project Manager: Lisa A. P. Bushey
Design Direction: Brian Salisbury

Printed in the United States of America

Last digit is the print number: 9 8 7 6 5 4 3 2 1

  Working together to grow libraries in developing countries

www.elsevier.com • www.bookaid.org

About the Author

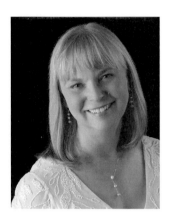

JoAnn Zerwekh has worked as a family nurse practitioner at Carondelet Health Care primary health care clinics in southern Arizona. She taught FNP students at the University of Phoenix and worked for a brief period of time as the advance practice consultant for the Arizona Board of Nursing. She is the author of numerous publications, including *Nursing Today: Transition & Trends, Illustrated Study Guides for the NCLEX-RN* and *PN* review books, and the popular *Memory Notecards of Nursing* and *Memory Notebooks of Nursing*. She is the President/CEO of Nursing Education Consultants and is the Director of Nursing Education for Picmonic, the visual learning community for nursing and medical students.

Contributors

WENDY L. BIDDLE, PHD, MSN, RN, FNP-BC
Program Director, MSN to FNP
South University;
Nurse Practitioner
Gastroenterology LTD
Virginia Beach, Virginia

JANEEN DAHN, PHD, FNP-C
Associate Director, Complaints and Investigations
Arizona State Board of Nursing
Chandler, Arizona;
Faculty
School of Nursing
University of Phoenix
Phoenix, Arizona;
Faculty
School of Nursing
Simmons University
Boston, Massachusetts;
Faculty
School of Nursing
Keiser
Fort Lauderdale, Florida

ASHLEY GARNEAU, PHD, RN
Faculty
Nursing Division
GateWay Community College
Phoenix, Arizona

MELLISA A. HALL, DNP, AGPCNP-BC, FNP-BC
Associate Professor
College of Nursing
University of Southern Indiana
Evansville, Indiana

THERESA J. FRIMEL, FNP-C
Provider
Arthritis Health Limited; Rheumatology
Scottsdale, Arizona

PETER G. MELENOVICH, PHD, RN, CNE
Faculty
Nursing Division
GateWay Community College
Phoenix, Arizona

LAURA PACHELLA, RN, MSN, AGPCNP-BC, AOCNP
Advanced Practice Registered Nurse
Thoracic and Cardiovascular Surgery
The University of Texas MD Anderson Cancer Center
Houston, Texas

RICHARD MATTHEW PRIOR, DNP, FNP-BC, FAANP
Associate Professor
College of Nursing
University of Cincinnati
Cincinnati, Ohio

KATHLEEN REEVE, DRPH, MSN, APRN, ANP-BC, FNP-C
Associate Dean
College of Nursing
University of Houston
Houston, Texas

MARYLOU ROBINSON, PHD, FNP-C
Associate Professor
School of Nursing
Pacific Lutheran University
Tacoma, Washington

ARTHUR ROTHSTEIN, MSN, FNP-C, AGACNP-BC
NextCare Urgent Care;
St. Joseph's Hospital Emergency Department
Phoenix, Arizona

DARYLE WANE, PHD, ARNP, FNP-BC
Nursing Program Director
Professor of Nursing BSN Faculty
Department of Nursing and Health Programs
Pasco-Hernando State College
New Port Richey, Florida

ERICH WIDEMARK, PHD, MSN, RN, FNP-BC
Curriculum and Instruction Developer
Chamberlain University, College of Nursing
Downers Grove, Illinois

Reviewers

DIANE DADDARIO, MSN, ANP-C, ACNS-BC, RN-BC, CMSRN
Adjunct Faculty, RN to BSN Program
Pennsylvania State University
University Park, Pennsylvania

WM. KENDALL WYATT, MD, RN, EMTP
Internal Medicine Resident Physician
West Virginia University
Charleston Area Medical Center
Charleston, West Virginia

Preface

With the proliferation of new DNP programs, there is an increasing need for additional reference information and study materials for the certification examinations. Nurse practitioners are playing a vital role in the health care delivery system in the United States. With the assistance of certified nurse practitioners and my editorial expertise in test item writing, the *Adult-Gerontology Primary Care Nurse Practitioner Certification Review* has been developed to assist the advanced practice nurse to prepare for the certification exam that tests clinical knowledge of young adults (including adolescents and emancipated minors), adults, and older adults (including young-old, middle-old, and oldest-old adults). Extensive efforts have been made to include current information that is representative of the content, based on the blueprints for both certification exams. This book of test questions is not intended to be an exhaustive review of the content but an adjunct to the review process.

Test-taking strategies are included in Chapter 1. As a candidate prepares for the exam, it is vitally important to be familiar with and to practice good testing strategies. Testing strategies can prevent the candidate from making mistakes and selecting the wrong answer. As the review process begins, a review of the test-taking strategies chapter and the practice of good testing strategies is critical. With many years of experience in the field of testing, I consistently have identified the importance that practice testing plays in the review process. Practice questions give the candidate an opportunity to review questions written from different perspectives. To enhance the review process, answers with complete rationales are provided at the end of each chapter. A bibliography of references list is provided. Not only does the candidate increase his/her knowledge of the subject area, but also, with more practice, testing skills become fine-tuned. Good testing skills make the candidate more comfortable and help decrease the stress associated with certification exams.

This book also includes chapters reviewing important concepts related to Growth & Development and Health Promotion & Maintenance. These chapters provide questions that test information related to growth and development, general health supervision, and health maintenance. The clinical chapters are developed using a systems approach (i.e., cardiovascular, respiratory, endocrine, etc.), including mental health. In each of these chapters, the test questions are divided into three areas: Physical Examination & Diagnostic Tests, Disorders, and Pharmacology. This format assists the candidate to easily locate specific questions. The last two chapters in the text are on Research & Theory and Professional Issues. The test questions in these chapters focus on professional competencies inherent in the role and function of the adult-gerontology primary care nurse practitioner.

My thanks to the many nurse practitioners across the country who provided questions and insight into the role of the nurse practitioner. I wish to thank Liz Kilgore, my editor at Elsevier, for her support and suggestions in the preparation of the manuscript. Thank you also goes to the nurse practitioners who took time from their busy schedules to review the questions for content correctness and clarity.

Acknowledgments

I want to express my appreciation to Lee Henderson at Elsevier and his "can-do" attitude that made the realization of this new adult gerontology primary care nurse practitioner edition possible.

I am especially grateful to the many people at Elsevier who assisted with this major revision effort, including the folks who have assisted with the online test bank and the alternate item formats. In particular, I want to thank Liz Kilgore in Content, Lisa Bushey in Production, Kristen Oyirifi in Marketing, and Brian Salisbury in Design.

I want to thank the contributors and reviewers for their assistance in the revision process. Your current practice and clinical expertise is surely noted in your contribution to updating this edition.

I am particularly appreciative to the many nurse practitioners who used the previous editions to pass their certification exams and faculty who have requested a new edition of this test question review book.

And lastly, I want to thank my husband, John Masog, for his tolerance and sense of humor as I continued to work on a revision of another book! Thank you so much for the awesome meals you prepare for us and snatching me away from the computer for a round of golf—I appreciate the balance you bring to my life.

A special note to my amazing grandchildren (Maddie and Harper Zerwekh; Ben Garneau; Brooklyn Parks; and Owen and Emmett Masog) who have such bright futures; you always put a smile on Grandma's face and make her proud.

Contents

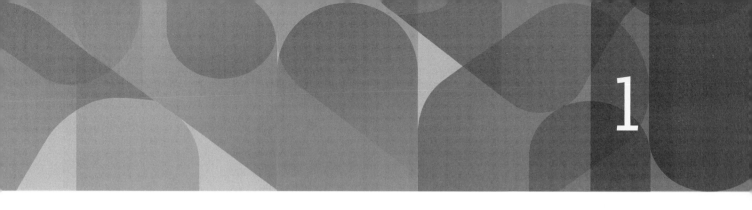

Test-Taking Strategies

Certification Exam Information

For the adult-gerontology primary care nurse practitioner certification exam, there are two credentialing bodies, the American Nurses Credentialing Center (ANCC) and the American Academy of Nurse Practitioners Certification Board (AANPCB). Both groups provide detailed information in handbooks available for download at their respective websites. This information includes the application process, testing procedure, test content outline, bibliography of references, and other relevant information for the exam candidate. Certification from both agencies is recognized by the U.S. Department of Veterans Affairs, Centers for Medicare & Medicaid (CMS), health insurance companies, the National Council State Boards of Nursing (NCSBN), and state boards of nursing. Both exams are computer based, and the candidate will schedule the exam at a designated testing center.

ANCC

The ANCC certification exam consists of multiple-choice test questions, drag and drop (ordered response or a proper sequence), hot spot (click on a particular feature or area of a graphic image), and multiple responses (asked to select a specific number of correct responses). There are a total of 200 questions on the adult-gerontology primary care nurse practitioner exam with 175 items scored and 25 pilot test items that do not count toward the final score. The passing score is a scale score of 350 or higher. The raw score (number of test items answered correctly, for example, 122 out of 175) is converted to a scale score using a conversion formula before the results are given to the exam candidate at the testing site. Candidates who successfully complete the ANCC certification exam may use the credential Adult-Gerontology Primary Care Nurse Practitioner-Board Certified (AGPCNP-BC).

AANPCB

Each AANPCB exam consists of 150 multiple-choice questions (135 test items are scored and 15 pretest items are not counted in the final score). A "preliminary" exam score is provided to the candidate at the completion of the exam. The scaled score ranges from 200 to 800 points, with a minimum passing score of 500.

Candidates who successfully complete the AANPCB certification exam may use the credential Nurse Practitioner-Certified (NP-C). Using a letter before (A-G for adult-gerontology) indicates a population specialty and may precede the NP-C credential. Use of these initials (AGNP-C), however, depends upon individual, state board of nursing, and/or employer preference.

Testing Strategies

Knowing how to take an exam is a skill that is developed through practice and experience. Being able to take an exam effectively is almost as important as the basic knowledge required to answer the question. Everyone has taken an exam only to find in the review of the exam that questions were missed because of inadequate testing skills.

Nurse practitioner programs provide the graduate student with a comprehensive base of knowledge; how you utilize this knowledge will determine your success on a certification exam. The certification exam is an objective test that covers knowledge, understanding, and application of professional nursing theory and practice.

Read the information in this chapter carefully and make sure you understand the strategies discussed. This chapter is designed to help you identify problem areas in testing skills and learn how to use strategy and judgment in selecting correct answers. It is important for you to practice testing skills if you are going to be able to utilize these skills on the certification exam.

1. **Do not read extra meaning into the question.** The question is asking for specific information; if it appears to be simple "common sense," then assume it is simple. Do not look for a hidden meaning in what appears to be an easy question.

> **EXAMPLE**
>
> The adult-gerontology primary care nurse practitioner (NP) understands that the most common form of facial paralysis in the adult patient is:
> 1. Facial nerve fasciitis.
> 2. Trigeminal neuralgia.
> 3. Bell palsy.
> 4. Herpes zoster.

The correct answer is Option #3. Be careful not to "read into" the question and add pain to the facial paralysis symptom. Instead, concentrate on the question's key words, "the most common form of facial paralysis," which is Bell palsy, a disorder that affects the facial nerve and is characterized by muscle flaccidity of the affected side of the face. Trigeminal neuralgia is a disorder of cranial nerve V that is characterized by an abrupt onset of pain in the lower and upper jaw, cheek, and lips. Herpes zoster affects the dermatomes and does not cause a paralysis, but rather pain, herpetic grouped skin vesicles, and possibly postherpetic neuralgia.

2. **Read the stem correctly.** Make sure you understand exactly what information the question is asking. It is important to understand the question before reviewing the options for the correct answer.

EXAMPLE

Cardiac auscultation of an older patient reveals a grade II/VI murmur that is heard best at the right second intercostal space. The murmur is louder with squatting. There is a small carotid pulse with a delayed upstroke. The patient's history is benign, and his activity tolerance is within normal limits for his age. The adult-gerontology primary care NP would interpret this murmur to be indicative of:
  1. Aortic regurgitation.
  2. Aortic stenosis.
  3. Mitral valve prolapse.
  4. Mitral regurgitation.

The test question asks you to determine what type of murmur based on a description of the assessment findings. When there is considerable assessment data presented, go back and reread the test question. In this instance, the assessment is consistent with aortic stenosis (correct answer Option #2). Aortic regurgitation is a diastolic murmur secondary to rheumatic heart disease, for which no history is given. Mitral valve disease is one of the most common valvular disorders. A small percentage of patients who have a mitral valve prolapse do experience autonomic dysfunction and complain of palpitations, atypical chest pain, orthostatic dizziness, near-syncope, cold extremities, throbbing headaches, and neurasthenia, and manifest tachydysrhythmias. Patients who have mitral regurgitation may remain asymptomatic for many years because the left ventricle dilates and adjusts well to the increase in volume load. Onset of dyspnea and fatigue may not occur for decades.

3. **Before considering the options, think about the characteristics of this condition and the critical concepts to consider.** Begin by assessing each option with regard to the concepts of the condition.

EXAMPLE

What therapeutic treatment option would be prescribed by the adult-gerontology primary care NP for an older adult patient who presents with several skin tears with no other contributory findings on physical examination?
  1. Diuretic therapy to prevent fluid accumulation.
  2. Use of topical emollients to hydrate skin.
  3. Baby aspirin to prevent cardiovascular disease.
  4. Antibiotic to prevent infection.

The correct answer is Option #2. Formulate in your mind critical information for the care of this patient. Think to yourself, "what are treatment options for skin tears?" Skin tears are seen in the older adult population and therapeutic treatment should focus on maintaining hydration of the skin. Diuretic therapy could lead to dehydration. Baby aspirin therapy is unrelated to the appearance of skin tears. Antibiotic therapy would only be used if infection was suspected or identified upon examination.

4. **Identify what type of response the question is asking.** A positive stem requires identification of three false items and one correct answer.

EXAMPLE

How soon after exposure is the earliest that patients who believe they have been exposed to human immunodeficiency virus (HIV) can have an HIV antibody test?
  1. The next day and 2 months later.
  2. 6 months after exposure and again at 12 months.
  3. 3–12 weeks after exposure and again at 3 months.
  4. 4 weeks and 12 weeks later.

The correct answer is Option #3. This question requires you to identify three incorrect responses and one correct response. The HIV antibody develops between 3 and 12 weeks after exposure. Because of the variability of antibody development, it is recommended that the test be repeated in 3 months to confirm the findings.

5. **Identify questions that require identification of something the adult-gerontology primary care NP should not or would not do** (that is, an unsafe action, contraindication, or inappropriate action).

EXAMPLE

An older adult patient is diagnosed with chronic open-angle glaucoma. The patient has a past history of bradycardia and first-degree atrioventricular block. In consideration of her treatment, what medication is to be avoided?
  1. Pilocarpine (Isopto Carpine).
  2. Timolol (Timoptic).
  3. Hydrochlorothiazide (HydroDiuril).
  4. Acetazolamide (Diamox).

The correct answer is Option #2. Topical beta blockers, such as timolol, lower intraocular pressure but can be absorbed systemically. The major side effects are similar to those associated with systemic beta-blocker therapy, which can include a worsening of heart failure, bradycardia, and heart block. Topical beta blockers are contraindicated in some patients who have cardiac or pulmonary disease.

6. **Questions may also be analytical.** These questions may ask the adult-gerontology primary care NP to identify findings and statements that are consistent or inconsistent with the patient's presenting problem, and/or differentiate between them.

EXAMPLE

An older adult patient is experiencing a recent onset of confusion. The adult-gerontology primary care NP is trying to determine whether the confusion is related to depression or dementia. In evaluating the patient, what specific assessment finding would be helpful in making this distinction?

1. Determining whether confusion worsens in the evening.
2. Assessing early morning agitation, hyperactivity, and insomnia.
3. Noting signs of anger, hostility, and loss of control.
4. Assessing reality distortions and preoccupation with family matters.

Before you examine the options in this question, it is important to think about the differences between confusion found in dementia and depression. The correct answer is Option #1. Confusion can occur in both dementia and depression. However, with dementia, symptoms worsen at night and are commonly referred to as sundowning. Additionally, the adult-gerontology primary care NP must also ensure that the increased confusion is not a result of an acute illness. Often the only sign or symptom the older adult may present with is confusion. Usually the culprit is a urinary tract infection. The adult-gerontology primary care NP should order a urine analysis (UA) to ensure that the confusion is not the result of an acute illness and is reversible.

7. **Identify key words that affect your understanding of the question.** Make sure you understand exactly what information the question is asking. Be aware of questions in the stem such as *except, contraindicated, avoid, least, not applicable,* and *does not occur.* These words change the direction of the question. It may help to rephrase the question in your own words to better understand what information is being requested.

EXAMPLE

A patient complains of intolerable itching in the pubic hair. On exam, the adult-gerontology primary care NP notes erythematous papules and tiny white specks in the pubic hair. The differential diagnosis includes all except:

1. Pediculosis pubis.
2. Scabies.
3. Impetigo.
4. Atopic dermatitis.

Rephrase the question and look for the three conditions associated with itching, "What are the three differential diagnoses for pruritus or itching in the pubic hair?" Intense itching is characteristic of pediculosis pubis, scabies, and atopic dermatitis. Impetigo starts out as a tender erythematous papule and progresses through a vesicular to a honey-crusted stage with no itching. The correct answer is Option #3, because impetigo is not in the differential diagnosis with conditions that are characterized by itching.

8. **As you read the options, eliminate the options you know are not correct.** This will help narrow the field of choice. When you select an answer or eliminate a distracter, you should have a specific reason for doing so. Do not try to predict a correct answer; it is distressing if the answer you want is not a selection.

EXAMPLE

An adult patient complains of knee pain while kneeling and a "clicking" noise when walking up steps. On exam, there is a slight knee effusion and tenderness when palpating the patella against the condyles. The diagnosis for this patient is:

1. Anterior cruciate tear. *(No, the patient generally cannot bear weight on the extremity without it buckling or giving way.)*
2. Dislocated patella. *(No, there would be considerable effusion and locking of the knee in flexion.)*
3. Chondromalacia patella. *(Yes, there is clicking and anterior knee pain around or under the kneecap, aggravated by knee extensor stress.)*
4. Patellar tendonitis. *(No, there would be no clicking sound with movement.)*

After systematically evaluating the options, Option #3 is the correct answer.

9. **Identify similarities in the distracters.** Frequently, three distracters will contain similar information, and one will be different. The different one may be the correct answer.

EXAMPLE

An older adult patient is encouraged to increase protein intake. The addition of which of these foods to 100 mL of milk will provide the greatest amount of protein?

1. 50 mL of light cream and 2 tbsp of corn syrup.
2. 30 g of powdered skim milk and 1 egg.
3. 1 small scoop (90 g) of ice cream and 1 tbsp of chocolate syrup.
4. 2 egg yolks and 1 tbsp of sugar.

Options #1, #3, and #4 all contain a simple sugar. The correct answer, Option #2, has the greatest amount of protein. Notice that three of the options are similar and the one that is different is the correct answer. This strategy is not a substitute for basic knowledge but may help you figure out the answer.

10. **Select the most comprehensive answer.** All options may be correct, but one will include the other three options or will need to be considered first.

EXAMPLE

The adult-gerontology primary care NP is planning to teach a client with newly diagnosed diabetes about his condition. Before the adult-gerontology primary care NP provides instruction, what is most important to evaluate? The patient's:

1. Required dietary modifications.
2. Understanding of carbohydrate counting.
3. Ability to administer insulin.
4. Present understanding of diabetes.

Options #1, #2, and #3 are certainly important considerations in diabetic education. However, they cannot be initiated until the adult-gerontology primary care NP evaluates the patient's knowledge of his or her disease state, which is the reason that Option #4 is the correct answer. When two options appear to say the same thing, only in different words, then look for another answer; that is, eliminate the options that you know are incorrect. Options #1 and #2 both refer to the client's understanding of nutrition.

11. **Select the best answer that is most specific to what the question asks.** All options may be correct, but one is more specific or essential to the question being asked.

EXAMPLE

An adult-gerontology primary care NP is reviewing a 72-year-old patient's history in the clinical setting. Which finding, if noted, requires a priority action in terms of health promotion and maintenance?
1. Patent is not current for flu vaccination.
2. Smoking history of 1 pack per day (PPD) for 10 years but has not smoked for 30 years.
3. Patient wears glasses for reading.
4. History of osteoarthritis bilaterally in knees.

Option #1 is the correct answer. The question is focusing on a priority action related to health promotion and maintenance. When reviewing an older patient's history in the clinical setting, it is important to assess whether the patient is current (up-to-date) with immunizations. Older patients are especially susceptible to seasonal flu, which may end up compromising their health. Past smoking history, even with a recorded PPD is not a priority assessment if it has been 30 years since active smoking. The fact that a patient wears reading glasses does not require a priority action. Similarly, a history of osteoarthritis does not require a priority action unless there are known deficits related to ambulation and/or increases in pain.

12. **Watch questions in which the options contain several items to consider.** After you are sure you understand what information the question is requesting, evaluate each part of the option. Is it appropriate to what the question is asking? If an option contains one incorrect item, the entire option is incorrect. All items listed in the selection must be correct if the option is to be the answer to the question.

EXAMPLE

Which diagnostic tests are typically abnormal when ruling in systemic lupus erythematosus (SLE) as a differential diagnosis?
1. Complete blood count (CBC), electrolyte panel, and erythrocyte sedimentation rate (ESR).
2. Chest x-ray and coagulation profile.
3. Antinuclear antibodies (ANA), ESR, and C-reactive protein.
4. CBC, urinalysis (UA), and chest x-ray.

The correct answer is Option #3. In a methodical evaluation of the diagnostic tests in the options, you can eliminate Options #1, #2, and #4. Although all tests included in the answer may be included in a complete physical exam, the laboratory test specific to the diagnosis of SLE includes the ANA, ESR, and C-reactive protein. During flares, ESR and C-reactive protein are elevated. The ANA titer in a patient with SLE is positive at a 1:80 ratio.

13. **Be alert to relevant information contained in previous questions.** Sometimes as you are answering questions, you will find information similar to the question being tested. Previous questions may assist you in identifying relevant information in the current question. This strategy is particularly helpful when the student is answering paper-and-pencil tests.

EXAMPLE

The Advisory Committee of Immunization Practices (ACIP) recommends that healthy older adults receive the Tdap vaccination:
1. Every 5 years.
2. At age 75.
3. At age 65.
4. Every 10 years.

The correct answer to this question is Option #3. On February 22, 2012, ACIP approved the use of Tdap for all adults aged 65 years and older. Boostrix should be used for adults aged 65 years and older; however, ACIP concluded that either vaccine (Boostrix or Adacel) administered to a person 65 years or older is immunogenic and would provide protection. In another question involving immunizations, you read the following question (See next example.):

EXAMPLE

In taking the history of an alert older adult, the adult-gerontology primary care NP determines the patient is an avid gardener and spends much time outside. The patient had a pneumococcal vaccination last year but cannot remember whether a tetanus vaccination was ever administered. A health maintenance recommendation for this patient would be to obtain:
1. Pneumococcal vaccine.
2. Tdap/Td vaccine.
3. Hepatitis B vaccine.
4. No recommendation.

The correct answer is Option #2. A clue to the correct answer may be found in the previous question. Older adults who enjoy gardening and outdoor activities should have a Tdap/Td booster once, as recommended by the ACIP. As part of standard wound management care to prevent tetanus, a tetanus toxoid–containing vaccine might be recommended for wound management in adults aged 19 years and older if 5 years or more have elapsed since last receiving the vaccine. If a tetanus booster is indicated, Tdap is preferred over Td for wound management in adults aged 19 years and older who have not received Tdap previously.

When you are taking the test on a computer, it is more difficult to remember previous questions because you may not be able to go back and change answers or review previous questions; therefore, this strategy is often most helpful for those students taking paper-and-pencil tests.

14. **Multiple-choice mathematical computations may be included in the exam.** Mathematical computations may include calculations of IM, PO, and IV dosages; determining creatinine clearance; and conversion of units of measurement.

EXAMPLE

The adult-gerontology primary care NP is calculating the creatinine clearance on an 80-year-old male patient. The patient's weight is 172 pounds. What is the patient's creatinine clearance?
1. 27 mL/min.
2. 57 mL/min.
3. 127 mL/min.
4. 1 mL/min.

The correct answer is Option #1. Using the Cockcroft-Gault formula for calculating creatinine clearance in a male patient, the value is calculated as 140 minus the patient's age in years times their weight in kilograms (times 0.85 for women), divided by 72 times the serum creatinine level in mg/dL.

Note: According to the National Kidney Foundation, the formula is not adjusted for body surface area. Because of this, the formula is no longer recommended for clinical use, as it has not been expressed using standardized creatinine values. However, for purposes of calculation practice, it is being provided in this example.

$$\text{Men}: \text{Creatinine clearance} = \frac{\text{Weight(kg}^*) \times (140 - \text{Age in years})}{72 \times \text{Serum creatinine (mg/dL)}}$$

*The patient's weight is 172 pounds, which is approximately 78 kg. The creatinine clearance is

$$\frac{78 \text{ kg} \times (140 - 80)}{72 \times 2.4 \text{ mg/dL}} = \frac{4680}{172.8} = 27.08 \text{ mL/min}$$

The normal range is 97–137 mL/min for men and 88–128 mL/min for women, which indicates that this patient does not have a healthy creatinine clearance. Here is a Medscape link with a calculator for creatinine clearance: http://reference.medscape.com/calculator/creatinine-clearance-cockcroft-gault

Another calculation example is as follows:

The adult-gerontology primary care NP writes the following prescription. How many days will the capsules last?

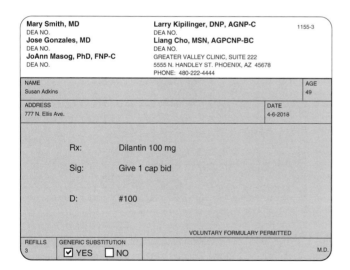

Mary Smith, MD	Larry Kipilinger, DNP, AGNP-C	1155-3
DEA NO.	DEA NO.	
Jose Gonzales, MD	Liang Cho, MSN, AGPCNP-BC	
DEA NO.	DEA NO.	
JoAnn Masog, PhD, FNP-C	GREATER VALLEY CLINIC, SUITE 222	
DEA NO.	5555 N. HANDLEY ST. PHOENIX, AZ 45678	
	PHONE: 480-222-4444	

| NAME | | AGE |
| Susan Adkins | | 49 |

| ADDRESS | DATE |
| 777 N. Ellis Ave. | 4-6-2018 |

Rx: Dilantin 100 mg

Sig: Give 1 cap bid

D: #100

VOLUNTARY FORMULARY PERMITTED

| REFILLS | GENERIC SUBSTITUTION | |
| 3 | ☑ YES ☐ NO | M.D. |

1. 20 days.
2. 40 days.
3. 50 days.
4. 100 days.

The correct answer is Option #3, which is 50 days. The number of days' supply can be calculated by dividing the number of capsules dispensed by the number of capsules used per day.

100 caps/2 caps per day = 50 days

15. **Evaluate priority questions carefully.** Frequently, all answers are appropriate to the situation. You need to decide which actions you should do first.

While hiking in a rural area, a young adult was bitten on the hand by a raccoon. At the rural clinic, the adult-gerontology primary care NP cleansed the wound. The next action is:

1. Administer tetanus antitoxin.
2. Contact local animal control authorities.
3. Administer rabies immune globulin (RIG) and human diploid cell vaccine (HDCV).
4. Teach the patient how to do hourly soaks to the hand using normal saline and peroxide.

The correct answer is Option #3. Any type of animal bite that might be associated with an animal that may harbor rabies (skunks, bats, raccoons, foxes, coyotes, rats) should be treated with both active and passive rabies immunization. The priority action is to prevent rabies. Tetanus antitoxin would be indicated if the young adult was not current on the immunization. Animal authorities would be called after the initial treatment to locate the animal and kill it if found, so that the brain can be examined for rabies.

Techniques to Increase Critical Thinking Skills

Memory aids and Mindmapping™ are tools that assist in drawing associations from other ideas with the use of visual images. **Mnemonics** are words, phrases, or other techniques that help you remember information. **Imagery** is a tool that helps you identify a problem and visualize a mental picture. Learning content that uses these techniques will assist you to recall information more effectively.

Mindmapping™ is a method of organizing important information that is in sharp contrast to the traditional outline format. A thought or concept is written in the center of the page, and images and color are added to information as ideas begin to flow from the center focus (see **Fig. 1.1**).

Acronyms help you recall specific information through word associations or letter arrangements. Examples of these are the "6-Ps" of dyspnea (see **Fig. 1.2**), the "6-Ps" of circulatory assessment (see **Fig. 1.3**), and the "ABCDE" of malignant melanoma (see **Fig. 1.4**).

Acrostics are catchy phrases in which the first letter of each word stands for something to recall. For example, in remembering the use of canes and walkers, think of "Wandering Wilma's Always Late" (**W**alker **W**ith **A**ffected **L**eg) (see **Fig. 1.5**). Everyone remembers the cranial nerve mnemonic (see **Fig. 1.6**).

Memory aids/images are pictures or caricatures that help you recall information more effectively (see **Fig. 1.7**).

Rhymes are phrases or words spoken in a rhythmic or musical manner that increase recall, such as the rhyme for hypoglycemia versus hyperglycemia (see **Fig. 1.8**). Another rhyme,

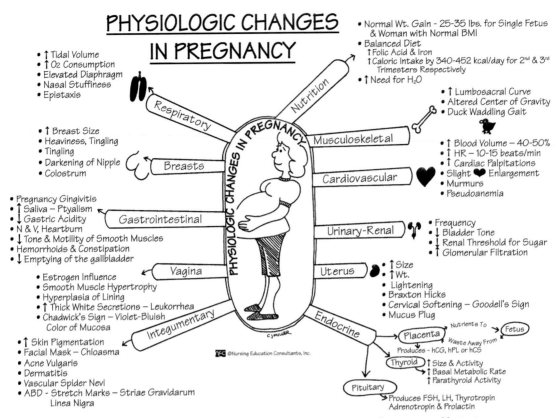

PHYSIOLOGIC CHANGES IN PREGNANCY

Respiratory
- ↑ Tidal Volume
- ↑ O₂ Consumption
- Elevated Diaphragm
- Nasal Stuffiness
- Epistaxis

Nutrition
- Normal Wt. Gain - 25-35 lbs. for Single Fetus & Woman with Normal BMI
- Balanced Diet
  ↑Folic Acid & Iron
  ↑Caloric Intake by 340-452 kcal/day for 2ⁿᵈ & 3ʳᵈ Trimesters Respectively
- ↑ Need for H₂O

Musculoskeletal
- ↑ Lumbosacral Curve
- Altered Center of Gravity
- Duck Waddling Gait

Breasts
- ↑ Breast Size
- Heaviness, Tingling
- Tingling
- Darkening of Nipple
- Colostrum

Cardiovascular
- ↑ Blood Volume – 40-50%
- ↑ HR – 10-15 beats/min
- ↑ Cardiac Palpitations
- Slight ♥ Enlargement
- Murmurs
- Pseudoanemia

Gastrointestinal
- Pregnancy Gingivitis
- ↑ Saliva – Ptyalism
- ↓ Gastric Acidity
- N & V, Heartburn
- ↓ Tone & Motility of Smooth Muscles
- Hemorrhoids & Constipation
- ↓ Emptying of the gallbladder

Urinary-Renal
- Frequency
- ↓ Bladder Tone
- ↓ Renal Threshold for Sugar
- ↑ Glomerular Filtration

Vagina
- Estrogen Influence
- Smooth Muscle Hypertrophy
- Hyperplasia of Lining
- ↑ Thick White Secretions – Leukorrhea
- Chadwick's Sign – Violet-Bluish Color of Mucosa

Uterus
- ↑ Size
- ↑ Wt.
- Lightening
- Braxton Hicks
- Cervical Softening – Goodell's Sign
- Mucus Plug

Integumentary
- ↑ Skin Pigmentation
- Facial Mask – Chloasma
- Acne Vulgaris
- Dermatitis
- Vascular Spider Nevi
- ABD - Stretch Marks – Striae Gravidarum Linea Nigra

Endocrine
- Placenta → Nutrients To → Fetus / Waste Away From
  - Produces - hCG, hPL or hCS
- Thyroid ↑Size & Activity
  ↑Basal Metabolic Rate
  ↑Parathyroid Activity
- Pituitary → Produces FSH, LH, Thyrotropin Adrenotropin & Prolactin

©Nursing Education Consultants, Inc.

Fig. 1.1 Example of Mindmapping™: Physiologic Changes in Pregnancy. (From: Zerwekh, J., Garneau, A., & Miller, C.J. (2017). *Digital Collection of the Memory Notebooks of Nursing.* 4ed., Chandler, AZ: Nursing Education Consultants, Inc.)

6-Ps OF DYSPNEA

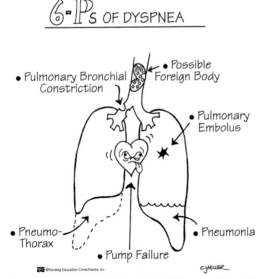

- Pulmonary Bronchial Constriction
- Possible Foreign Body
- Pulmonary Embolus
- Pneumo-Thorax
- Pump Failure
- Pneumonia

©Nursing Education Consultants, Inc.

Fig. 1.2 Acronym Memory Aid: The "6-Ps" of Dyspnea. (From: Zerwekh, J., Garneau, A., & Miller, C.J. (2017). *Digital Collection of the Memory Notebooks of Nursing.* 4ed., Chandler, AZ: Nursing Education Consultants, Inc.)

"fingers, nose, penis, toes," identifies the areas where lidocaine with epinephrine is contraindicated as a local anesthetic. "Two is too much" may help you remember toxic levels of lithium, digoxin, and theophylline, which have a narrow margin of safety (see **Fig. 1.9**). Books and electronic resources are available on these helpful aids (see References at the end of this chapter).

NEUROVASCULAR ASSESSMENT

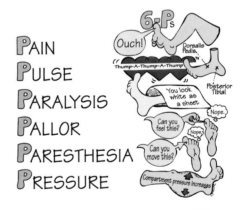

PAIN
PULSE
PARALYSIS
PALLOR
PARESTHESIA
PRESSURE

©Nursing Education Consultants, Inc.

Fig. 1.3 The "6-Ps" of Circulation Assessment. (From: Zerwekh, J., Garneau, A., & Miller, C.J. (2017). *Digital Collection of the Memory Notebooks of Nursing.* 4ed., Chandler, AZ: Nursing Education Consultants, Inc.)

Testing Skills for Paper-and-Pencil Tests

Because your certification exams are available on computer, the following skills are applicable for ***paper-and-pencil tests***, which you may encounter as a student in your program.

1. Go through the exam and mark all answers that you know are correct. This ensures you have adequate time to answer

MALIGNANT MELANOMA
(SIGNS OF)

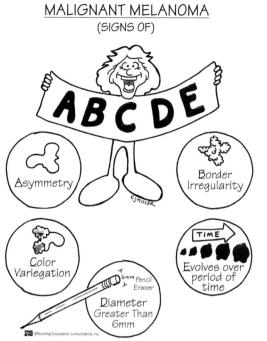

Fig. 1.4 Indications of Possible Malignant Melanoma: "ABCDE." (From: Zerwekh, J., Garneau, A., & Miller, C.J. (2017). *Digital Collection of the Memory Notebooks of Nursing.* 4ed., Chandler, AZ: Nursing Education Consultants, Inc.)

CANES AND WALKERS

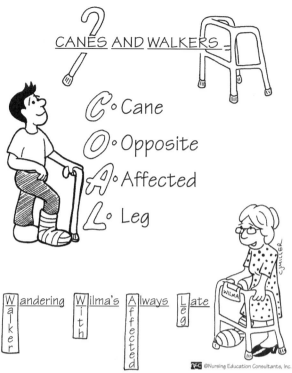

C • Cane
O • Opposite
A • Affected
L • Leg

Wandering Wilma's Always Late
Walker With Affected Leg

Fig. 1.5 Mnemonics for Canes ("COAL") and Walkers ("WWAL"). (From: Zerwekh, J., Garneau, A., & Miller, C.J. (2017). *Digital Collection of the Memory Notebooks of Nursing.* 4ed., Chandler, AZ: Nursing Education Consultants, Inc.)

CRANIAL NERVE MNEMONIC

S = Sensory	M = Motor	B = Both

O	Olfactory	O	On	S	Some
O	Optic	O	Old	S	Say
O	Oculomotor	O	Olympus	M	Marry
T	Trochlear	T	Towering	M	Money
T	Trigeminal	T	Tops	B	But
A	Abducens	A	A	M	My
F	Facial	F	Finn	B	Brother
A	Acoustic	A	And	S	Says
G	Glossopharyngeal	G	German	B	Bad
V	Vagus	V	Viewed	B	Business
S	Spinal	S	Some	M	Marry
H	Hypoglossal	H	Hops	M	Money

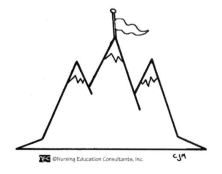
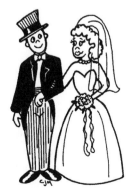

Fig. 1.6 Cranial Nerve Mnemonic. (From: Zerwekh, J., Garneau, A., & Miller, C.J. (2017). *Digital Collection of the Memory Notebooks of Nursing.* 4ed., Chandler, AZ: Nursing Education Consultants, Inc.)

HYPERTHYROIDISM

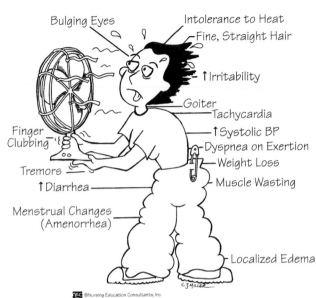

Fig. 1.7 Image as Memory Aid for the Signs/Symptoms of Hyperthyroidism. (From: Zerwekh, J., Garneau, A., & Miller, C.J. (2017). *Digital Collection of the Memory Notebooks of Nursing.* 4ed., Chandler, AZ: Nursing Education Consultants, Inc.)

BLOOD SUGAR MNEMONIC

HOT & DRY = SUGAR HIGH

COLD & CLAMMY = NEED SOME CANDY

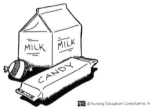

Fig. 1.8 Blood Sugar Rhyme. (From: Zerwekh, J., Garneau, A., & Miller, C.J. (2017). *Digital Collection of the Memory Notebooks of Nursing.* 4ed., Chandler, AZ: Nursing Education Consultants, Inc.)

the questions you know. Then, go back and evaluate those questions for which you did not readily recognize the answer.

2. Do not indiscriminately change answers. If you go back and change an answer, you should have a specific reason for doing so. You may remember information and realize

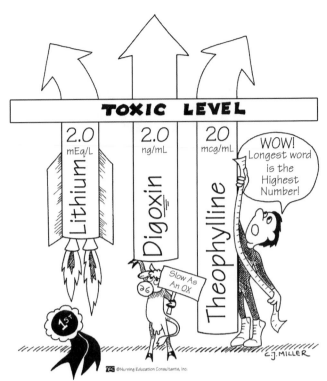

Fig. 1.9 "Two is Too Much": Toxic Levels of Lithium, Digoxin, and Theophylline. (From: Zerwekh, J., Garneau, A., & Miller, C.J. (2017). *Digital Collection of the Memory Notebooks of Nursing.* 4ed., Chandler, AZ: Nursing Education Consultants, Inc.)

you answered the question incorrectly. Frequently, test-takers "talk themselves out of" the correct answer and change it to an incorrect one.

3. After you have completed the exam, go back and check your booklet and make sure all questions are answered. Be sure to answer all questions, even if you must guess at some.

Successful Test Taking

1. Listen carefully to the instructions given at the beginning of the exam. Make sure you understand all information given and exactly how to mark your answers and/or how to use the keyboard and mouse. Adjust the computer screen for optimum viewing.

2. Watch your timing. Do not spend too much time on one question. It is very important that you practice your timing on the sample exams. You may not be able to review your questions and answers on completion of the computerized test; therefore, watch your timing on the computerized tests and make use of a computer clock if it is available.

3. Be aware of your "first hunch" because it is frequently the correct answer. Sometimes information is processed by the brain without your awareness. If something about an

answer "feels right" or if you have a "gut feeling" about an answer, pay attention to it.

4. Eliminate options that assume the patient "would not understand" or "is ignorant of" the situation or those that "protect them from worry." For example, "The patient should not be told she has cancer because it would upset her too much."

5. Be aware of options that contain the words *always* and *never*.

6. There is no pattern of correct answers. Both computerized and paper-and-pencil exams are compiled by a computer and the position of the correct answers is selected at random.

7. Watch the length of the options to consider. The number of words required to adequately state the correct answer is sometimes longer than the other options.

Decrease Anxiety

Your activities on the day of the exam strongly influence your level of anxiety. By carefully planning ahead, you will be able to eliminate some anxiety-provoking situations. If you are a diabetic or have special needs, contact the certification agency ahead of time to make arrangements to have accommodations that you may require.

1. Visit the exam site before the day of the exam. Evaluate travel time, parking, and time to reach the designated area. Be sure to get an early start to allow for extra time.

2. If you have to travel some distance to the exam site, try to spend the night in the immediate vicinity.

3. Do something pleasant the evening before the exam. This is not the time to "crash study."

4. Anxiety is contagious. If those around you are extremely anxious, avoid contact with them before the exam.

5. Make your meal before the test a light, healthy one.

6. Avoid eating highly spiced or different foods. This is not the time for a gastrointestinal upset.

7. Wear comfortable clothes. This is not a good time to wear tight clothing or new shoes.

8. Wear clothing of moderate weight. It is difficult to control the temperature to keep everyone comfortable. Take a sweater or wear layered clothes. You may not be allowed to remove any garments once you are seated for the exam.

9. Wear soft-soled shoes; this decreases the noise in the testing area.

10. Make sure you have the papers and proper identification that are required to gain admission to the exam site. If you wear reading glasses, do not forget to bring them with you.

11. Do not take study materials to the exam site. You will not be able to take such materials with you into the exam area.

12. Do not panic when you encounter content with which you are unfamiliar in a question. Use good test-taking strategies, select an answer, and continue. Remember, you are not going to know all of the correct answers.

13. Reaffirm to yourself that you know the material. It is not time for any self-defeating behavior or negative self-talk. You will pass! Build your confidence by visualizing yourself in 6 months working in the area you desire. Create that mental picture of where you want to be and who you want to be—a certified adult-gerontology primary care NP. Use your past successes to bring positive energy and "vibes" to your certification. You can do it!

Study Habits
Enhancing Study Skills

- Decide on a realistic study schedule; write it down and stick with it.
- Divide the review material into segments—pediatrics, well woman, cardiac, and so forth.
- Prioritize the segments; review first the areas in which you seem deficient or weak.
- Identify areas that will require additional review.
- Establish a realistic schedule; study in short segments or "bursts." Avoid marathon sessions.
- Plan on achieving your study goal several days before the exam.
- Do not study when you are tired or when there are frequent distractions or interruptions.
- Review general concepts of practice from a variety of resources.

Group Study

- Keep the group limited to three to five people.
- Group members should be mature and serious about studying.
- The group should agree on the planned study schedule.
- If the group makes you anxious, or if you do not think the group meets your study needs, do not continue to participate.

Testing Practice

- Include testing practice in your schedule.
- Select about 50 questions for a practice testing session of 1 hour. This will allow you to evaluate the pace of the exam (that is, approximately one question per minute).

- Try to answer the questions as if you were taking the real exam. Do not look up the correct answer immediately after answering the question. Complete all questions you have selected, then go back and grade the questions.
- Utilize the testing strategies described in this chapter.
- Evaluate the practice exam for problem areas: testing skills and knowledge base.
- Evaluate the questions you answer incorrectly. Review the rationale for the right answer and understand why you missed it.
- Utilize the questions at a later point to review the information again.

REFERENCES

Academy of Nurse Practitioners Certification Program (AANPCB), 2016. Candidate Handbook and Renewal of Certification Handbook. Retrieved from http://www.aanpcert.org/.

American Nurses Credentialing Center (ANCC), 2016. Certification: general Testing and Renewal Handbook. Retrieved from http://nursecredentialing.org/Exam61-AdultGeroPrimaryCareNP-TCO.

Beitz, J., 1997. Unleashing the power of memory: the mighty mnemonic. Nurse Educator 22 (2), 25–28.

Bloomingfield, R., 1982. Mnemonics, Rhetorics, and Poetics for Medics. Harbinger Medical Press, Salem, NC.

Zerwekh, J., 2016. Test-taking strategies. In: NCLEX-RN®: A Comprehensive Study Guide, ninth ed. Elsevier, St. Louis, pp. 1–22.

Zerwekh, J., Garneau, A., Miller, C.J., 2017. Digital Collection of the Memory Notebooks of Nursing, fourth ed. Nursing Education Consultants Publishing, Chandler, AZ.

2

Growth & Development

Physical Assessment

1. What are common findings noted when assessing the skin of an older adult patient? Select two findings.
   1. Petechiae.
   2. Thick, brittle nails.
   3. Senile lentigines.
   4. Sebaceous gland hyperplasia.
   5. Chloasma.

2. Which statement is accurate about frailty?
   1. Frailty is an uncommon syndrome in older adults.
   2. Sarcopenia occurs because of increased lean body mass.
   3. There is increased tolerance for exertion and physical activity.
   4. Assessment findings include low grip strength and slowed walking speed.

3. Which statement is accurate about conducting a physical exam on an older adolescent?
   1. Provide a previsit screening tool or questionnaire to allow the adolescent to identify and write down concerns prior to the start of the visit.
   2. Have the adolescent's parent remain in the room during the health history and review of systems.
   3. Explain to the adolescent that everything that is discussed will remain confidential.
   4. Use a gentle confrontational approach when the adolescent is silent or unable to express specific words about physical changes occurring.

4. The adult-gerontology primary care NP is assessing immediate recall or new learning. A healthy adult patient should be able to repeat a series of how many numbers?
   1. More than 15 numbers.
   2. 10–14 numbers.
   3. 5–8 numbers.
   4. 3–5 numbers.

5. **QSEN** The adult-gerontology primary care NP selects which assessment tool to evaluate balance and gait problems in older adult patients?
   1. Lawton & Brody Balance and Coordination Scale.
   2. Tinetti Balance and Gait Evaluation.
   3. Instrumental Activities of Daily Living Scale.
   4. Index of Independence of Activities of Daily Living.

6. **QSEN** As part of a Medicare annual wellness visit, screening for cognitive deficits or impairment is an important component of the visit. Which three tests can be used to assess the progression of cognitive impairment?
   1. Short Portable Mental Status Questionnaire.
   2. Folstein Mini–Mental State Examination.
   3. Index of Independence of Activities of Daily Living.
   4. Katz Index.
   5. AD8 Dementia Screening Interview.
   6. 15 Minute Screen (15MS).

7. The adult-gerontology primary care NP is constructing a pedigree chart during a clinical visit. What is the purpose of obtaining a pedigree diagram?
   1. Record of growth and development milestones.
   2. Sexual orientation (LGBT) and sexual development.
   3. Genetic and familial health problems.
   4. Cultural variation and ethnic background.

8. In assessing the nutritional status of an older adult patient, the adult-gerontology primary care NP identifies the common physiologic change in the gastrointestinal system to be:
   1. Increased peristalsis.
   2. Decreased absorption of iron.
   3. Maintenance of normal fat metabolism.
   4. Overgrowth of certain bacteria.
   5. Increased elasticity of the stomach.

9. When an 88-year-old patient who has short-term memory loss is interviewed, the patient states that she cannot remember what she ate for breakfast a few hours later. What would be an appropriate action for the adult-gerontology primary care NP?
   1. Order lab work and stop all medications.
   2. Consult with the patient's family member and/or caregivers to validate the patient's concerns.
   3. Refer the patient to a neurologist.
   4. Consider the short-term memory loss finding as a normal age-related change associated with aging.

10. **QSEN** Which of these clinical findings would indicate a deviation from the normal age-related changes in the neurologic system that may have some diagnostic significance for the older patient?
    1. Decreased sense of touch.
    2. Diminished ankle tendon reflex.
    3. Decreased short-term memory.
    4. Decreased ability to maintain balance.

11. Which statement is accurate about pain assessment in the very old adult?
    1. Pain perception varies from what is usually expected in the adult patient.
    2. Pain symptoms are more dramatic and specific as the patient ages.
    3. Older adults often exaggerate pain symptoms.
    4. Dull pain is often felt as sharp, stabbing pain.

12. Which statement is accurate about common changes occurring because of aging that are considerations during a physical assessment?
    1. Tenting of the skin is a good indicator of hydration status.
    2. The whispered voice test is a helpful aid in screening for loss of hearing.
    3. Third and fourth heart sounds are uncommon.
    4. Increased sensitivity to touch and exaggerated vibratory sense in the lower extremities is noted.

13. **QSEN** During the physical exam of an older patient, the adult-gerontology primary care NP indicates an understanding of deviations in the neurologic system from the normal aging process with which clinical finding?
    1. Decrease in short-term memory.
    2. Decrease in deep tendon and superficial reflexes.
    3. Decreased sense of touch.
    4. Positive Romberg sign.

14. An adult-gerontology primary care NP is interviewing an older adult with a physical disability, for which the patient requires a wheelchair. What are important considerations? Select three responses.
    1. Have an uncluttered surrounding, so that the patient has room to maneuver the wheelchair.

2. Start the interview with a written questionnaire and have the patient take notes on the form.
3. Speak clearly and with higher volume because of the patient' significant hearing impairment.
4. Face the patient at eye level while communicating.
5. Use a conversational tone of voice to promote a sense of ease with the patient.

15. **QSEN** An adult-gerontology primary care NP is assessing a 47-year-old patient who has come to the office for an annual physical examination. One of the first physical signs of aging is:
    1. Having more frequent aches and pains.
    2. Diminished eyesight, especially close vision.
    3. Increasing loss of muscle tone.
    4. Diminished hearing or taste.

16. The adult-gerontology primary care NP is asking questions during a review of systems and understands that constitutional symptoms include:
    1. Increased heart rate, bounding pulse, dizziness.
    2. Pruritic rash, malaise, diminished visual acuity.
    3. Weight, height, body mass index.
    4. Pain, fever, malaise.

17. Which of the following tools are available to assist with evaluating polypharmacy in the older adult patient? Select three tools.
    1. Medication Appropriateness Index (MAI).
    2. Screening Tool to Alert Medical Practitioners (STAMP).
    3. Katz Index.
    4. Screening Tool of Older Persons' Potentially Inappropriate Prescriptions (STOPP).
    5. Beers List.

18. Which physical assessment finding is a normal physiologic change of the respiratory system that occurs with aging?
    1. Decreased residual lung volume.
    2. Hyperresonance.
    3. Increased forced vital capacity.
    4. Increased tactile fremitus.

19. When assessing the dehydration status of an older adult, which finding resulting from aging may provide unreliable physical assessment evidence?
    1. Poor skin turgor.
    2. Slight elevated temperature.
    3. Very dry mucous membranes.
    4. Swollen, furrowed tongue.

20. An adult patient with cerebral palsy and minimal cognitive dysfunction is seen at the clinic. The adult-gerontology primary care NP understands that health history information should:
    1. Be obtained only from the past medical record.

2. Be obtained from the patient's family member and/or caregiver.
3. Involve the patient to the limit of their ability.
4. Involve the community group home where the patient resides.

21. The adult-gerontology primary care NP indicates an understanding of the normal aging process with which documentation of the gastrointestinal (GI) system in the physical examination?
    1. Increase in the size of the liver (16 cm).
    2. Absent bowel sounds.
    3. Femoral bruit.
    4. Increased adipose tissue.

22. **QSEN** Which functional assessment tool should the adult-gerontology primary care NP use to evaluate the safety of a patient who had a stroke and is planning to return to a home environment?
    1. OARS ADL Scale.
    2. Bennet Social Isolation Scale.
    3. Mini–Mental State Examination.
    4. Norton Scale.

23. When communicating with adolescents, the adult-gerontology primary care NP needs to be sensitive to the adolescent's:
    1. Reluctance to talk.
    2. Desire to be in control.
    3. Need for detailed instructions.
    4. Urge to communicate.

24. Which of the following is *not* considered a common geriatric syndrome?
    1. Polypharmacy.
    2. Failure to thrive.
    3. Falls.
    4. Muscular hypertrophy.

Aging

25. As an individual ages, dehydration becomes a more prevalent problem. The adult-gerontology primary care NP understands this issue is related to which normal aging changes? Select two answers.
    1. Increased glomerular filtration.
    2. Ineffective water conservation.
    3. Decreased solute/water ratio.
    4. Decreased thirst drive.
    5. Increased vasopressin release.

26. In the older adult population, which group is considered the fastest growing cohort?
    1. 60–64 years old.
    2. 65–74 years old.

3. 75–84 years old.
4. 85 years and older.

27. As an individual ages, which physiologic change would affect responses to pharmacologic agents?
    1. Increased gastric emptying.
    2. Increased glomerular filtration rate.
    3. Decreased percentage of body fat.
    4. Decreased albumin concentration.

28. **QSEN** Although driving is an important task that allows the older adult to be mobile and independent, it is important when counseling an older adult driver to include the following:
    1. Drive only during the day when it is bright and sunny.
    2. Drive with headlights on at dusk and at night.
    3. Avoid driving in inclement weather.
    4. Use the bright headlights when driving at night.

29. **QSEN** The number one cause of accidental death in patients older than 65 years of age is:
    1. Motor vehicle accidents.
    2. Poisoning.
    3. Falls.
    4. Drowning.

30. What are the normal physiologic changes in the thyroid gland that occur with aging?
    1. Hypertrophy with a decrease in triiodothyronine (T_3) and thyroxine (T_4).
    2. Normal size with increase in thyroid-stimulating hormone (TSH) and decrease in T_4.
    3. Atrophy of the gland with a decrease in TSH, T_3, and T_4.
    4. Increase in nodularity with normal TSH and T_4.

31. The aging process causes what normal physiologic changes in the heart?
    1. Heart size stays the same, and the valves thicken and become rigid secondary to fibrosis and sclerosis.
    2. Cardiomegaly occurs along with the prolapse of the mitral valve and regurgitation.
    3. Dilation of the right ventricle with sclerosis of pulmonic and tricuspid valves.
    4. Hypertrophy of the right ventricle with decreasing capacity and compromised efficiency of the coronary arteries.

32. Which pulmonary physiologic change is commonly associated with the aging process?
    1. Increased cough response.
    2. Decrease in vital capacity.
    3. Decreased AP diameter of the thorax.
    4. Increase in residual Po_2.

33. As patients age, it becomes particularly important to encourage an increased intake of (select three nutrients):
    1. Vitamin D.
    2. Iron and folic acid.
    3. Vitamin C.
    4. B vitamins.
    5. Omega-3 fatty acids.

34. During a teaching session, the adult-gerontology primary care NP instructs the patient regarding normal skin lesions in the older population. These would include:
    1. Seborrheic dermatitis.
    2. Senile keratosis.
    3. Senile lentigo.
    4. Squamous cell.

35. As an individual ages, which three findings are associated with normal age-related visual changes?
    1. Increased sensitivity to glare and sunlight.
    2. Loss of peripheral vision.
    3. Diminished color discrimination with colors appearing faded.
    4. Difficulty in focusing on objects far away.
    5. Decreased tear production.

36. **QSEN** The adult-gerontology primary care NP understands which factor is most influential in the driving ability of an older adult?
    1. Ability to coordinate a clutch transmission.
    2. Acuity of vision.
    3. Comprehension of the details of road rules.
    4. Reaction times.

37. Based on changes in hepatic function in older adult patients, which adjustment should the adult-gerontology primary care NP expect for oral medications that undergo extensive first-pass metabolism?
    1. The interval between doses should be increased.
    2. The metabolism of the oral medication will not be affected.
    3. A higher dose should be used with the same time schedule.
    4. The interval between doses should be reduced.

38. As an individual ages, which physiologic change would affect sleep?
    1. Decreased REM sleep.
    2. Increased delta or stage IV sleep.
    3. Decreased nocturnal awakenings.
    4. Decreased sleep latency.

39. What is a general principle regarding drug absorption in the older adult?
    1. Rate of absorption is slowed.
    2. Amount or percentage of absorption is greatly reduced.
    3. Absorption responses are enhanced.
    4. Absorption and bioavailability are increased.

40. When treating an infection in the older adult, the adult-gerontology primary care NP must consider that:
    1. Thymus-derived immunity is increased.
    2. Immune function declines with age.
    3. Immune function increases with age.
    4. Antibody production increases.

41. The diminished immunity of the older adult can be attributed to a decline in:
    1. B-cell function.
    2. T-cell production.
    3. B-cell production.
    4. T-cell function.

42. Which two statements are accurate regarding pharmacokinetics in the older adult patient?
    1. Older adults are less sensitive to drugs than younger adults.
    2. Reduced renal function, with resultant drug accumulation, is the most important cause of adverse drug reactions in older adults.
    3. The rate of absorption is increased.
    4. Reduced liver function may prolong drug effects.
    5. Serum creatinine tests should be performed on all medications primarily eliminated by the kidneys.

43. Which physiologic factor of aging contributes to incontinence in older adults?
    1. Decreased vascularity of the bladder mucosa.
    2. Increased urethral closing pressure.
    3. Increased ability to concentrate urine.
    4. Decreased bladder capacity.

44. What is the pathophysiologic age-related change that predisposes an older adult to dehydration?
    1. A decrease in body fat along with a significant decrease in lean muscle mass makes the older adult more susceptible to minute changes in blood volume.
    2. Thirst is normally experienced when there is a loss of 2% of the client's body weight or when osmolality is increased; this mechanism is significantly diminished in the older adult.
    3. With aging, the glomeruli reduce in number, which leads to a corresponding increase in glomerular filtering surface, which causes the kidney to increase its ability to concentrate urine in the older adult.
    4. Antidiuretic hormone (ADH) increases as the kidney loses function, leading to diminished ability to maintain osmolality.

45. Normal physiologic changes in the respiratory system of the geriatric patient include:
    1. Increased residual volume.
    2. Increased ciliary action, resulting in a more forceful and recurrent cough.

3. Increase in number of smaller alveoli with decreased residual capacity.
4. Decrease in AP diameter of rib cage with decreased lung expansion.

46. The adult-gerontology primary care NP understands that as the patient ages changes occur in the cells of the immune system. Which statement reflects these changes?
    1. The cells are able to proliferate as they would in the younger patient.
    2. The total number of T cells is decreased.
    3. There is an increased ability to respond to infections with previously produced "remembered" antibodies.
    4. The immune system is able to respond to antigenic stimulation as in the younger patient.

2 Growth & Development Answers & Rationales

Physical Assessment

1. Answer: 3, 4

   Rationale: Both structural and functional changes occur in the skin. Older adults often have senile lentigines (liver spots), which are brown macules found on the backs of the hands, forearms, and face caused by localized mild epidermal hyperplasia in association with increased numbers of melanocytes and increased melanin production. Sebaceous gland hyperplasia is found especially on the forehead and nose, with a raised area from 1 to 3 mm in size with a central pore. Petechiae are reddish, purple spots (usually 1–2mm) of bleeding under the skin that may occur from numerous causes but is not affected by age. The nails become thin and brittle, with marked ridging. Senile purpura is commonly found, characterized by purple macules (not petechiae) appearing on the backs of the hands or on the forearms that result from blood that has extravasated through capillaries due to a loss of skin elasticity. Chloasma is hyperpigmentation occurring on the face of a pregnant woman.

2. Answer: 4

   Rationale: Frailty (also known as failure to thrive) is a common clinical syndrome in older adults. Common findings with the condition of frailty are low grip strength, slowed walking speed, low physical activity, unintentional weight loss, decreased lean body mass (sarcopenia), osteopenia, cognitive impairment, and anemia. Frailty can leave a patient vulnerable to falls, functional decline, disability, disease, and death.

3. Answer: 1

   Rationale: Providing a previsit screening tool or questionnaire to allow the older adolescent to identify and write down concerns prior to the start of the visit is a helpful open-ended approach to assist the adult-gerontology primary care NP to phrase questions in an appropriate way to promote a sense of partnership that encourages communication. Adolescents may be reluctant to talk, and have a clear need for confidentiality. All adolescent patients should be given the opportunity to discuss their concerns privately. Every effort should be made to maintain confidentiality; however, it is important to explain that there are limits on what can be kept confidential during the clinical visit. It should be explained that information that suggests that the adolescent's safety or the safety of another is at risk may be reasons for the adult-gerontology primary care NP to "break" confidentiality. Adolescents do not respond well to confrontation or any type of "forced" conversation to express how they are feeling.

4. Answer: 3

   Rationale: When assessing immediate recall or new learning, a healthy adult patient without cognitive decline should be able to repeat a series of 5–8 numbers.

5. Answer: 2

   Rationale: The Tinetti Balance and Gait Evaluation is an activity-based test that asks the patient to perform tasks, such as sitting and rising from a chair, turning, and bending. It requires no more than 15 to 20 minutes to perform. Another appropriate test for the assessment of falls is the timed "Up and Go" test, which assesses balance and gait speed. The Instrumental Activities of Daily Living Scale assesses complex tasks such as shopping, laundry, and food preparation. The Index of Independence of Activities of Daily Living helps identify daily activities with which the patient needs assistance.

6. Answer: 1, 2, 5

   Rationale: The following tests can be used to assess cognitive impairment and dementia: the Folstein Mini–Mental State Examination, the Mini-Cog screen for dementia, the Short Portable Mental Status Questionnaire, the AD8 Dementia Screening Interview, and the Montreal Cognitive Assessment (MoCa). The Index of Independence of Activities of Daily Living helps identify daily activities with which the patient needs assistance, as does the Katz Index. The Seven Minute Screen (7MS) (not 15 minute) is a quick and common test used to assess temporal orientation, enhanced cued recall, clock drawing, and verbal fluency. The 7MS has been shown to be useful for detecting Alzheimer disease in a patient with memory problems.

7. Answer: 3

   Rationale: A pedigree chart is a diagram of family information using a standardized set of symbols (squares representing males and circles females). A dark symbol is used to indicate someone affected with a genetic condition, and unfilled symbols for those who are unaffected; carriers of a condition are often indicated by a gray symbol. The pedigree chart should have at least three generations noted. The pedigree chart is an important component of a family history and can provide information regarding diseases that are transmitted or occur in family generations. It can be used as a diagnostic tool to help guide decisions about genetic testing for the patient and at-risk family members.

8. Answer: 2, 4

Rationale: Decreased hydrochloric acid, which occurs with aging, leads to decreased absorption of iron and vitamin B12. Excessive growth of certain bacteria (bacterial overgrowth syndrome) becomes more common with age and can lead to pain, bloating, and weight loss. Bacterial overgrowth may also lead to decreased absorption of certain nutrients, such as vitamin B12, iron, and calcium. The stomach cannot accommodate as much food (because of decreased elasticity), and the rate at which the stomach empties food into the small intestine decreases with aging. Fat absorption will decrease, as would peristalsis.

9. Answer: 2

Rationale: Older adults may be confused or experience recent memory loss. Recent memory for important events and conversations is usually not impaired. Consultation with the patient's family member and/or caregivers to validate the patient's concerns is important to determine if this is an isolated incident or a pattern of decline of memory loss. Although a careful review of medications is important, as changes in memory can be associated, for instance, with use of opiates, benzodiazepines, antidepressants, corticosteroids, and muscle relaxants, the patient's medications should not be stopped until further assessment is obtained. Loss of immediate and recent memory with retention of remote memory suggests dementia. Referral to a neurologist would be appropriate after concerns of the patient's memory loss are validated with the family member and/or caregiver.

10. Answer: 4

Rationale: Decreased ability to maintain balance may indicate a cerebellar complication. The other findings (decreased sense of touch, diminished ankle tendon reflex, and decreased short-term memory are normal age-related changes.

11. Answer: 1

Rationale: Pain is both highly prevalent and undertreated in the older adult population. Pain may be unreliably reported because, with age, its perception varies from the expected. Pain symptoms may be less dramatic, vague, or nonspecific. The severe pain usually associated with pancreatitis, for example, may be perceived as a dull ache, and the perception of pain during a cardiac event (myocardial infarction) may be minimal. Some patients may not report chronic pain symptoms because they attribute them to getting older or feel that nothing can be done to relieve the pain, especially since they have lived with the chronic pain for such a long time that it becomes part of their daily living.

12. Answer: 2

Rationale: High-frequency hearing loss (presbycusis) is a common age-related change with hearing. The whispered voice test is a simple test that can be useful in hearing assessment during a clinic visit, if older patients do not identify that they have difficulty hearing. It is the only test that does not require any equipment. Older adult patients with sensorineural hearing loss will have difficulty with the whispered voice test because their hearing loss is usually in the high frequency range. A whisper is a high-frequency sound and is used to detect high-tone loss. Because of thinning of the skin, tenting is not a good indicator of hydration status. Fourth heart sounds are common. There is a decreased or absent vibratory sense of the lower extremities, testing unnecessary.

13. Answer: 4

Rationale: Romberg sign indicates the inability to maintain balance, which indicates a need for further evaluation. A decrease in short-term memory, deep tendon and superficial reflexes, and sense of touch are normal age-related changes. If it affects the patient's functional ability, a decrease in short-term memory would be considered a deviation. Also, the testing strategy of looking for similarities in the options applies here, as the three incorrect responses all relate to a decrease in a body function with age.

14. Answer: 1, 4, 5

Rationale: When interviewing an older adult that uses a wheelchair because of a physical disability, it is important to have the environment setting for the interview conducive to making the patient comfortable. This means having an uncluttered room that the patient can easily move around in a wheelchair, facing the patient at eye level to assist with eye contact while communicating, and using a conversational tone of voice to promote a sense of ease with the patient. It is not necessary to speak loudly, but better to face the patient while talking. Written questionnaires may be useful, but should be given in advance of the interview visit.

15. Answer: 2

Rationale: Refractive errors are the most frequent eye problems in the United States. Blurred vision results from an inappropriate length of the eye and/or shape of the eye or cornea, and almost all errors—myopia (nearsightedness), hyperopia (farsightedness), astigmatism (distorted vision at all distances), and presbyopia (a form of farsightedness that usually occurs between 40 and 45 years of age)—can be corrected by eyeglasses, contact lenses, or, in some cases, surgery.

16. Answer: 4

Rationale: A constitutional symptom is defined as a symptom that affects the general well-being or general status of a patient. Examples include weight loss, shaking, chills, fever, pain, and vomiting. Constitutional symptoms tend to be nonspecific to a particular disease and because of this, they are not useful in diagnosis of conditions as nonconstitutional symptoms.

17. Answer: 1, 4, 5

Rationale: The following screening tools are available for the adult-gerontology primary care NP to use to assess for polypharmacy in the older adult patient: Medication Appropriateness Index (MAI), Screening Tool of Older Persons' Potentially Inappropriate Prescriptions (STOPP), and the most familiar and recommended—Beers List. It is updated by experts in geriatric care (American Geriatrics Society) and pharmacology using Institute of Medicine standards. The Katz Index helps identify daily activities where the patient needs assistance.

18. Answer: 2

Rationale: A normal age-related change is an increase in the AP diameter that results in hyperresonance. Age-related changes result in an increase in the residual lung volume (RV) and decrease in the forced vital capacity (FVC). An increased tactile fremitus is a deviation that is of diagnostic significance.

19. Answer: 1

Rationale: Because of changes in skin collagen and loss of skin elasticity with aging, poor skin turgor, which is often used as a sign of dehydration in younger individuals, is unreliable in older adults. The patient's body temperature may be elevated due to dehydration or the elevation may be a result of an inflammatory or infectious process. Mucous membranes are often not noticeably dry until severe dehydration is present. The tongue may be swollen and furrowed in the older adult who is dehydrated.

20. Answer: 3

Rationale: The patient with a history of cerebral palsy with minimal cognitive dysfunction should be fully involved in the health history interview to the best of their ability. Support from the patient's family and/or caregiver may be encouraged; however, the focus should be on the patient by speaking directly to them. Additional information from past medical records and the community group home can be obtained either prior to (preferable) or following the health history interview.

21. Answer: 4

Rationale: Common age-related changes in the GI system include increased adipose tissue, decreased liver size, reduced motility and peristalsis, decreased acid secretions and motor activity of the stomach, and decreased glomerular filtration rate. Absence of bowel sounds after five full minutes and bruits are deviations of clinical significance.

22. Answer: 1

Rationale: The Older Americans Resources and Services (OARS) Activities of Daily Living (ADL) Scale is the more appropriate screening tool for identifying at-risk populations. The Bennet Social Isolation Scale would be appropriate to evaluate social interactions and resources. The Mini–Mental State Examination is used to evaluate memory, orientation, and attention. The Norton Scale is used to evaluate pressure ulcer risk.

23. Answer: 1

Rationale: Adolescents may be reluctant to talk with a health care provider and if they are willing to communicate, they often have a need for confidentiality. All adolescent patients should be given the opportunity to discuss their concerns privately. Explain to the adolescent and parent that during the clinical visit, you will be asking the parent to leave the room to provide an opportunity for the adolescent to communicate confidentially. It is important with motivational interviewing to show concern for the adolescent's perspective, as often it has not been acknowledged, which leads to a desire to be in control. Avoid assumptions, judgments, and lectures. When possible, ask open-ended questions beginning with less sensitive issues and then proceeding to more sensitive ones.

24. Answer: 4

Rationale: There are several complex, multicausal geriatric syndromes that are common, which are polypharmacy, cognitive impairment, dehydration, falls, failure to thrive, urinary incontinence, and elder abuse. Muscle atrophy, not hypertrophy, occurs in the older adult.

Aging

25. Answer: 2, 4

Rationale: The thirst response is diminished, which results in an increased solute/water ration. Decreased renal plasma flow (glomerular filtration) leads to reduced ability to concentrate urine. The inability to concentrate urine prevents the body from retaining fluid leading to dehydration. Vasopressin release is decreased because of low fluid volume. These changes lead to ineffective water conservation.

26. Answer: 4

Rationale: The fastest growing cohort is the oldest-old with the number of centenarians (over the age of 100) increasing the fastest. Age ranges are as follows: adult age range, 18 to 64 years; young-old, 65 to 74 years; middle-old, 75 to 84 years; oldest-old, 85 years and older.

27. Answer: 4

Rationale: Medications are often protein bound (not fat bound); albumin decreases with age. A low albumin level decreases the number of protein-binding sites, causing an increase in the amount of free drug in the plasma. Drug overdose may occur in older adult patients. Gastric emptying and glomerular filtration rate *decrease* with the aging process.

28. Answer: 3

Rationale: It is important to have the older driver recognize unsafe driving conditions, which include inclement weather, driving in bright sunlight or at dusk, and driving at night. Older adults should avoid interstate driving and driving long distances.

29. Answer: 3

Rationale: Falls are the major cause of morbidity and mortality in the older adult. A fall is often the precipitating event for a cascade of problems leading to death. Complications from falls include fractures, pneumonia, pressure ulcers, pain, and immobility.

30. Answer: 4

Rationale: There is usually adequate secretion of TSH and a normal serum concentration of T_4. Aging may produce fibrosis and increased nodularity, but overall the thyroid function remains within normal limits.

31. Answer: 1

Rationale: The heart does not increase in size with normal aging. An enlarged heart is a result of cardiac dysfunction. Dilation of the left ventricle occurs with myocardial infarction and altered cardiac functioning secondary to cardiac disease, not from normal aging. The aging process does cause fibrosis and sclerosis of the cardiac valves; all valves are equally affected.

32. Answer: 2

Rationale: A decrease in the vital capacity, along with a 50% increase in residual volume, occurs during the aging process. Other aging changes include a less effective cough, impaired ciliary action, and weaker respiratory muscles. Increased AP diameter is associated with aging and in chronic obstructive pulmonary disease. Po_2 usually decreases, but Pco_2 usually remains unchanged or slightly increased.

33. Answer: 1, 2, 4

Rationale: Decreased hydrochloric acid, which occurs with aging, leads to decreased absorption of iron and vitamin B12 and is related to loss of intrinsic factor. Older adults are considered at risk for vitamin D deficiency, which contributes to osteoporosis. Bone loss that occurs with aging is related to low calcium. There are no particular recommendations for the older adult to increase the intake of vitamin C or omega-3 fatty acids in the diet.

34. Answer: 3

Rationale: The senile lentigo is a gray-brown, irregular, macular lesion on sun-exposed areas of the face, arms, and hands that are normal skin lesions. The other lesions are common abnormal skin lesions in the older adult.

35. Answer: 1, 3, 5

Rationale: Normal vision changes that occur with aging include increased sensitivity to glare and sunlight, diminished color vision with colors appearing faded, difficulty in focusing on objects close-up, need for more light for reading, and decreased tear production. Any sudden decrease or loss of peripheral vision can be indicative of a detached retina, which requires immediate treatment by an ophthalmologist.

36. Answer: 2

Rationale: The most age-dependent factor is sensory change. The older adult being assessed for driving capacity should use any prescribed corrective devices for optimal performance. Poor hearing by itself is generally not a limiting factor for motor vehicle operation, and vision assessment has received the greatest emphasis in assessing older drivers. Documenting the best-corrected binocular visual acuity, color perception, and dark vision is basic in assessing driving visual acuity. Laboratory performance studies have not clearly demonstrated that the other factors are highly applicable to the on-the-road skills of the older adult driver.

37. Answer: 1

Rationale: In the older adult patient liver function is diminished, which may increase the half-lives of certain drugs, leading to prolonged responses. Responses to oral drugs that ordinarily undergo extensive first-pass metabolism may be enhanced because fewer drugs are inactivated prior to entering the systemic circulation. Consequently, the interval between doses should be increased.

38. Answer: 1

Rationale: REM sleep begins approximately 120 minutes from sleep onset and recurs in three or four regularly spaced, 10- to 15-minute cycles. REM sleep, associated with skeletal muscle atonia and dreaming, decreases with aging. Delta sleep, or stage IV, is deep sleep and also decreases with age. Nocturnal wakening and sleep latency increase. Sleep is generally less efficient in older adults, who spend more time in bed and less time sleeping.

39. Answer: 1

Rationale: With aging, the rate of absorption is slowed due to delayed gastric emptying and reduced splanchnic blood flow. Amount or percentage of absorption does not usually change with age. Drug responses are delayed, not enhanced because of aging. Bioavailability is the degree to which a drug or other substance becomes available to the target tissue after administration.

40. Answer: 2

Rationale: Immune function declines with age, making the older adult more susceptible to infection. The older adult has less thymus-derived immunity because of the shrinking of the thymus gland, thus making it more difficult for the older adult to produce antibodies.

41. Answer: 4

Rationale: The older adult has diminished cell-mediated immunity because of a decline in T-cell function. The T cells have a decreased ability to produce cytokines, which are needed to facilitate B-cell growth and maturation, and have a decreased ability to proliferate in response to an antigen.

42. Answer: 2, 4

Rationale: Older adult patients are generally more sensitive to drugs than are younger adults, and they show wider individual variation. Drug accumulation secondary to reduced renal excretion is the most important cause of adverse drug reactions in older adults. In older adults, the proper index of renal function is creatinine clearance, not serum creatinine levels. Serum creatinine levels do not adequately reflect kidney function in older adults because the source of serum creatinine—lean muscle mass—declines in parallel with the decline in kidney function. Consequently, serum creatinine levels may be normal even though renal function is greatly reduced. The rate of absorption is slowed due to delayed gastric emptying and reduced splanchnic blood flow. Rates of hepatic drug metabolism tend to decline with age due to reduced hepatic blood flow, reduced liver mass, and decreased activity of some hepatic enzymes, which may prolong the drug effects.

43. Answer: 4

Rationale: Decreased bladder capacity, decreased ability to concentrate urine, and decreased urethral closing pressure after menopause lead to incontinence. Other factors are depression, decreased mobility, decreased vision, and lack of attention to bladder cues of feelings of fullness.

44. Answer: 2

Rationale: The older adult experiences significant hypodipsia and diminished thirst sensations, which leads to problems associated with adequate fluid intake. The older adult has increased body fat and less lean muscle mass. In addition, the quantity of total body water as a proportion of body weight decreases. The functional decline of the aging kidney leads to a gradual loss of glomeruli that results in a diminished filtering surface. The kidney does not concentrate urine effectively, and there is a decreased effect of ADH.

45. Answer: 1

Rationale: With aging, the number of alveoli decreases. The alveoli become rigid and lose their recoil and elasticity, which affects the patient's ability to exhale effectively. This increases a patient's residual volume (the amount of air left in the chest after expiration). Residual volume increases, whereas basilar inflation and ability to expel foreign matter decrease. The AP diameter of the chest increases, as seen in patients with kyphosis.

46. Answer: 3

Rationale: Older adult patients are able to respond to infections with previously produced "remembered" antibodies, but they are less able to respond to antigenic stimulation (new antigens) than younger patients. In the older adult patient, the cells of the immune system also are less likely to proliferate. The total number of T cells remains the same with age, but T-cell function decreases and cells have decreased cytotoxicity.

Health Promotion & Maintenance

1. The adult-gerontology primary care NP is preparing to provide an education class on medication compliance to a group of older adult individuals. Which strategies could lead to potential barriers that would affect the group's ability to receive the information?
   1. Assume that mental deficits exist in the group; therefore, repetition of information should be strongly encouraged.
   2. Use handouts that contain easily understood language.
   3. Provide pill boxes as a demonstration technique to help engage the audience.
   4. Ensure that the room in which the teaching session is taking place has good lighting.

2. **QSEN** The adult-gerontology primary care NP is assessing an older adult patient using the STEADI (Stopping Elderly Accidents, Deaths, & Injuries) initiative algorithm: Algorithm for Fall Risk Assessments & Interventions. Which documentation is representative of moderate risk?
   1. The patient has not fallen within the past year, no gait, balance, or strength deficits.
   2. The patient has sustained more than two falls within the past year with injuries.
   3. The patient has fallen once in the past year without injury, gait, and balance deficits present.
   4. The patient indicates that she is concerned about falling but doesn't exhibit balance problems upon ambulation.

3. What is an example of a secondary level of prevention measure for an older adult patient?
   1. Dietary counseling.
   2. Focus on preventing complications related to disease processes.
   3. Assessment of vitamin D level.
   4. Identification of smoking based on self-report of patient.

4. What are the current American Cancer Society (ACS) dietary recommendations for cancer prevention?
   1. Maintaining a desirable body weight and eating a variety of foods, including fruits and vegetables as well as foods that are high in fiber.
   2. Increasing the amount of protein in the diet.
   3. Alcohol use in small to moderate amounts.
   4. Increase in consumption of fresh fruits, fish, and dairy products.

5. The adult-gerontology primary care NP is aware that adolescents who have a history of being unsupervised after school are more likely to (select three items):
   1. Have no symptoms of depression.
   2. Use alcohol and smoke marijuana.
   3. Adjust and perform well in school.
   4. Be involved in risky behavior.
   5. Smoke tobacco.

6. In the presence of dyslipidemia and diabetes, the National Cholesterol Education Program guidelines set the goals for lipid levels as follows:
   1. LDL <100 mg/dL and triglyceride levels <150 mg/dL.
   2. LDL <160 mg/dL and triglyceride levels <240 mg/dL.
   3. LDL <100 mg/dL and triglyceride levels <180 mg/dL.
   4. LDL <150 mg/dL and triglyceride levels <220 mg/dL.

7. Which of the following is recommended as an annual screening test for colorectal cancer in a patient who is 51 years old?
   1. Guaiac-based fecal occult blood test (gFOBT) at-home test.
   2. Digital rectal exam.
   3. Sigmoidoscopy.
   4. Stool sample (gFOBT) collected at the office.

8. The American Diabetes Association recommends screening adults starting at age 45 with a fasting plasma glucose (FPG) test every:
   1. 1 year.
   2. 3 years.
   3. 5 years.
   4. 10 years.

9. What are tertiary prevention activities for an older adult woman who has had a stroke?
   1. Annual influenza vaccination.
   2. Physical therapy program.
   3. Annual mammogram.
   4. Annual ophthalmologic examination to evaluate for glaucoma.

10. Considering primary prevention of Alzheimer disease (AD) in the older adult population, the adult-gerontology primary care NP would acknowledge which statement as being supported by research findings?
    1. Age is an independent risk factor that is not aligned with clinical diagnosis.
    2. Genetics plays a strong role in presentation of cases independent of other comorbidities.
    3. History of nonparticipation in cognitive performance activities.
    4. History of increased physical activity.

11. A patient is continuing his recovery at home after an extensive surgery. The adult-gerontology primary care NP would instruct the patient to increase intake of which foods to promote healing?
    1. Tomatoes, rice, and whole-bran cereal.
    2. Milk, poultry, and yellow vegetables.
    3. Red meat, oranges, and green beans.
    4. Liver, corn, and eggs.

12. Patients with low health literacy are at risk for which of the following? Select three responses.
    1. Keeping appointments for yearly exams.
    2. Misunderstanding forms to complete for a health assessment.
    3. Lower hospitalization and morbidity rates.
    4. Increased visits to urgent care clinics and emergency departments.
    5. Engaging actively in self-care and chronic disease management.
    6. Not using preventive health measures, such as screenings and immunizations.

13. For an older adult patient who has an alteration in the sensory-perceptual function of hearing, which plan would be most appropriate for the adult-gerontology primary care NP to implement during a health promotion session?
    1. Increase the pitch of the voice.
    2. Stand behind the patient when speaking.
    3. Speak in a tone that does not include shouting.
    4. Use typical complex sentences to prevent insulting the patient.

14. **QSEN** Which of the following management plans demonstrates an understanding of primary prevention of falls among older adults?

    1. Evaluate the need for assistive devices for ambulation after the patient has been injured in a fall.
    2. Provide resources to correct hazards that contributed to falling in the home environment.
    3. Reinforce the need to use prescribed eyeglasses to prevent further injury resulting from falls.
    4. Provide information about medications, side effects, and interactions.

15. Which of these health promotion screenings should be completed annually for the patient who is over age 50?
    1. Chest x-ray.
    2. Pneumococcal vaccination.
    3. Colonoscopy.
    4. gFOBT.

16. According to the Older Americans Act (OAA), which recommendation is made to help support nutritional intake of older individuals?
    1. Milk intake is preferred as the main source of calcium.
    2. Meals can be served at other times than typically scheduled.
    3. Congregate meals are served at identified sites.
    4. Salt shakers should not be placed on tables.

17. While teaching a class to a group of senior citizens, which would be most important for the adult-gerontology primary care NP to consider during the presentation?
    1. Provide increased overhead lighting to enhance visualization.
    2. Provide handouts on blue paper with black print.
    3. Review a video narrated by a woman.
    4. Recognize that past life experiences are beneficial in learning new information.

18. Select two instruments that assess health literacy in the primary care setting.
    1. New Dale-Chall readability formula.
    2. SMOG Index.
    3. Flesch-Kincaid readability test.
    4. Rapid Estimate of Adult Literacy in Medicine–Short Form (REALM-SF).
    5. Newest Vital Sign.

19. **QSEN** What is the most common occupationally related health problem?
    1. Repetitive motion injury.
    2. Hearing loss.
    3. Lung disease.
    4. Cancer.

20. The adult-gerontology primary care NP is scheduled to provide health promotion teaching on oral health for a group of older patients who reside in an assisted living community. Which four content areas should be included in the discussion?

1. Excessive salivation.
2. Periodontal irritation.
3. Tooth loss.
4. Decreased taste perception.
5. Maintaining hydration.

21. Which of the following best describes the benefit of sports screening physicals?
    1. Screening for undiagnosed cardiomyopathy.
    2. Assessment of drug and alcohol use.
    3. Estimation of aerobic capacity.
    4. Identification of risk for an adverse cardiovascular event.

22. According to U.S. Department of Health and Human Services guidelines, which test is considered an important screening test to be done every 2 years for women between the ages of 50 and 64?
    1. HIV test.
    2. Colonoscopy.
    3. Mammogram.
    4. Chlamydia test.

23. A 48-year-old man presents to the clinic after having his cholesterol checked at a health fair. He states that his results were over 300 mg/dL and that he needs to see his primary care provider for further testing. Appropriate interventions for the adult-gerontology primary care NP include:
    1. Prescribing a cholesterol-lowering agent.
    2. Ordering an electrocardiogram (ECG) and an exercise stress test.
    3. Starting the patient on an exercise program.
    4. Performing a thorough history and physical and drawing a lipid profile.

24. The adult-gerontology primary care NP understands that some cultures believe that a patient should not be told of a diagnosis of a terminal disease, such as metastatic cancer. Select two cultural groups where informing the patient would be discouraged:
    1. Hispanics.
    2. Italian Americans.
    3. Navajo Native Americans.
    4. People from the Middle East.
    5. African Americans.

25. In preparing a patient for a colorectal screening, the adult-gerontology primary care NP should instruct the patient to:
    1. Eat at least two servings of meat daily before collecting samples.
    2. Avoid aspirin, iron, and anti-inflammatory medications.
    3. Avoid taking extra vitamin and mineral supplements before the test.
    4. Eat extra servings of high-fiber foods and water to ensure good samples.

26. **QSEN** The adult-gerontology primary care NP is performing an annual Medicare exam on a 77-year-old patient. Which recommendation below would be of greatest benefit in maintaining optimal health?
    1. "Exercise your arms and legs as much as you can each day."
    2. "Sleeping at least 9 hours will improve your energy level."
    3. "Urinate every 2 hours while awake to prevent accidents."
    4. "You should avoid soda and other types of junk food."

27. According to ChooseMyPlate, which two foods are included in the vegetable group?
    1. Chickpeas.
    2. Quinoa.
    3. Beans.
    4. Popcorn.
    5. Wild rice.

28. Which three acronyms can the health history be organized around when performing an assessment on an adolescent?
    1. FAST.
    2. GENES.
    3. HEADSS FIRST.
    4. CRAFTT.
    5. PLISSIT.

29. At what age should a routine screening mammography begin for women who have average risk of breast cancer, according to the USPSTF 2016 recommendations?
    1. 30 years old.
    2. 35 years old.
    3. Begin at age 40.
    4. After age 50.

30. Which of the following components should be included when taking a history from a patient who is new to the clinic?
    1. Past medical and surgical history, family medical and surgical histories, psychosocial history, diet and exercise habits, chemical use, sexual practices, and review of systems.
    2. Interval history, past medical history, family medical history, dietary habits, substance use, and sexual practices.
    3. Past medical and surgical histories, family medical history, psychosocial history, physical activity, tobacco and other substance use, and sexual practices.
    4. The history listed on the form provided to patients for completion before the physical exam is sufficient, and no interview needs to be done.

31. **QSEN** To promote safety when prescribing a narcotic analgesic to an 82-year-old patient who lives alone, the adult-gerontology primary care NP should do which of the following? Select three responses.
    1. Determine if the patient has constipation.
    2. Conduct an assessment of the patient's cognitive and motor abilities.
    3. Start with a low dose of analgesic and increase slowly, if needed.
    4. Assess the patient's usual waking and sleeping patterns.
    5. Evaluate for polypharmacy before ordering the analgesic.

32. A 50-year-old woman presents to the clinic for a first-visit checkup. She states that she is in good health and takes no medications. She was adopted and does not know her family history. She is 62 inches tall and weighs 175 lb. She is a secretary and admits to a sedentary lifestyle. She does not smoke and drinks four to five alcoholic beverages per week. Which of the following interventions would be most appropriate for the adult-gerontology primary care NP to recommend in this patient's plan of care?
    1. Recommend that she start an exercise program that includes jogging and weight training.
    2. Prescribe vitamin supplements to incorporate into her diet while she eliminates alcoholic beverages.
    3. Discuss possible job changes that that will increase her daily amount of exercise.
    4. Suggest that she keep a daily record of her food intake and bring it to her next visit.

33. Which group is at greatest risk for alterations in immune functions related to nutritional status?
    1. Young adults.
    2. Adults.
    3. Adolescents.
    4. Older adults.

34. An adult-gerontology primary care NP is examining a 78-year-old man in an assisted-living facility who has exhibited decreased food intake for 1 day but is still taking fluids. Which priority assessment would alert the adult-gerontology primary care NP to perform?
    1. Review medication profile, looking for potential adverse effects of medications that would lead to decreased food intake.
    2. Prescribe enteral nutritional support to maintain caloric intake.
    3. Inspect the patient's oral cavity to determine if there are any structural or infectious processes.
    4. Switch the patient to a pureed diet.

35. The adult-gerontology primary care NP is discussing making lifestyle changes that will decrease the older adult's risks for cardiovascular disease. Which of the following is most important to include in this discussion?
    1. Decrease smoking, increase vitamin supplements, and increase protein intake.

2. Control hypertension, stop smoking, maintain normal weight, and exercise regularly.
3. Maintain normal levels of serum blood sugar and decrease cholesterol intake.
4. Have a yearly physical examination, increase fiber in the diet, and exercise regularly.

36. **QSEN** The adult-gerontology primary care NP is seeing an 86-year-old patient diagnosed with postural hypotension. Which intervention would be recommended to reduce the patient's fall risk?
    1. Avoid excessive foot movement prior to standing.
    2. Encourage exercise in the early morning.
    3. Recommend wearing support stockings.
    4. Recommend walking away from the table within 10 minutes of eating.

37. Which of the following is an example of a community health promotion activity?
    1. High school–based family planning clinic.
    2. Work-site urgent care clinic.
    3. Asthma follow-up clinic in an elementary school.
    4. Employer-sponsored multiphasic health screening.

38. Which of the following two guidelines should the adult-gerontology primary care NP follow when developing educational materials?
    1. Present the most important material first, using all capital letters for emphasis.
    2. Provide the information in English along with three other languages.
    3. Keep sentences short and to the point, using graphic images for clarification.
    4. Keep the readability no higher than an eighth-grade level.
    5. Use only brightly colored paper and boldface type to enhance learning.

39. An older adult client reports being forgetful. The adult-gerontology primary care NP is planning a possible drug regimen. Which of the following would promote adherence to the drug regimen? Select three responses.
    1. Time doses of medications to mealtime.
    2. Choose medications that are similar in size and color.
    3. Prescribe the smallest number of medications.
    4. Order medications that are dosed once daily whenever possible.
    5. Provide detailed written instructions for each medication.
    6. Teach the patient to reduce the dose if side effects occur.

40. In explaining the purpose of primary prevention programs to a group of nursing students, the adult-gerontology primary care NP states that primary prevention programs:
    1. Work to lower the incidence of birth defects.

2. Emphasize early diagnosis and treatment of pediatric anomalies.
3. Minimize the handicapping effect of mental retardation.
4. Focus on the prevention of complications and rehabilitation.

41. A father (height 74 inches, onset of puberty at age 16) is concerned that his 15-year-old son is going to be short. In a physical exam, the adult-gerontology primary care NP finds the son is Tanner stage II, height 62 inches, and the results of the rest of the exam are essentially normal for a well-nourished adolescent. After reviewing his growth records, which indicate a growth pattern of height at the fifth percentile, the most likely diagnosis is:
    1. Constitutional growth delay.
    2. Familial short stature.
    3. Hypopituitarism.
    4. Idiopathic gonadotropin deficiency.

42. In the preparation of reading and educational materials for patients and parents, the adult-gerontology primary care NP is aware that the reading level of most adults is at the:
    1. 12th-grade level.
    2. 10th-grade level.
    3. Sixth-grade level.
    4. Fourth-grade level.

43. Which of the following is found in the LGBTQ young adult, as compared with a heterosexual young adult? Select two responses.
    1. Increased rate of substance abuse.
    2. Increased rate of smoking tobacco.
    3. Increased anxiety and manic-type behavior.
    4. Decreased rates of suicide and depression.
    5. Decreased rate of drinking alcohol.

44. Which lifestyle modifications are most effective in controlling hypertension in the older adult patient?
    1. Maintain normal weight, decrease sodium in diet, and exercise regularly.
    2. Increase dietary protein, decrease weight, and use stress-reduction techniques.
    3. Consume a high complex carbohydrate, low-sodium diet and decrease stress.
    4. Reduce weight, increase vitamin supplements, and exercise regularly.

45. An adult-gerontology primary care NP is reviewing a 72-year-old patient's history in the clinical setting. Which finding, if noted, requires a priority action in terms of health promotion and maintenance?
    1. Patient is not current for flu vaccination.
    2. Smoking history of one pack per day (PPD) for 10 years but has not smoked for 30 years.
    3. Patient wears eyeglasses for reading.
    4. History of osteoarthritis bilaterally in the knees.

46. When screening for intimate partner violence (IPV), it is important for the adult-gerontology primary care NP to understand that the following statement is true:
    1. Only men with psychological problems abuse women.
    2. IPV occurs in a small percentage of the population.
    3. Only people who come from abusive families end up in abusive relationships.
    4. One-fourth of all women experience IPV.

47. The adult-gerontology primary care NP has been asked by a local high school to provide an education program on teaching adolescents about social networking and texting on phones. The adult-gerontology primary care NP understands (select four responses):
    1. Mobile access to the Internet has become widespread among adolescents.
    2. Multitasking and using multiple media types at the same time have been associated with late nights and sleep deprivation in adolescents.
    3. Adolescents do not use the online social environment to interact with the same peers they spend their day with at school.
    4. Adolescent "sexting" has been linked to risky sexual behaviors in a few research studies.
    5. Adolescents texting on the phone while driving is outlawed in many states.
    6. Texting and emailing do not create opportunities for cyberbullying.

48. The adult-gerontology primary care NP who volunteers at a senior citizens center is planning activities for the members who attend the center. Which activity would best promote and maintain health for these senior citizens?
    1. Gardening every day for 1 hour.
    2. Cycling three times per week for 20 minutes.
    3. Sculpting once per week for 40 minutes.
    4. Walking three to five times per week for 30 minutes.

Immunizations

49. According to the Centers for Disease Control and Prevention (CDC), which two immunizations are recommended as primary prevention for adults ages 60 and above?
    1. Flu.
    2. Shingles.
    3. Yearly tetanus prophylaxis.
    4. Adult who has had previous allergic reaction to an immunization.

50. The mother of an older adolescent who has not had chickenpox is concerned and wants her daughter to be vaccinated. The recommendation is:
    1. Not recommended for children over age 12.
    2. One-time dose.
    3. Two doses at least 28 days apart.
    4. Three doses at 2 months apart.

51. Which of the following immunizations makes epiglottitis less likely?
    1. Epstein-Barr virus.
    2. *Haemophilus influenzae* type B (Hib).
    3. *Streptococcus pyogenes*.
    4. Coxsackievirus.

52. The influenza vaccination is recommended annually for high-risk groups. The adult-gerontology primary care NP knows that the greatest need for this vaccination is for:
    1. Adults with chronic disease.
    2. Residents of long-term care facilities.
    3. Dialysis patients.
    4. Healthcare employees.

53. The adult-gerontology primary care NP understands that the only contraindication to hepatitis B vaccination is:
    1. Pregnancy and lactation.
    2. History of poliomyelitis.
    3. Prior anaphylaxis or severe hypersensitivity.
    4. Mild viral illness.

54. A female college student develops symptoms of hepatitis A virus (HAV) about 5 weeks after receiving a vaccination for HAV. The adult-gerontology primary care NP explains to the patient (select three responses):
    1. HAV infections in the United States are most often acquired during travel to HAV-endemic countries.
    2. HAV vaccine is effective only after the second dose.
    3. Unprotected intercourse is the primary mode of transmission.
    4. Symptoms occur primarily after consuming food or water contaminated with HAV or via direct contact with a person with HAV infection with poor hygiene.
    5. A prevaccine exposure to HAV could be the reason for the patient's symptoms.

55. Immunizations and chemoprophylaxis offered routinely to patients 65 years of age or older are:
    1. Tdap/Td, influenza, shingles, and pneumococcal vaccine.
    2. Td, varicella, or shingles vaccine.
    3. Td and influenza; for those with a weakened immune system, offer the shingles vaccine.
    4. Offer influenza and Td vaccines to those who have not had these vaccines in the last 10 years.

56. Based on 2017 recommendations for immunizations for individuals who are over the age of 65, which schedule may be recommended on the basis of individual risk assessment?
    1. MMR.
    2. Chickenpox (varicella-zoster virus).
    3. Hepatitis B virus.
    4. Pneumococcal.

57. Which of the following patient situations requires the use of inactivated (not live) vaccines?
    1. History of nonspecific allergies.
    2. Immunocompromised adult.
    3. Concurrent antimicrobial therapy.
    4. Mild acute illness.

58. The adult-gerontology primary care NP performs a physical exam on a 75-year-old patient who is healthy. The patient remembers having chickenpox as a child and reports remembering a mild case of shingles on her back that occurred when she was in her 40s, with no postherpetic neuralgia. She has had no further episodes of shingles. What should the adult-gerontology primary care NP do?
    1. Administer the Zostavax vaccine.
    2. Order a varicella titer.
    3. Administer Twinrix vaccine.
    4. Do nothing, because the patient reports having had chickenpox.

59. In taking the history of a healthy 50-year-old man, the adult-gerontology primary care NP determines the patient is an avid gardener and spends much of his time enjoying outdoor activities. A health maintenance recommendation for this patient is to obtain a:
    1. Pneumococcal vaccine.
    2. Tdap/Td vaccine.
    3. Hepatitis B vaccine.
    4. Varicella vaccine.

60. At which patient age should the adult-gerontology primary care NP's recommend routine use of the pneumococcal vaccination?
    1. 65 years of age or older.
    2. 60 years of age or older.
    3. 55 years of age or older.
    4. 50 years of age or older.

61. The ACIP recommends that healthy older adults receive the Td or tetanus booster vaccination:
    1. Every 5 years.
    2. Every 10 years.
    3. At age 65.
    4. At age 50.

62. A 65-year-old woman inquires about her vaccination requirements regarding the pneumococcal vaccine. She received a single Pneumovax 23 (PPSV23) vaccination at age 57 because of the presence of risk factors. She has never received any other pneumococcal vaccinations. Which of the following should the adult-gerontology primary care NP recommend?
    1. Administer Pneumovax 23 (PPSV23) vaccine now.
    2. No further vaccination is necessary.
    3. Administer Prevnar (PCV13) vaccine now.
    4. Administer Pneumovax 23 (PPSV23) vaccine at age 67.

63. Which statement most correctly describes tetanus toxoid?
    1. Tetanus toxoid is a bacterial toxin that has been changed to a nontoxic form.
    2. DTaP and DT are safe to give to adults.
    3. The recommended dose of tetanus toxoid for adults is 1 mL intramuscularly.
    4. Tetanus toxoid provides immunity from *Corynebacterium diphtheriae.*

64. Immunizations recommended for healthy young adults include:
    1. Measles, rubella, varicella, and hepatitis B.
    2. Pneumovax, influenza, and rubella.
    3. Tetanus, influenza, varicella, Pneumovax, and hepatitis B.
    4. Influenza, hepatitis B, rubella, measles, and tetanus.

65. An elderly patient comes to your office 2 days after receiving the pneumococcal conjugate vaccine (PCV13). He complains of pain at the injection site and difficulty raising his arm without pain. He has a fever of 100.4°F (38°C). You recognize that:
    1. This is a serious reaction to the immunization and that he may need hospitalization.
    2. The fever and the vaccination are likely unrelated.
    3. It is somewhat common to get a fever and localized reaction to this vaccine.
    4. The patient may be allergic to eggs.

66. Primary prevention of neonatal abstinence syndrome (NAS) includes:
    1. Prescribing a reliable form of birth control for a patient being treated for chronic pain with opioids.
    2. Universally screening pregnant women for substance abuse and making referrals for treatment when appropriate.
    3. Never prescribing opioids to a woman of childbearing age.
    4. Obtaining a patient's records from the state prescription drug monitoring program if you suspect she is getting opioids from another provider.

67. Smallpox vaccine is offered to certain members of the military in anticipation of possible exposure due to bioterrorism. What are two common side effects of smallpox vaccination?
    1. Myocarditis and pericarditis.
    2. Dime-sized blister lesion at the injection site that forms a scab and leaves a scar.
    3. Severe allergic reaction.
    4. Fatigue.
    5. Severe skin conditions.

68. The human papilloma virus (HPV) vaccine should be recommended to:
    1. A 28-year-old man who did not finish the vaccine series as a teen.
    2. Young men through the age of 21.
    3. Any man who has sex with men.
    4. Men with compromised immune systems (including HIV infection) through age 30 if they did not get the HPV vaccine when they were young.

69. The following person should not receive the shingles vaccine:
    1. A 62-year-old patient who previously had chickenpox.
    2. A 45-year-old patient who was exposed to chickenpox.
    3. A 60-year-old patient who had the vaccine at 50 years old.
    4. A person being treated with corticosteroids.

70. An adult who works as a veterinarian has been administered a rabies vaccination. What are four possible side effects and risks of receiving the vaccination?
    1. Hives, fever, and joint pain.
    2. Soreness and redness at the injection site.
    3. Headache and dizziness.
    4. Abdominal pain and gastric distress.
    5. Diplopia and confusion.
    6. Severe allergic reaction.

71. Immunizations recommended for a healthy 40-year-old adult who has had his childhood series include:
    1. Measles, rubella, varicella, and hepatitis B.
    2. Pneumovax, influenza, and rubella.
    3. Tetanus, influenza, varicella, Pneumovax, OPV, and hepatitis B.
    4. Influenza, hepatitis A, hepatitis B, varicella, MMR, and tetanus.

3 Health Promotion & Maintenance Answers & Rationales

1. Answer: 1

Rationale: With the older adult population, there are normal changes associated with aging that may lead to potential sensory deficits (sensory losses) that can prove to be a barrier in providing and receiving information. Although information may have to be repeated, the assumption that this is due to mental deficits associated with aging is a form of implicit bias. Handouts that contain easily understood language, providing examples to use in demonstration of content, and ensuring that the room in which teaching/learning occurs has good lighting will help to promote educational learning.

2. Answer: 3

Rationale: Any patient with gait, balance, or sensory deficits is considered moderate or high risk, regardless of fall history. A patient with gait, balance, or sensory deficits who has not fallen, or a patient who has fallen 1 time without injury is classified as moderate risk. A patient who has fallen once with injury or fallen two or more times is considered at high risk. Only patients without gait and balance issues without a history of falls are classified as low risk and may need further evaluation with other assessment tools. A patient who had concerns about falling but didn't exhibit any balance or ambulation problems would be considered at low risk.

3. Answer: 3

Rationale: Secondary prevention measures focus on detection and management of potential disease states through diagnostic testing and scheduled examinations; thus, detection of vitamin D levels helps to establish a baseline. Dietary counseling and identifying smoking are examples of primary level of prevention measures because they focus on preventing the occurrence of disease and identifying relevant risk behaviors. Focusing on preventing complications related to disease is an example of a tertiary level of prevention because the disease process is already established.

4. Answer: 1

Rationale: The ACS recommends maintenance of a desirable body weight; research has shown an association between increased mortality resulting from various cancers and varying degrees of being overweight. Another recommendation is to eat a wide variety of foods, consistent with the ChooseMyPlate guide of the U.S. Department of Agriculture and U.S. Department of Health and Human Services. A variety of fruits and vegetables should be included in the daily diet (make half your plate fruits and vegetables) because research has shown an association between lower cancer rates and high fruit and vegetable consumption. High-fiber foods are also recommended; a lower risk of colon cancer is seen in those who consume a high-fiber diet. Currently, there are no recommendations to increase the amount of protein in the diet. Because of the high consumption of red meat in the American diet, many people are already receiving large quantities in their current diets. It is recommended that red meat and processed foods should be limited. The ACS recommends limiting the daily consumption of alcohol to two drinks for males, one drink for females, and no drinks for pregnant females. They also state that ideally, no alcohol should be consumed; regular alcohol consumption has been shown to increase the risk of various cancers.

5. Answer: 2, 4, 5

Rationale: Adolescents most likely to smoke, abuse substances, perform poorly in school, be depressed, and engage in risky behavior are those who have a history of being unsupervised after school.

6. Answer: 1

Rationale: The recommendation is LDL <100 mg/dL and triglyceride levels <200 mg/dL for individuals with risk factors for coronary heart disease (CHD). Although 150 mg/dL is the ideal goal for triglyceride, treatment is started at >200 mg/dL in the diabetic and almost all other patients with risk factors. In a diabetic patient, LDL goal is independently <100 mg/dL. If the patient has triglycerides >200 mg/dL, then the goal is <130 mg/dL non-LDL cholesterol. All other choices have inaccurate goals.

7. Answer: 1

Rationale: The U.S. Preventive Services Task Force (USPSTF) recommends screening for colorectal cancer using high-sensitivity gFOBT, sigmoidoscopy, or colonoscopy beginning at age 50 years and continuing until age 75 years. Of course, a colonoscopy is the best test and it is okay to have a standalone screening of gFOBT, as long as colonoscopy is recommended first. The multiple gFOBT stool take-home test should be used. One gFOBT test obtained by the adult-gerontology primary care NP in the office is not adequate for testing. A colonoscopy should be scheduled if the gFOBT test result is positive.

8. Answer: 2

Rationale: The American Diabetes Association recommends screening adults starting at least by age 45 and repeating the FPG every 3 years. This is for all patients and screening is indicated at 3 year intervals for patients with >25 BMI or other risk factors at any age for an adult. The USPSTF recommends screening for abnormal blood glucose as part of cardiovascular risk assessment in adults aged 40 to 70 years who are overweight or obese.

9. Answer: 2

Rationale: Tertiary prevention refers to reducing the impact of an ongoing illness or injury. The physical therapy program will assist the older adult woman in restoring her optimum level of functioning after a stroke. An annual influenza vaccination is a primary prevention activity nonspecific to the care of a patient with a stroke. An annual mammogram and ophthalmologic examination to evaluate for glaucoma are examples of secondary prevention activities nonspecific to the care of a patient with a stroke.

10. Answer: 3

Rationale: Research literature has been focused on several primary risk factors for the development of AD being related to advancing age, low education levels, lack of cognitively stimulating activities, family history, specific genotypes, and head trauma. Research has shown that with continued physical activity, cognitive deficits are prevented.

11. Answer: 3

Rationale: The patient needs an increased intake of protein and vitamin C to promote healing. Red meat, citrus fruits, and green vegetables will give the highest amounts of these elements among the selections offered.

12. Answer: 2, 4, 6

Rationale: Health literacy is the degree to which a person has the capacity to obtain, discuss, process, and understand health information and systems and to use that knowledge to make informed, appropriate decisions. Low health literacy affects people's ability to navigate the healthcare system, including filling out complex forms, locating providers and services, keeping appointments, and engaging in appropriate self-care and chronic disease management. Other risks associated with low health literacy are higher hospitalization rates and urgent care clinic and emergency department visits, as well as not using preventive health measures, such as screenings and immunizations. Older adults, racial and ethnic minorities, individuals who have less than a high school degree or GED (general educational development) certificate, individuals living in poverty and having low income levels, non-native speakers of English, and people with compromised health status are associated with low health literacy.

13. Answer: 3

Rationale: Shouting increases the pitch of the voice. In presbycusis, or hearing loss in older adults, high-pitched consonant sounds are the first to be affected, and the change may occur gradually. The adult-gerontology primary care NP should face the patient when speaking. If the nurse needs to stand behind the patient, touch is used to get the patient's attention. Simple sentences should be used to facilitate understanding.

14. Answer: 4

Rationale: The information about side effects and interactions of medication will prevent complications that may result in a fall. Evaluating for assistive devices following a fall and providing resources to correct hazards in the home are appropriate for tertiary prevention. Reinforcing the need to wear prescribed eyeglasses is appropriate for secondary prevention, which is intended to prevent the patient from experiencing another fall.

15. Answer: 4

Rationale: The guaiac-based fecal occult blood test (gFOBT) will assist in identifying any problems with intestinal bleeding, polyps, and cancer and is recommended to be started at age 50. Pneumococcal vaccination is not a screening test. A colonoscopy is recommended at age 50 and then every 10 years thereafter, not annually. Annual chest x-rays are recommended for adults ages 55–80 years who have a 30 pack-year smoking history and currently smoke or have quit within the past 15 years.

16. Answer: 2

Rationale: The Older Americans Act (OAA) functions at the state level and provides rules to assist with nutritional well-being for the older adult. Toward that end, meals can be delivered at other nonscheduled times to facilitate engagement. Other sources of dietary calcium can be used because milk is not the preferred dietary source. Congregate meals can be served at nontraditional locations, and salt shakers can be provided at the table.

17. Answer: 4

Rationale: Using past life experiences applies the concept of adult educational principles. Overhead lighting may produce an increase in the glare, which can decrease visualization. There is an alteration of color perception (for example, blue appears green-blue) as an individual ages. As individuals age, the ability to hear women's and children's voices decreases because these are generally at a higher pitch. The video would not enhance the program because the patients frequently have presbycusis as a result of the normal aging process.

18. Answer: 4, 5

Rationale: The REALM-SF and Newest Vital Sign are two instruments that can easily be used in the primary care setting to assess health literacy. The REALM-SF tests the subject's comprehension as well as pronunciation of health-related or medical terminology in either English or Spanish, takes only 2–3 minutes to perform, and requires minimal training. The Newest Vital Sign instrument, also known as the ice cream label test, tests literacy skills for both numbers and words. The patient is asked to read and analyze the nutrition label on an ice cream container and then answer six questions. The SMOG Index, Flesch-Kincaid readability test, and New Dale-Chall readability formula are instruments that measure the readability of text and can assist with determining at what grade level information is written.

19. Answer: 3

Rationale: All these disorders can be associated with workplace exposure, but lung disease is currently still the most common occupationally related disease. Representing approximately 10% of the chronic occupational diseases, lung disease has been named as 1 of 10 leading work-related disease and injury categories by the National Institute for Occupational Safety and Health. Musculoskeletal injuries are on the rise.

20. Answer: 2, 3, 4, 5

Rationale: The older patient is at risk for oral health problems, and health promotion teaching should be focused on periodontal irritation, tooth loss, decreased taste perception, and maintaining hydration. Excessive salivation is typically not seen in the older patient; rather, dry mouth occurs because of decreased salivation.

21. Answer: 4

Rationale: The primary goal and benefit of a sports screening physical exam is to identify athletes at risk for an adverse cardiovascular event. The physical exam also screens for athletes at risk for orthopedic injuries secondary to previously unresolved injuries; however, this is not the primary benefit. Even with a thorough history obtained from the screening exam, performing the exam is unlikely to completely eliminate injuries or be able to identify all underlying health problems. The other options (assessing drug and alcohol use and estimating aerobic capacity) are not the benefit of the sports screening physical.

22. Answer: 3

Rationale: Starting at age 50, a screening mammogram should be performed every 2 years through age 74. At ages 75 and older, the patient needs to check with the doctor or adult-gerontology primary care NP to see if screening is re-

quired because of previous findings and current risk factors. Patients should be tested for chlamydia or HIV if they are sexually active and at increased risk. Starting at age 50, a patient should be screened for colorectal cancer every 10 years unless there are increased risk factors or polyps are present.

23. Answer: 4

Rationale: The patient's history and physical exam will reveal the presence of any CHD risk factors (age, family, history of CHD, diabetes, current cigarette smoking, blood pressure, height/weight, cardiovascular exam). A lipid profile is also recommended to assess the level of risk and consists of total cholesterol, high-density lipoprotein, LDL, and triglyceride levels. It would be prudent to have a precise cholesterol measurement done because the previous measurement was done at a screening health fair, and no written record was taken. These parameters should be assessed first, before a cholesterol-lowering agent, ECG, or stress test is ordered. An exercise program is also important but should be done only after a history is taken and a physical exam is done, as well as after lipid profile results are known. If the lipid profile or the history and physical exam results are abnormal, stress testing may be appropriate before undertaking a new exercise program.

24. Answer: 3, 4

Rationale: Navajo Native Americans and individuals from Middle Eastern cultures embrace the practice of not informing a patient of a terminal disease. With the Navajo culture, it is believed that a person's thought and language have the power to shape reality; therefore, talking about a possible negative outcome is thought to ensure the outcome. The other cultural groups do not share this attitude.

25. Answer: 2

Rationale: Screening for colorectal cancer includes annual fecal occult blood screening for individuals over age 50. Avoiding medications that can cause gastrointestinal irritation and bleeding can help avoid false-positive results. Rare meat and vegetables that are high in peroxidase will cause false-positive results, whereas vitamin C can cause false-negative results.

26. Answer: 1

Rationale: Maintaining muscle strength reduces the risk of immobility. Immobility is a predictor of loss of independence, depression, reduced quality of life, falling, institutionalization, and death. Sleeping long hours is not associated with improved energy. Optimal nutrition and urinary incontinence are not as great a threat to loss of independence as immobility is. Fall reduction is a Healthy People 2020 goal.

27. Answer: 1, 3

Rationale: Beans and peas are legumes, which are included in the vegetable group and are excellent sources of plant proteins. Quinoa, popcorn, and wild rice belong to the grains group.

28. Answer: 3, 4, 5

Rationale. The correct answers are HEADSS FIRST, CRAFTT, and PLISSIT. The mnemonic HEADSS FIRST refers to **h**ome, **e**ducation, **a**ctivities, **d**rugs, **s**exual activity, **s**uicide or depression, **f**riends, **i**mage, **r**ecreation, **s**afety issues, and **t**hreats. These are six areas for the adult-gerontology primary care NP to focus questions on after determining the adolescent's dietary practices as well as elimination and sleep habits. If there is acknowledgement by the adolescent regarding the use of street drugs or alcohol, the CRAFTT acronym can be used to further explore the areas of **c**ars, **r**elax, **a**lone, **f**orget, **f**riends, **t**rouble, which provide the first letters of six screening questions. The CRAFTT screening questions are as follows:

- Ever ridden in a **car** driven by someone who was high or had been using drugs (including yourself)?
- Ever use alcohol or drugs to **relax**, feel better about yourself, or fit in?
- Ever use alcohol or drugs while you are **alone**?
- Ever **forget** things you did while using alcohol or drugs?
- Do family or **friends** ever tell you to cut down on your drinking or drug use?
- Ever in **trouble** while using alcohol or drugs?

The PLISSIT acronym describes a model for four levels of interventions used in primary care addressing sexual concerns: **p**ermission, **l**imited **i**nformation, **s**pecific **s**uggestions, and **i**ntensive **t**herapy. The acronym FAST (**f**ace, **a**rm, **s**peech, **t**ime) is used as a way of identifying the signs of a stroke. The acronym GENES may be useful in identifying red flags in a family history. The G represents groups of anomalies, the E represents early or extreme presentation of common diseases, the N represents neurodevelopmental or neurodegenerative conditions, the E represents exception or unusual pathology, and the S represents surprising laboratory findings—any of which may be indicative of an underlying genetic condition.

29. Answer: 3

Rationale: According to the 2016 U.S. Preventive Services Task Force (USPSTF) recommendations, screening mammography in women prior to age 50 years should be an individual decision. Women may choose to begin biennial screening between the ages of 40 and 49 years. Biennial screening mammography is recommended for women aged 50-74 with average risk. The American Cancer Society (2015) recommendations are that women aged 40-44 years should have the choice to start annual breast cancer screening with mammograms if they wish to do so, and women aged 45-54 years should get mammograms every year and switch to every 2 years at the age of 55.

30. Answer: 1

Rationale: All areas are important to probe in the initial interview of a new patient. The history will help to determine the necessary components of the physical exam and lab or radiologic studies that are ordered as well as the counseling that is done during the appointment.

31. Answer: 2, 3, 5

Rationale: The adult-gerontology primary care NP should identify specific methods to improve safe use of medications in the older adult by conducting a thorough assessment of the patient's cognitive and motor abilities and presence of polypharmacy. Although many analgesics can contribute to constipation, it is assessment of kidney function that is most important because the older adult is less able to eliminate drugs, owing to glomerular filtration rate gradually declining by about 40% from ages 20 to 80 years. The golden rule in prescribing to the older adult is to start with the lowest dose possible and titrate the medication dose slowly on the basis of the renal and hepatic function of the patient. Determining sleeping patterns does not focus on promoting drug safety in the older adult.

32. Answer: 4

Rationale: An account of the patient's usual food intake is necessary so that problem areas can be identified. Before beginning any exercise program, a physical exam should be done to assess the patient's physical condition and to aid in the proper selection of a specific exercise plan. A dietary assessment needs to be completed before recommending vitamin and protein supplements; the patient may already be receiving adequate amounts in her diet. A more active job would be ideal; however, most people do not have options regarding their choice of job, so increasing her activity outside of work would be most appropriate.

33. Answer: 4

Rationale: The older adult is at greatest risk for altered immune function related to nutrition. The older adult often does not receive enough nutrition for a variety of reasons, including altered taste, eating alone, ability to prepare meals, and malabsorption. Adequate nutrition in the older adult has been shown to improve immune status and antibody response to influenza vaccine.

34. Answer: 3

Rationale: Because the patient is experiencing a decrease in food intake but still taking fluids, there is no immediate need to prescribe enteral nutritional support or switching of diet. Best practice would be to inspect the oral cavity to see if there is any structural or infectious process that is preventing ingestion of food. Reviewing the medication profile of the patient may be needed but would not be the priority assessment at this time.

35. Answer: 2

Rationale: Hypertension, smoking, and hyperlipidemia are the major risk factors in the development of cardiovascular disease. Controlling hyperglycemia, increasing high dietary fiber intake, and taking vitamin supplements assist in maintaining a healthy lifestyle, but they are not as important in preventing cardiovascular disease.

36. Answer: 3

Rationale: Support stockings improve blood return to the central circulation, improving cardiac output and cerebral perfusion. Dorsiflexion of the feet and leg movement help improve cardiac output. Exercise should be postponed until later in the afternoon or evening, when blood pressure is higher. Waiting for 20 minutes or longer to stand from the table helps reduce orthostatic hypotension following meals.

37. Answer: 4

Rationale: Multiphasic health screening is a form of periodic health surveillance in which participants undergo a battery of laboratory or diagnostic tests to determine risk factors and disease detection. The other three settings described are not examples of community health promotion activities; they are secondary care settings. The locations of the two clinics are in community settings.

38. Answer: 3, 4

Rationale: The average adult in the United States reads at about the sixth- to eighth-grade level. Printed materials must be written at a level of readability so that they can be understood. Do not use all capital letters or all-boldface type, because such words are difficult to read. In addition, it is helpful to write in the active versus the passive voice, to use one- and two-syllable words, to avoid complex grammatical structures, and to express only one idea in each sentence. Well-chosen and easily understood graphics can significantly enhance the literature, as can the selection of paper on which to print the material.

39. Answer: 1, 3, 4

Rationale: To promote patient adherence in prescribing medications, the following are effective measures: prescribe the lowest dose and the smallest number of medications with the simplest dose regimens, providing simple verbal and written instructions for each medication and what it is for. The scheduling of medications that is best for the patient who is forgetful is a once-a-day dose and timing the doses to mealtimes to support the older adult in remembering to take the medication. If side effects occur, the patient should be told to call the adult-gerontology primary care NP. The patient should not be taught to reduce or alter the dose of the medication without guidance from the adult-gerontology primary care NP. Medications that are similar in size and color can be difficult for the older adult to discriminate because of reduced vision or being forgetful.

40. Answer: 1

Rationale: Primary prevention programs exist to prevent disease, malfunctioning, or maladaptation from occurring (for example, work to lower the incidence of birth defects). Examples of these types of programs include the promotion of a healthy diet, practice of safe sex, and avoidance of alcohol and tobacco. Secondary prevention is early diagnosis and treatment (for example, screening for tuberculosis or sickle cell disease, breast and testicular self-examination). Tertiary prevention is the prevention of complications and rehabilitation after the disease or condition has occurred (for example, cardiac rehabilitation, complete blood count done before chemotherapy).

41. Answer: 1

Rationale: Familial short stature is not indicated in this case, because the father is of normal height. Hypopituitarism would be associated with other findings (micropenis, small testes, immature facies, olfactory defects). Gonadotropin deficiency might be a possibility, but considering all findings in the situation and based on the father having a pubertal onset at age 16 and achieving an average height, the more likely diagnosis is constitutional growth delay.

42. Answer: 3

Rationale: The reading level of most American adults is between grades 6 and 8; therefore, the sixth-grade level would be the most appropriate answer among the choices given.

43. Answer: 1, 2

Rationale: LGBTQ is a common acronym that typically refers to lesbian, gay, bisexual, transgender, and queer or questioning individuals. LGBTQ young adults have increases rates of smoking, drinking alcohol, and substance abuse as compared with their heterosexual peers. In addition, they also have increased rates of eating disorders, anxiety, depression, and suicidal thoughts.

44. Answer: 1

Rationale: Maintaining normal weight, decreasing sodium in the diet, and exercising regularly are three modifications that are most effective in maintaining normal blood pressure in the older adult.

45. Answer: 1

Rationale: When reviewing an older patient's history in the clinical setting, it is important to assess whether the patient is current (up-to-date) with immunizations. Older patients are especially susceptible to seasonal flu, which may end up compromising their health. Past smoking history, even with a recorded PPD, is not a priority assessment if it has been 30 years since active smoking. The fact that a patient wears reading glasses does not require a priority action. Similarly, a history of osteoarthritis does not require a priority action, unless there are known deficits related to ambulation and/or increases in pain.

46. Answer: 4

Rationale: One-fourth of all women experience IPV. IPV can occur in any adult-gerontology primary care setting. Most abused women report that their partner was the first person to abuse them. Many batterers are successful professionals, including politicians, ministers, physicians, and lawyers.

47. Answer: 1, 2, 4, 5

Rationale: The use of social media and access to the Internet are very prominent and widespread among adolescents. This promotes opportunities for developing interpersonal skills and in some environments (rural areas, adolescents with rare health conditions or shyness) provides an avenue for the adolescent to interact with others like themselves. Many states have outlawed the use of handheld mobile devices while an adolescent is actively driving a car. Sexting is the sending of sexually explicit or suggestive pictures or messages online and has been linked to risky sexual behaviors. Adolescents actually do use the online social environment to interact with the same peers they spend their day with at school and in extracurricular activities. The online environment can create opportunities for cyberbullying. Cyberbullying is the communication of insults, harassment, and publicly humiliating statements via social media, that is, emails, online chat rooms, or texting on cell phones.

48. Answer: 4

Rationale: Exercise and activity are essential for health promotion and maintenance in the older adult and to achieve an optimal level of functioning. About half of the physical deterioration of the older patient is caused by disuse rather than by the aging process or disease. One of the best exercises for an older adult is walking, progressing to 30-minute sessions, three to five times each week. Swimming and dancing are also beneficial.

Immunizations

49. Answer: 1, 2

Rationale: The CDC recommends that adults ages 60 and over should receive immunizations for seasonal flu and herpes zoster. Yearly tetanus prophylaxis is not indicated, because the required time interval for a booster is every 10 years and/or in response to an injury. An adult who has had a previous allergic reaction to an immunization should be further evaluated to determine potential adverse reactions to specific components before any immunization schedule is started.

50. Answer: 3

Rationale: Adolescents over the age of 13 years who have not had chickenpox and have not previously been immunized are recommended to have two doses at least 28 days apart for effective immunity.

51. Answer: 2

Rationale: Hib makes infection less likely. Hib vaccine successfully decreases the possibility of epiglottitis. A wide variety of viruses, bacteria, and even fungi can cause epiglottitis. There are no vaccines for Epstein-Barr virus, *Streptococcus pyogenes, or coxsackievirus.*

52. Answer: 2

Rationale: Influenza outbreaks may affect 60% of those in long-term care, and mortality rates are high. All the other groups listed are appropriate for the influenza vaccine but are not as high a priority.

53. Answer: 3

Rationale: Prior anaphylaxis and severe hypersensitivity would be considered a contraindication; a mild viral illness would not. The patient who is pregnant or lactating may be immunized.

54. Answer: 1, 4, 5

Rationale The primary transmission is fecal-oral; bloodborne transmission is rare. Men who have sex with men is a risk factor. The incubation period is 2–6 weeks (mean 4 weeks). Infection occurs primarily after consuming food or water contaminated with HAV or via direct contact with a person with HAV infection with poor hygiene. The Advisory Committee on Immunization Practices (ACIP) recommends that one dose of single-antigen HAV vaccine administered at any time before travel departure may provide adequate protection for most healthy persons. In this patient situation, prevaccine exposure to HAV was present.

55. Answer: 1

Rationale: Pneumococcal and annual influenza immunizations are recommended for those who are age 65 and older, along with shingles. Tdap for all adults aged 65 years and older is recommended for those who never received a Tdap as an adult, because then they would just get Td booster every 10 years since this is recommended at all ages >19 years. Boostrix should be used for adults aged 65 years and older; however, the ACIP concluded that either vaccine (Adacel or Boostrix) administered to a person 65 years or older is immunogenic and provides protection. Shingles vaccine is contraindicated in women who are pregnant and in individuals who have a weakened immune system.

56. Answer: 3

Rationale: A hepatitis B series *may be* recommended for adults who are 65 years of age and older on the basis of clinical risk assessment. MMR vaccination would not be required or recommended for this age group. Chickenpox (varicella-zoster virus) and pneumococcal immunization *would be* recommended for this age group.

57. Answer: 2

Rationale: The live vaccine can produce serious disseminated disease in patients with immunocompromised status (for example, leukemia, lymphoma, HIV/AIDS) and in those undergoing cancer chemotherapy. Mild acute illness, concurrent antimicrobial therapy, and a history of nonspecific allergies are not contraindications for use of a live vaccine.

58. Answer: 1

Rationale: People 60 years of age or older should get a shingles vaccine (Zostavax). They should get the vaccine regardless of whether they recall having had chickenpox. There is no maximum age for getting a shingles vaccine. Twinrix is a combined HAV and hepatitis B virus vaccine that can be given to adults. There is no reason to order a varicella titer.

59. Answer: 2

Rationale: All adults (not just the ones who enjoy gardening and outdoor activities) should have a Tdap/Td booster once, as recommended by the ACIP. As part of standard wound management care to prevent tetanus, a tetanus toxoid–containing vaccine might be recommended for wound management in adults aged 19 years and older if 5 years or more have elapsed since last receiving a Td vaccine. If a tetanus booster is indicated, Tdap is preferred over Td for wound management in

adults aged 19 years and older who have not received Tdap previously. A pneumococcal vaccine is recommended for adults aged 65 or older and for those with a chronic illness or in an immunosuppressed state. Most older adults had chickenpox as a child and do not require the vaccine.

60. Answer: 1

Rationale: The pneumococcal polysaccharide vaccine Pneumovax 23 (PPSV23) is recommended in patients without risk factors starting at age 65. PPSV23 vaccination is indicated only for those ages 2–64 if additional risk factors or comorbidities are present, including smoking, immunosuppression, or serious disease.

61. Answer: 2

Rationale: Td is usually given as a booster dose every 10 years but it can also be given earlier after a severe and dirty wound or burn. For adults aged 19 through 64 years who previously have not received a dose of Tdap, a single dose of Tdap should replace a single decennial (occurring every 10 years) Td booster dose. Persons aged 65 years and older (e.g., grandparents, child-care providers, and health-care practitioners) who have or who anticipate having close contact with an infant aged less than 12 months and who previously have not received Tdap should receive a single dose of Tdap to protect against pertussis and reduce the likelihood of transmission. For other adults aged 65 years and older, a single dose of Tdap vaccine may be administered instead of Td vaccine in persons who previously have not received Tdap. Boostrix should be used for adults aged 65 years and older; however, the ACIP concluded that either vaccine (Boostrix or Adacel) administered to a person aged 65 years or older is immunogenic and would provide protection.

62. Answer: 3

Rationale: Patients who have received any pneumococcal vaccination require investigation regarding the time of administration and type of vaccine administered. Ideally, patients without additional risk factors should be administered the PCV13 (Prevnar) vaccine at age 65 or older, followed by PPSV23 1 year later. A patient with risk factors and a previous PPSV23 vaccination history should be administered the PCV13 vaccine at age 65, but no less than 1 year after the PPSV23 was administered. Continued revaccination with the PPSV23 is indicated on the basis of type and severity of risk factors.

63. Answer: 1

Rationale: Tetanus toxoid is a bacterial toxin that has been changed to nontoxic form and produces persistent antitoxin antibody titers because the patient's immune system is stimulated to manufacture antitoxins (that is, antibodies directed against the bacterial toxin). *C. diphtheriae* is the organism that causes diphtheria, not tetanus. DTaP and DT are for use in children under age 7 years and should *not* be used in adults. DT does not contain pertussis and is given as a substitute for children who cannot tolerate the DTaP vaccine, which contains pertussis. The recommended dose of tetanus toxoid alone for an adult is 0.5 mL IM. To help you remember, look closely at the letters and keep the following in mind:

- Upper case "T" means there is about the same amount of tetanus in DTaP, Tdap, and Td. (DTaP is given to children, usually infants, under age 7.)
- Upper case "D" and "P" mean there is more diphtheria and pertussis in DTaP than in Tdap and Td; lower case letters ("d" and "p") mean there is less. (Tdap is a booster given at age 11 years and throughout life, usually every 10 years, and is recommended as a booster after age 65.)

64. Answer: 4

Rationale: A percentage of young adults (5% to 20%) are susceptible to measles and/or rubella. Influenza and hepatitis B vaccinations are recommended for young adults who have exposure to a large number of people. Tetanus is recommended every 10 years, especially in high-risk situations (young adults who participate in outdoor sports). Pneumovax is indicated in a young adult who has a chronic disease (for example, diabetes, chronic pulmonary disease, chronic cardiovascular disease) and is also indicated for young adults who are immunocompromised.

65. Answer: 3

Rationale: According to the CDC, one of three patients develops a mild fever and localized pain at the injection site. There is no indication that this patient requires hospitalization at this time. The fever is likely related to the vaccination. There is no contraindication about receiving this vaccine with an allergy to egg.

66. Answer: 1

Rationale: Pregnancy prevention is the primary prevention strategy for NAS. Universal screening and referrals for treatment are recommended, but they do not prevent NAS. There will be times when women of childbearing age must be prescribed opioids. Although consulting the drug monitoring program does help decrease "doctor shopping," it does not prevent NAS.

67. Answer: 2, 4

Rationale: The smallpox vaccination has the following common side effects: itching, swollen lymph nodes, sore arm resulting from the injection, fever, headache, body ache, mild rash, and fatigue. The injection site lesion starts as a red and itchy bump forming at the vaccination site within 2–5 days, then in the next few days, the bump becomes a blister and fills with pus. During the second week, the blister dries up, and a scab forms. The fluid from the lesion and the crust are contagious until a scab forms. The scab falls off after 2–4 weeks, leaving a scar. Serious side effects include heart problems (myocarditis and pericarditis), severe allergic reaction, swelling of the brain or spinal cord, and severe skin diseases.

68. Answer: 2

Rationale: All boys and girls ages 11 or 12 years should get vaccinated. Catchup vaccines are recommended for males through age 21 and for females through age 26. The vaccine is also recommended for gay and bisexual men (or for any man who has sex with a man) through age 26. It is also recommended for men and women with compromised immune systems (including people living with HIV infection) through age 26 if they did not get fully vaccinated when they were younger.

69. Answer: 4

Rationale: A person should not receive the shingles vaccine if immunosuppressed or receiving medications that suppress the immune system, such as corticosteroids. Other situations when a person should not receive the immunization include pregnancy, untreated tuberculosis, allergy to gelatin or neomycin, or receiving chemotherapy or radiation therapy. Anyone 60 years of age or older should receive the vaccine, regardless of whether they can recall having received the vaccine. Exposure to chickenpox in a 45-year-old patient does not warrant vaccination at this time. Adults receiving the vaccine before the age of 60 might not be protected when their risk for shingles and its complications are greatest.

70. Answer: 1, 2, 3, 4

Rationale: The risk of the rabies vaccine causing serious harm or death is extremely small. Serious problems arising from the rabies vaccine are very rare, according to the CDC. The adult-gerontology primary care NP recognizes the following as a mild problem following immunization: soreness, redness, swelling, or itching where the shot was given; headache; nausea; abdominal pain; muscle aches; and dizziness. Moderate problems following vaccination include hives, pain in the joints, and fever. Diplopia, confusion, and severe allergic reactions are not typical side effects or reactions.

71. Answer: 4

Rationale: It would be important to start the hepatitis B series, considering his age, because this was not included as part of his childhood vaccination series. Hepatitis A is also recommended, especially if the person travels to foreign countries, along with varicella because these immunizations were not available during his childhood. An MMR immunization is required for adults born in 1957 or later who have no laboratory proof of immunity or documentation of either previous vaccination or a physician-documented case of measles. Tetanus vaccination is recommended every 10 years, especially in high-risk situations (adults who participate in outdoor sports). Pneumovax is indicated for an adult who has a chronic disease, such as diabetes, chronic pulmonary disease, or chronic cardiovascular disease, and it is also indicated for adults who are immunocompromised. If the adult did not receive the OPV series as a child, it is recommended to vaccinate the adult with injectable enhanced-potency inactivated polio virus vaccine because the risk of vaccine-associated poliomyelitis is lower.

Cardiovascular

4

Physical Examination & Diagnostic Tests

1. The adult-gerontology primary care NP is taking a history and performing a physical examination on a female patient who is complaining of chest pain. Which technique would be best practice for the following finding that would increase suspicion for determination of a cardiac event?
   1. Patient denies drug use.
   2. Presence of adventitious lung sounds.
   3. Absent T waves on electrocardiogram (ECG).
   4. Absence of jaw pain.

2. The adult-gerontology primary care NP is providing instructions to a patient who is scheduled for a transthoracic echocardiogram (TTE). Which instruction should be included in the teaching session?
   1. Do not eat or drink for at least 12 hours prior to testing.
   2. Do not take any medication prior to the test, unless it considered to be a cardiac medication.
   3. Take all regularly scheduled medications prior to testing.
   4. Increase fluids prior to testing.

3. The adult-gerontology primary care NP is performing a physical examination on a healthy adult male. On auscultation, the stethoscope would be placed in which areas to best hear the characteristic heart sounds S_1 and S_2?
   1. S_1 is best heard at the apex and S_2 at the base of the heart.
   2. Both are heard equally well at the right midclavicular line.
   3. On the left side, S_1 is at the area of the pulmonic valve and S_2 at the aortic valve.
   4. Both sounds are best heard at Erb point.

4. On the basis of a general assessment of an adult patient, the adult-gerontology primary care NP determines the presence of the apical impulse at the point of maximal impulse (PMI) on the patient's chest wall. Where on the chest wall is the PMI normally found?
   1. Second intercostal space at the midclavicular line on the left side.
   2. Right lower sternal border, fifth intercostal space.
   3. Left side at the fifth intercostal space on the midclavicular line.
   4. Left fifth intercostal space, lateral to the midclavicular line.

5. The adult-gerontology primary care NP is auscultating the carotid arteries for bruits. What is the correct procedure?
   1. Use the diaphragm of the stethoscope.
   2. Use the bell of the stethoscope.
   3. Place the stethoscope 1 inch off the area above the sternocleidomastoid muscle.
   4. Position the patient at a 30-degree angle and press firmly, using the bell of the stethoscope.

6. When inspecting the precordium, the adult-gerontology primary care NP's primary purpose in doing this inspection is to examine for:
   1. Scars and anatomic landmarks.
   2. Pulsations and retractions.
   3. Heaves and cardiac dullness.
   4. Pericardial friction rub and lifts.

7. While examining a patient in a left lateral position, the adult-gerontology primary care NP auscultates a third heart sound (S_3). The adult-gerontology primary care NP knows:
   1. This sound is considered normal in children and young adults.
   2. This rarely is associated with myocardial failure in the older adult.
   3. This patient should be immediately referred to a cardiologist for evaluation.
   4. This is considered a normal splitting of the S_2 during inspiration.

8. The adult-gerontology primary care NP knows that the correct auscultatory site for the aortic area is the:
   1. Midclavicular line, fifth interspace, left side.
   2. Left fourth interspace close to the sternum.
   3. Right second interspace close to the sternum.
   4. Midclavicular line, second interspace, left side.

9. The adult-gerontology primary care NP should include which statement in patient teaching when ordering a lipid profile on a patient? Eat a typical diet over the next week and:
   1. Eat a normal breakfast the morning of the lipid profile blood draw.
   2. Fast for 8–12 hours as directed before the lipid profile is drawn.
   3. There are no restrictions on alcohol consumption for this blood test.
   4. Take any current medications with a few sips of water before the blood test.

10. When auscultating the heart sounds of a 72-year-old patient with a history of hypertension, the adult-gerontology primary care NP notes a fourth heart sound (S_4). This finding could indicate:
    1. Normal variant in people ages 65 years and older.
    2. Beginning of ventricular failure.
    3. Decreased resistance to ventricular filling.
    4. Severely failing heart.

11. Which of the following is an appropriate blood pressure goal for a 65-year-old male with no comorbidities?
    1. SBP <150 mm Hg/DBP <90 mm Hg.
    2. SBP <140 mm Hg/DBP <90 mm Hg.
    3. SBP <140 mm Hg/DBP <80 mm Hg.
    4. SBP <150 mm Hg/DBP <90 mm Hg.

12. The adult-gerontology primary care NP is examining a patient with a history of rheumatic fever who is being followed for the development of carditis. During cardiac auscultation, where on the chest wall is the stethoscope placed to determine the most common murmur associated with this condition?
    1. At the left sternal border, fourth left intercostal space.
    2. Fifth intercostal space, left side, at the midclavicular line.
    3. Second or third intercostal space at the left of the sternal border.
    4. Second intercostal space on the right of the sternal border.

13. A patient presents with unusual coolness in the left hand compared with the right hand. What is the next step in the exam?
    1. Palpate the radial pulse on both hands for a full minute.
    2. Perform the Allen test on both hands.
    3. Feel the forearms with the backs of the fingers.

4. Hold the hand in a dependent position and then reexamine.

14. The first (S_1) and second heart sounds (S_2) are identified when the adult-gerontology primary care NP auscultates for cardiac sounds. The physiology responsible for the production of these heart sounds is:
    1. Closure of atrioventricular (AV) valves produces S_1; closure of semilunar valves forms S_2.
    2. Closure of the aortic valve produces S_2; opening of the mitral valve produces S_1.
    3. Opening of AV valves produces S_1; closure of semilunar valves produces S_2.
    4. Opening of the tricuspid valve produces S_1; closure of the pulmonic valve forms S_2.

15. The adult-gerontology primary care NP is assessing a cardiac patient who is experiencing an atrial dysrhythmia. The patient's pulse rate is irregular at 110 beats/min, and there is concern regarding a pulse deficit. How is a pulse deficit determined in this patient?
    1. A 12-lead ECG is necessary to determine the presence and length of the PR intervals.
    2. The apical pulse is counted, and then the radial pulse is counted; the pulse deficit is determined by the difference between the two rates.
    3. The apical pulse is counted, and an increase or decrease is correlated with the phases of the respiratory cycle.
    4. The apical pulse and radial pulse are determined simultaneously; a pulse deficit is established if the apical rate is higher than the radial rate.

16. The adult-gerontology primary care NP notes a Grade V systolic murmur while examining a patient's precordium. Which characteristic describes this type of murmur?
    1. Barely audible; faintly heard with the bell of the stethoscope.
    2. Heard only with the diaphragm of the stethoscope.
    3. Heard with the stethoscope partly off the chest.
    4. Heard without the aid of the stethoscope.

17. Normal physiologic changes in the geriatric population that affect conductivity and contractility of the myocardium include:
    1. Increased automaticity and excitability.
    2. Increased contractility and conductivity.
    3. Decreased excitability and conductivity.
    4. Decreased automaticity and contractility.

18. When assessing the temperature of an extremity as part of a patient's peripheral vascular assessment, which part of the hand is the most sensitive for assessing temperature?
    1. Palm.
    2. Fingertips.
    3. Back of the wrist.
    4. Back of the fingers.

19. A 45-year-old male patient's lipid profile results are sent to the adult-gerontology primary care NP with the following levels: total cholesterol, 287 mmol/L; HDL, 30 mg/dL; and LDL, 165 mg/dL. On the basis of interpretation of these findings, the adult-gerontology primary care NP should do which of the following?
    1. Initiate treatment with low-dose statins.
    2. Discuss adherence to a heart-healthy diet and regular aerobic physical activity.
    3. Assess the 10-year arteriosclerotic cardiovascular disease (ASCVD) risk.
    4. Refer to cardiologist.

20. A patient returns to the chest pain clinic 3 weeks post-myocardial infarction (post-MI) complaining of pericardial pain and elevated temperature. A physical exam reveals a pericardial friction rub. What diagnostic studies are indicated?
    1. 24-hour Holter monitoring.
    2. Echocardiogram.
    3. Complete blood count (CBC) with differential.
    4. Cardiac enzymes with myoglobin.

21. On assessment of an older adult patient, the adult-gerontology primary care NP notes bilateral pulsations and distention of the jugular veins when the patient's head is elevated 45 degrees. What further assessment needs to be done at this time?
    1. Estimate the level of venous pressure by measuring from the sternal angle to the highest level of venous pulsations.
    2. Place the patient in a supine position and determine the effect of position change on distention and pulsations of the jugular vein.
    3. Measure carotid pulses because of the increased left ventricular pressure.
    4. Have the patient hold his or her breath to facilitate evaluation for the presence of carotid bruits.

22. The adult-gerontology primary care NP is examining a woman with a known history of mitral valve disease. What type of murmur heard on auscultation supports a history of mitral valve stenosis?
    1. Diastolic murmur, heard loudest at the apex with the patient on her left side.
    2. Midsystolic ejection murmur heard loudest over the left lower sternal border.
    3. Holosystolic murmur, heard loudest over the apex and left axillary area.
    4. Diastolic murmur, heard loudest with the patient in a sitting position, leaning forward.

23. The adult-gerontology primary care NP is doing an assessment of a patient who is 2 weeks post-MI affecting the left ventricle. The adult-gerontology primary care NP would pay particular attention to what area of the physical assessment?
    1. Lower extremities and the jugular vein.
    2. Area on the chest where the PMI is heard.
    3. Presence of dyspnea and auscultation of crackles in the lungs.
    4. Level of dependent edema and fluid intake over the past 24 hours.

24. Which symptoms would indicate to the adult-gerontology primary care NP that the patient is experiencing intermittent claudication?
    1. Petechiae and itching of the lower part of the leg.
    2. Extensive discoloration and edema of the upper leg.
    3. Profuse rash and discoloration from the trunk down to the feet.
    4. Complaints of pain on walking, relieved by sitting down.

25. Stress testing, or the exercise tolerance test, is the most widely used diagnostic test in ischemic heart disease. It is most accurate, up to 98%, in what patient population?
    1. Males under age 40 with atypical angina pectoris.
    2. Asymptomatic premenopausal females without risk factors.
    3. Males over age 50 with typical angina pectoris.
    4. Males receiving digitalis with typical angina pectoris.

26. When palpating for the apical impulse of a 46-year-old female, the adult-gerontology primary care NP feels a hyperkinetic impulse. The nurse would auscultate for which additional finding?
    1. Pericardial friction rub.
    2. Pansystolic murmur.
    3. Pulsus paradoxus.
    4. Decreased intensity of heart sounds.

27. Which three predictor variables are included in the Thrombolysis in Myocardial Infarction (TIMI) risk score?
    1. Lipid profile.
    2. Aspirin use.
    3. CK-MB level.
    4. ST segment elevation ≥0.5.
    5. Warfarin use.

28. While assessing a patient with a history of recent MI, the adult-gerontology primary care NP notes pulsus alternans. The nurse would assess for other assessment changes most likely caused by:
    1. Unstable angina.
    2. Cardiogenic shock.
    3. Recurrent MI.
    4. Left-sided heart failure.

Disorders

29. With regard to cardiovascular disorders, which three factors would the adult-gerontology primary care NP include as having an impact on healthcare economic costs?
    1. Decrease in reimbursement for health promotion/prevention measures.
    2. Increase in healthcare costs directly affecting a patient's ability to access resources.
    3. Potential for morbidity/mortality because of the aging process.
    4. Altered quality-of-life measurements.
    5. Newer diagnostic procedures leading to improved outcomes regardless of physiologic status.

30. Which priority critical assessment should the adult-gerontology primary care NP include when performing an initial cardiac workup on an adult patient who is thought to have cardiovascular disease (CVD)?
    1. Perform a Mini–Mental State Examination to secure a baseline.
    2. Obtain height and weight measurements to calculate body mass index (BMI).
    3. Ask questions about family history.
    4. Obtain BP using Dinamap equipment.

31. A 70-year-old woman comes to the clinic with a complaint of severe aching of her legs after standing for 10 minutes. What other assessment finding of the lower extremities would support the adult-gerontology primary care NP's tentative diagnosis of chronic venous insufficiency?
    1. Pitting edema of 3+ and cyanosis on dependency.
    2. Shiny skin and dusky red appearance on dependency.
    3. Minimal hair and pallor on elevation.
    4. Pulses 1+ and ulceration involving the toes.

32. The diagnosis of hypertension (HTN) should be established on the basis of:
    1. At least three hypertensive readings in 1 week.
    2. At least five readings 1 month apart.
    3. One reading of 140 mm Hg SBP and 90 mm Hg DBP or higher.
    4. One reading taken in three different positions.

33. A patient has a 2-year history of hypertensive heart disease. The adult-gerontology primary care NP expects the major pathophysiologic change to be:
    1. Right ventricular hypertrophy.
    2. Left atrial dilation.
    3. Left ventricular hypertrophy.
    4. Right atrial dilation.

34. A 60-year-old female presents to the clinic for ongoing management of hypertension. Which physical finding, if noted by the adult-gerontology primary care NP, would warrant further inquiry?
    1. 20/20 vision screening.
    2. Presence of nosebleeds.
    3. Brisk capillary refill bilaterally.
    4. Occasional nonproductive cough in response to self-identified seasonal allergies.

35. Of the following descriptions, which data most clearly describe atrial tachycardia?
    1. Heart rate of 96 beats/min, P waves present on each QRS complex, T wave present on every other beat.
    2. P waves present on every other beat, heart rate of 100 beats/min, and irregular rhythm.
    3. Heart rate of 110 beats/min, P waves present before each QRS complex, and regular rhythm.
    4. P waves for every third QRS complex, adequate PR interval, heart rate of 90 beats/min.

36. Which clinical manifestation of a myocardial infarction (MI) is frequently not present in the older adult cardiac patient?
    1. Prolonged, severe chest pain.
    2. Diaphoresis, pallor, and syncope.
    3. Dyspnea and increasing anxiety.
    4. Gastrointestinal distress and orthopnea.

37. The adult-gerontology primary care NP is performing an assessment on a patient who is having difficulty controlling his left-sided heart failure. The adult-gerontology primary care NP understands that the primary symptoms associated with this type of heart failure are:
    1. Systemic venous congestion.
    2. Dyspnea and pulmonary congestion.
    3. Increased peripheral edema and anorexia.
    4. Atrial fibrillation with a heart rate around 110 beats/min.

38. The adult-gerontology primary care NP is concerned that a post-MI patient is developing a problem of constrictive pericarditis. What is a characteristic finding with constrictive pericarditis, and how is it evaluated?
    1. Cardiac tamponade, identified by muffled heart sounds and a paradoxical pulse.
    2. Pericardial triphasic friction rub, best heard at the apical area of the heart.
    3. Mitral valve prolapse, characterized by late systolic murmur at apex and left sternal borders.
    4. Altered waves on jugular venous pulse, as determined with a light directed tangentially to illuminate the shadows of the pulsations.

39. An older adult patient has a diagnosis of left-sided heart failure (HF). The adult-gerontology primary care NP would identify what common condition associated with HF?
    1. Peripheral vascular disease.
    2. Untreated hypertension.
    3. Ventricular dysrhythmias.
    4. Chronic obstructive pulmonary disease (COPD).

40. In evaluating the effectiveness of cardiopulmonary resuscitation (CPR) on the adult patient, the adult-gerontology primary care NP would note:
    1. Dilated pupils.
    2. Palpable carotid pulse.
    3. Capillary refill.
    4. Pink and warm skin.

41. The adult-gerontology primary care NP is evaluating an ECG of a patient who presented at the clinic with complaints of weakness and fainting. The patient's ECG reveals a cardiac rate of 52 beats/min, identifiable P waves, regular QRS complex, and T waves present after each QRS complex. What is the best interpretation of this information?
    1. Normal ECG; need to further evaluate patient's complaints of weakness.
    2. Third-degree block with junctional escape rhythm; transfer patient to emergency room for cardiology consult.
    3. First-degree block; need to further evaluate patient related to cardiac medications.
    4. Administer sublingual nitroglycerin and refer patient for a cardiology consult.

42. The adult-gerontology primary care NP is conducting a follow-up examination on a patient with CAD and a history of pericarditis. What is a characteristic physical finding in pericarditis, and how is it evaluated?
    1. Paradoxical pulse, identified by evaluating the changes in the amplitude of arterial pulse pressure associated with the respiratory cycle.
    2. Pulse deficit, as determined by counting the radial pulse and apical pulse at the same time and evaluating the difference.
    3. Pericardial friction rub, best heard using the diaphragm of the stethoscope and loudest to the left of the sternum at the fourth or fifth intercostal space.
    4. An S_4 is present, usually heard at the apex with the bell of the stethoscope and the patient in a left lateral position.

43. The symptoms of MI usually experienced by the older adult patient include:
    1. Dyspnea and diaphoresis.
    2. Back pain and muscle cramping.
    3. Numbness and tingling of the left arm.
    4. Epigastric pain and nausea.

44. What are the risk factors predisposing females to cardiovascular disease?
    1. Absence of estrogen adversely affects lipoprotein metabolism.
    2. Fat deposited on the hips mobilizes, raising serum cholesterol.

    3. Coronary arteries are longer and wider in diameter.
    4. Resting ejection fraction is lower.

45. The adult-gerontology primary care NP is planning the treatment of an older adult patient newly diagnosed with HTN. What parameters are most important in determining the appropriate pharmacologic therapy?
    1. Determine medications and dosage on the basis of the patient's weight, age, and drug availability.
    2. Begin step method using diuretics and beta-adrenergic blockers.
    3. Initiate lifestyle changes before beginning medications.
    4. Determine other medical conditions for which the patient is being treated.

46. Which statement accurately describes coronary artery disease (CAD) in geriatric patients?
    1. Cardiovascular disease is increased in the female patient receiving estrogen replacement therapy.
    2. A major risk factor for cardiovascular disease in females and males is chronic HTN.
    3. The majority of geriatric patients with CAD also have type 2 diabetes.
    4. Males over 60 years old continue to experience the highest level of CAD.

47. A patient with a history of COPD comes to the clinic for his annual checkup with complaints of increasing difficulty breathing. Assessment findings include S_3 gallop; early systolic ejection click; and increased P-wave amplitude in leads II, III, and aVF of the ECG. The adult-gerontology primary care NP would expect to observe which change on the chest x-ray film?
    1. Hypertrophy of the left ventricle.
    2. Hypertrophy of the right ventricle.
    3. Hypertrophy of the left atrium and ventricle.
    4. Hypertrophy of the right atrium and ventricle.

48. When cardiac output falls in HF, the body attempts to compensate. What electrolyte imbalances result from this response?
    1. Hypernatremia and hyperkalemia.
    2. Hyponatremia and hypokalemia.
    3. Hypophosphatemia and hypercalcemia.
    4. Hyperphosphatemia and hypocalcemia.

49. When assessing the carotid pulse of a 72-year-old patient at a community-based clinic, the adult-gerontology primary care NP notes a bounding pulse with rapid rise and sudden collapse. The adult-gerontology primary care NP would include which additional assessment to support this finding?
    1. Auscultation for a diastolic murmur.
    2. Auscultation for paradoxical pulse.
    3. BP in both arms while lying, sitting, and standing.
    4. BP for an auscultatory gap.

50. The adult-gerontology primary care NP understands that the pain experienced with angina pectoris or MI is caused by irritation of the myocardial nerve fibers by the increase in:
    1. Blood glucose.
    2. Lactic acid.
    3. Serum potassium.
    4. Serum magnesium.

51. New York Heart Association Functional Class III for patients with cardiac disease is characterized by:
    1. Symptoms present at rest, with any activity leading to increased discomfort.
    2. Slight limitation in ordinary activity, resulting in fatigue, palpitations, dyspnea, or angina.
    3. No physical limitation in activity.
    4. Marked limitation in activity, comfortable at rest, but ordinary activity leads to symptoms.

52. During the history and physical examination of a patient with suspected early HF, which is the most prominent finding?
    1. Moist crackles in the lung bases bilaterally.
    2. Anorexia with weight loss of 3 lb in 1 week.
    3. Increased urine output and peripheral edema.
    4. Facial edema and distended neck veins.

53. Chest pain that is sudden and severe, described as "tearing," and accompanied by a decrease in peripheral pulses may indicate a diagnosis of:
    1. Angina.
    2. Acute myocardial infarction (AMI).
    3. Aortic dissection.
    4. Pericarditis.

54. Which of the following would be appropriate dietary therapy recommendations for a patient with hyperlipidemia?
    1. Limiting intake of salt, sweets, and sugar-sweetened beverages.
    2. Increasing the average daily protein intake to 70 g/day.
    3. Decreasing total fat to <37% of the daily total calories per day.
    4. Limiting carbohydrate intake.

55. The most frequent life-threatening dysrhythmia experienced by a patient with AMI is:
    1. Atrial fibrillation.
    2. Ventricular tachycardia.
    3. Third-degree heart block.
    4. Ventricular fibrillation.

56. In an overweight older adult female patient with an elevated cholesterol level and abnormal lipoprotein profile, the first step in treatment includes:
    1. Prescribing a bile acid sequestrant agent.
    2. Initiation of a diet and exercise program.
    3. Estrogen replacement therapy.
    4. Referral to a cardiologist.

57. Patients with chronic atrial fibrillation are at risk for which condition?
    1. Sudden cardiac death.
    2. Stroke.
    3. Ventricular tachycardia.
    4. Acute myocardial infarction.

58. The adult-gerontology primary care NP understands that the most common symptom of HF in adults is:
    1. Anorexia.
    2. Dependent edema.
    3. Dyspnea.
    4. Weakness.

59. The adult-gerontology primary care NP teaches the cardiac patient to avoid foods high in saturated fats, which include:
    1. Nuts, legumes, and seeds.
    2. Fish, shellfish, and mussels.
    3. Palm oil, coconut oil, and butter.
    4. Peanut oil, soybean oil, and olive oil.

60. An older adult male patient is complaining of chest pain. A parameter to assist the adult-gerontology primary care NP to differentiate the chest pain of angina from that of an MI is:
    1. Myocardial pain with an infarction is more severe.
    2. Anginal pain is more substernal and does not radiate to other areas.
    3. Anginal pain is frequently relieved by nitroglycerin.
    4. Pain from an infarction is always associated with other symptoms.

61. The adult-gerontology primary care NP is evaluating a patient in the office who is complaining of chest pain. The patient's BP is 86/52 mm Hg, and ECG results show some signs of ischemia. The patient is to be transferred to the emergency department. What drug might the adult-gerontology primary care NP give the patient while awaiting transfer?
    1. Furosemide (Lasix) 40 mg IV.
    2. Morphine sulfate 5–10 mg IV.
    3. Nitroglycerin 0.3 mg SL.
    4. Aspirin 81 mg PO.

62. Which would *not* be considered as contributing to the development of thrombophlebitis?
    1. Excessive use of oral anticoagulants.
    2. Blow to the leg or arm.
    3. Recent intravenous therapy.
    4. Secondary to pregnancy.

63. An older adult patient is being evaluated for a complaint of dizziness. What symptom/observation will make the adult-gerontology primary care NP consider that this is a life-threatening event?
    1. The dizziness occurs in certain positions.
    2. It is accompanied by tinnitus.
    3. The symptoms worsen when standing.
    4. It is preceded by rapid breathing.

64. A 28-year-old male presents to the adult-gerontology primary care NP with a history of chest pain that has been increasing over the past several days. The patient states that the pain worsens on lying down and denies any shortness of breath, cough, or radiation of the pain. The patient gives a history of a recent infection with coxsackievirus. An examination shows that the patient has a cardiac friction rub. One probable diagnosis considered by the adult-gerontology primary care NP is:
    1. Acute myocardial infarction (AMI).
    2. Pleural effusion.
    3. Pericarditis.
    4. Esophageal reflux.

65. The adult-gerontology primary care NP would most likely suspect which differential diagnosis for an older adult patient presenting with atrial fibrillation and functional decline along with memory loss?
    1. Hyperthyroidism.
    2. Hypothyroidism.
    3. Sick sinus syndrome.
    4. HF.

66. Which assessment made by the adult-gerontology primary care NP for an older patient would be a deviation from the normal changes of aging?
    1. Decreased exercise tolerance.
    2. Grade II/VI systolic ejection murmur.
    3. Prolongation of PR intervals on an ECG.
    4. JVP of 14 cm H_2O.

67. Cardiac auscultation of an older patient reveals a grade II/VI murmur that is heard best at the right second intercostal space. The murmur is louder with squatting. There is a small carotid pulse with a delayed upstroke. The patient's history is benign, and his activity tolerance is within normal limits for his age. The adult-gerontology primary care NP would interpret this murmur to be indicative of:
    1. Aortic regurgitation.
    2. Aortic stenosis.
    3. Mitral valve prolapse.
    4. Mitral valve regurgitation.

68. What is the most frequently diagnosed valvular heart problem in older adult patients?
    1. Aortic stenosis.
    2. Mitral valve stenosis.
    3. Mitral valve regurgitation.
    4. Aortic regurgitation.

69. A middle-aged man with no known risk factors for coronary artery disease presents with a total cholesterol level of 255 mg/dL. The adult-gerontology primary care NP would:
    1. Start him on a HMG-CoA reductase inhibitor.
    2. Reevaluate the total cholesterol in 8 weeks.
    3. Repeat the total cholesterol and obtain HDL and calculated LDL levels.
    4. Do nothing because this patient demonstrates no coronary risk factors other than male sex.

70. Infective endocarditis prophylaxis may be required for adolescents with congenital heart defects in which of the following procedures?
    1. Dental procedures such as simple adjustment of orthodontic appliances.
    2. Cardiac catheterization.
    3. Tonsillectomy and/or adenoidectomy.
    4. Endotracheal intubation.

71. **QSEN** For the young adult with congenital heart disease and a permanent pacemaker, electrical safety precautions include avoidance of:
    1. Cellular phones.
    2. Microwave ovens.
    3. Household electrical appliances.
    4. Metal detectors.

72. A young adolescent is having a workup for rheumatic fever. The physical findings are temperature of 103.6°F (39.8°C); swollen, painful joints; and increased ESR. According to the Jones criteria, what is essential for the diagnosis of rheumatic fever?
    1. History of group A beta-hemolytic streptococcal throat infection.
    2. Carditis.
    3. Sydenham chorea.
    4. History of erythema marginatum for the past 3 days.

Pharmacology

73. An adult patient who is being treated for hyperlipidemia prefers to take a "natural" medication approach. On the basis of this patient's request, the adult-gerontology primary care NP would order which medication?
    1. Ezetimibe (Zetia).
    2. Gemfibrozil (Lopid).
    3. Colesevelam (Welchol).
    4. Niacin (Niaspan).

74. An adult-gerontology primary care NP is reviewing a female patient's medication profile during her annual wellness examination. The patient's past medical history includes recent treatment for HTN that began 8 months ago with lisinopril (Prinivil) 10 mg PO daily. The patient now states that she may be considering having a child. Which action should be taken by the adult-gerontology primary care NP at this time?
    1. Immediate direct referral of the patient to a women's healthcare NP.
    2. Maintain dosage of prescribed beta blocker.
    3. Discontinue lisinopril (Prinivil).
    4. Decrease the dosage of prescribed angiotensin-converting enzyme (ACE) inhibitor.

75. A 75-year-old male patient presents to the office complaining of "not feeling well." He has a history of chronic lung disease and HF. His vital signs are pulse 78 beats/min and irregular, respiration 26 breaths/min, and BP of 158/100 mm Hg. An ECG indicates sinus rhythm and confirms the rate. The PR interval is 0.28 second, P waves are present, and each is followed by a QRS complex. There are frequent premature atrial beats. The patient is taking digitalis, potassium, theophylline, hydrochlorothiazide, and a calcium channel blocker. What is the next best action to take?
    1. Obtain serum theophylline, digitalis, and potassium levels.
    2. Increase dosage of calcium blocker and diuretic.
    3. Order pulmonary function studies.
    4. Refer the patient to a cardiologist.

76. A 49-year-old female was started on a thiazide diuretic for HTN 1 month ago. She arrives in the clinic complaining of muscle cramps and dizziness. Physical exam findings are BP 132/88 mm Hg (previously 186/112 mm Hg), pulse 112 beats/min, respiration 24 breaths/min, tenting positive, skin turgor decreased, neck veins flat, sodium 114 mEq/L, chloride 92 mEq/L, potassium 3.0 mEq/L, and blood glucose 201 mg/dL. Initial treatment for this patient should include fluid replacement:
    1. Orally with free water and a potassium supplement.
    2. Intravenously with normal saline and regular insulin subcutaneously.
    3. Intravenously with 1000 mL of normal saline at 100 mL/hr with a 100-mL piggyback of 40 mEq of KCl at 50 mL/hr.
    4. Intravenously with 1000 mL of lactated Ringer solution at 250 mL/hr.

77. A patient is recovering from an acute episode of thrombophlebitis and is being treated with warfarin (Coumadin) 5 mg PO daily. In reviewing the patient's medication information, the adult-gerontology primary care NP would include what information in her teaching?
    1. Do not take a multivitamin supplement.
    2. Limit dairy products.
    3. Aerobic exercises are the most effective.
    4. Maintain a daily record of intake and output.

78. The adult-gerontology primary care NP is evaluating a patient who is "not feeling good." He has a history of CAD and HF. His vital signs are pulse 72 beats/min, respiration 20 breaths/min, BP 130/88 mm Hg, and temperature normal. The patient has no complaints of chest pain or difficulty breathing. The patient has had some nausea but no vomiting over the past 2 days. His lower extremities are negative for edema. The patient states that he has been able to take his medications. His current medications are digoxin (Lanoxin) 0.5 daily, hydrochlorothiazide (HydroDIURIL) 100 mg twice daily, potassium (Micro-K) 10 mEq daily, and nitroglycerin transdermal patches. What is the priority of care for this patient?
    1. Immediate ECG and WBC count.
    2. Arterial blood gases and oxygen at 4 L/min.
    3. Serum digoxin and potassium levels.
    4. Serial cardiac enzymes now and q6h ×2.

79. A 77-year-old female patient with a history of nonvalvular AF has been treated historically with warfarin (Coumadin) titrated to obtain an INR between 2 and 3. What action should the adult-gerontology primary care NP take during the office visit for evaluation of anticoagulation?
    1. Consider discontinuing warfarin (Coumadin) and switching to aspirin therapy.
    2. Continue anticoagulation therapy because the patient has a CHA_2DS_2-VASc score of 2 or more.
    3. Provide follow-up order for activated partial thromboplastin time/INR in 3 months because target value has been reached.
    4. Schedule patient for an echocardiogram and stress test.

80. The adult-gerontology primary care NP has prescribed losartan (Cozaar) 50 mg PO daily. This medication promotes vasodilation by:
    1. Blocking the action of angiotensin II.
    2. Promoting release of aldosterone.
    3. Promoting synthesis of prostaglandin.
    4. Inhibiting calcium influx into smooth muscle cells.

81. The adult-gerontology primary care NP, in using best practice, should discuss which medication for patients who are over age 40 with a history of cardiovascular disease risk factors?
    1. ACE inhibitor medication and potassium chloride.
    2. Loop diuretic and beta blocker.
    3. Aspirin 81 mg daily in conjunction with statin.
    4. Beta blocker and thiazide diuretic.

82. Which medication would be prescribed by the adult-gerontology primary care NP for a 50-year-old female adult patient with no history of cardiac disease (a calculated 10-year risk of a cardiovascular event >10%) who was placed on lisinopril (Zestril) 3 months ago for trended BP readings of 150/92 mm Hg on two separate occasions that have responded to treatment?
    1. HMG-CoA reductase inhibitor.
    2. Loop diuretic.
    3. Low-molecular-weight heparin.
    4. Antihistamine.

83. A patient with a history of HTN is started on spironolactone (Aldactone) 50 mg PO daily. The adult-gerontology primary care NP instructs the patient to call the clinic if which symptoms are experienced?
    1. Increased irritability, abdominal cramping, and lower extremity weakness.
    2. Decreased reflex response, nausea, and vomiting.
    3. Muscle twitching, numbness, tingling, burning sensations of the limbs, and diarrhea.
    4. Weight gain, excessive thirst, and fever.

84. A patient with a history of unstable angina is seen in the cardiac clinic for a checkup. The assessment reveals increased weight of 10 lb, distended jugular neck veins, and S_3. What changes in the pharmacologic treatment should be initiated?
    1. Discontinue beta blockers and calcium channel blockers.
    2. Initiate thrombolytic therapy.
    3. Discontinue nitrate and aspirin therapy.
    4. Initiate diuretic and vasoconstrictor therapy.

85. A patient arrives at the emergency room of a small, rural hospital complaining that he "feels like my heart is racing." He is connected to a cardiac monitor, which reveals supraventricular tachycardia at a rate of 184 beats/min, QRS complex of <0.10 second, and BP of 112/62 mm Hg. Which treatment modality is indicated?
    1. Synchronized cardioversion with 50 J.
    2. Defibrillation with 100 J.
    3. Adenosine 6 mg IV push.
    4. Lidocaine 1 mg/kg IV push.

86. An 80-year-old patient with a history of glaucoma develops unstable angina. He is started on diltiazem (Cardizem) 30 mg PO qid daily and aspirin 325 mg PO daily in addition to timolol ophthalmic solution (Timoptic) one drop in the right eye twice daily. This patient would have an increased risk for:
    1. Bleeding episodes.
    2. Fainting episodes and falls.
    3. Rebound supraventricular tachycardia.
    4. Blurred vision.

87. A patient with a serum cholesterol level of 256 mg/dL, HDL of 38 mg/dL, and LDL of 172 mg/dL is instructed on dietary modifications and taking niacin (nicotinic acid) 1 g by mouth three times daily. Specific instructions include:
    1. Limiting daily fluid intake.
    2. Taking measures to minimize flushing.
    3. Administering the drug 1 hour after eating.
    4. Avoid exposure to direct sunlight.

88. When monitoring for the therapeutic effects of verapamil (Calan SR), the adult-gerontology primary care NP would assess for:
    1. Increase in heart rate.
    2. Decrease in systemic vascular resistance.
    3. Increase in BP.
    4. Decrease in ventricular premature beats.

89. A 45-year-old African-American male patient with essential HTN is treated by the adult-gerontology primary care NP with sodium restriction and chlorothiazide (Diuril) 25 mg PO daily. After 3 months of therapy, the patient's BP is measured at 160/110 mm Hg. At this point, the adult-gerontology primary care NP would:
    1. Begin enalapril (Vasotec) 5 mg daily.
    2. Begin 50 mg of metoprolol (Toprol XL) daily.
    3. Add 5 mg of amlodipine (Norvasc) daily.
    4. Discontinue Diuril and change to captopril (Capoten) 50 mg tid.

90. When prescribing antihypertensive drug therapy for older adult patients, the adult-gerontology primary care NP recognizes that which class of antihypertensive agents should be avoided in the older adult?
    1. Calcium channel blockers.
    2. Diuretics.
    3. Beta blockers.
    4. ACE inhibitors.

91. Medications used in managing ischemic heart disease include:
    1. Beta blockers, sedatives, and aspirin.
    2. Nitrates, beta blockers, calcium channel blockers, and aspirin.
    3. Vasoconstrictors, aspirin, and anxiolytics.
    4. Nitrates, ACE inhibitors, aspirin, and lipid-lowering drugs.

92. The adult-gerontology primary care NP initiates antihypertensive therapy for a middle-aged nonsmoking male. One week later, the patient returns for a follow-up visit and complains of a recurrent dry cough since initiating the medications. This is most likely a side effect of:
    1. Beta blocker.
    2. Thiazide diuretic.
    3. ACE inhibitor.
    4. Calcium channel blocker.

93. The role of digoxin in the management of HF is indicated for patients with:
    1. Atrial fibrillation.
    2. Mitral valve stenosis.
    3. Normal ejection fraction.
    4. Pericarditis.

94. The adult-gerontology primary care NP should monitor the older adult patient for which of the most common adverse reactions of digoxin?
    1. Blurred vision.
    2. Confusion.
    3. Diarrhea.
    4. Eating disorder.

95. The adult-gerontology primary care NP has been treating an older patient's HTN successfully with diet, exercise, and hydrochlorothiazide (HydroDIURIL) 25 mg PO daily for 5 months. During today's clinic visit, the patient's BP was 154/90 mm Hg and temperature was 99.9°F (37.7°C). The patient's physical exam revealed clear breath sounds; S_1 and S_2 with no murmurs, gallops, or rubs; and no JVD. The patient denied syncope, headaches, or visual changes; there was a tender and edematous right ankle. Which laboratory values would be most appropriate for evaluation?
    1. Blood urea nitrogen and sodium.
    2. Serum cholesterol and serum calcium.
    3. Serum potassium and CBC.
    4. Serum uric acid and CBC.

96. An older adult white male with a long history of COPD has recently developed HTN. Which class of antihypertensive agents should the adult-gerontology primary care NP avoid for this patient?
    1. ACE inhibitors.
    2. Beta blockers.
    3. Calcium channel blockers.
    4. Diuretics.

97. Which class of pharmacologic agents would the adult-gerontology primary care NP select for an older adult patient who has HTN and is newly diagnosed with HF?
    1. ACE inhibitors.
    2. Beta blockers.
    3. Calcium channel blockers.
    4. Diuretics.

98. A male patient who is mildly hypertensive and takes hydrochlorothiazide presents with red, painful swelling of the great toe. In addition to treating the gout, the adult-gerontology primary care NP also knows to:
    1. Order laboratory studies for diabetes.
    2. Explore for possible alcohol abuse.
    3. Advise him to lose weight.
    4. Change his thiazide antihypertensive medication.

99. An older adult male was diagnosed 3 months ago with systolic HTN and presents for follow-up care. He is on a no-added-salt diet and has lost 8 lb in 3 months. Weekly BP checks at a senior center average in the 180s/70s. The patient's health history includes benign prostatic hyperplasia, diet-controlled type 2 diabetes, and CAD with an MI 8 years ago. His chief complaint includes periodic angina, occasional heartburn, slowed urine stream with some dribbling, and decreasing energy level. His BP today is 188/78 mm Hg. His current medications are cimetidine (Tagamet) 200 mg as needed, aspirin 325 mg daily, nitroglycerin, and aluminum hydroxide/magnesium hydroxide (Maalox) as needed. The patient is married and sexually active. Which medication would the adult-gerontology primary care NP initiate after a complete physical, including an ECG and all indicated blood work?
    1. ACE inhibitor.
    2. Diuretic.
    3. Alpha-1-adrenergic blocker.
    4. Beta-adrenergic blocker.

100. An older adult patient has been on procainamide (Pronestyl) for 4 years to control his cardiac dysrhythmias. The adult-gerontology primary care NP would evaluate for which side effect in the chronic use of this medication?
    1. Elevated liver function tests.
    2. Appearance of antinuclear antibodies.
    3. Shortened AV interval.
    4. Tachycardia.

101. Secondary prophylaxis for acute rheumatic fever in a 25-year-old schoolteacher who experienced carditis includes:
    1. Penicillin V 125–250 mg PO twice daily indefinitely.
    2. Erythromycin 800 mg PO twice daily.
    3. One-time dose of 2.0 million units of benzathine penicillin G, combined with penicillin G procaine (Bicillin C-R) IM.
    4. No medication prophylaxis is needed after a patient reaches the early 20s.

102. A patient has been prescribed lisinopril (Prinivil) 5 mg by mouth daily for HTN. He has developed an intractable cough that is unrelated to HF. Which of the following medications can be substituted for this medication?
    1. Calcium channel blocker.
    2. Digoxin.
    3. ACE inhibitor.
    4. ARB.

103. A 60-year-old male with a history of unstable angina comes to the clinic complaining of increased pain that is not relieved by his nitroglycerin. During the assessment, the adult-gerontology primary care NP notes elevation of the ST segment on the patient's ECG. Oxygen therapy is administered, and an intravenous line is inserted. What other therapy should be initiated while arranging transfer to an acute care facility?
    1. Lidocaine drip at 2 mg/min.
    2. Metoprolol (Toprol) 100 mg PO.
    3. Morphine 2 mg IV push.
    4. Aspirin 162 mg PO.

104. A 54-year-old patient with type 2 diabetes has been diagnosed with HTN. Which antihypertensive drug is the recommended choice to treat HTN in patients with diabetes?
    1. Beta blocker.
    2. Diuretic.
    3. Calcium channel blocker.
    4. ACE inhibitor.

105. A 68-year-old patient with a history of MI who has experienced atrial fibrillation for 2 years comes to the clinic with a complaint of "increasing difficulty breathing and occasionally awakening at night with a feeling of smothering." Which pharmacologic therapy would be appropriate?
    1. Digitalis and ACE inhibitor.
    2. Loop diuretic and beta blocker.
    3. Thiazide diuretic and calcium channel blocker.
    4. Alpha-1-adrenergic blocker and nitrate.

106. A patient with CAD has a serum cholesterol level of 278 mg/dL and a triglyceride level of 300 mg/dL. The adult-gerontology primary care NP initiates therapy with lovastatin (Mevacor) 20 mg daily. The patient is instructed to take the lovastatin daily:
    1. In the morning with breakfast.
    2. 30 minutes before eating breakfast.
    3. In the evening.
    4. Around noon.

107. A 70-year-old white female is a resident of a long-term care facility where the adult-gerontology primary care NP makes rounds on a weekly basis. The nurse is reviewing recent laboratory results and notices the following: serum potassium of 5.9 mEq/L, serum sodium of 144 mEq/L, serum of chloride 111 mEq/L, BUN of 28 mg/dL, and creatinine of 1.8 mg/dL. Her current medications include furosemide (Lasix) 20 mg PO daily, potassium chloride (Klor-Con) 40 mEq PO daily, captopril (Capoten) 25 mg PO daily, and citalopram (Celexa) 10 mg PO daily. There have been no changes in her medications. What is the likely cause of her elevated serum potassium?
    1. Furosemide (Lasix).
    2. Potassium chloride.
    3. Captopril (Capoten).
    4. Citalopram (Celexa).

4 Cardiovascular Answers & Rationales

Physical Examination & Diagnostic Tests

1. Answer: 2

   Rationale: With regard to gender, female patients may present with atypical findings associated with chest pain that may indicate a cardiac event. In this situation, the presence of adventitious lung sounds is a key indicator that the patient may be experiencing pulmonary edema, which would increase the likelihood of a cardiac event. Denial of drug use, absent T waves, and absence of jaw pain would be considered pertinent negative findings.

2. Answer: 3

   Rationale: There are no specific preprocedure instructions for a transthoracic echocardiogram (TTE), because it is considered to be a noninvasive diagnostic test. Patients should be advised to wear comfortable clothing that can be removed easily and to take their regularly scheduled medications.

3. Answer: 1

   Rationale: S_1 is heard loudest at the apex (characteristic "lub" sound) and S_2 at the base (characteristic "dub" sound). Each sound should be assessed carefully regarding the intensity of the sound in each area. The S_2 second heart sound has two components: A_2 is produced by aortic valve closure, and P_2 is produced by pulmonic valve closure.

4. Answer: 3

   Rationale: The PMI represents the thrust and contraction of the left ventricle (LV). The LV lies behind the right ventricle (RV) and extends to the left, forming the left border of the heart.

5. Answer: 2

   Rationale: The correct procedure is to listen for carotid bruits with the bell of the stethoscope, which brings out low-frequency sounds and filters out high-frequency sounds. The bell should be placed very lightly on the neck with just enough pressure to seal the edge.

6. Answer: 2

   Rationale: The purpose of inspection and palpation of the precordium is to determine the presence and extent of normal and abnormal pulsations. A slight retraction of the chest wall just medial to the midclavicular line in the fifth interspace is a normal finding, whereas marked or active retraction of the rib is abnormal and may indicate pericardial disease. Pericardial friction rubs are heard by auscultation.

7. Answer: 1

   Rationale: The splitting during inspiration refers to S_1 and S_2. The S_3 is normal in children, young adults up to age 40, and pregnant women. In the older adult with heart disease, this often signifies myocardial failure or left ventricular enlargement.

8. Answer: 3

   Rationale: The right side of the chest close to the sternal border at the second intercostal space is the correct area to auscultate the aortic valve. The mitral valve is auscultated at the fifth left intercostal space at the midclavicular line. The tricuspid valve is auscultated at the fourth left intercostal space at the sternal border. The pulmonic valve is auscultated at the second left intercostal space at the sternal border.

9. Answer: 2

   Rationale: An 8- to 12-hour fast is recommended because of the influence of intake on cholesterol levels, which may increase. A normal diet for the 7 days before drawing the lipid profile is recommended so that an accurate picture of the patient's normal life is obtained. Alcohol should not be consumed for 48 hours before the test, because it may increase cholesterol, HDL, LDL, and triglyceride levels. If possible, all medications should be withheld until the blood test is drawn, especially corticosteroids, diuretics, beta blockers, oral contraceptives, and estrogens.

10. Answer: 1

    Rationale: An S_4 is a normal variant in people ages 65 years and older and may result from increased resistance to ventricular filling during atrial contraction.

11. Answer: 1

    Rationale: Based on the Joint National Committee 8 report (JNC 8) hypertension treatment guidelines, an appropriate BP goal for a patient aged 60 years or older is SBP <150 mm Hg/DBP <90 mm Hg. Patients younger than 60 years old, or patients at any age with diabetes or chronic kidney disease (CKD), should have BP goals set at SBP <140 mm Hg/DBP <90 mm Hg.

12. Answer: 2

Rationale: Acute rheumatic fever would most likely affect the aortic and mitral valves first, and because these murmurs are difficult to auscultate, the mitral valve would be the best choice among the options given. The fifth intercostal space at the midclavicular line on the left side is the best place to auscultate the closure sounds of the mitral valve. Auscultating at the left sternal border, fourth left intercostal space, describes the area of the tricuspid valve. Auscultating at the second or third intercostal space at the left of the sternal border describes the pulmonic valve area. The aortic valve area is auscultated at the second intercostal space on the right of the sternal border.

13. Answer: 3

Rationale: It is important to determine whether the coolness extends proximally from the hand, so feeling the forearms with the backs of the fingers is appropriate. Next, it would be important to palpate the radial pulses. The Allen test relates to arterial blood gas collection and is not indicated. Holding the hand in a dependent position would facilitate perfusion but would not help to determine bilateral comparison of extremities.

14. Answer: 1

Rationale: The mitral and tricuspid valves are considered AV valves. Closure of the AV valves produces the first heart sound (S_1). This marks the beginning of systole and emptying of both ventricles. The aortic and pulmonic valves are semilunar valves. At the end of systole, closure of the semilunar valves produces the second heart sound (S_2).

15. Answer: 4

Rationale: The apical and radial pulses must be evaluated simultaneously to determine whether all the apical beats are being reflected in the radial pulse. If there is an apical rate of 100 and a radial rate of 94, the patient is said to have a pulse deficit of 6. This is usually done with two people counting simultaneously over the same period.

16. Answer: 3

Rationale: A grade V heart murmur is very loud and can be heard with the stethoscope partly off the chest wall with a thrill that is easily palpable. A grade I murmur is barely audible in a quiet room or very faintly heard with the bell of the stethoscope. A grade II murmur is quiet but clearly audible. A grade III murmur is moderately loud. A grade IV murmur is loud and associated with thrill. A grade VI murmur is the loudest, is audible with the stethoscope removed from contact with the chest wall, and is accompanied by a thrill that is palpable and visible.

17. Answer: 4

Rationale: The normal aging process impairs automaticity, conductivity, and contractility. Ischemic changes and degeneration decrease sinus node automaticity and conduction velocity, resulting in bradycardic rhythms or atrial fibrillation. The poor myocardial contractility, usually related to hypertension or valvular disease, causes decreased ventricular emptying and increased filling pressures. These changes predispose the older adult patient to heart failure.

18. Answer: 4

Rationale: The most sensitive area for temperature on the examiner's hand is the back of the fingers. The fingertips should be used to assess texture and moisture.

19. Answer: 3

Rationale: The Adult Treatment Panel (ATP IV) cholesterol guidelines no longer recommend treatment adjusted to a specific target lipid value. The patient's 10-year ASCVD risk should be calculated, and determination should be made whether the patient falls into a pharmacologic treatment benefit group. A heart-healthy diet, lifestyle modifications, and regular aerobic physical activity should always be included in the treatment regimen. Referral to a cardiologist is not appropriate at this time.

20. Answer: 3

Rationale: Dressler syndrome (post-MI syndrome) may develop 1–4 weeks post-MI and is characterized by pericarditis with effusion, fever, and markers of inflammation such as leukocytosis. Dressler syndrome is caused by antigen–antibody reactions. Laboratory findings include elevated white blood cell (WBC) count and erythrocyte sedimentation rate (ESR). Treatment includes NSAIDs and colchicine.

21. Answer: 1

Rationale: Jugular vein distention (JVD) is common in older adult patients. If JVD is present when the patient's head is elevated 45 degrees, further examination is necessary regarding the venous pressure, which reflects pressure in the right-side heart chambers. The supine position will increase venous pressure and does not provide valid information in this situation. Auscultation for carotid bruits is an important part of assessment but is not significant in evaluating JVD.

22. Answer: 1

Rationale: Mitral valve stenosis is a diastolic murmur of low intensity heard at the apex of the heart. Midsystolic ejection murmur heard loudest over the left lower sternal border describes characteristics of a murmur with aortic stenosis. A holosystolic murmur is characteristic of mitral valve regurgitation, which allows for backflow of blood from ventricles into the atrium and is heard loudest over the apex and left axillary area. A diastolic murmur, heard loudest with patient in a sitting position and leaning forward best describes aortic regurgitation.

23. Answer: 3

Rationale: The patient had a left ventricular MI. One of the most common complications is left-sided HF. This would manifest first as pulmonary congestion (crackles in lungs) and difficulty breathing.

24. Answer: 4

Rationale: Classically, intermittent claudication is described as pain in the lower extremity on activity that is relieved by stopping the activity. During exercise, there is an increased demand for blood supply to the extremity that cannot be met. Subsequently, there is a buildup of lactic acid and other metabolites in the muscle, which causes the tightening or cramping discomfort in the calf muscles.

25. Answer: 3

Rationale: A positive result on stress testing indicates the likelihood of coronary artery disease (CAD) with 98% accuracy in males over age 50. Results are progressively lower in asymptomatic persons, with false-positive results increased in asymptomatic men under age 40, premenopausal women without risk factors, and patients taking digitalis.

26. Answer: 2

Rationale: A hyperkinetic impulse (increased amplitude) is caused by pressure overload of the left ventricle. Causes include hyperthyroidism, severe anemia, or mitral valve regurgitation. A pansystolic murmur is a classic finding of mitral valve regurgitation.

27. Answer: 2, 3, 4

Rationale: The TIMI risk score is a well-known tool used to identify risk for patients with unstable angina and non–ST-segment elevation myocardial infarction. Seven predictor variables are each given 1 point and include age ≥65, aspirin use in the last 7 days, at least three risk factors for coronary artery disease (CAD), severe symptoms of angina within the previous 24 hours, elevated cardiac markers (CK-MB or cardiac-specific troponin level), ST-segment elevation ≥0.5 mm, and prior CAD with ≥50% stenosis. Low risk is from 0 to 2 points, with 5 to 7 points considered as high risk. Warfarin use and a lipid profile are not part of the risk score. There are other risk scores using troponin-only levels (HEART [history, ECG, age, risk factors, and troponin], Global Registry of Acute Coronary Events [GRACE], Emergency Department Assessment of Chest Pain Score [EDACS]) that provide better risk stratification.

28. Answer: 4

Rationale: Pulsus alternans (weak pulse alternating with strong pulse) is most often caused by left ventricular failure (strong and weak ventricular contractions), is usually accompanied by an S_3 heart sound, and is seen in patients with left-sided HF. It may be present in severe acute aortic insufficiency (AI), but it is unusual in patients with chronic AI.

Disorders

29. Answer: 2, 3, 4

Rationale: Cardiovascular disorders represent increased financial costs to patients, based on therapeutic management, morbidity and mortality, and altered quality-of-life measurements. Reimbursement for health promotion/prevention measures is typically included in most insurance-based plans to prevent potential hospitalizations. The impact of increased morbidity/mortality associated with cardiovascular disorders plays a significant role in financial stressors affecting the patient and family members. Although newer diagnostic procedures may help to provide more accurate clinical diagnoses, the test itself is impacted by each patient's physiological status; thus, improved outcomes are not mutually exclusive.

30. Answer: 3

Rationale: The adult-gerontology primary care NP, when performing an initial cardiac workup on an adult patient who is thought to have CVD, should pay specific attention to the significance of family history. Family history serves as a primary indicator for the development of atherosclerosis. Performing a Mini–Mental State Examination would be indicated for neurologic assessment. Height and weight measurements to help calculate BMI, although important, would not be the priority critical assessment. Obtaining BP using a manual sphygmomanometer would provide a more reliable estimate of the patient's BP.

31. Answer: 1

    Rationale: This assessment reflects changes caused by chronic venous insufficiency, which includes edema, varicose veins, chronic skin changes, dependent cyanosis, and skin ulceration. The other assessment findings reflect chronic arterial insufficiency.

32. Answer: 1

    Rationale: A diagnosis of HTN based on a single measurement of BP elevation should not be done. A minimum of three readings with an average greater than or equal to SBP of 140 mm Hg and DBP of 90 mm Hg establishes the diagnosis. In October 2015, the U.S. Preventive Services Task Force (USPSTF) updated the guidelines for BP measurement and now recommends that a BP reading should be obtained outside the clinic setting prior to initiating treatment for HTN. An average of two or more readings taken at each of two or more visits should follow an initial screening. The patient should be seated with the arm at heart level. No caffeine or nicotine ingestion should be allowed for 30 minutes before the reading. The room should be quiet for at least 5 minutes, and an appropriate cuff should be used. Another high reading should be confirmed within 2 months.

33. Answer: 3

    Rationale: In the early stages of hypertensive heart disease, when there is an increased peripheral resistance to blood flow, the most significant change occurring in the heart is left ventricular hypertrophy. This is associated with an increase in the size of the myocardial cells without a corresponding increase in cell number (hyperplasia). Over time, all other options listed occur in the heart.

34. Answer: 2

    Rationale: Clinical confirmation of nosebleeds in a patient who already has a diagnosis of HTN may be significant. As such, the adult-gerontology primary care NP should follow this physical symptom for its potential impact on the patient's vascular status. 20/20 vision screening and brisk capillary refill bilaterally are normal findings. An occasional nonproductive cough in response to the patient's self-identified seasonal allergies is considered a normal abnormal finding.

35. Answer: 3

    Rationale: Sinus or atrial tachycardia is characterized by a heart rate of 100 beats/min or greater, P waves present for each QRS complex, PR interval <0.20 seconds, T wave after each QRS complex, and regular rhythm.

36. Answer: 1

    Rationale: The classic chest pain associated with a MI may not be present in the older adult patient because of altered pain perception and diminished pain sensation.

37. Answer: 2

    Rationale: Respiratory symptoms are predominant in patients with left-sided heart failure. Venous congestion and peripheral edema are associated with right-sided heart failure.

38. Answer: 1

    Rationale: Cardiac tamponade occurs as a complication of pericarditis. An excessive accumulation of fluids between the pericardium and myocardium interferes with effective cardiac contraction and produces a paradoxical pulse. The triphasic friction rub is common to pericarditis but is not indicative of a complication of constrictive pericarditis. Jugular venous pressure (JVP) is used to determine levels of venous distention.

39. Answer: 2

    Rationale: Untreated hypertension causes significant increased work of the left ventricle, eventually causing left-sided HF.

40. Answer: 2

    Rationale: Palpable carotid pulse with each compression is the best sign of effective CPR. The other answers are appropriate but not the best indicators of effective resuscitation efforts.

41. Answer: 2

    Rationale: This is a description of complete heart block with hemodynamic consequences and a junctional escape rhythm. The patient should be seen immediately by a cardiologist for possible pacemaker insertion. First-degree block has characteristic P waves and a long PR interval >0.20 seconds.

42. Answer: 3

    Rationale: A triphasic friction rub or pericardial rub occurs in the majority of patients with pericarditis. Paradoxical pulse may occur if constrictive pericarditis and cardiac tamponade are present. Pulse deficits and presence of S_4 are not characteristic of problems with pericarditis.

43. Answer: 1

    Rationale: Older adults experience atypical symptoms of MI, including dyspnea, diaphoresis, vomiting, syncope, confusion, and weakness.

44. Answer: 1

Rationale: Risk factors predisposing women to cardiovascular disease include smaller body size, declining estrogen level, heart and thoracic cavity smaller and lighter, coronary arteries smaller in diameter, shorter PR interval, and a higher resting ejection fraction. Increased body fat percentage and fat distributed in the abdomen may be mobilized more easily in response to stress. This may raise serum cholesterol and blood glucose levels.

45. Answer: 4

Rationale: The adult-gerontology primary care NP must consider the geriatric patient's other medical problems and treatment along with race before prescribing medications for HTN. Frequently, geriatric patients cannot take beta blockers because of chronic pulmonary conditions; they may already be taking diuretics for problems of fluid retention. Step therapy is appropriate if there is no other significant medical history. Lifestyle changes should be initiated and medications adjusted as changes are made.

46. Answer: 2

Rationale: HTN is considered a major factor in the development of CAD in the geriatric patient. Female patients have an increased incidence of CAD after menopause; estrogen replacement therapy appears to have cardioprotective effects on the heart, thus decreasing the incidence of CAD. Although patients with diabetes have an increased incidence of CAD, most patients with CAD do not have diabetes.

47. Answer: 4

Rationale: Cor pulmonale is characterized by hypertrophy of the right ventricle secondary to pulmonary HTN (resistance) and central pulmonary artery enlargement noted on an x-ray. The increased P-wave amplitude (P pulmonale) occurs as the right atrium enlarges. The best test to identify cor pulmonale is echocardiography.

48. Answer: 2

Rationale: The compensatory mechanism (activation of the renin-angiotensin-aldosterone system) causes excess secretion of aldosterone that predisposes to potassium excretion. Total body sodium content will be above normal, but the excessive secretion of antidiuretic hormone (ADH) causes greater retention of water, diluting the serum level. ADH is continually secreted because of the presence of low pressure at the carotid sinus baroreceptors, directly related to low cardiac output.

49. Answer: 1

Rationale: Water-hammer pulse, also known as Corrigan or hyperkinetic pulse (bounding pulse with a rapid rise and sudden collapse), results from an increase in pulse pressure and may be caused by increased stroke volume, decreased peripheral vascular resistance, or both. Because the adult-gerontology primary care NP suspects either aortic regurgitation or patent ductus arteriosus (primarily in children), auscultation for a diastolic murmur is indicated.

50. Answer: 2

Rationale: Occlusion of the coronary arteries deprives the myocardial cells of glucose needed for aerobic metabolism. Anaerobic metabolism occurs, which causes the accumulation of lactic acid. Lactic acid irritates the myocardial nerve fibers, sending pain messages to the cardiac nerves and upper thoracic posterior roots located in the left shoulder and arm.

51. Answer: 4

Rationale: Marked limitation in activity, comfortable at rest, but ordinary activity leading to symptoms is noted as Functional Class III. Symptoms present at rest, with any activity leading to increased discomfort, characterizes Functional Class IV. Slight limitation in ordinary activity, resulting in fatigue, palpitations, dyspnea, or angina is defined as Functional Class II. Functional Class I is characterized by no physical limitation in activity.

52. Answer: 1

Rationale: The moist crackles (rales) heard in the bases of the lung are the most prominent physical examination findings of early HF. They are caused by transudation of fluid into the alveoli and the airways. Later findings include distended neck veins, peripheral edema, hepatomegaly, and ascites (rather than weight loss).

53. Answer: 3

Rationale: Aortic dissection almost invariably begins with a sudden onset of severe chest pain that is tearing or ripping in quality and is accompanied by absent or decreased peripheral pulses and neurologic deficits. The pain of angina and AMI is usually described as "pressure." Pericarditis produces pain that is more gradual in onset.

54. Answer: 1

Rationale: The ATP IV, the American College of Cardiology, and American Heart Association (AHA) cholesterol guidelines recommend lifestyle modifications for patients with hyperlipidemia, including increasing vegetables, fruits, and whole grains and limiting sodium, sweets and sugar-sweetened drinks, red meats, and saturated fats, and should include <10% of unsaturated fat. The amount of fat in the average diet should be between 20% and 35% of the total calories. Daily protein intake should be between 10% and 35%. Carbohydrate intake should be monitored in the maintenance of a healthy weight.

55. Answer: 4

Rationale: Although the other dysrhythmias may occur after MI, the most life-threatening is ventricular fibrillation. The vast majority of deaths resulting from ventricular fibrillation occur within the first 24 hours, and more than half of these occur in the first hour. The majority of out-of-hospital deaths resulting from MI are caused by ventricular fibrillation.

56. Answer: 2

Rationale: Diet and exercise are the mainstays of any treatment program and would be used initially in all cases. A bile acid sequestrant agent or estrogen replacement therapy may eventually be necessary if no improvement is seen with diet and exercise therapy. Referral to a cardiologist is not necessary, unless the patient develops symptoms or shows resistance to treatment.

57. Answer: 2

Rationale: A stroke is often the outcome of chronic atrial fibrillation because of the blood pooling in the quivering atria. As a result, a blood clot can be formed in this pooling blood, which then travels to the brain and causes an ischemic stroke. For this reason, warfarin (Coumadin) should be maintained at an international normalized ratio (INR) of 2–3 or other anticoagulants, such as dabigatran (Pradaxa), rivaroxaban (Xarelto), and apixaban (Eliquis) may be prescribed.

58. Answer: 3

Rationale: Dyspnea is the most common symptom of HF. Initially, it is present only with moderate exertion, but as the severity of HF increases, dyspnea may occur on mild exertion or at rest. Fatigue is another common complaint. Right-sided HF is associated with weakness, anorexia, nausea, and dependent edema. Chronic left ventricular failure usually leads to right ventricular failure.

59. Answer: 3

Rationale: Palm and coconut oils, along with butter, are very high in saturated fats and should be avoided. The other selections are moderately high in fat content but are mainly unsaturated fats.

60. Answer: 3

Rationale: Anginal pain is difficult to differentiate from the pain of an infarction. One of the most characteristic symptoms of angina pain is relief with the administration of sublingual nitroglycerin.

61. Answer: 4

Rationale: Aspirin helps prevent the formation of platelet-aggregating substances and may help the occlusion of narrowed coronary arteries. Although furosemide and morphine have a role in treating acute MI, aspirin can readily be given in the typical primary care office. Nitroglycerin should not be given, because the patient's SBP is <90 mm Hg.

62. Answer: 1

Rationale: Superficial inflammation of a vein may be caused by trauma (for example, blow to the arm or leg) or recent intravenous therapy with irritating fluids, or it may occur secondary to pregnancy, especially during the postpartum period, because of the increase in clotting factors (thromboplastin). Excessive use of oral anticoagulants can lead to bleeding but not to thrombophlebitis. Deep vein thrombosis associated with thrombophlebitis results from prolonged bed rest, major surgical procedures, injury to the blood vessel wall, and hypercoagulable states, such as use of oral contraceptives (especially in women who smoke or have cancer) and polycythemia vera.

63. Answer: 3

Rationale: Dizziness that improves when lying down and worsens when standing is symptomatic of cardiac involvement and may indicate serious cardiac dysrhythmias. If it occurs in certain positions, the dizziness suggests benign positional vertigo, which is common in older adults. Dizziness accompanied by tinnitus is common in acute labyrinthitis and, if preceded by rapid breathing, may be caused by hyperventilation.

64. Answer: 3

Rationale: The stated history of a recent coxsackievirus infection, pain that worsens when supine, and a friction rub is classic for viral pericarditis. The patient's age makes an AMI unlikely, and the pain is not typical for pleural effusion or esophageal reflux.

65. Answer: 1

Rationale: Signs and symptoms of hyperthyroidism in the older adult include progressive functional decline, atrial fibrillation, MI, tachycardia, weakness, fatigue, weight loss, anorexia, diarrhea, nervousness, tremor, pruritus, memory loss, and heat intolerance. Symptoms of hypothyroidism include arthralgia; weakness; decreased mental function; depression; constipation; weight loss; dry, coarse skin with a yellowish cast; dry, sparse hair; and masklike puffy face with periorbital edema. Bradycardia would be assessed with sick sinus syndrome. Sick sinus syndrome is often associated with the "bradycardia-tachycardia" syndrome.

66. Answer: 4

Rationale: JVP of 14 cm H_2O is a sign of HF (normal JVP is 3–10 cm H_2O). Decreased exercise tolerance is a normal sign of aging. A grade II/VI systolic ejection murmur is a result of sclerosing of the aorta, which occurs with aging. Prolongation of PR intervals on an ECG is expected with the aging process.

67. Answer: 2

Rationale: This assessment is consistent with aortic stenosis. Aortic regurgitation is a diastolic murmur secondary to rheumatic heart disease, for which no history is given. Mitral valve disease is one of the most common valvular disorders. A small percentage of patients who have a mitral valve prolapse do experience autonomic dysfunction and complain of palpitations, atypical chest pain, orthostatic dizziness, near-syncope, cold extremities, throbbing headaches, and neurasthenia, and they manifest tachydysrhythmias. Patients who have mitral valve regurgitation may remain asymptomatic for many years because the left ventricle dilates and adjusts well to the increase in volume load. Onset of dyspnea and fatigue may not occur for decades.

68. Answer: 1

Rationale: Aortic stenosis is the most frequently diagnosed valvular heart problem and is caused by aortic valve thickening and calcification. The symptoms include syncope, angina, and dyspnea on exertion. Patients may develop aortic stenosis earlier in life if they have a congenital valve abnormality, such as a bicuspid valve, or if they have a history of rheumatic valve disease.

69. Answer: 3

Rationale: The adult-gerontology primary care NP needs to repeat the cholesterol and obtain HDL and LDL values before initiating any treatment. The HDL and LDL will help stratify risks and aid in the determination of recommended management.

70. Answer: 3

Rationale: Procedures for which endocarditis prophylaxis is recommended include dental procedures known to induce gingival bleeding. It is also recommended for surgical procedures that involve respiratory mucosa tonsillectomy/adenoidectomy. Endocarditis prophylaxis is not recommended for insertion of tympanostomy tubes, cardiac catheterization, simple dental procedures, or endotracheal intubation. Cardiac catheterizations are done under sterile conditions, and prophylactic treatment is not recommended because of a very low incidence of infection.

71. Answer: 4

Rationale: Metal detectors have an electromagnetic field that could alter the pacemaker's function temporarily. In addition, the alarm will be set off as a result of the metal in the pacemaker. For the adolescent with a pacemaker, an electric shock may irreparably damage the pacemaker, and immediate surgical replacement would be necessary. There is no risk of electromagnetic interference between the permanent pacemaker and household items such as electrical appliances, radios, electronic equipment, cellular phones, or microwave ovens. Ovens and pacemakers have filtering systems that prevent interference with the pacemaker's function.

72. Answer: 1

Rationale: According to the Jones criteria, in addition to two major manifestations (carditis, polyarthritis, Sydenham chorea, erythema marginatum, and subcutaneous nodules) or one major and two minor manifestations (arthralgia, fever, elevated ESR, C-reactive protein, and prolonged PR interval), a diagnosis of rheumatic fever is highly likely if there is evidence of a previous group A beta-hemolytic streptococcal infection.

Pharmacology

73. Answer: 4

Rationale: Niacin (Niaspan) is also known as vitamin B_3 and as such would be considered to be a "natural" medication approach. The other medications represent medication classes: a cholesterol absorption inhibitor (Zetia), a fibric acid derivative (Lopid), and a bile acid sequestrant (Welchol).

74. Answer: 3

Rationale: A female patient who is being treated with lisinopril (Prinivil), an ACE inhibitor, which is contraindicated in women who are pregnant and/or who wish to become pregnant. Therefore, the medication should be discontinued at this time. An immediate direct referral to a women's healthcare NP is not indicated at this time, because the patient is not pregnant but is discussing potential concerns at this time. A change in BP medication is warranted at this time on the basis of the patient's voiced concerns.

75. Answer: 1

Rationale: This patient is presenting with symptoms of digitalis toxicity—first-degree block and increasing cardiac irritability. If the patient's potassium level is low, it may be precipitating the toxicity. Also, it is important to determine that serum theophylline levels remain within the therapeutic range. No evidence indicates that the pulmonary disease is progressing. BP may be adequately controlled for this patient; further information should be obtained before adjusting the medications. On the basis of the information presented, referral to a cardiologist is not appropriate at this time.

76. Answer: 3

Rationale: Thiazide diuretics inhibit sodium reabsorption, promoting the excretion of sodium, chloride, and water. As the extracellular fluid volume decreases, plasma renin activity and aldosterone levels increase, resulting in potassium loss. Treatment is given to restore the volume with normal saline and correct the potassium depletion. If the sodium is increased too rapidly, irreversible neurologic damage can occur.

77. Answer: 1

Rationale: Vitamin K is an antidote for warfarin. Increased intake of green leafy vegetables could cause an increase in vitamin K levels and decrease the effectiveness of the medication. Also, multivitamin supplements may contain additional vitamin K.

78. Answer: 3

Rationale: The patient presents with the classic profile of digitalis toxicity, which is frequently related to hypokalemia, especially because the potassium replacement is rather low for an adult and the patient has a history of poor eating and nausea. The actions listed in the other options may be taken, but it is important to determine the presence of hypokalemia and digitalis toxicity so that these may be addressed immediately.

79. Answer: 2

Rationale: Women who are above the age of 75 should remain on warfarin (Coumadin) therapy because age in itself indicates a CHA_2DS_2-VASc score of 2 and being female a score of 1, giving the woman over 75 a score of 3. A patient with a score of 2 or greater is at "moderate-high" risk and should otherwise be an anticoagulation candidate. Aspirin is ineffective in preventing strokes in patients older than 75. The CHA_2DS_2-VASc score is the most commonly used method to predict thromboembolic risk in atrial fibrillation. CHA_2DS_2-VASc stands for (**c**ongestive heart failure, **h**ypertension, **a**ge (>65 = 1 point, >75 = 2 points), **d**iabetes (yes = 1 point), previous **s**troke/transient ischemic attack (yes = 2 points). **VASc** stands for vascular disease (peripheral arterial disease, previous MI, aortic atheroma; yes = 1 point) and sex category (female = 1 point; male = 0 points). Switching to aspirin therapy would not be appropriate on the basis of evidence-based practice guidelines. There is no indica-

tion for additional diagnostic or laboratory testing at this time.

80. Answer: 1

Rationale: Angiotensin II receptor blockers (ARBs), such as losartan (Cozaar), block access of angiotensin II to its receptors in blood vessels, the adrenals, and all other tissues. By blocking the action of angiotensin II, losartan relaxes muscle cells and dilates blood vessels (arterioles and veins), thereby reducing BP. By blocking angiotensin II receptors in the adrenals, ARBs decrease release of aldosterone, which increases renal excretion of sodium and water. Sodium and water excretion is further increased through dilation of renal blood vessels.

81. Answer: 3

Rationale: Best practice for patients with a history of CVD risk factors is to start low-dose aspirin therapy in conjunction with a statin to help reduce the risk of potential cardiac events. Initiating an ACE inhibitor medication and potassium chloride would be contraindicated because the mechanism of action of an ACE inhibitor would lead to hyperkalemia. Initiation of a loop diuretic and beta blocker or a beta blocker and a thiazide diuretic would not be warranted, unless there is specific clinical evidence to support this therapy.

82. Answer: 1

Rationale: Treatment regimens for patients with HTN should include initiation of statin therapy to decrease cardiovascular risk if three criteria are met according to the USPSTF: (1) aged 40–75 years, (2) presence of one or more CVD risk factors (that is, dyslipidemia, diabetes, HTN, or smoking), and (3) calculated 10-year risk of a cardiovascular event of 10% or greater. Unless there is specific clinical evidence of fluid retention (or edema), a loop diuretic would not be indicated. Anticoagulation therapy would not be indicated, because there is no clinical evidence to support increased cardiovascular risk. An antihistamine would not be indicated in this case, unless there is specific clinical evidence of seasonal allergies and/or nasal congestion.

83. Answer: 3

Rationale: Aldactone is a potassium-sparing diuretic. Patients should be instructed on the early signs of hyperkalemia, which include muscle twitching, numbness, tingling, and burning sensations of the limbs, diarrhea, palpitations, and skipped heartbeats. Hypokalemia symptoms are characterized by irritability, confusion followed by lethargy, abdominal cramping, distention, and constipation, and lower extremity weakness.

84. Answer: 1

Rationale: Beta blockers are myocardial depressants that suppress heart rate and contraction (negative inotropic). Calcium channel blockers decrease AV conduction, which suppresses heart rate. Both drugs are contraindicated with the onset of left ventricular dysfunction. The increase in JVD and a 10-lb weight gain are associated with right-sided HF. The presence of S_3 indicates left ventricular dysfunction, especially when associated with signs and symptoms of right-sided HF.

85. Answer: 3

Rationale: The American Heart Association advanced cardiac life support guidelines recommend adenosine as the drug of choice for emergency treatment of supraventricular tachycardia when a patient is hemodynamically stable.

86. Answer: 2

Rationale: The use of beta-adrenergic blocking agents (for example, timolol), whether systemic or ophthalmic, may result in bradycardia and/or hypotension.

87. Answer: 2

Rationale: Niacin can cause vasodilation, leading to intense flushing of the face, neck, and ears. The flushing can be mitigated by gradually increasing the dose, taking the medication with food, or by taking 325 mg of aspirin 30 minutes prior to each dose. Aspirin reduces flushing by preventing synthesis of prostaglandins, which mediate the flushing response. Antihyperlipidemic drugs may cause constipation. Antihyperlipidemic effectiveness is enhanced when the drug is taken before or with meals.

88. Answer: 2

Rationale: Calcium channel blockers (1) depress the rate of discharge from the sinoatrial node and conduction velocity through the AV node, causing a decrease in heart rate; (2) relax the coronary and systemic arteries, producing vasodilation (decrease in afterload and BP); and (3) decrease myocardial contractility (negative inotropic effect).

89. Answer: 3

Rationale: According to the JNC 8, African-American males without diabetes or CKD should be prescribed calcium channel blockers alone or in combination with a thiazide-type diuretic in the treatment of HTN. Enalapril and captopril are ACE inhibitors, which are not appropriate for this patient. Metoprolol is a beta blocker and not recommended in the JNC 8 guidelines for the treatment of HTN.

90. Answer: 3

Rationale: Beta blockers are not appropriate in normal doses for older adults because of decreased beta-receptor sensitivity in these patients. Larger doses may also result in depression, impotence, fatigue, and declining mental function. Older adult patients are especially likely to experience HF and peripheral vascular insufficiency resulting from beta-adrenergic blocker toxicity. BP should be lowered cautiously by using smaller doses of calcium channel blockers, ACE inhibitors, or diuretics in older adult patients.

91. Answer: 2

Rationale: Nitrates are venous and arterial dilators that decrease myocardial oxygen demand. Beta blockers have an antianginal effect and reduce myocardial oxygen demand. Calcium channel blockers relieve myocardial ischemia by reducing myocardial oxygen demand and dilate coronary arteries. Aspirin is effective for secondary prevention of MI. Unless contraindicated, small doses of aspirin (81–325 mg daily) should be prescribed for patients with angina. Patients remaining symptomatic when treated with nitrates, beta blockers, or calcium channel blockers should be treated with a beta blocker plus another agent. Appropriate combinations are a nitrate or beta blocker plus a calcium channel blocker other than verapamil. Combination therapy does not include sedatives, vasoconstrictors, ACE inhibitors, or lipid-lowering drugs.

92. Answer: 3

Rationale: Adverse side effects of ACE inhibitors include cough (1% to 30% of patients), headache, dizziness, and hyperkalemia. Patients who experience a cough side effect should be switched to a different medication. Adverse effects of calcium channel blockers include peripheral edema, dizziness, headache, nausea, and tachycardia. Adverse effects of thiazide diuretics include nausea, vomiting, diarrhea, dizziness, and headache. Side effects of beta blockers include fatigue, bradycardia, impotence, depression, and shortness of breath.

93. Answer: 1

Rationale: Digoxin, once a first-line drug for all patients with HF, is now used in patients with atrial fibrillation, other tachycardias, and left ventricular dysfunction. By controlling the ventricular rate in the patient with atrial fibrillation or tachycardias, cardiac output increases. In cases of diastolic dysfunction with a sinus rhythm, digitalis is of no benefit. Digoxin is of relatively little value in most forms of cardiomyopathy, myocarditis, mitral valve stenosis, and chronic constrictive pericarditis.

94. Answer: 2

Rationale: Noncardiac adverse reactions include a change in mental status. Although visual disturbances, diarrhea, anorexia, nausea, and vomiting are also adverse reactions, they are not the most common in older adult patients.

95. Answer: 4

Rationale: The assessments indicate gout. A side effect of hydrochlorothiazide is hyperuricemia. Blood for a CBC should be drawn before therapy. The other options do not address the assessment of a tender and edematous right ankle. The cardiac assessments were benign. No evidence indicates a concern for hypo- or hypernatremia or hypo- or hyperkalemia.

96. Answer: 2

Rationale: Beta blockers increase peripheral vascular resistance, a phenomenon that already occurs with normal aging, so these drugs can precipitate or worsen symptoms of asthma, COPD, peripheral vascular disease, sexual dysfunction, or HF. The other drug classes have no effect or decrease the effect on peripheral resistance.

97. Answer: 1

Rationale: ACE inhibitors have been shown to prolong life in patients with HF by improving overall cardiac function. Beta blockers and calcium channel blockers should be contraindicated in patients with HF. Although the use of diuretics may be correct, diuretics are not a priority over ACE inhibitors.

98. Answer: 4

Rationale: The most likely precipitating cause of this patient's gout is the thiazide diuretic used to control his HTN, because it blocks the excretion of uric acid, leading to hyperuricemia. Although gout may be more common in obese, alcoholic, and diabetic patients, these conditions are not indicated here.

99. Answer: 1

Rationale: The ACE inhibitor will preserve renal function and have less impact on sexual function. The adult-gerontology primary care NP must monitor the patient's potassium and carefully follow renal status for change. The ACE inhibitor has fewer negative side effects or interactions with this patient's other medical conditions.

100. Answer: 2

Rationale: Of the patients receiving long-term procainamide therapy, 80% develop antinuclear antibodies, and 23% of these develop a lupus-like syndrome.

101. Answer: 1

Rationale: Secondary prevention or preventing the recurrent attacks of acute rheumatic fever is controversial. Some authorities identify (1) reaching the early 20s and (2) 5 years since the last attack as the criteria for stopping the use of prophylactic penicillin, unless the patient is at increased risk of exposure to streptococcal infections, as are schoolteachers and health professionals. Other authorities recommend lifelong prophylactic drug therapy, depending on cardiac damage. Although erythromycin is an alternative medication for penicillin-sensitive individuals, the dose of 800 mg is for a patient having a dental or surgical procedure. The secondary prophylactic dose for erythromycin is 250 mg by mouth twice daily.

102. Answer: 4

Rationale: An annoying, untoward effect of ACE inhibitors is an intractable cough. Lisinopril is an ACE inhibitor. ARBs can be substituted as long as the cough is not related to HF. Antidysrhythmic agents, calcium channel blockers, and NSAIDs should be avoided.

103. Answer: 4

Rationale: The AHA recommends that aspirin (162–325 mg by mouth once) be administered as soon as possible whenever a patient is suspected of having an MI. The decreased platelet aggregation effect of aspirin helps limit the size of the myocardial damage.

104. Answer: 4

Rationale: ACE inhibitors enhance renal function in patients with diabetes and slow the progression of kidney injury.

105. Answer: 1

Rationale: This patient with atrial fibrillation is exhibiting symptoms of left ventricular failure. Treatment recommendations include enhancing contractility with a positive inotropic agent (digitalis), and ACE inhibitors have been shown to slow LV dilation. Beta blockers, ARBs, and aldosterone antagonists are also recommended.

106. Answer: 3

Rationale: Because most cholesterol is synthesized between midnight and 3:00 AM, HMG-CoA reductase inhibitors (lovastatin) are best taken in the evening.

107. Answer: 2

Rationale: The likely cause of the patient's elevated serum potassium is the potassium chloride. The adult-gerontology primary care NP should hold the potassium chloride (Klor-Con) and order daily serum potassium monitoring until the patient's serum potassium levels return to normal. The patient is taking furosemide, which is a potassium-wasting diuretic, and the amount of potassium given to compensate for the anticipated losses apparently was too much. This often occurs as a result of the changes of aging. Once serum potassium returns to normal, the level is monitored again at 1 week. With the low dose of furosemide and with captopril (an ACE inhibitor that may retain potassium), the patient may not need to have potassium chloride restarted.

Respiratory

5

Physical Examination & Diagnostic Tests

1. When examining a patient, the adult-gerontology primary care NP suspects a small pleural effusion. The most sensitive diagnostic test to determine a small effusion would be:
   1. Chest ultrasound.
   2. Chest radiograph.
   3. Spirometry testing.
   4. Ventilation/perfusion scan.

2. The adult-gerontology primary care NP is assessing a patient who is complaining of shortness of breath and chest discomfort. His respirations are shallow at 26 breaths/min. When evaluating the diaphragmatic excursion, it is determined that the diaphragm on the right is slightly higher than on the left side. The best interpretation of these findings is:
   1. This is normal because the liver is located on the right side.
   2. There may be atelectasis in the right lower lobe.
   3. Consolidation is present in the right lower lobe.
   4. This indicates the presence of severe chronic obstructive lung disease.

3. The adult-gerontology primary care NP knows that normal breath sounds that have a low pitch, soft intensity, and that are heard best on inspiration over the posterior lung fields are called:
   1. Bronchial.
   2. Vesicular.
   3. Bronchovesicular.
   4. Rhonchi.

4. A diagnostic evaluation for chronic obstructive pulmonary disorder will include:
   1. Chest x-ray.
   2. CBC with differential.
   3. Pulmonary function test.
   4. Arterial blood gas.

5. When auscultating for vocal resonance in a patient with possible consolidation of lung tissue, the adult-gerontology primary care NP tells the patient to say "ninety-nine," and the voice remains loud and distinct over the area of suspected consolidation. This is called:
   1. Tactile fremitus.
   2. Bronchophony.
   3. Whispered pectoriloquy.
   4. Egophony.

6. The adult-gerontology primary care NP understands that in percussion of the lungs, hyperresonance is:
   1. A normal finding in the adult patient.
   2. Common when the lungs are hyperinflated, like with chronic emphysema.
   3. Characterized by soft intensity, high pitch, short duration, and extremely dull quality.
   4. Characterized by loud intensity, high pitch, medium duration, and dull quality.

7. What is the correct procedure when percussing the anterior and posterior chest?
   1. Percuss the entire right side of the anterior chest and move to the left side.
   2. Begin at the upper left side of the posterior chest and compare with the respective anterior side, moving from front to back.
   3. Percuss systematically and symmetrically the intercostal spaces of the anterior chest, moving from the left to the right side, and then percuss the posterior chest.
   4. Percuss the posterior chest, and then measure for diaphragmatic excursion on the anterior chest.

8. The adult-gerontology primary care NP understands that pleural friction rubs are:
   1. Auscultated in the lower anterolateral chest.
   2. Heard best at the end of expiration.
   3. Characterized by a continuous, low-pitched, snoring sound that is heard early in inspiration.
   4. Noted when the patient says "e-e-e" and the examiner hears through the stethoscope "a-a-a."

9. An older adult patient who recently travelled outside the country is presenting to your office with significant dyspnea. The patient recently returned from Japan on a 12-hour flight. The patient's lungs are clear, heart rate and blood pressure are mildly elevated, and oxygen saturation is 88%. The patient has bilateral 1+ pedal edema. The most important diagnostic study to complete emergently includes:
   1. ECG.
   2. Ventilation/perfusion (V/Q) scan.
   3. Chest radiograph.
   4. Spiral CT scan.

10. When assessing for tactile fremitus, the adult-gerontology primary care NP knows that increased fremitus:
    1. Occurs when there is an obstruction in the transmission of vibrations.
    2. Occurs with consolidation or compression of lung tissue.
    3. Is the symmetric transmission of vibration through the chest wall.
    4. Is found in emphysema.

11. On assessment of the patient's respiratory status, crepitation is felt over the third rib at the midaxillary line on the left side. What is the interpretation of this finding?
    1. There is consolidation of fluid in the left lower lobe of the lung.
    2. Severe inflammation is present on the visceral pleural surfaces of the left lung.
    3. An increase in pressure has occurred in the pleural cavity of the right lung.
    4. Air is present in the subcutaneous tissue.

12. An important anatomic landmark on the anterior thoracic wall is the angle of Louis. Where on the thorax is this landmark present?
    1. The midnipple line on either side of the manubrium.
    2. At the manubriosternal junction.
    3. Midline at the base of the suprasternal notch.
    4. Just below the clavicle, but above the manubrium.

13. During the assessment of an older adult patient's respiratory status, the adult-gerontology primary care NP determines increased tactile fremitus posteriorly at the second intercostal space. The best interpretation of this finding is:
    1. Increased air trapping in the alveoli on the affected side.
    2. Presence of fluid or solid mass within the lungs.
    3. Increased pressure in the bronchial tree.
    4. Presence of reactive airway disease.

14. When the lateral diameter of the chest is the same size as the anterior-posterior (AP) diameter, the adult-gerontology primary care NP correctly identifies this finding as:
    1. A normal finding in a younger adult.
    2. Pectus carinatum.
    3. Pectus excavatum.
    4. Suggestive of obstructive lung disease.

15. The adult-gerontology primary care NP is planning a community screening program for lung cancer in older adult patients. The current evidence-based practice suggests that:
    1. Bronchoscopy with biopsy for cytology should be done every 2–3 years for smokers.
    2. Low-dose computed tomography be used in high-risk individuals.
    3. Routine screening for lung cancer does not decrease mortality in high-risk populations.
    4. Chest x-ray with comparison of previous x-ray is a sensitive test for lung cancer.

16. An adult male patient comes to the clinic with the chief complaint of "coughing up blood" and night sweats. He has no history of respiratory or cardiac problems. His vital signs are pulse of 96 beats/min, respirations of 28 breaths/min, BP of 140/92 mm Hg, and a temperature of 99°F (37.2°C) orally. The initial diagnostic evaluation of this patient includes:
    1. Electrocardiogram, pulmonary function studies, and sputum cytology.
    2. Complete blood count, chest x-ray, and sputum smear for acid-fast bacillus.
    3. ABG studies, complete blood count, and chest x-ray.
    4. Referral for direct bronchoscopy with biopsy and complement fixation antibody titer.

17. An adult male patient comes into the clinic complaining of increased fatigue and irritability. He has gained approximately 20 pounds over the last year. Although he sleeps through the night, his spouse says he seems somewhat restless. Based on these symptoms, what else should be determined?
    1. Presence of ongoing daytime sleepiness.
    2. History of depression.
    3. Fluctuations in blood pressure.
    4. Recent changes in medications.

18. When assessing the pulmonary function studies of a patient, which assessment finding is seen in chronic obstructive disease, such as in emphysema?
    1. Decreased forced vital capacity (FVC) and decreased forced expiratory volume in 1 second (FEV_1).
    2. Decreased functional residual capacity (FRC) and residual volume (RV).
    3. Decreased RV and increased total lung capacity (TLC).
    4. Increased FEV_1 and TLC.

19. When interpreting purified protein derivative (PPD) skin tests in patients at a long-term care facility, the adult-gerontology primary care NP identifies positive results in individuals with:
    1. Redness or erythema at the site.
    2. Induration reaction ≥ 5 mm.
    3. Induration reaction ≥ 10 mm.
    4. Induration reaction up to 15 mm.

20. A 65-year old obese female presents to the clinic with difficulty breathing. Upon examination, there is a low suspicion of a pulmonary embolus. Which of the following should the adult-gerontology primary care NP use to rule out the likelihood of a pulmonary embolus?
    1. Decreased platelets.
    2. Normal fibrin D-dimer.
    3. Normal chest x-ray.
    4. Normal aPTT.

21. The adult-gerontology primary care NP knows that screening for lung cancer includes:
    1. Sputum sample in those with a diagnosis of chronic bronchitis.
    2. Annual CT scan of the chest in asymptomatic individuals between the ages of 55 and 80 who have a 30-pack-year smoking history or greater and continue to smoke or have quit less than 15 years ago.
    3. Chest x-ray in all current smokers.
    4. Pulmonary function testing in those exposed to second hand smoke for more than 20 years and who have a 5-pack-year smoking history between the ages of 40 and 80 years.

22. The adult-gerontology primary care NP is auscultating a patient's chest and asks the patient to say "ninety-nine." With the stethoscope, a clear transmission of the words is heard indicating increased lung density. This describes which voice sound:
    1. Egophony.
    2. Pleural friction rub.
    3. Rhonchal fremitus.
    4. Bronchophony.

Disorders

23. A patient with severe COPD says he experiences fatigue and dyspnea with activity. In determining his activity level, the adult-gerontology primary care NP understands:
    1. Patients with moderate to severe COPD should avoid strenuous activity and conserve their energy.
    2. Pulmonary rehabilitation has been shown to improve functional exercise capacity and quality of life.
    3. It is important to first maximize pharmacologic therapy before increasing any type of activity level.
    4. Supplemental oxygen would be the best, most cost-effective choice for this patient.

24. In treating a patient with acute bronchitis lasting more than 5 days, the adult-gerontology primary care NP understands:
    1. Most patients will need antibiotic therapy.
    2. There is strong evidence to support the use of OTC preparations.
    3. A beta agonist should always be prescribed.
    4. Symptom management should be the primary focus of treatment.

25. A patient was hit in the chest. Which assessment finding would suggest a serious respiratory complication requiring immediate attention?
    1. Complaints of increased pain over the affected area.
    2. Oximetry readings consistently about 90%.
    3. Decreased breath sounds on the affected side.
    4. Fever of 102°F (38.9°C) and increased sputum production.

26. A patient with COPD smokes 1 pack of cigarettes daily. In approaching the patient about smoking cessation, the adult-gerontology primary care NP knows:
    1. Transitioning to e-cigarettes is a safe and effective alternative to smoking cessation.
    2. Smoking cessation does not significantly change the course of COPD.
    3. Counseling does not significantly increase quit rates over other strategies.
    4. Smoking cessation counseling should be done at every clinic visit.

27. The adult-gerontology primary care NP understands that the following characteristic is more likely to occur when the adult patient has pneumonia (due to *Streptococcus pneumoniae*) rather than bronchitis:
    1. Purulent sputum production.
    2. Nonproductive cough.
    3. Dyspnea.
    4. Wheezing.

28. **QSEN** A young adult is recovering from tuberculosis. What information should be included in a teaching plan for home care?
    1. It is critical for the young adult to take medications at the prescribed time; do not skip doses or allow the supply to run out.
    2. Respiratory isolation procedures need to be carried out at home; the young adult should avoid contact with immediate adult-gerontology primary care members.
    3. It will be necessary for the young adult to return to the clinic every week to have his or her sputum checked for viable bacteria.
    4. The young adult may experience a rash along with nausea and vomiting from the medications; if this occurs, he or she should decrease the dosage.

29. When questioning a patient about her risk factors for lung cancer, the adult-gerontology primary care NP knows that:
    1. 90% of all lung cancers present with symptoms.
    2. Only half of all cases of lung cancer are related to tobacco use.
    3. The risk of lung cancer is not any higher than the general population.
    4. There is a higher risk than the general population for cancer given second-hand smoke exposure.

30. What would be a priority intervention for a patient experiencing respiratory arrest, who has a pulse?
    1. Starting chest compressions at 30 compressions followed by two breaths.
    2. Starting rescue breathing, which is 1 breath every 5–6 seconds or about 10–12 breaths/min.
    3. Giving oxygen using a rebreathing mask at 10 L/min.
    4. Pinching the nose and giving two breaths.

31. A patient comes to the adult-gerontology primary care practice clinic complaining of difficulty breathing. What is most important to establish initially in this patient?
    1. Type of activity that produces the dyspnea.
    2. Presence of consolidation on chest x-ray.
    3. ABGs with respect to oxygen pressures.
    4. Presence of bilateral breath sounds over the lower lobes.

32. A patient's history strongly suggests the possibility of a foreign body in the bronchi. What observation would contribute to the documentation of this problem?
    1. Coughing and unilateral wheezing.
    2. Presence of crepitation on the anterior chest wall.
    3. Retraction of the lower chest wall with decreased breath sounds.
    4. A friction rub heard over the area of the bronchi.

33. A 22-year-old male comes to the office complaining of chest pain and shortness of breath. He states the problems started suddenly after running sprints in basketball practice. He states he has no past history of pulmonary problems. He is about 72 inches tall and 145 lb, with pulse rate of 118 beats/min, respiratory rate of 30 breaths/min, decreased breath sounds, and hyperresonance over the left lung. Based on these findings, what is the best diagnosis for the patient?
    1. Spontaneous pneumothorax.
    2. Exercise-induced asthma.
    3. Pulmonary edema.
    4. Acute bronchiectasis.

34. A young woman presents at the clinic with complaints of tingling in her face and hands, sudden shortness of breath, and vague chest discomfort. She appears very anxious and denies any history of respiratory problems. On examination, her hands are cool to the touch; her vital signs are respirations of 34 breaths/min, pulse regular at 100 beats/min, BP 110/76 mm Hg, and normal temperature. Respiratory examination reveals bilateral breath sounds with tachypnea, no adventitious sounds, and normal percussion and visual examination of the chest. What is the best immediate treatment?
    1. Relaxation techniques and encouraging controlled diaphragmatic breathing.
    2. Two puffs of short-acting bronchodilator (albuterol) with metered-dose inhaler (MDI).
    3. Oxygen at 4 L and ABGs after 30 minutes.
    4. Rebreathing into paper bag to increase $Paco_2$ levels.

35. A patient with newly diagnosed COPD is being discharged from the hospital. The adult-gerontology primary care NP is discussing home care with the patient. What information is important for the adult-gerontology primary care NP to include in the home care teaching?
    1. Use the bronchodilator before exercising.
    2. Maintain bed rest for the first few days at home.
    3. Decrease the amount of fluid intake to prevent fluid overload.
    4. Use the inhaled corticosteroid inhaler only when significantly short of breath.

36. Age-associated changes that increase the risk for respiratory symptoms in the older adult patient include an increase in:
    1. Compliance of the chest wall.
    2. Diameter of the trachea and bronchi.
    3. Lung parenchyma.
    4. Cough forcefulness.

37. An adult patient arrives at the family practice clinic complaining of difficulty breathing, a cough, and chest pain. History indicates that she was discharged from the hospital 2 days ago, after a cesarean section and has a 15-pack per year smoking history. What would be an appropriate action?
    1. Obtain a sputum specimen for culture and sensitivity.
    2. Order a chest x-ray, pulmonary CT scan, and angiogram.
    3. Perform spirometry testing.
    4. Immediately transfer to the emergency department.

38. The adult-gerontology primary care NP is aware that the flu or influenza:
    1. Can be caused by receiving a live attenuated influenza vaccine when one's resistance is low.
    2. Is characterized by a slow, insidious onset of chills, fever, and muscle aches.
    3. In older adults, may persist for weeks and increase the prevalence of bacterial pneumonia.
    4. Is primarily contagious in the early autumn and spring.

39. An adult patient with a history of asthma calls to tell the adult-gerontology primary care NP that she is achieving 55% of her personal best on the peak flow meter. She is talking in phrases and sounds calm. What advice would the adult-gerontology primary care NP give this patient?
    1. Call an ambulance immediately.
    2. Use a bronchodilator now and come in for evaluation in the office today.
    3. Use an inhaled corticosteroid inhaler now and every 4 hours as needed.
    4. Refer to a pulmonologist.

40. An older adult patient is evaluated by the adult-gerontology primary care NP for a complaint of cough, fever, pleuritic chest pain, and sputum production. In gathering a history on this patient, it is most important to know if the patient has:

1. Received the pneumococcal vaccine.
2. Traveled out of the country.
3. Pets in the household.
4. Recently changed or started new medications.

41. An older adult patient presents with signs and symptoms that make the adult-gerontology primary care NP suspect the diagnosis of community-acquired pneumonia (CAP). Which assessment would the adult-gerontology primary care NP most likely evaluate specific to an older adult patient during the examination?
    1. Chest pain with inspiration.
    2. Confusion/disorientation with or without a low-grade fever.
    3. Productive cough.
    4. Fever with leukocytosis.

42. In developing a plan for an older patient with typical pneumonia, the adult-gerontology primary care NP understands that 60%–65% of community-acquired pneumonia is caused by which organism?
    1. *Haemophilus influenzae.*
    2. *Klebsiella pneumoniae.*
    3. *Mycobacterium tuberculosis.*
    4. *Streptococcus pneumoniae.*

43. What would be most appropriate to include in the health promotion plan for an older adult patient who is at risk for developing pneumonia?
    1. Administer the pneumococcal vaccination annually.
    2. Administer the pneumococcal vaccination and yearly influenza immunization.
    3. Sputum culture annually along with a chest x-ray.
    4. PPD skin test every 3–5 years.

44. The adult-gerontology primary care NP evaluates an older adult patient with a current history of alcoholism. The patient presents with an elevated temperature, congested cough with rusty sputum, and occasional chills. The suspected diagnosis is bacterial pneumonia. The Gram-stained sputum smear would most likely reveal which organism?
    1. *Haemophilus influenzae.*
    2. *Klebsiella pneumoniae.*
    3. *Staphylococcus aureus.*
    4. *Pseudomonas aeruginosa.*

45. An older adult patient residing in a nursing home has recently been exposed to tuberculosis (TB). During the contact investigation, the adult-gerontology primary care NP interprets the initial PPD skin test to be negative. Which plan would be most appropriate at this time?
    1. Evaluate the patient in another year.
    2. Repeat PPD test in 8–10 weeks.

3. Ignore results and immediately begin ethambutol.
4. Evaluate the patient in 6 months because the patient is asymptomatic at this time.

46. Which two statements are accurate regarding sarcoidosis?
    1. Is a noninfectious, multisystem granulomatous disease.
    2. Affects only the lungs.
    3. May resolve spontaneously.
    4. Commonly affects the older and frail adult.
    5. High dose oral steroids are always prescribed.

47. The adult-gerontology primary care NP knows that Horner syndrome, a condition that can cause unilateral pupillary constriction and anhidrosis, is often associated with:
    1. Chronic bronchitis.
    2. Pulmonary tuberculosis.
    3. Pulmonary sulcus (Pancoast) tumor.
    4. Pulmonary embolism.

48. An adult patient who smokes presents with complaints of orthopnea. The adult-gerontology primary care NP notes on examination dilated blood vessels on the chest and mild edema of the head and supraclavicular area. The adult-gerontology primary care NP recognizes this condition as:
    1. Thyroid abnormality.
    2. Chronic bronchitis with mild heart failure.
    3. Asthma with fluid retention.
    4. Superior vena cava syndrome.

49. An older adult patient presents with postural hypotension and laboratory studies reveal hyponatremia. The patient is currently not taking any medications that may cause this. Which condition is likely the cause of these findings?
    1. Respiratory acidosis.
    2. Blunt chest trauma.
    3. Bronchogenic carcinoma.
    4. Bronchitis.

50. The adult-gerontology primary care NP knows the following about asthma in older adult patients:
    1. Subcutaneous epinephrine is standard therapy.
    2. It is usually of the allergic type.
    3. It can be confused with ischemic heart disease.
    4. Clinical presentation is usually dyspnea, costal retraction, and fever.

51. Clinical signs and symptoms of late-phase antigen exposure in asthma include:
    1. Bronchoconstriction refractory to bronchodilator therapy.
    2. Sneezing, watery eyes, and cough.
    3. Wheezing and increased sputum production.
    4. Bronchodilation secondary to the release of histamine.

52. The adult-gerontology primary care NP is assessing a patient for asthma. What is a common clinical manifestation of asthma?
    1. Pruritus.
    2. Diffuse crackles.
    3. Nocturnal exacerbation.
    4. Chronic hypoxemia.

53. During a routine follow-up visit for a patient with asthma, the patient states that she has been doing fine except that, when she goes out for dinner, she has increased bronchospasm and wheezing. Which of the following would be an appropriate response by the adult-gerontology primary care NP?
    1. "Have you been taking your medication?"
    2. "Do you usually have wine with dinner?"
    3. "I recommend you do not go out for dinner."
    4. "Does going out to dinner make you feel stressed?"

54. The adult-gerontology primary care NP is evaluating an adult with symptoms characteristic of obstructive sleep apnea. An overnight polysomnography (PSG) is ordered. What is the characteristic result of this study that would be indicative of sleep apnea?
    1. Loud snoring all night long.
    2. Oxygen desaturation and 10-second periods of apnea.
    3. Frequent periods of brief arousal during sleep.
    4. Periods of 5-second apnea with brief arousal.

55. The adult-gerontology primary care NP is screening older adult patients for problems related to obstructive sleep apnea (OSA). What risk factors are typically associated with this condition?
    1. Usage of sleep aids.
    2. Weight loss.
    3. Frequent nighttime sleep disturbance.
    4. Daytime hyperactivity.

56. A patient comes to the clinic complaining of difficulty breathing, lethargy, and coughing up blood in his sputum. He has no history of chronic illness or major health problems. The adult-gerontology primary care NP orders diagnostic tests to determine the problem. What diagnostic test results would require immediate treatment of this patient?
    1. Positive sputum smear for acid-fast bacillus.
    2. Sputum culture positive for *Pneumocystis carinii*.
    3. Presence of hemolysis on complement fixation test.
    4. Oxygen saturation 94%, leukocyte count >5000 WBCs/mm^3.

57. When determining the classification of asthma control in an adult patient who has symptoms less than 2 days per week, no interference with normal activity, reports no nighttime awakening, and using a short-acting β_2 agonist 2 times per week, the adult-gerontology primary care NP would classify the patient as:
    1. Well controlled.
    2. Partly controlled.
    3. Uncontrolled.
    4. Out of control.

58. When examining the chest x-ray of patient with an initial tuberculosis infection, you would expect to see changes in what part of the lung?
    1. Trachea.
    2. Upper lobes.
    3. Bronchi.
    4. Lower lobes.

59. An adult, who has an FEV1 greater than 80%, has been experiencing nighttime awakenings (4–5 times per week) and using a short-acting β_2 agonist 3–4 times per week, and reports minimal limitation to normal activity would be classified as:
    1. Well-controlled.
    2. Partly controlled.
    3. Uncontrolled.
    4. Severe persistent.

Pharmacology

60. When selecting a pharmacologic agent to assist in smoking cessation the adult-gerontology primary care NP recognizes a medication that binds potently with nicotine receptors is:
    1. Nortriptyline (Pamelor).
    2. Nicotine transdermal patch (Nicoderm).
    3. Bupropion (Zyban).
    4. Varenicline (Chantix).

61. **QSEN** The adult-gerontology primary care NP is following up on a patient who is experiencing acute asthma problems. Albuterol (Proventil) by metered-dose inhaler (MDI; 2 puffs) has been ordered as treatment. Which patient response would indicate to the adult-gerontology primary care NP that the patient understands how to take the medication?
    1. "I will take 1 puff of the medication, and then wait a minute before taking the second puff."
    2. "I will take 2 puffs of the medication every 4 hours, even if I am not short of breath."
    3. "It is important for me to take this medication on a regular cycle to prevent future attacks."
    4. "I will take 2 puffs, one right after the other, whenever I begin to get short of breath."

62. A patient with COPD complains of increased dyspnea and sputum volume over the last two days. The patient presents with a respiratory rate of 20 breaths/min, resting oxygen saturation of 88% on room air, and no cyanosis or peripheral edema. The patient is currently taking salmeterol (Serevent) 50 mcg diskus one puff every 12 hours

with tiotropium (Spiriva Handihaler) 18 mcg inhaled two puffs daily. To improve lung function and recovery time, the adult-geriatric primary NP starts:
1. Supplemental oxygen therapy.
2. Azithromycin (Zithromax) 250 mg 2 tablets now and 1 tablet daily for 4 days.
3. Prednisone 40 mg daily for 5 days.
4. Theophylline 300 mg daily for 7 days.

63. A patient who was recently diagnosed with tuberculosis calls the clinic because her urine is reddish orange. She is taking isoniazid (INH), rifampin (Rifadin), and pyrazinamide (PZA). What would be an appropriate response for the adult-gerontology primary care NP to make?
    1. "This is a urinary tract infection symptom; drink plenty of fluids."
    2. "This is a normal response to the rifampin."
    3. "This often is an indication of liver toxicity. Stop the medications."
    4. "This is indicative of bleeding. You must see a physician immediately."

64. A patient with a history of bronchial asthma is seen in the clinic for increased episodes of difficulty breathing. He has been taking theophylline 100 mg PO tid. He is 40 years old and obese with an 18-pack-year history of cigarette smoking and excessive intake of coffee daily. He eats a low-carbohydrate, high-protein diet. Which identified factors decrease the therapeutic effects of the theophylline?
    1. Age and sex.
    2. Coffee intake and weight.
    3. Age and weight.
    4. Smoking history and diet.

65. **QSEN** An adult male comes to the clinic with complaints that he is experiencing increased difficulty breathing over the past few days. He has a history of asthma and coronary artery disease. He was recently diagnosed with hypertension. Examination reveals no jugular vein distention and no productive cough. Breath sounds are present, but expiratory wheezes are noted bilaterally, and he denies any chest pain. His vital signs are pulse of 72 beats/min, respirations of 34 breaths/min, and BP of 170/100 mm Hg. His current medications are albuterol (Proventil) inhaler 2 puffs every 4 hours prn for wheezing, nitroglycerin transdermal patch for coronary artery disease, and propranolol (Inderal) 60 mg PO bid for his hypertension. What is the best treatment for this patient?
    1. Discontinue propranolol and begin amlodipine (Norvasc) 5 mg PO daily.
    2. Start a Prednisone burst with dosage taper over 1 week.
    3. Discontinue propranolol (Inderal) and begin atenolol (Tenormin) 50 mg PO daily.
    4. Start beclomethasone (Beclovent) inhaler 2 puffs 3 to 4 times daily.

66. The recommended range for maintaining serum theophylline levels is:
    1. 0.05–2 mcg/mL.
    2. 10–20 mcg/mL.
    3. 20–25 mcg/mL.
    4. 30–40 mcg/mL.

67. An otherwise recently healthy nonsmoking patient presents with a dry cough for the last 5 months. She has a history of hypertension and gastroesophageal reflux disorder. She is on ranitidine (Zantac) 150 mg PO bid and lisinopril (Zestril) 20 mg PO daily. The treatment that may yield the highest probability of success includes:
    1. Discontinuing ranitidine.
    2. Starting albuterol (Proventil) inhaler, 90 mcg every 4 to 6 hours as needed.
    3. Starting dextromethorphan 20 mg every 4 hours as needed.
    4. Discontinuing lisinopril.

68. **QSEN** An immunocompromised patient in a long-term facility whose roommate has been diagnosed with active tuberculosis should be started on latent tuberculosis infection (LTBI) treatment:
    1. As soon as possible and initiated at the time of the tuberculosis skin testing.
    2. In 72 hours after PPD skin test results are obtained.
    3. Only if PPD skin test results are positive.
    4. In 3 months if the repeated skin test is positive.

69. In adults with asthma, the most common reason outpatient treatment fails, resulting in hospitalization, is:
    1. Exposure to allergens.
    2. Increased use of steroids.
    3. Improper inhaler technique.
    4. Use of cromolyn inhalers.

70. Which can elevate theophylline levels?
    1. Concomitant treatment with cimetidine (Tagamet).
    2. Intravenous ampicillin.
    3. Heavy smoking.
    4. History of seizure disorder.

71. A patient with a long history of COPD has noticed an increase in dyspnea and a change in sputum over the past few days, with increased amounts of thick, yellow-green mucus and congestion. What would be the appropriate therapy?
    1. Loratadine (Claritin) 10 mg PO daily.
    2. Amoxicillin/clavulanate (Augmentin) 500 mg/125 mg PO three times daily for 10 days.
    3. Acetaminophen with codeine 300 mg/30 mg PO every 6 hours as needed.
    4. Beclomethasone (Qvar) 40 mcg MDI 2 puffs every 4 hours as needed.

72. Which medication is most effective in promoting a decrease in airway inflammation as well as providing long-term medication coverage in a patient with asthma?
    1. Montelukast (Singulair).
    2. Beclomethasone (Vanceril; Beclovent).
    3. Albuterol (Proventil; Ventolin).
    4. Salmeterol (Serevent).

73. The adult-gerontology primary care NP is planning regular daily treatment for a patient with asthma. Which is the preferred medication for the asthmatic patient who is not currently experiencing an exacerbation?
    1. Antibiotic.
    2. Inhaled corticosteroid.
    3. β_2 agonist.
    4. Leukotriene receptor antagonist.

74. Patients with asthma need to be instructed to:
    1. Begin inhaled corticosteroids as soon as symptoms appear.
    2. Take 1 to 2 puffs of β_2 agonist as needed using MDI.
    3. Use inhaled corticosteroids when they experience bronchospasm.
    4. Start antibiotic regimen when they experience bronchospasm.

75. The adult-gerontology primary care NP understands that one of the following over-the-counter preparations in high doses can cause euphoria, disorientation, paranoia, and hallucinations and has been known to be abused by adolescents.
    1. Pseudoephedrine.
    2. Diphenhydramine.
    3. Guaifenesin.
    4. Dextromethorphan.

76. An adult patient with chronic asthma is seen in the clinic complaining of vomiting and stomach cramps. He is confused and unsure what medications he is currently taking. His vital signs are BP of 158/92 mm Hg, pulse of 152 beats/min and irregular, and respirations of 28 breaths/min and shallow. What STAT diagnostic study should be obtained?
    1. Serum electrolytes.
    2. Digoxin level.
    3. Theophylline level.
    4. Arterial blood gases.

77. An adult patient is seen in the clinic complaining of increased difficulty breathing and an intermittent productive cough that worsens in the evening. The history reveals that the patient has a 20-pack-year history of smoking. Breath sounds are clear to auscultation, there is no evidence of fever, and chest radiography is within normal limits. The adult-gerontology primary care NP instructs the patient concerning the importance of smoking cessation and fluid therapy then prescribes:

    1. Erythromycin 500 mg PO qid × 14 days.
    2. Albuterol 2 mg PO tid.
    3. Acetylcysteine (Mucomyst) 10 mL 10% solution nebulized q4h prn.
    4. Cough, cold, and antiinflammatories for symptom control.

78. When initiating preventive care to decrease the incidence of pneumonia in patients in an extended-care facility, the adult-gerontology primary care NP would identify patients receiving immunosuppressive therapy, frequent antibiotic use, sedation, and:
    1. β_1 adrenergic blockers.
    2. Calcium channel blockers.
    3. Diuretics.
    4. Histamine (H_2) antagonists.

79. An older adult patient presents with new complaints of dyspnea, cough, fatigue, and dependent edema that has been worsening over the past few days. In planning treatment, the adult-gerontology primary care NP considers:
    1. Levofloxacin (Levaquin) 750 mg PO bid for 7 days.
    2. Referral for hospitalization for evaluation of heart function.
    3. Furosemide (Lasix) 40 mg PO daily.
    4. Addition of a calcium channel blocker to the patient's medications.

80. **QSEN** A patient with a history of Parkinson disease has an initial positive tuberculosis (TB) skin test, and INH is ordered for treatment of latent tuberculosis infection. Before beginning INH, it is important for the adult-gerontology primary care NP to determine:
    1. If the patient's Parkinson condition is being treated with levodopa (Larodopa).
    2. How long the patient has been diagnosed with Parkinson disease.
    3. How much respiratory compromise the patient is currently experiencing.
    4. The adequacy of urine output and renal function.

81. An adult white male with a history of COPD presents to the clinic with increased dyspnea, temperature of 102°F (39°C), pulse of 104 beats/min, respirations of 44 breaths/min, and O_2 saturation of 84%. Physical examination reveals diffuse rales and rhonchi bilaterally. Medications include atenolol (Tenormin) 25 mg PO daily, prednisone (Deltasone) 10 mg PO daily, ipratropium bromide (Atrovent) 1 to 2 puffs 18 mcg qid prn, and fluticasone and salmeterol (Advair Diskus 100/50) 2 puffs bid. The adult-gerontology primary care NP's preliminary diagnosis is pneumonia, pending chest x-ray results. Which medication puts this patient at risk to become immunocompromised?
    1. Atenolol.
    2. Prednisone.
    3. Ipratropium.
    4. Fluticasone and salmeterol.

82. The pharmacologic treatment shown to be superior in multiple studies for the treatment of COPD by reducing exacerbation, lowering cost, and improving lung function and quality of life is:
    1. Albuterol (Proventil) metered dose inhaler.
    2. Theophylline (Theo-24).
    3. Ipratropium bromide (Atrovent) metered dose inhaler.
    4. Ipratropium bromide and albuterol (Proventil) combined.

83. An adult female comes to the clinic with complaints of cough, clear rhinorrhea, and a low-grade fever for 2 days. The adult-gerontology primary care NP diagnoses acute bronchitis. The adult-gerontology primary care NP knows that with acute bronchitis:
    1. The patient will likely need antibiotics.
    2. A cough can last for 10–20 days.
    3. Routine sputum cultures are helpful because of nasopharyngeal colonization.
    4. Only 5%–10% of acute bronchitis cases have a viral etiology.

84. The adult-gerontology primary care NP has diagnosed an adult patient with community-acquired pneumonia (CAP). In this healthy patient with no comorbidities, and no previous antibiotic use within the past 3 months, the adult-gerontology primary care NP should prescribe:
    1. Doxycycline 100 mg PO bid for 10 days.
    2. Amoxicillin (Amoxil) 500 mg PO tid for 10 days.
    3. Azithromycin (Zithromax) 500 mg PO once, and then 250 mg daily for 4 days.
    4. Ciprofloxacin (Cipro) 500 mg PO daily for 7 days.

85. An adult male comes into office with a complaint of a chronic cough. The cough has persisted for 6 weeks and continued following resolution of his upper respiratory infection. The adult-gerontology primary care NP understands that:
    1. This cough is chronic and is likely caused by cigarette use or exposure to second-hand smoke.
    2. This is a subacute cough and is likely postinfectious.
    3. The cough has lasted longer than 3 weeks, which means it is not related to past infection.
    4. The patient should be worked up for gastroesophageal reflux (GERD).

86. **OSEN** An adult male is started on ciprofloxacin (Cipro) 500 mg PO bid daily for 60 days for possible exposure to anthrax. Five days later, upon return to the clinic, he notes increased pain in his posterior ankle. Understanding the potential complications with fluoroquinolone therapy, the adult-gerontology primary care NP knows:
    1. The posterior ankle pain is an unrelated condition.
    2. This is a known side effect and the ciprofloxacin (Cipro) should be continued as prescribed.

    3. This is a known adverse reaction and the ciprofloxacin (Cipro) should be discontinued.
    4. Ciprofloxacin (Cipro) should not be used empirically to treat anthrax exposure.

87. An adult teacher comes to the office with a loud cough starting 2 days before. She says that several children in her fourth-grade class have been out sick because of whooping cough. There is a high probability of exposure to *Bordetella pertussis*. The adult-gerontology primary care NP elects the best treatment option to be:
    1. Watchful, waiting to see if the cough clears up in the next few days.
    2. Doxycycline 100 mg PO bid daily for 7 days.
    3. Azithromycin (Zithromax) 500 mg PO once, and then 250 mg PO daily for 4 days.
    4. Oseltamivir (Tamiflu) 75 mg PO bid daily for 5 days.

88. According to the 2017 Global Initiative for Chronic Obstructive Lung Disease (GOLD) guidelines, COPD should be considered in a patient presenting with which 3 findings:
    1. Smoking history.
    2. Chronic cough.
    3. Shortness of breath.
    4. FEV_1/FVC ratio of 0.75.
    5. History of alcohol and drug abuse.

89. During a first-time office visit, the adult-gerontology primary care NP sees an adult female with a history of asthma. She had been using albuterol (Proventil) metered dose inhaler (MDI) one inhalation twice monthly over the past several years. More recently, she has been using her MDI inhaler 5 to 7 times per week. Based on the Global Initiative for Asthma (GINA) guidelines, the adult-gerontology primary care NP diagnoses partly controlled asthma and starts her on "Step 2" therapy which includes:
    1. Fluticasone and salmeterol (Advair) 250 mg/50 mg one inhalation bid.
    2. Fluticasone (Flovent) 44 mcg two inhalations daily.
    3. Fluticasone and salmeterol (Advair) 100 mg/50 mg one inhalation bid.
    4. Salmeterol (Serevent) 42 mcg one inhalation bid.

90. An older adult female comes in for a follow-up for COPD. She notes an increased frequency of morning headaches and daytime somnolence. A complete blood count notes that her hematocrit is 52%. The adult-gerontology primary care NP understands that a common, but not always recognized complication of COPD this patient could have is:
    1. Acute respiratory failure.
    2. Cor pulmonale.
    3. Depression.
    4. Nocturnal oxygen desaturation.

91. An adult patient in the adult-gerontology primary care NP's office has been diagnosed with community-acquired pneumonia (CAP). According to the Infectious Disease Society of America and American Thoracic Society (IDSA/ATS) joint guidelines for CAP, criteria indicating the probable need for immediate admission to an inpatient facility includes which 3 findings:
    1. White blood cell count of 2500 cells/mm³.
    2. Temperature of 96.2°F (36.8°C).
    3. Respiratory rate of 30 breaths/min.
    4. Platelet count of 165,000 cells/mm³.
    5. BUN of 32 mg/dL.

92. **QSEN** The adult-gerontology primary care NP is teaching a patient about the role of medications in the treatment of asthma. Which statement by the patient would require further teaching?
    1. "My albuterol is my quick-relief medication."
    2. "The salmeterol that I take provides me with long-term control."
    3. "I do not need to use a spacer with my MDI."
    4. "I need to use my peak flow meter to self-monitor how I am doing."

93. A 15-year-old adolescent comes to the emergency department (ED) with complaints of extreme shortness of breath. The patient is confused, and the past medical history is not available. Vital signs are pulse of 124 beats/min, respirations of 32 breaths/min, BP of 124/80 mm Hg, and temperature normal. Physical examination reveals diffuse expiratory wheezes, hyperresonance on percussion, and prolonged expiratory phase. The best treatment for this patient includes:
    1. Aminophylline by mouth.
    2. Beclomethasone (Beclovent) inhaler.
    3. Epinephrine by injection.
    4. Albuterol (Proventil) by MDI.

94. The adult-gerontology primary care NP understands that an appropriate medication regimen for an adolescent with drug-susceptible pulmonary tuberculosis (TB) is:
    1. Montelukast (Singulair) therapy with rifampin (Rifadin).
    2. Streptomycin, pyrazinamide, and rimantadine (Flumadine).
    3. Isoniazid (INH), pyrazinamide, and rifampin.
    4. Montelukast therapy with pyrimethamine (Fansidar).

95. A young adult is taking isoniazid (INH) prophylactically for exposure to TB complains of headache, palpitations, rash, and diarrhea. Management would be based on:
    1. Avoidance of foods containing tyramine and histamine.
    2. Addition of pyridoxine to the diet.
    3. Change in therapy from INH to rifampin.
    4. Evaluation for hepatic impairment.

96. Which two medications are prescribed and used in smoking cessation?
    1. Cetirizine (Zyrtec).
    2. Valacyclovir (Valtrex).
    3. Varenicline (Chantix).
    4. Bupropion (Zyban).
    5. Lisinopril (Zesteril).

97. An adolescent male is experiencing problems with wheezing, coughing, and shortness of breath about 4 hours after basketball practice. He has normal respirations and only experiences the problems after exercise. He is experiencing no other respiratory problems, and the physical findings are within normal limits. What is the treatment of choice for this patient?
    1. Albuterol (Ventolin) 2 puffs MDI 20–30 minutes before exercise.
    2. Cromolyn sodium (Intal) 2 puffs each morning.
    3. Theophylline (Theo-24; methylxanthine) 100 mg PO bid.
    4. Beclomethasone (Beclovent) 2 puffs 3–4 times daily.

5 Respiratory Answers & Rationales

Physical Examination & Diagnostic Tests

1. Answer: 1

Rationale: A pleural effusion should always be confirmed by ultrasonography as this will detect effusions as low as 5 mL to 50 mL, as will a CT scan. A chest radiograph does not always detect small effusions. Spirometry testing will suggest restrictive lung disease, but will not identify the potential cause. A ventilation-perfusion scan will identify lung perfusion, but not lung effusion.

2. Answer: 1

Rationale: This is a normal finding because of the anatomical location of the bulk of the liver. Atelectasis and consolidation present with normal diaphragmatic movement, but with dullness to percussion over the affected area. Severe obstructive lung disease results in hyperinflation and limited diaphragmatic excursion, but is bilateral.

3. Answer: 2

Rationale: Vesicular breath sounds are normal low pitched, low intensity sounds heard in the peripheral lung fields. Inspiration is 2.5 times longer than the expiratory phase. Bronchial breath sounds, normally heard over the trachea and larynx, are high-pitched loud sounds with a shortened inspiratory and lengthened expiratory phase. Bronchovesicular breath sounds that are heard mainly where fewer alveoli are located, which is over the second intercostal space anteriorly and between the scapulae posteriorly, have a moderate pitch and intensity with equal duration of expiratory and inspiratory sounds. Rhonchi are abnormal breath sounds that are low pitched with a snoring quality.

4. Answer: 3

Rationale: Pulmonary function test (spirometry) is used to determine the degree of restriction that leads to the diagnosis of chronic obstructive pulmonary disease (COPD). Chest x-ray can determine the physical finding of COPD without the functional status. CBC will show anemia, a possible consequence of chronic COPD. Arterial blood gas will show active changes in the oxygenation of the blood.

5. Answer: 2

Rationale: Greater clarity and increased loudness of spoken sounds are defined as bronchophony. If bronchophony is extreme (e.g., in the presence of consolidation of the lungs), even a whisper can be heard clearly and intelligibly through the stethoscope (whispered pectoriloquy). Bronchophony or bronchiloquy is a type of pectoriloquy

normally heard as a soft, muffled, indistinct voice. When you ask the patient to say "ninety-nine," during auscultation, you will hear an abnormally clear distinct sound of "ninety-nine," if there is lung consolidation. Whispered pectoriloquy is exaggerated bronchophony and is heard through a stethoscope when the patient whispers a series of words (e.g., "one-two-three"). In egophony, the spoken voice has a nasal or bleating quality when heard through a stethoscope, and the spoken "e-e-e" sounds like "a-a-a." Tactile fremitus is a palpable vibration of the thoracic wall that is produced when the patient speaks.

6. Answer: 2

Rationale: Hyperresonance is a percussion assessment finding suggestive of air trapping, which can be found in obstructive lung conditions like emphysema. It is characterized by very loud intensity, very low pitch, long duration, and a booming quality. It is not a normal finding.

7. Answer: 3

Rationale: Both the anterior and posterior chest should be percussed systematically and symmetrically at 4–5-cm intervals over the intercostal spaces, moving from left to right. Care is needed to ensure percussion is done in the intercostal spaces. Diaphragmatic excursion is usually only measured on the posterior chest.

8. Answer: 1

Rationale: Pleural friction rubs are loud, dry, creaking or grating sounds produced by the rubbing together of inflamed and roughened pleural surfaces. Rubs are heard best during the latter part of inspiration and the beginning of expiration, and in the lower anterolateral chest where the lung expands the most. A continuous, low-pitched, snoring sound that is heard early in inspiration is characteristic of sonorous rhonchi. Egophony is noted when the patient says "e-e-e" and the examiner hears through the stethoscope "a-a-a.", and is suggestive of lung consolidation.

9. Answer: 4

Rationale: Given the patient's recent 12-hour flight, the patient is at high risk for deep vein thrombosis and subsequent pulmonary embolism. The best test choice that would show a pulmonary embolism is the spiral CT scan. A V/Q scan is only useful in patients with a normal chest x-ray, which would need to be completed before V/Q scan. An ECG may have some nonspecific changes, but is not diagnostic. A chest radiograph may likely be normal. Spirometry may be abnormal, but not specific. The patient will need emergent care.

10. Answer: 2

Rationale: Consolidation or compression of lung tissue will cause an increase in fremitus, which is noted with lobar pneumonia. Decreased fremitus occurs with obstruction of vibration, like in emphysema, pneumothorax, or obstructed bronchus. Symmetric transmission of vibration is a normal finding.

11. Answer: 4

Rationale: Crepitation or crepitus (also called subcutaneous emphysema) usually results from air bubbles under the skin caused by a leakage of air into the subcutaneous tissue. Infection by a gas-producing organism is a less common cause. Crepitation always requires attention. Severe inflammation of the pleural surface would not have a palpable abnormality. Fluid consolidation would cause an increased asymmetric fremitus on palpation.

12. Answer: 2

Rationale: This landmark can be used to determine the position of the second rib and intercostal space and corresponding spaces below that level. The angle of Louis (manubriosternal junction) is a visible and palpable angle of the sternum at the point where the second rib attaches to the sternum.

13. Answer: 2

Rationale: Fluid or a solid mass will increase the transmission of vibration. Increased air trapping decreases or masks the transmission of vibration. A reactive airway results in wheezing due to mucous and inflamed airways. Increased pressure in the bronchial tree is not measurable and will not cause asymmetric vibratory changes.

14. Answer: 4

Rationale: The adult chest is usually symmetrical and the anterior-posterior (AP) diameter is often half the lateral diameter. Pigeon chest (pectus carinatum) is a forward protrusion of the sternum with the ribs sloping back. Funnel chest (pectus excavatum) is a depression of the sternum. Barrel chest occurs when the AP diameter equals the transverse diameter and is usually a sign of advancing obstructive lung disease.

15. Answer: 2

Rationale: According to 2013 guidelines, the U.S. Preventive Services Task Force (USPSTF) recommends an annual screening for lung cancer with low-dose computed tomography (LDCT) in adults aged 55 to 80 years who have a calculated smoking history of 30 packs per year and currently smoke or have quit within the past 15 years. This should be discontinued after they have stopped smoking after 15 years. Current evidence-based research does support routine screening for lung cancer in the general population. There is insufficient evidence that lung cancer screening by x-ray or sputum cytology reduces mortality. Bronchoscopy with biopsy is a diagnostic test, not a screening test.

16. Answer: 2

Rationale: The patient should be initially evaluated for tuberculosis, which includes a chest x-ray, sputum smear for acid-fast bacillus, and a complete blood count (CBC). Pulmonary function studies, arterial blood gas (ABG) studies, and bronchoscopy are not indicated initially. Complement fixation studies are done to diagnose atypical pneumonia.

17. Answer: 1

Rationale: A male patient with recent weight gain and restless sleep is at risk for having obstructive sleep apnea (OSA). Ongoing daytime sleepiness is the hallmark sign of OSA. While reoccurring depression could be a cause, a provider should consider physical causes of presenting symptoms first. Fluctuations in blood pressure, including hypertension, can be seen in OSA, but would not cause the fatigue and nighttime restlessness. Recent changes in medication should be evaluated, but is unlikely to cause all his symptoms.

18. Answer: 1

Rationale: Hyperinflation due to air trapping causes an increase in functional residual capacity (FRC), residual volume (RV), and total lung capacity (TLC), which may be twice normal. A corresponding decrease in forced vital capacity (FVC) and forced expiratory volume in second (FEV_1) occurs. This causes a flattening of the diaphragm, decreased inspiratory efficiency, and increased work of breathing.

19. Answer: 3

Rationale: Positive interpretation of purified protein derivative (PPD) skin test results are as follows, based on the 2012 criteria from the Centers for Disease Control and Prevention:

INDURATION	POSITIVE PPD SKIN TEST RESULT
≥5 mm	Individuals with human immunodeficiency virus (HIV) infection
	Individuals in recent close contact with persons who have active tuberculosis (TB)
	Individuals with chest x-ray indicating healed TB
≥10 mm	Medically underserved individuals
	Intravenous drug users
	Residents in long-term care facilities and health care workers
≥15 mm	All individuals

20. Answer: 2

Rationale: Fibrin D-dimer is normally <500 ng/mL and is elevated when plasmin crosslinks fibrin and creates degradation products in the blood. Unless the suspicion of a pulmonary embolism is high a D-dimer level of <500 can be used to rule out pulmonary embolism. D-dimer is sensitive but not specific and cannot be used to diagnose pulmonary embolism.

21. Answer: 2

Rationale: Current recommendations (December, 2013) for lung cancer screening from the U.S. Preventative Services Task Force (USPSTF) is for individuals (ages 55–80) to have a low-dose computed tomography (LDCT) who have a 30-pack-year smoking history and currently smoke or have quit within the past 15 years. This has proven to be the most effective in decreasing lung cancer related deaths. Screening should be discontinued once a person has not smoked for 15 years or develops a health problem that substantially limits life expectancy or the ability or willingness to have curative lung surgery.

22. Answer: 4

Rationale: Bronchophony is the clear loud transmission of sound usually through abnormally consolidated lung tissue. Extreme bronchophony results in the ability to hear whispered words over the involved area (whispered pectoriloquy). With normal voice transmission, sound is soft, muffled, and indistinct; the sound can be heard through the stethoscope but cannot be distinguished as to what is being said. Egophony is a change to a more nasal quality of the sound best demonstrated by asking the patient to say long set of "e-e-e" sounds. Normally these sounds are clearly heard through the stethoscope; with consolidation or compression, the "e-e-e" sounds change to a bleating long "a-a-a" sound (similar to a goat sound). A pleural friction rub is a dry, crackly, grating, low pitched sound suggesting pleural inflammation. Rhonchal fremitus is vibration felt when inhaled air passes through thick secretions in the larger bronchi.

Disorders

23. Answer: 2

Rationale: According to the 2017 Global Initiative for Obstructive Lung Disease (GOLD) standards, pulmonary rehabilitation has been shown to improve exercise capacity and quality of life across all levels of severity in COPD. It has shown to be the most cost-effective treatment strategy available. COPD patients should not avoid physical activity, because this will only add additional immobility issues. While it is important to optimize pharmacologic therapy, pulmo-nary rehabilitation is beneficial with any COPD patient. Supplemental oxygen should not be prescribed routinely even in patients who moderately desaturate with activity.

24. Answer: 4

Rationale: Most cases of acute bronchitis rely on symptom management as the primary treatment choice. In most cases, antibiotics are discouraged due to increase resistance and lack of evidenced-based efficacy. There is no significant evidence for or against the usage of OTC preparations. While a beta agonist has been shown to resolve cough faster in those with underlying wheezing, there is nothing recommending wide use.

25. Answer: 3

Rationale: The most common respiratory complication after a traumatic injury to the chest is pneumothorax caused from a fractured rib. Oximetry readings below 90% and increased pain are expected at this point and may not be indicative of a problem. Although fever and increased sputum are problems, they are not associated with early manifestations of blunt trauma chest injury.

26. Answer: 4

Rationale: According to the GOLD 2017 standards, there is no current research supporting the safe use of e-cigarettes in smoking cessation. Smoking cessation has the strongest ability to influence the natural course of COPD. There is a strong relationship between counseling and cessation success. Every tobacco user should be offered smoking cessation advice at every visit.

27. Answer: 1

Rationale: Community-acquired pneumonia (CAP) due to *Streptococcus pneumoniae* often presents abruptly with high fever, shaking chills (rigor), cough productive of purulent sputum, and pleuritic chest pain. In acute bronchitis, cough is the primary symptom and initially is dry and nonproductive. Fever, dyspnea, wheezing, and possible mucoid sputum production are also characteristic of acute bronchitis.

28. Answer: 1

Rationale: On discharge, a patient must understand the importance of taking medications as prescribed. Missed doses increase mutation of the tubercle bacillus and decrease the medication's effectiveness. Respiratory isolation at home is not necessary, and if the patient experiences problems of rash, nausea, and vomiting, he or she should contact the health care provider. A patient should never change a medication dosage without first consulting with a health care provider. Weekly sputum checks are not necessary.

29. Answer: 4

Rationale: Between 5% and 15% of lung cancers are asymptomatic. It is suggested that over 80%–90% of all cases of lung cancer are attributed to tobacco use. Exposure to environmental tobacco has shown to increase the risk for cancer. In one 2007 meta-analysis, wives of husbands who smoked had a 27% increased risk.

30. Answer: 2

Rationale: According to the American Heart Association, the protocol for respiratory arrest (has a pulse) is rescue breathing, which is to give 1 breath every 5–6 seconds or about 10–12 breaths/min. Pulse should be checked every 2 minutes, if no pulse, then begin CPR with 30 chest compressions followed by 2 breaths.

31. Answer: 1

Rationale: It is most important to obtain information about the dyspnea. Is it present during rest or does it occur with activity? What level of activity precipitates dyspnea? This information is necessary to determine the severity of the patient's complaint. A chest x-ray gives only limited information and may be normal in conditions like asthma. An ABG result is abnormal when the symptoms are severe. Presence of bilateral breath sounds over the lower lobes is a normal finding.

32. Answer: 1

Rationale: The most common area for a foreign body obstruction is the right bronchus, which produces a unilateral retraction of the right chest wall and leads to cough and unilateral wheezing with diminished breath sounds to that area. Retraction of the lower chest occurs with lower respiratory problems, such as asthma. A pleural friction rub is heard when there is inflammation between the viscera and parietal pleura. Crepitation is present when air is leaking into the subcutaneous tissue.

33. Answer: 1

Rationale: Spontaneous pneumothorax occurs in healthy, thin young adults, especially after strenuous exercise; predominant symptoms include sudden pain, dyspnea, and asymmetric chest expansion. The clinical hallmark of asthma is wheezing; with pulmonary edema, there is frequently coughing, frothy sputum, and crackles heard on auscultation. Bronchiectasis is most often chronic and is characterized by moist crackles and wheezing on auscultation; cough is usually present.

34. Answer: 1

Rationale: The situation described is hyperventilation syndrome (HVS); treatment should be concentrated on patient education through reassurance and suggested breathing and relaxation techniques. Albuterol, oxygen, and arterial blood gases (ABGs) are not appropriate initial treatments. Breathing into a paper bag is not recommended because significant hypoxemia and death has occurred in the past from this treatment.

35. Answer: 1

Rationale: To prevent dyspnea on activity, the bronchodilator should be used before walking or increased physical activity. The patient should not stay in bed and should be encouraged to increase activity gradually. Fluid intake of 2–3 L/day should be encouraged, unless there are cardiac problems. An inhaled corticosteroid inhaler should be used at regular intervals as ordered and is not meant for rescue during periods of acute dyspnea.

36. Answer: 2

Rationale: Age-associated physiologic changes include decreased compliance of the chest wall, making deep inspiration difficult. Increased trachea and bronchi diameters that increase dead space and result in a decreased volume of air reaching the alveoli. An increase in small airway closure results in decreased vital capacity and increased residual volume. Less elastic lung parenchyma results in decreased function of the alveoli. Shallow breathing and less forceful cough occurs because respiratory muscles weaken.

37. Answer: 4

Rationale: The patient is at risk for a pulmonary embolism, as a result of hypercoagulation related to giving birth, smoking, and vascular injury (recent surgery). Immediate testing and treatment is critical to survival of someone with a pulmonary embolism, so they should be referred or transferred to the highest level of care available. Assessment reveals common symptoms of a pulmonary embolism: dyspnea, cough, and pleuritic pain. Diagnostic tests include D-dimer test, chest x-ray, ventilation/perfusion (V/Q) scan, CT scan, and/or pulmonary angiogram, which would be ordered at the emergency department.

38. Answer: 3

Rationale: The flu or influenza is a highly contagious respiratory infection that occurs epidemically during the winter months and may increase the prevalence of bacterial pneumonia. It is characterized by a sudden onset of chills, elevated temperature (101°–104°F [38.3°–40°C]), headache, fatigue, muscle pain, dry cough, laryngitis, rhinorrhea, and red eyes occurring 24–48 hours after exposure directly through respiratory droplets from an infected person or indirectly by drinking from a contaminated glass. Flu vaccines do not cause the flu; they are made with a live attenuated (nasal vaccine) or killed virus (injection).

39. Answer: 2

Rationale: According to the Global Initiative for Asthma (2016) guidelines, this patient does not need immediate transfer to an acute care facility because she is achieving greater than 50% of personal best on her peak flow meter, remains calm, and is speaking in phrases. The patient should use her bronchodilator immediately and be evaluated urgently. If she does not improve or becomes worse, she will need emergency intervention. Inhaled corticosteroids are used for maintenance therapy and are a poor choice for "rescue" symptoms. A referral to a pulmonologist may be necessary at some point, but not immediately.

40. Answer: 1

Rationale: The pneumococcal vaccine is recommended for older adult patients because their immune system is less efficient. The symptoms of fever, chest pain, and sputum production suggest pneumonia.

41. Answer: 2

Rationale: Confusion/disorientation with or without a low-grade temperature may be the first sign that the older adult patient has an infection. The patient may not have a fever or leukocytosis; however, leukopenia may suggest severe CAP and require hospitalization. The patient may not experience any discomfort or a cough with the onset of infection.

42. Answer: 4

Rationale: *Streptococcus pneumoniae* is the most common cause of community-acquired and nursing home-acquired bacterial pneumonia. *Haemophilus influenzae* is common in older adult patients with underlying chronic diseases (e.g., COPD, diabetes). *Klebsiella pneumoniae* and other gram-negative bacteria are pathogens in patients with alcoholism, immunocompromised hosts, and hospitalized patients. *Mycobacterium tuberculosis* is an infrequent cause of pneumonia.

43. Answer: 2

Rationale: The pneumococcal vaccination should be given to all adults 65 years or older and yearly influenza immunization will decrease complications and hospitalizations for the older adult patient. The pneumococcal vaccination is not administered annually. There is no evidence to support the use of an annual sputum culture or chest x-ray for pneumonia prevention. The purified protein derivative (PPD) skin test should be done annually for high-risk patients and only detects exposure to tuberculosis.

44. Answer: 2

Rationale: *Klebsiella pneumoniae* is an important pathogen in patients with alcoholism. *Staphylococcus aureus* generally affects older adult patients recovering from influenza and is also common in hospitalized patients with

diabetes and in IV drug users. *Pseudomonas aeruginosa* is most likely found in someone with structural lung disease (e.g., bronchiectasis).

45. Answer: 2

Rationale: If a person is infected, a delayed-type reaction may occur 2–8 weeks after infection. In a contact exposure, if the initial PPD skin test is negative, a repeat purified protein derivative (PPD) test 8–10 weeks later is recommended in all patients. A patient should not be treated empirically for tuberculosis (TB) exposure. Six months is too long to wait for someone who could have active TB. A yearly evaluation should be reserved for those who work or live in high-risk environments, but have not been exposed.

46. Answer: 1, 3

Rationale: Sarcoidosis is a noninfectious, multisystem granulomatous disease that may affect almost any organ system; however, 90% of affected individuals have pulmonary involvement. It most commonly affects young and middle-aged adults, with 80% of the presenting patients between age 20 and 45. The majority of patients have a spontaneous resolution within 2 years. NSAIDs and low dose steroids are used to treat symptoms; however, many patients are asymptomatic and do not require medication. Higher dose steroids are prescribed when patients have acute respiratory failure, cardiac, neurologic, or ocular disease.

47. Answer: 3

Rationale: Horner syndrome, which is a paralysis of the cervical sympathetic nerves that results in ptosis, loss of sweating, pupillary constriction, and sometimes enophthalmos, is often associated with malignant tumors in the upper lung, leading to nerve compression (e.g., pulmonary sulcus [Pancoast] tumor or superior sulcus tumor).

48. Answer: 4

Rationale: Over 70% of the cases of superior vena cava syndrome (SVCS) occur as a complication of lung malignancy involving the mediastinum. This is considered an oncologic emergency and requires immediate referral. Although chronic bronchitis or heart failure may cause orthopnea, upper extremity edema is usually not present. A thyroid abnormality usually results in unilateral or bilateral thyroid enlargement in the neck. Asthma does not cause fluid retention.

49. Answer: 3

Rationale: Hyponatremia results from an overproduction of antidiuretic hormone and can be caused by ectopic production from a bronchogenic tumor (e.g., small cell lung carcinoma). Blunt chest trauma could result in hemorrhage and fluid loss, causing hypernatremia. Bronchitis and respiratory acidosis do not usually cause sodium abnormalities.

50. Answer: 3

Rationale: In older individuals, asthma can be confused with ischemic heart disease or left ventricular failure. Asthma symptoms can be discounted as old age or a lack of fitness. It is rarely allergic, and costal retraction and fever are not usually seen. Subcutaneous epinephrine is not standard treatment for asthma at any age, but may be indicated in emergency situations.

51. Answer: 1

Rationale: Late-phase asthma occurs at 8–12 hours after the initial or acute bronchoconstrictive phase. The inflammatory response is the result of mast cell degranulation and the release of inflammatory mediators, including histamines and leukotrienes. The mediators act on the lung by causing bronchoconstriction, vascular permeability, and vasodilation. In late-phase asthma, bronchoconstriction is refractory to most bronchodilator therapy.

52. Answer: 3

Rationale: Nocturnal exacerbation of asthma is a clinical sign. It is linked to variations in circulating cortisol, epinephrine, inflammatory mediators, and vagal tone. Chronic hypoxemia and diffuse crackles are seen in the patient with chronic bronchitis. Pruritus is often seen in contact allergic reactions.

53. Answer: 2

Rationale: Asking the patient about the consumption of wine with dinner is the most appropriate response. Many wines, especially white wines, contain sulfites, which can trigger a mild allergic response.

54. Answer: 2

Rationale: Desaturation and 10-second periods of apnea that occur 10–15 times per hour is considered clinically significant of obstructive sleep apnea. Loud snoring at night, frequent arousals during the night, and sleeping during the day are characteristic of the problem, but are not diagnostic.

55. Answer: 1

Rationale: Frequent substance use, including alcohol, benzodiazepines, sleep aids, opiates, and muscle relaxants, can exacerbate obstructive sleep apnea. Obesity, weight gain, nasal allergies, and polyps are common factors associated with this condition. Most patients with sleep apnea will not report nighttime sleep disturbances even though a spouse may witness nighttime restlessness. Snoring, daytime sleepiness, and fatigue are frequently reported symptoms. Men are more likely than premenopausal women to have obstructive sleep apnea.

56. Answer: 1

Rationale: The positive sputum for acid-fast bacillus is indicative of active tuberculosis. *Pneumocystis carinii* is a common organism in healthy respiratory tracts; it becomes a problem if the patient is immunocompromised. Hemolysis on a complement fixation test is a negative finding. When oxygen saturation is low and white blood cell (WBC) count is within normal range, treatment is not as important as it is with tuberculosis.

57. Answer: 1

Rationale: According to the Global Initiative on Asthma (2016), the level of control is based on the most severe impairment or risk category. This patient is well-controlled. The components of well-controlled asthma are daytime symptoms ≤2 times/week, no nighttime awakening, no interference with normal activity, using a short-acting β_2 agonist ≤2 times/week.

58. Answer: 4

Rationale: The initial tuberculosis infection is seen more often in the lower lobes of the lung. The local lymph nodes are infected and enlarged. An asymptomatic period usually follows the primary infection and can last for years or decades before clinical symptoms develop. When there a reactivation of the disease in a previously infected person, this scenario is more likely to occur in situations when defenses are lowered, such as with older adults and people with HIV disease. The upper lobes are the most common site of reactivation.

59. Answer: 3

Rationale: According to the Global Initiative on Asthma (2016), asthma control is evaluated based on the presence or absence of symptoms. Symptoms suggesting the asthma is not well controlled include daytime symptoms more than twice per week, night waking due to asthma, any activity limitation due to asthma, and usage of an asthma reliever (i.e., short-acting beta agonist) more than twice weekly. One to two of the criteria being true suggest the asthma is partly controlled, more than two being true suggests uncontrolled asthma.

Pharmacology

60. Answer: 4

Rationale: Varenicline (Chantix) prevents nicotine stimulation of mesolimbic dopamine system associated with nicotine addiction. Varenicline stimulates dopamine activity but to a much smaller degree than nicotine, resulting in decreased craving and withdrawal symptoms.

61. Answer: 1

Rationale: A 1-minute lapse between the two puffs is necessary for the medication to be most effective. The first puff opens the upper airways, allowing more effective penetration of the lower tract with the second puff. Albuterol (Proventil) should not be use as maintenance therapy. Only inhaled corticosteroids should be taken on a regular schedule.

62. Answer: 3

Rationale: According to GOLD 2017, 80% of COPD exacerbations are managed on an outpatient basis. Systemic corticosteroids (1 mg/kg/day commonly 40 mg daily for 5 days) are used for an acute exacerbation because they improve lung function, oxygenation, and short recovery time. While oxygen is a key component of exacerbation treatment in the hospital, it is not an appropriate first choice in this patient. Antibiotics are recommended when a patient has increased dyspnea, increased sputum volume, and increased sputum purulence, which is not the case here. Methylxanthines like theophylline are not recommended for exacerbations due to increased side effect profile.

63. Answer: 2

Rationale: Urine color change is a normal side effect of rifampin, and is not a reason for the patient to stop taking their medication. Also, soft contact lenses may become discolored.

64. Answer: 4

Rationale: Because tobacco increases the metabolism of theophylline, a higher dose is required in smokers than in nonsmokers. A high-protein, low-carbohydrate diet increases the metabolism of theophylline and decreases serum concentrations. Coffee (and other xanthine-containing beverages) may increase the central nervous system effects of xanthine derivatives.

65. Answer: 1

Rationale: Beta blockers (propranolol, atenolol) are known to exacerbate chronic respiratory problems, especially reactive airway disease. Another antihypertensive, such as a calcium channel blocker (amlodipine), should be considered. The patient's pulse is 72 beats/min and blood pressure remains elevated, which indicates the beta blocker is probably not effective in decreasing blood pressure in this patient. Prednisone is not indicated unless other medications are not effective. Although beclomethasone may be appropriate to start, discontinuing the beta blocker, which is likely exacerbating the problem, is the better choice.

66. Answer: 2

Rationale: Therapeutic plasma levels range from 10 to 20 mcg/mL. Drug levels of ≥20 mcg/mL are associated with toxicity.

67. Answer: 4

Rationale: The most likely causes of subacute cough include postinfection, GERD, or asthma. This patient has been healthy and is currently being treated for GERD symptoms. A likely cause of this cough is lisinopril, an ACE inhibitor. Albuterol and dextromethorphan may be good options if the cough doesn't clear within 4 weeks of discontinuing the lisinopril in favor of a different antihypertensive medication.

68. Answer: 1

Rationale: Latent tuberculosis infection (LTBI) treatment is initiated at the time of the tuberculosis skin testing (TST). TST should be repeated in 3 months if initial test results are negative. If the second TST is negative, LTBI treatment can be discontinued.

69. Answer: 3

Rationale: One of the most common causes of outpatient treatment failure is improper inhaler technique. Exposure to allergens may trigger an asthma attack, but proper use of inhalers will control the attacks in many cases. Use of both steroids and cromolyn inhalers has decreased the severity of asthma attacks.

70. Answer: 1

Rationale: Theophylline is used in the treatment of chronic lung disease and can accumulate in toxic levels. Cimetidine decreases the hepatic clearance of theophylline. Nicotine and some antiseizure drugs may actually increase clearance, and ampicillin does not change the clearance.

71. Answer: 2

Rationale: In someone with COPD, antibiotic therapy is indicated when there is a change in color, consistency, or amount of sputum and increased symptoms of COPD exacerbation. Antitussives are not recommended in stable COPD. Inhaled corticosteroids should be taken on a schedule and not ordered as needed.

72. Answer: 2

Rationale: Beclomethasone is a long-acting corticosteroid that stabilizes mast cells and greatly reduces mast-cell degranulation when exposed to allergens. Albuterol is a short-acting bronchodilator used as a rescue medication. Salmeterol is a long-acting bronchodilator most useful in controlling nocturnal asthma symptoms. Montelukast, a leukotriene receptor antagonist, inhibits bronchoconstriction and is used as an adjunct to bronchodilators and corticosteroids.

73. Answer: 2

Rationale: Preferred, regular daily treatment (long-term treatment) of the patient with asthma includes inhaled corticosteroid for their antiinflammatory effects. Antibiotics are indicated if there is a concurrent infection, such as acute bronchitis. β_2 agonists are used for their bronchodilator effects and rapid onset of action when a patient may need "rescue" or acute treatment of symptoms with quick-relief medications. Leukotriene receptor antagonist is another option, but not preferred to inhaled corticosteroid for regular daily treatment.

74. Answer: 2

Rationale: Patients with asthma should be instructed to keep their inhaled β_2 agonists with them at all times in case of bronchospasm and use them as necessary (prn). The β_2 agonists are effective in reversing bronchospasm. Inhaled corticosteroids are long acting and will not give immediate relief, so the patient should be instructed to use them as prescribed. Antibiotics are not indicated for acute bronchospasm.

75. Answer: 4

Rationale: Dextromethorphan is a widely used cough suppressant and is found in many cough and cold remedies. At low doses used for cough suppression, dextromethorphan lacks psychologic effects. However, at doses 5 to 10 times higher, dextromethorphan can cause euphoria, disorientation, paranoia, and altered sense of time, as well as visual, auditory, and tactile hallucinations. Guaifenesin is an expectorant; pseudoephedrine a decongestant; and diphenhydramine an antihistamine.

76. Answer: 3

Rationale: The drug therapy regimen for chronic asthma may include theophylline. Symptoms of toxicity include anorexia, nausea, vomiting, confusion, restlessness, tachycardia, dysrhythmias, and seizures.

77. Answer: 4

Rationale: Most patients with acute bronchitis benefit from symptomatic treatment with antiinflammatory, cough, and cold preparations. Because underlying asthma and pneumonia differential diagnoses have been eliminated, current clinical guidelines do not support routine bronchodilator use or antibiotic therapy for acute bronchitis. Research has demonstrated that antibiotic-susceptible organisms rarely cause acute bronchitis.

78. Answer: 4

Rationale: Histamine H_2 antagonists neutralize the normal gastric acid barrier, allowing for an increased colonization of gram-negative bacilli and *Staphylococcus aureus*.

79. Answer: 2

Rationale: Worsening dyspnea and fatigue with increasing cough may indicate early pulmonary edema. Patients with pulmonary edema require hospitalization with oxygen therapy, IV furosemide (Lasix), and morphine. Patients suspected of having new-onset pulmonary edema **should not** be treated as outpatients. Calcium channel blockers are of little benefit in heart failure and can make dependent edema worse. Empirical antibiotics are not indicated in this situation and may delay proper diagnosis of a serious condition.

80. Answer: 1

Rationale: INH requires concurrent administration of vitamin B_6 to prevent problems of optic neuritis. Vitamin B_6 will decrease the effectiveness of levodopa. If the patient is to receive INH, his anti-Parkinson medication needs to be reevaluated.

81. Answer: 2

Rationale: Prednisone is a corticosteroid that suppresses immune response and puts the patient in an immunocompromised state, increasing susceptibility to infections. Patients on prednisone therapy should be educated about the risk for developing infections and the need to seek medical attention if they suspect illness. Atenolol is a beta blocker used as an antihypertensive. Ipratropium is an anticholinergic used in the acute treatment of asthma. Fluticasone propionate and salmeterol is a combination of inhaled corticosteroid and a long-acting beta agonist. Although inhaled corticosteroids can suppress immune response, absorption is considerably less than oral prednisone.

82. Answer: 4

Rationale: Multiple studies show that the combination of anticholinergic and beta agonist, particularly ipratropium bromide and albuterol, reduce exacerbation, lower cost, improve lung function, and quality of life.

83. Answer: 2

Rationale: Most cases of acute bronchitis are of viral etiology and do not require antibiotic therapy. Approximately 5%–10% of acute bronchitis is bacterial. A cough can last for at least 10–20 days, but routine sputum cultures are not helpful.

84. Answer: 3

Rationale: In the absence of drug-resistant *Streptococcus pneumoniae* (DRSP) or other comorbidities, the Infectious Disease Society of America (IDSA) guidelines suggest azithromycin (Zithromax) is the best choice with Level I Evidence, and doxycycline is a weak recommendation (Level III). If a beta-lactam like amoxicillin is used, a macrolide should also be prescribed for better coverage. A respiratory fluoroquinolone is recommended in instances of comorbid conditions or the presence of additional risk factors for DRSP, and ciprofloxin (Cipro) is not a respiratory fluoroquinolone. Moxifloxacin, levofloxacin, gemifloxacin are respiratory fluoroquinolones.

85. Answer: 2

Rationale: The patient most likely has a subacute, postinfectious cough, which can last up to 8 weeks. After 8 weeks, it would more likely be a chronic cough related to environmental factors like smoking, asthma exacerbation, or gastroesophageal reflux.

86. Answer: 3

Rationale: Posterior ankle pain is suggestive of Achilles tendonitis. Tendon ruptures are a known adverse reaction to fluoroquinolone therapy, and there have been a significant number of cases in the United States. If tendon inflammation or pain occurs, the fluoroquinolone should be discontinued immediately. Ciprofloxacin (Cipro) is recommended for 60 days as part of empiric treatment of anthrax, as postexposure prophylaxis.

87. Answer: 3

Rationale: In patients with high probability of exposure to *Bordetella pertussis,* first-line therapy with a macrolide antibiotic will improve symptoms if started within 5 to 7 days of symptom onset. Doxycycline is not a first-line choice for *Bordetella pertussis.* Waiting delays the possibility of limiting the spread and treatment of *Bordetella pertussis.* Oseltamivir (Tamiflu) is an antiviral and will not be effective against *Bordetella pertussis.*

88. Answer: 1, 2, 3

Rationale: Exposure to risk factors that include tobacco use, chronic cough, and family history all suggest chronic obstructive pulmonary disease (COPD). A postbronchodilator ratio FEV_1/FVC of >0.70 is **not** diagnostic; however, a postbronchodilator ratio FEV_1/FVC of <0.70 is diagnostic and required to establish a diagnosis.

89. Answer: 2

Rationale: According to the Global Initiative for Asthma (GINA) guidelines, "Step 2" therapy should start with a low-dose inhaled corticosteroid (ICS). Flovent is an ICS and would be the most appropriate therapy to start, based on GINA guidelines. Fluticasone and salmeterol (Advair) is a combination ICS and long-acting β_2 agonist (LABA) used when reaching "Step 3", and should not be used for initial therapy. Salmeterol (Serevent) is a LABA and should not be used initially.

90. Answer: 4

Rationale: Although acute respiratory failure, cor pulmonale, and depression are common complications of chronic obstructive pulmonary disease (COPD), they are less likely to cause the patient's current symptoms. Elevated hematocrit, morning headaches, and daytime somnolence are all potential signs of decreased oxygen saturation at night, and would be an indication for home overnight oxygen monitoring or sleep disorder specialist referral.

91. Answer: 1, 3, 5

Rationale: Criteria for severe community-acquired pneumonia (CAP) includes white blood cell count less than 4000 cells/mm³, temperature less than 36°C, respiratory rate greater than or equal to 30 breaths/min, arterial oxygen pressure/fraction of inspired oxygen (Pao_2/Fio_2) ratio less than 250, platelet count less than 100,000 cells/mm³, and uremia (blood, urea, and nitrogen) greater than 20 mg/dL.

92. Answer: 3

Rationale: It is important to emphasize how to take medications correctly. The MDI usually has three parts: mouthpiece, cap that goes over the mouthpiece, and a canister of medicine. A spacer device will help to avoid getting less medication in mouth. The spacer connects to the mouthpiece. The inhaled medicine goes into the spacer tube first. The patient takes two deep breaths to get the medicine into the lungs; waiting a full minute between the two breaths. Using a spacer wastes a lot less medicine than spraying the medicine into the mouth. MDI technique is important, as well as understanding the use of the devices, such as the prescribed valved holding chamber (VHC), spacer, and nebulizer.

93. Answer: 4

Rationale: Beta agonist (albuterol) by MDI is the first line of treatment to decrease airflow obstruction. Aminophylline by mouth would take too long to be effective. Epinephrine is used predominantly for anaphylactic reaction. Beclovent is a steroid inhaler that is most effective when used prophylactically rather than in acute episodes.

94. Answer: 3

Rationale: These are the common drugs used for combination therapy for the treatment of tuberculosis in adolescents. Rimantadine is an antiviral; pyrimethamine is an antimalarial. Montelukast therapy is not indicated because of the virulence of the tubercle bacillus.

95. Answer: 2

Rationale: Pyridoxine (vitamin B_6) is added to prevent peripheral neuropathy. Foods containing tyramine and histamine (e.g., tuna; aged cheese; yeast; vitamin supplements) cause interaction with monoamine oxidase (MAO) inhibitors. Anorexia, jaundice, malaise, and fatigue would be signs of hepatic involvement.

96. Answer: 3, 4

Rationale: Bupropion originally marketed as an antidepressant and later for smoking cessation under the trade name of Zyban is thought to reducing cravings for nicotine and symptoms of withdrawal, because of its capacity to block neural reuptake of the neurotransmitters, dopamine and norepinephrine. Varenicline (Chantix) interferes with nicotine receptors in the brain, which decreases the pleasurable effects of the nicotine and reduces symptoms of nicotine withdrawal. Valacyclovir (Valtrex) is used in the treatment of herpes virus infections, including shingles, cold sores, and genital herpes. Lisinopril (Zesteril) is an ACE inhibitor used to treat high blood pressure and heart failure. Cetirizine (Zyrtec) is an antihistamine used to relieve allergy symptoms.

97. Answer: 1

Rationale: Medications should be taken only when the patient is planning to exercise and anticipates respiratory difficulty or exercised-induced bronchospasm. Cromolyn and beclomethasone are used for asthma management and do not provide immediate relief. Theophylline should be avoided unless symptoms progressively worsen and cannot be controlled with standard recommended asthma therapies.

Immune & Allergy

6

Physical Examination & Diagnostic Tests

1. When taking the history of a patient with known atopic disorder, what is the most important information to determine?
   1. Specific reaction.
   2. Drug allergies.
   3. Food allergies.
   4. Environmental exposure.

2. Which test is used to determine the concentration of gamma globulins that contain the majority of the immunoglobulins?
   1. C-reactive protein (CRP).
   2. Complement fixation.
   3. Protein electrophoresis.
   4. Antinuclear antibody (ANA).

3. Which diagnostic studies are typically abnormal when ruling in systemic lupus erythematosus (SLE) as a differential diagnosis?
   1. CBC, CMP, and ESR.
   2. Chest radiograph and coagulation profile.
   3. ANA, ESR, and C-reactive protein.
   4. CBC, urinalysis, and chest radiograph.

4. Which tests are appropriate for the adult-gerontology primary care NP to order in an initial workup for asymptomatic patients at risk for HIV infection?
   1. CD4 count and HIV enzyme-linked immunosorbent assay (ELISA).
   2. Serology for cytomegalovirus, herpes simplex virus, and Epstein-Barr virus.
   3. HIV-1/HIV-2 antigen/antibody combination immunoassay and HIV-1/HIV-2 antibody differentiation immunoassay.
   4. Hepatitis C virus screen and Western blot analysis.

5. The adult-gerontology primary care NP would identify which two laboratory findings as most significant in a patient with joint pain, malar rash, photosensitivity, weight loss, and fever?
   1. Presence of antinuclear antibodies (ANAs).
   2. Positive serum complement level.
   3. Decreased red blood cells (RBCs).
   4. Thrombocytopenia.
   5. Glycosuria.
   6. Negative LE cell preparation.

6. When assessing a patient for angioedema, the adult-gerontology primary care NP would examine the:
   1. Neck and ears.
   2. Lower extremities.
   3. Torso.
   4. Eyes and mouth.

7. How soon after exposure should patients who believe they have been exposed to HIV have an HIV antibody test?
   1. The next day and 2 months later.
   2. 6 months after exposure and again at 12 months.
   3. 3–12 weeks after exposure and again at 3 months.
   4. 4 weeks and 12 weeks after exposure.

8. Which two tests are the most reliable for detecting the presence of specific immunoglobulin E (IgE) antibody?
   1. Skin testing.
   2. Nasal smear for eosinophils.
   3. Complete blood count.
   4. Serum ImmunoCAP testing.
   5. Western blot analysis.

9. To diagnose allergic rhinitis and treat symptoms that do not respond to treatment, the adult-gerontology primary care NP would consider:
   1. Obtain a nasal smear for eosinophils.
   2. Order a total serum IgE.
   3. Referral for skin testing.
   4. Order a serum radioallergosorbent testing (RAST).

10. The adult-gerontology primary care NP is evaluating the tuberculosis (TB) skin test of an adult who has no risk factors for TB. The PPD is considered positive for this patient when it measures:
    1. 5 mm.
    2. 10 mm.
    3. 15 mm.
    4. 20 mm.

Disorders

11. A 44-year-old female presents to the clinic with a complaint of a red rash that has been appearing beneath a new ring she recently purchased. She is confused because she has never experienced this problem previously. Which type of hypersensitivity reaction most likely causes this reaction?
    1. Type I hypersensitivity.
    2. Type II hypersensitivity.
    3. Type III hypersensitivity.
    4. Type IV hypersensitivity.

12. A young adult presents to the clinic with a 10-day history of fever, myalgia, sore throat, and measles-like rash. The patient is not taking any medications. Which viral syndrome is characterized by a measles-like rash?
    1. Influenza.
    2. Varicella.
    3. HIV.
    4. Mononucleosis.

13. **QSEN** A young woman presents to the urgent care center reporting that a male "date" vaginally raped her last night. She is treated today for *Chlamydia* infection, gonorrhea, and syphilis and is started on a 28-day course of medications to prevent HIV. She wants to know why she needs the HIV therapy because no one she knows has AIDS. What is the basis for the adult-gerontology primary care NP's counseling?
    1. The patient should assume that the man was not HIV positive.
    2. She probably does not need the therapy, but it is a good idea to take the medications.
    3. More than 15% of HIV-infected individuals are unaware that they are infected.
    4. HIV is not easily transmitted.

14. **QSEN** A patient tells the adult-gerontology primary care NP that her husband's sister has HIV but that now she is "cured." She takes medications, and "her doctor cannot find the virus in her blood." Which response would be appropriate?

    1. "Oh, I'm so sorry, but she must be mistaken; AIDS is not curable."
    2. "That is wonderful news, but are you sure?"
    3. "You must be very happy; I didn't know that was possible."
    4. "I've heard that the new medications are very good at lowering the virus counts."

15. **QSEN** A co-worker has just stuck herself with a needle while performing a phlebotomy. She asks the adult-gerontology primary care NP for help and requests that the nurse manager not be informed about the incident. What should be the adult-gerontology primary care NP's initial response?
    1. Send the co-worker to the nurse manager.
    2. Sit with her and calm her down.
    3. Have the co-worker wash the needlestick area with soap and water.
    4. Put on gloves and pour povidone-iodine (Betadine) on the area.

16. An adult patient presents to the clinic with fatigue, sore throat, and myalgia. On examination, the adult-gerontology primary care NP finds axillary lymphadenopathy and a slightly enlarged spleen. Based on the history, the nurse adds acute HIV infection to the differential diagnosis. Which STAT laboratory result increases concern about HIV infection?
    1. Hypochromic, normocytic anemia.
    2. Leukopenia and thrombocytopenia.
    3. Elevated lymphocyte count.
    4. Elevated neutrophil count.

17. A woman comes to the clinic for the first time in the seventh month of her pregnancy. She states that she has a history of a positive HIV test but has never been treated. Physical examination includes Doppler ultrasound of the fetal heart, a prenatal panel, and a urine specimen. The adult-gerontology primary care NP discusses the patient's urgent need for obstetric and prenatal care, and the patient refuses, saying that it is too late and that she "knows" her baby is infected. The adult-gerontology primary care NP's response is based on the following information:
    1. All infants contract HIV from their mothers, unless the mother takes medications.
    2. It is not too late to begin antiviral medications to decrease the risk to the baby.
    3. The mother's viral load is probably high, and the baby may already be HIV positive.
    4. HIV is nearly always fatal to infants who contract it.

18. A new mother tells the clinic nurse that her infant was born HIV-positive. She asks the adult-gerontology primary care NP about her baby's condition. Which of the following two items should be the basis of the adult-gerontology primary care NP's response?
    1. Maternal HIV antibody crosses the placenta and will be detectable in all HIV-exposed newborns.
    2. If antibodies are present at birth, the infant has AIDS in an active form.
    3. Because the infant is HIV positive, the child will develop full-blown AIDS within 3 years.
    4. HIV virologic testing should be performed at 14–21 days of life and at ages 1–2 months and 4–6 months.
    5. There is no risk of HIV transmission from breast milk.

19. Patient education regarding common antigens of anaphylaxis includes:
    1. Oats.
    2. Egg albumin.
    3. Dust mites.
    4. Animal dander.

20. The adult-gerontology primary care NP understands that HIV infection results in a reduction of:
    1. Helper T cells.
    2. Suppressor T cells.
    3. Killer T cells.
    4. Suppressor B cells.

21. Which assessment findings are typically associated with a diagnosis of systemic lupus erythematous (SLE)?
    1. Excitability, diarrhea, and vomiting.
    2. High fever, measles-like rash on limbs, and weight loss.
    3. Joint pain, malar rash, and photosensitivity.
    4. Weight loss, diarrhea, and generalized abdominal pain.

22. After a repeat HIV antibody test, a patient continues to test positive but is asymptomatic. Which is important for the adult-gerontology primary care NP to understand regarding the transmission of the virus by this patient?
    1. The patient is infectious when symptoms are active.
    2. The patient may remain infectious for life.
    3. The dormant virus is not infectious while the patient is asymptomatic and the T-cell count is high.
    4. Laboratory tests should be done every 4–6 weeks to identify the infectious periods of the disease process.

23. **QSEN** A young woman has just received news of a positive HIV test. She does not want her sexual partner to be informed. What is the adult-gerontology primary care NP's most appropriate response?
    1. Respect for her decision because she is the patient.
    2. Informing her that she has a legal responsibility to inform her partner and to notify the health department of her positive HIV test.

    3. Educate her about the importance of notifying all sexual partners and that it is the nurse's legal and ethical responsibility to report her case to the health department.
    4. Document her decision in the record for future reference.

24. The adult-gerontology primary care NP has been assigned a new patient. The problem list indicates that this patient has CREST syndrome (**C**alcinosis, **R**aynaud phenomenon, **E**sophageal dysfunction, **S**clerodactyly, **T**elangiectasia). The adult-gerontology primary care NP will be following this patient for what condition?
    1. Scleroderma.
    2. Dental caries.
    3. Systemic lupus erythematosus.
    4. Rheumatoid arthritis.

25. A patient presenting with complaints of fatigue, malaise, arthralgias, oral ulcers, malar rash, and a positive ANA test would most likely be diagnosed as having:
    1. Chronic fatigue syndrome.
    2. Fibromyalgia.
    3. Scleroderma.
    4. Systemic lupus erythematosus (SLE).

26. What are the most common clinical manifestations of Sjögren syndrome?
    1. Corneal dryness and lack of saliva.
    2. Increased urination and hunger.
    3. Abdominal discomfort and thickening of the epidermis.
    4. Joint destruction and alopecia.

27. An older adult female patient presents to the adult-gerontology primary care NP with a low-grade temperature and a unilateral throbbing headache. She also reports scalp sensitivity and some visual disturbances. Laboratory results show a greatly elevated ESR and anemia. She has been relatively healthy except for a recent history of polymyalgia rheumatica (PMR). Which condition should be diagnosed based on this clinical presentation?
    1. Bacterial meningitis.
    2. Primary angle closure glaucoma (PACG).
    3. Giant cell (temporal) arteritis.
    4. Subdural hematoma.

28. A middle-aged female patient presents with weight loss, heartburn, dysphagia, dry cough, pain, stiffness of the fingers and knees, and Raynaud phenomenon. The adult-gerontology primary care NP recognizes these as the symptoms of:
    1. Rheumatoid arthritis.
    2. Systemic lupus erythematosus (SLE).
    3. Barrett esophagus.
    4. Scleroderma.

29. The erythematous confluent macular eruption of the face known as the "butterfly rash" is characteristic of:
    1. Allergic drug eruption.
    2. Systemic lupus erythematosus (SLE).
    3. Rosacea.
    4. Seborrheic dermatitis.

30. The adult-gerontology primary care NP is discussing general health care with a female patient who has systemic lupus erythematosus (SLE) and is in remission. What are important points to include in the teaching?
    1. Daily weight checks to assess for fluid retention.
    2. Decrease physical and psychological stress.
    3. Avoid isometric exercise.
    4. Maintain diet low in fat and high in carbohydrates.

31. A 50-year-old male patient presents with complaints of frequent sinus infections, decrease in ability to hear, and arthralgia. Laboratory findings are mild normochromic/normocytic anemia, elevated ESR, mild hypergammaglobulinemia (elevated IgA), proteinuria, and hematuria with granular or cellular casts. Physical findings include mild conjunctivitis, vasculitis dermatitis, chronic cough, chest pain, dyspnea, paranasal sinus pain, occasional epistaxis, and imbalance of intake and output. What would be a tentative diagnosis?
    1. Connective tissue disease.
    2. Granulomatosis with polyangiitis (Wegener granulomatosis).
    3. Pulmonary neoplasm.
    4. Infectious granulomatous disease.

32. A patient presents with sneezing, watery eyes, postnasal drip, and sore throat. What diagnosis do these symptoms most likely suggest?
    1. Acute sinusitis.
    2. Allergic rhinitis.
    3. Vasomotor rhinitis.
    4. Influenza.

33. A 70-year-old woman presents with complaints of morning headache, malaise, and anorexia. What condition would the adult-gerontology primary care NP suspect?
    1. Pneumonia.
    2. Giant cell (temporal) arteritis.
    3. Anemia of chronic disease.
    4. Acute sinusitis.

34. When teaching a patient about risk factors and prevention of transmission of HIV, which statement is most appropriate?
    1. HIV can be transmitted by casual kissing.
    2. Unprotected oral sex with an infected partner may result in transmission.

3. Sharing an office with an HIV-positive person increases the risk of HIV exposure.
4. Using the same bathroom as an infected adult-gerontology primary care member puts one at risk of HIV exposure.

35. Signs and symptoms that alert the adult-gerontology primary care NP to identify a patient who is at an increased risk for HIV infection include:
    1. Frequent emergency department visits for urinary tract infections (UTIs).
    2. Malaise and fatigue.
    3. Frequent sexually transmitted infections (STIs).
    4. Swollen glands and diarrhea.

36. What is an appropriate classification for HIV?
    1. Cytomegalovirus.
    2. Herpetic virus.
    3. Papillomavirus.
    4. Retrovirus.

37. What are the most frequently occurring symptoms of systemic lupus erythematous (SLE)?
    1. Splenomegaly and Raynaud syndrome.
    2. Pulmonary effusions and hepatomegaly.
    3. Butterfly rash on the face and lymphadenopathy.
    4. Fever, arthritis, arthralgia, and weight loss.

38. A systemic IgE-mediated antigen-antibody response resulting in a life-threatening massive release of mediators is:
    1. Recurrent urticaria.
    2. Allergic rhinitis.
    3. Anaphylaxis.
    4. Contact dermatitis.

39. The release of histamine results in:
    1. Bronchospasm, vasodilation, and vascular permeability.
    2. Bronchodilation, vasodilation, and vascular permeability.
    3. Smooth muscle contraction, decreased vascular permeability, and vasoconstriction.
    4. Pain, increased vascular permeability, and bronchodilation.

40. After a bone marrow transplant (BMT), the adult-gerontology primary care NP understands the following about acute graft-versus-host disease (GVHD) and would select which 2 responses?
    1. The most common sites include skin, GI tract, and liver.
    2. GVHD develops within 100 days posttransplant.
    3. The prevention strategy includes prophylactic immunosuppressive medication.
    4. GVHD develops more than 100 days posttransplant.
    5. Acute GVHD is graded from 0 to 3, with 3 being the most severe.

41. A patient who has a history of recent bone marrow transplant (BMT) presents to the clinic. The adult-gerontology primary care NP identifies signs and symptoms of graft-versus-host disease (GVHD) that include:
    1. Fever, headache, and mental status changes.
    2. Chills, fever, and urticaria over the flank area.
    3. Increased serum bilirubin level and presence of maculopapular rash and abdominal cramping.
    4. Decreased red blood cells (RBCs), hematocrit, and hemoglobin, as well as presence of petechiae.

42. The pathogenesis of systemic lupus erythematosus (SLE) is characterized by autoantibody development. This results in:
    1. Increased T-suppressor cells.
    2. B-cell increase.
    3. Polyclonal hypogammaglobulinemia.
    4. Decreased T-suppressor cells and inhibited cellular activity.

43. Which blood cell type is responsible for the activation of the immune response?
    1. Band neutrophil.
    2. T4 lymphocyte.
    3. Segmented neutrophil.
    4. B lymphocyte.

44. A 22-year-old male presents with breathlessness, weight loss, nonproductive cough, temperature of 100.4°F (38°C), pulse of 124 beats/min, respiration of 36 breaths/min, BP of 120/78 mm Hg, and a history of positive HIV serum test. Based on this information, which is the most accurate diagnosis?
    1. *Klebsiella pneumoniae* infection.
    2. *Mycoplasma pneumoniae* infection.
    3. *Pneumocystis jirovecii* pneumonia.
    4. Community-acquired pneumonia.

45. **QSEN** A nurse who has never been vaccinated against HBV experiences a needlestick at the clinic from a patient with known hepatitis B. What postexposure prophylaxis (PEP) should be administered?
    1. IgE.
    2. IgA.
    3. Pegylated interferon (PEG-IFN).
    4. Hepatitis B immune globulin (HBIG).

46. Which sign/symptom is indicative of a type I hypersensitivity reaction?
    1. Contact dermatitis.
    2. Immediate wheal and flare reaction.
    3. Hematuria.
    4. High fever.

47. Which patient is at highest risk for developing HIV/AIDS?
    1. Immunocompromised patient.
    2. Sexually active teenager.
    3. Middle-aged adult.
    4. Marijuana user.

48. What are the cardiovascular effects of anaphylactic shock?
    1. ST-segment and T-wave changes.
    2. Hypertension.
    3. Prolonged PR intervals with elevated QT segment.
    4. Elevated serum cardiac enzyme levels.

49. When assessing a patient for systemic lupus erythematous (SLE), what ophthalmologic findings would the adult-gerontology primary care NP determine to be consistent with this condition?
    1. Retinal hemorrhage.
    2. Conjunctivitis.
    3. Cotton-wool spots.
    4. Arteriovenous (AV) nicking.

50. What information does the adult-gerontology primary care NP include in the education for the patient with allergic rhinitis?
    1. Monitor air quality and the allergy index.
    2. Use a surgical-type mask when going outdoors.
    3. Remain inside during allergy season.
    4. Avoid working in the garden or yard.

51. **QSEN** A nurse from the operating room (OR) comes into the clinic with complaints of shortness of breath, itching, reddened hands, and wheezing. He says that he does not seem to have the symptoms when he is not working. Based on the history and symptoms, the adult-gerontology primary care NP would evaluate for:
    1. Indoor toxic mold exposure.
    2. Bronchitis.
    3. Latex allergy.
    4. Contact dermatitis.

52. Which statement is true regarding latex allergy?
    1. It usually only produces symptoms of contact dermatitis and allergic rhinorrhea.
    2. It is a progressive disorder that worsens with continued exposure.
    3. It affects less than 5% of the health care population.
    4. It is an autoimmune response.

53. Young adults who have seasonal allergic rhinitis often present with clinical symptoms that include:
    1. Mouth breathing and "skier's nose."
    2. Allergic "shiners" and Dennie-Morgan lines.
    3. Thick nasal discharge and sneezing.
    4. Flushed face and fever.

54. An adult patient is concerned that she has a significant reaction to poison ivy every spring with a rash that appears on the ventral surfaces of the arms in the antecubital fossa. The rash is flat and erythematous and comes on suddenly with exposure to grass. Which statement would best describe the trigger of this dermatologic symptom?
    1. Poison ivy is very common in the spring, and exposure results in immediate onset of symptoms.
    2. Plants that flower in the spring are laden with pollen that most likely will cause this type of symptom.
    3. Type IV hypersensitivity reactions are common in the spring with direct exposure to the allergen.
    4. Type I hypersensitivity reactions result in immediate symptoms upon exposure to the allergen.

Pharmacology

55. An adult patient comes to the urgent care clinic with nausea, vomiting, and acute abdominal pain. His history is significant for HIV infection, and for the last month, he has been taking didanosine (Videx) 400 mg daily, lopinavir/ritonavir (Kaletra) 400 mg/100 mg bid, and lamivudine (Epivir) 150 mg bid. After the examination, the adult-gerontology primary care NP determines that didanosine can cause pancreatitis and lactic acidosis. What laboratory tests would be ordered?
    1. CBC, CD4 count, viral load, and electrolytes.
    2. CBC with differential, lipase, lactic acid, electrolytes, BUN, creatinine, and liver function tests (LFTs).
    3. Amylase, lipase, and lactic acid.
    4. Lipase, amylase, and liver function tests (LFTs).

56. Which drugs have been associated with a lupus-like syndrome?
    1. Sulfonamides (Septra DS) and penicillin (Pen-Vee K, Penicillin G).
    2. Progestin/estrogen oral contraceptives.
    3. Nonsteroidal antiinflammatory drugs (NSAIDs; ibuprofen [Motrin]).
    4. Procainamide (Pronestyl) and hydralazine (Apresoline).

57. A 46-year-old male presents to the health care clinic for a follow-up visit after a bicycle injury requiring an immediate splenectomy. He has no other medical problems, and he states he received all vaccinations as a child but hasn't visited a medical provider prior to his injury for over 20 years. Select two items that should be considered by the adult-gerontology primary care NP for this patient.
    1. HPV vaccination.
    2. HAV vaccination.
    3. Trimethoprim-sulfamethoxazole prophylaxis.
    4. Meningococcal vaccination.
    5. Penicillin prophylaxis.

58. A patient is diagnosed with giant cell (temporal) arteritis. What is the medication of choice?
    1. Prednisone (Deltasone).
    2. Ibuprofen (Motrin).
    3. Indomethacin (Indocin).
    4. Azathioprine (Imuran).

59. A patient with a bacterial infection that is susceptible only to meropenem (Merrem) requires treatment. The patient reports urticaria and pruritus when administered meropenem in the past. Which of the following is the best action by the adult-gerontology primary care NP when no other medications are available?
    1. Administer ciprofloxacin (Cipro).
    2. Inform the patient there is no medication available.
    3. Begin desensitization therapy.
    4. Administer normal-dose meropenem (Merrem).

60. Which four medications are used for malaria prophylaxis?
    1. Ampicillin (Omnipen).
    2. Doxycycline (Vibramycin).
    3. Ceftriaxone (Rocephin).
    4. Chloroquine phosphate (Aralen).
    5. Mefloquine (Lariam).
    6. Primaquine.

61. Which medications are used in the treatment of allergic rhinitis?
    1. Antihistamines, corticosteroids, and environmental control.
    2. Antihistamines, analgesics, and allergen control.
    3. Anticholinergics, antibiotics, and oral prednisone.
    4. Nasal saline rinses, corticosteroids, and antibiotics.

62. Development of an adverse drug reaction depends on which factors?
    1. Patient age, prior drug reactions, genetic factors, and degree of exposure.
    2. Patient gender, oral route of administration, and history of atrophic disease.
    3. Patient age, gender, and genetic factors.
    4. Genetic factors, prior drug reactions, and patient gender.

63. Treatment of a patient with chronic urticaria has failed with multiple antihistamine medications over the past 3 months. The patient has a history of TB and was compliant with all medical treatment 5 years ago. Which of the following medications is the most appropriate choice by the adult-gerontology primary care NP for long-term control of symptoms?
    1. Topical corticosteroids.
    2. Systemic corticosteroids.
    3. Omalizumab (XOLAIR).
    4. Adalimumab (HUMIRA).

64. A medication frequently used for the prophylaxis as well as initial treatment of *Pneumocystis jirovecii* pneumonia is:
    1. Fluconazole (Diflucan).
    2. Amphotericin B (Fungizone).
    3. Trimethoprim-sulfamethoxazole (TMP-SMX; Septra).
    4. Acyclovir (Zovirax).

65. The adult-gerontology primary care NP should advise an adult patient with idiopathic chronic urticaria controlled by cetirizine (Zyrtec) to avoid which of the following medications?
    1. Ibuprofen (Motrin).
    2. Celecoxib (Celebrex).
    3. Penicillin.
    4. Cephalexin (Keflex).

66. When instructing patients with allergic rhinitis about the use of nasal decongestants, it is important for them to understand:
    1. The condition is self-limiting and will resolve in a matter of weeks, regardless of whether the patient is reexposed to the allergen.
    2. A nasal decongestant used continuously for more than 3 days can result in a worsening of the symptoms.
    3. It is not necessary to avoid exposure to the allergen once therapy has been initiated.
    4. Allergic rhinitis is seen only in the spring and fall; the condition requires treatment during these seasons only.

67. The adult-gerontology primary care NP should exercise caution with a patient taking azathioprine (Imuran) regarding the addition of which of the following medications?
    1. Levothyroxine (Synthroid).
    2. Esomeprazole (Nexium).
    3. Insulin glargine (Lantus).
    4. Allopurinol (Zyloprim).

68. What is the major advantage of using second-generation antihistamines, such as cetirizine (Zyrtec) and loratadine (Claritin)?
    1. Decreased cost.
    2. Increased anticholinergic activity.
    3. Delayed absorption.
    4. Do not cross the blood-brain barrier.

69. What is the desired action of sympathomimetics (adrenergics) when used in the treatment of allergic rhinitis?
    1. Promote vasoconstriction in the nasal mucosa.
    2. Block mast cell degranulation.
    3. Decrease the effect of histamines.
    4. Increase mast cell degranulation.

70. In the older adult patient, histamine H_1 blockers may cause which side effects?
    1. Ataxia.
    2. Nausea.
    3. Bradycardia.
    4. Gastrointestinal upset.

71. What information is important for the adult-gerontology primary care NP to include when teaching a patient about the use of antihistamines?
    1. Use of topical antihistamines is safe and has relatively few side effects.
    2. Do not use over-the-counter (OTC) medications without consulting the health care provider.
    3. Constipation and urinary retention are expected side effects and do not need to be reported.
    4. Once antihistamine therapy has been taken for 3 days, avoidance of allergens is not necessary.

72. A primary advantage of using loratadine (Claritin) in treating a patient with seasonal allergies is that it:
    1. Is prudent to take only as needed.
    2. May be prescribed for once-a-day (daily) dosing.
    3. Costs considerably less than other medications.
    4. Effectively decreases nasal secretions.

73. What medications are drugs of choice for the secondary treatment of patients with an anaphylactic reaction?
    1. Antibiotics and anticholinergics.
    2. NSAIDs and decongestants.
    3. Decongestants and expectorants.
    4. Antihistamines and corticosteroids.

74. A 46-year-old female is being evaluated for Raynaud phenomenon. Which of the following medications should the adult-gerontology primary care NP prescribe for symptomatic treatment in addition to lifestyle changes?
    1. Hydralazine.
    2. Amlodipine (Norvasc).
    3. Lisinopril (Zestril).
    4. Nitroglycerin.

75. Patients newly presenting with signs and symptoms of systemic lupus erythematous (SLE) should have their medication profile reviewed to determine whether they are taking any medication that may have caused drug-induced lupus. Which drug should the adult-gerontology primary care NP most suspect?
    1. Digoxin (Lanoxin).
    2. Procainamide (Pronestyl).
    3. Trimethoprim-sulfamethoxazole (TMP-SMX).
    4. Cimetidine (Tagamet).

76. An adult patient presents at the clinic, and his adult-gerontology primary care states that he has a history of anaphylactic reactions. What signs and symptoms indicate to the adult-gerontology primary care NP that the patient is experiencing another reaction?
    1. Cough, wheezing, and urticaria.
    2. Severe malaise, pallor, stridor, and dyspnea.
    3. Anxiety, nasal congestion, and tachycardia.
    4. Rhinorrhea, nausea, and gastrointestinal pain.

77. A 56-year-old female has been prescribed hydroxychloroquine (Plaquenil) to treat symptoms of Sjögren syndrome. Which of the following complications should the adult-gerontology primary care NP monitor during therapy?
    1. Hyperglycemia.
    2. Liver failure.
    3. Vision changes.
    4. Hypokalemia.

78. An adult reports receiving several bee stings while gardening and comes to the clinic because of difficulty breathing. Which medication should the adult-gerontology primary care NP have available for the patient's initial care?
    1. Lidocaine topical ointment.
    2. Epinephrine.
    3. Prednisone.
    4. Diphenhydramine (Benadryl) elixir.

79. What is an appropriate antihistamine to recommend for a college student with allergic rhinitis?
    1. Diphenhydramine (Benadryl).
    2. Chlorpheniramine (Chlor-Trimeton).
    3. Brompheniramine (Dimetane).
    4. Loratadine (Claritin).

6 Immune & Allergy Answers & Rationales

Physical Examination & Diagnostic Tests

1. Answer: 1

Rationale: The reaction to each allergen is most important to know. Often patients state that they have an "allergy" to a particular food or medication, such as nausea, stomach pain, or diarrhea, which they regard as an allergy. The signs and symptoms of the reaction, speed of onset, duration, and successful treatments used in the past are also important information. Medication side effects must be distinguished from true allergic reactions to drugs, so patient statements of drug or food allergies should be thoroughly explored.

2. Answer: 3

Rationale: In protein electrophoresis, proteins are electrically separated on a strip. It is a screening test to measure various proteins in body fluids, usually serum or urine. It assists in screening for diseases characterized by an increase or decrease in immunoglobulins. Serum and urine protein electrophoresis are also used to identify occult malignancy in a patient with failing health when no cause can be found. Immunofixation electrophoresis determines the presence of a heavy-chain immunoglobulin (IgG, IgM or IgA). Complement fixation and antinuclear antibodies (ANAs) are diagnostic studies for rheumatoid problems. C-reactive protein (CRP) is a blood test used to diagnose bacterial infectious disease and inflammatory disorders.

3. Answer: 3

Rationale: Although all tests listed may be included in a complete physical examination, laboratory tests ordered related to the diagnosis of systemic lupus erythematous (SLE) include antinuclear antibody (ANA), erythrocyte sedimentation rate (ESR), and C-reactive protein. The antinuclear antibodies (ANAs) has high sensitivity, but it has low specificity for SLE, and an elevation can indicate a number of disorders. The anti–double-stranded DNA (dsDNA) and anti-Smith antibodies have high specificity for SLE and are usually ordered if there is suspicion of SLE. During flares, ESR and C-reactive protein are elevated.

4. Answer: 3

Rationale: Based on recommendations from the CDC (2014), initial testing for HIV should be an antigen/antibody combination immunoassay to test for established HIV-1 or HIV-2 infection and for acute HIV-1 infection. No further testing is required for specimens that are nonreactive on the initial immunoassay. Specimens with a reactive antigen/antibody combination immunoassay result (or repeatedly reactive, if repeat testing is required by regulatory authorities) should be tested with an antibody immunoassay that differentiates HIV-1 antibodies from HIV-2 antibodies. Reactive results on the initial antigen/antibody combination immunoassay and the HIV-1/HIV-2 antibody differentiation immunoassay should be interpreted as positive for HIV-1 antibodies, HIV-2 antibodies, or HIV antibodies, undifferentiated.

5. Answer: 1, 4

Rationale: The majority of patients with systemic lupus erythematosus (SLE) have antinuclear antibodies (ANAs) present in their blood with leukopenia, thrombocytopenia, lymphopenia, anemia, positive LE cell preparation, elevated sedimentation rate (ESR), and positive C-reactive protein. Proteinuria with cellular casts is often noted.

6. Answer: 4

Rationale: Angioedema is edema of the mucous membrane tissue and is most easily seen in the eyes and mouth. It also affects the tongue, feet, hands, and genitalia. Diffuse erythema may be seen in the upper body parts. Gastrointestinal symptoms (e.g., vomiting, cramping, diarrhea) may occur. African American patients are more likely to experience angioedema when given ACE inhibitors (e.g., lisinopril, captopril).

7. Answer: 3

Rationale: The HIV antibody develops between 3 and 12 weeks after exposure. A known exposure and the best test to identify earliest antibodies would be fourth-generation enzyme immunoassays, which detect IgM, IgM antibody, and p24 antigen and demonstrate positive results in as little as 15–20 days. Because of the variability of antibody development, it is recommended that the test be repeated in 3 months to confirm the findings.

8. Answer: 1, 4

Rationale: The most reliable tests for the presence of the specific immunoglobulin E (IgE) antibody is the skin test and the serum ImmunoCAP test, which can provide quantitative measurement of IgE and accurately determine whether patients have allergies and determine what they are allergic to. The smear for eosinophils and complete blood count (CBC) are not specific for IgE antibody. Western blot analysis is used as a follow-up test to confirm the presence of an antibody and to help diagnose a condition, such as HIV or Lyme disease.

9. Answer: 3

Rationale: A referral to an allergist for skin testing would be appropriate to identify the allergen for immunotherapy to treat the condition. A nasal smear for eosinophils is not recommended as routine practice to be performed in an office setting. Many patients who have uncomplicated allergic rhinitis have a normal serum immunoglobulin E (IgE). Skin-prick testing should be performed by allergy-trained providers only. Radioallergosorbent testing (RAST) determines serum levels of allergen-specific IgE titers, but skin testing is more sensitive and is the preferred diagnostic method.

10. Answer: 3

Rationale: A positive purified protein derivative (PPD) test result for an immunocompetent adult is 15 mm. An adult who is HIV positive, immunocompromised, or exposed to an active case of TB is considered positive for TB at 5 mm. The adult who has chronic disease or has been exposed to HIV-positive individuals, persons born in a foreign country, or an IV drug abuser is considered positive for TB at 10 mm.

Disorders

11. Answer: 4

Rationale: Type IV hypersensitivity reactions are caused by delayed T-cell activation and often appear several days after the initial exposure to an allergen. Heavy metals, including nickel, are often causes of contact dermatitis. Treatment involves avoiding exposure to the offending agent.

12. Answer: 3

Rationale: Acute HIV infection is characterized by a history of prolonged fever and a red, raised, discrete skin eruption described as morbilliform ("measles-like"). Neither influenza nor mononucleosis typically presents with a rash. Varicella (chickenpox) presents with a vesicular skin eruption.

13. Answer: 3

Rationale: Treating a woman who has been raped requires time for patient education and postexposure prophylaxis (PEP) should be offered and recommended. The patient should not assume that the man was HIV negative. Evidence based on PEP in health care workers and infants supports its effectiveness. Traumatic sex increases the risk of sexually transmitted disease (STD), including HIV.

14. Answer: 4

Rationale: Repeating what the patient has said along with more information about how HIV medications can lower

viral counts is appropriate. The other responses do not address the patient's comments.

15. Answer: 3

Rationale: It is important after a needlestick injury that the person wash the area with soap and water and then report the incident to the immediate supervisor and immediately seek medical treatment for postexposure prophylaxis. Sending the co-worker to the nurse manager does not address the medical need of washing the needlestick site. Talking with the co-worker and providing support is necessary, but not until the adult-gerontology primary care NP addresses the need to wash the site immediately.

16. Answer: 2

Rationale: Acute, primary HIV infection depletes the CD4 cells, which produces leukopenia and depletes platelets. A hypochromic, normocytic anemia is present more often in advanced HIV. Elevated lymphocyte counts are more likely in other viral illnesses, and elevated neutrophil counts are seen in bacterial infections.

17. Answer: 2

Rationale: Not all infants contract HIV from their mothers during pregnancy. It is recommended that all HIV-positive pregnant women be started on antiretroviral therapy as soon as possible. Also, HIV may not be fatal in children with access to effective antiretroviral therapy. The immune system in some individuals with HIV keeps the viral load under control for many years.

18. Answer: 1, 4

Rationale: It is important to give the mother as much hope as possible but still be realistic about the infant's condition. Maternal HIV antibody crosses the placenta and will be detectable in all HIV-exposed newborns. HIV virologic testing should be performed at 14–21 days of life and at ages 1–2 months and 4–6 months. Two positive virologic HIV tests constitute a diagnosis of HIV infection. Many experts confirm HIV-negative status with an HIV antibody test at age 12–18 months. Persistence of HIV antibodies can occasionally occur at or beyond age 18 months. There is no way to tell when or if the infant will convert to active AIDS. Many infants seroconvert to HIV-negative status. HIV-infected women should not breastfeed their infants.

19. Answer: 2

Rationale: Egg albumin is one of many identified common antigens that may result in an anaphylactic reaction, most commonly in children. Other common antigens include vaccines, allergen extracts, sulfonamides, penicillins, hormones, legumes (especially peanuts), berries, nuts, seafood, and venom bites (bee, wasp, yellow jacket).

20. Answer: 1

Rationale: There is a severe, life-threatening reduction of helper T cells along with an increase in suppressor T cells. The helper T cells help amplify or increase the production of antibody-forming cells from B lymphocytes after an encounter with an antigen. Killer T cells are produced after mature helper T cells interact with an antigen. Suppressor T cells suppress the formation of antibody-forming cells from B lymphocytes, which, when their numbers are increased, have a detrimental effect on the immunity and ability of the patient with HIV to make antibody-forming cells.

21. Answer: 3

Rationale: The symptoms most often experienced with SLE are arthritis, arthralgias, fatigue, Raynaud phenomenon, chronic low-grade or recurrent fever, sun sensitivity, hair loss, weakness, butterfly (malar) facial rash, and weight loss. Typically, the pulmonary, cardiac, renal, and central nervous systems are involved, which may cause multisystem failure and contribute to mortality in patients systemic lupus erythematous (SLE).

22. Answer: 2

Rationale: HIV infection creates a chronic infectious state in the body that is transmitted through blood or body fluids and transplacentally throughout the patient's life.

23. Answer: 3

Rationale: Educate the patient about the importance of notifying all sexual partners and that the adult-gerontology primary care NP is required by law to report the positive HIV test result to the health department. It is still up to the patient to give names of sexual partners to the health department, which the patient can refrain from doing. *Only* if the patient has been adequately counseled or the provider believes that the patient will not disclose the information and will place others at risk can the provider disclose the patient's HIV-positive status. Ethical response and behavior include notification of all persons at risk so that early intervention and treatment can be initiated.

24. Answer: 1

Rationale: CREST syndrome (**C**alcinosis, **R**aynaud phenomenon, **E**sophageal dysfunction, **S**clerodactyly, **T**elangiectasia) is associated with a slow, progressive form of scleroderma.

25. Answer: 4

Rationale: The patient is presenting with 4 of the 11 criteria necessary for diagnosing systemic lupus erythematous

(SLE) using the 1997 American College of Rheumatology classification for SLE. No single test exists for SLE, but these characteristics plus laboratory results (antinuclear antibody [ANA], erythrocyte sedimentation rate [ESR], C-reactive protein) can differentiate the diagnosis.

26. Answer: 1

Rationale: Corneal dryness and lack of saliva are the most common clinical manifestations of Sjögren syndrome. Patients may also have joint inflammation, but this rarely leads to joint destruction.

27. Answer: 3

Rationale: About 40% of patients with giant cell (temporal) arteritis have a history of polymyalgia rheumatica (PMR). The other diagnoses may have some of these symptoms, but only arteritis has all symptoms listed for this patient. It is especially crucial to note visual disturbances because these patients can develop sudden blindness. Definitive diagnosis is confirmed by biopsy. Prior to confirmation of disease, immediate treatment is important for patients where there is any strong clinical suspicion. Treatment typically consists of increasing the patient's prednisone to 40–60 mg daily in single or divided doses for 4 weeks and then gradually tapering alongside ESR monitoring.

28. Answer: 4

Rationale: The symptom of Raynaud phenomenon differentiates this as scleroderma. Esophageal dysfunction is often an initial complaint in scleroderma, which affects women four times more often than men. Barrett esophagus is diagnosed in patients with long-term gastroesophageal reflux disease (GERD) and is associated with an increased risk of developing esophageal cancer.

29. Answer: 2

Rationale: The butterfly (malar) rash is one of the characteristic symptoms of systemic lupus erythematous (SLE). Allergic drug eruptions are characterized by an erythematous rash or hives. Rosacea is characterized by redness and small, red, pus-filled bumps. Seborrheic dermatitis is characterized by scaly patches and red skin, mainly on the scalp.

30. Answer: 2

Rationale: Because systemic lupus erythematous (SLE) is considered an autoimmune disorder, psychological and physical stress can exacerbate the condition. A balanced diet helps limit the side effects of some medications, and regular exercise helps reduce arthralgia and myalgia associated with SLE. It is not necessary to check weight daily.

31. Answer: 2

Rationale: Granulomatosis polyangiitis (Wegener granulomatosis) is a multisystem disorder that occurs more often in males. Peak occurrence is between 40 and 60 years of age. The disease usually targets the upper respiratory tract, lungs, and kidneys. Connective tissue disease, pulmonary neoplasm, and infectious granulomatous disease would be considered in the differential diagnosis.

32. Answer: 2

Rationale: The signs and symptoms presented are classic for allergic rhinitis. Acute sinusitis would present with sinus pressure and pain, perhaps with tooth pain and fever. Vasomotor rhinitis typically does not present with ocular symptoms and occurs in response to environmental triggers, such as cold air, strong smells, irritants, changes in weather, some medications (ACE inhibitors, beta blockers), stress, exercise, and certain foods. Influenza presents with acute onset, fever, chills, and general malaise.

33. Answer: 2

Rationale: The adult-gerontology primary care NP should suspect giant cell (temporal) arteritis, an inflammatory disorder of unknown etiology that affects large- and medium-sized arteries. It occurs two times more frequently in women than in men and most frequently in older adults, but rarely in the African American population. The clinical findings would reveal temporal tenderness and temporal bruits. About 40% of the patients who have been diagnosed with polymyalgia rheumatica (PMR) also have temporal arteritis, and the older adult patient may be relating some of her arthralgia and myalgia to normal changes of aging rather than PMR. The adult-gerontology primary care NP should also check the patient's ESR and consider referring the patient to a rheumatologist.

34. Answer: 2

Rationale: Unprotected oral sex with an HIV-positive person puts one at risk for exposure to the virus. Human contact, such as casual kissing or sharing an office or bathroom, does not transmit the virus. The virus is transmitted in body fluids and secretions.

35. Answer: 3

Rationale: Frequent sexually transmitted infections (STIs) would alert the adult-gerontology primary care NP to the patient's lack of protected sex and the possibility of multiple partners. Night sweats, malaise, fatigue, swollen glands, and diarrhea may be associated with many other illnesses. Urinary tract infections (UTIs) are not always diagnostic of frequent sexual activity.

36. Answer: 4

Rationale: HIV is a retrovirus. It contains an enzyme, reverse transcriptase, that copies ribonucleic acid (RNA) into deoxyribonucleic acid (DNA). When it binds to a CD4 receptor, the virus inserts its RNA and enzymes into the cell, where a copy of its RNA is made and enters the cell nucleus. As the infected host cell reproduces, HIV DNA is duplicated and passed on in the infectious cycle.

37. Answer: 4

Rationale: Although any of the clinical symptoms listed may be present in patients with systemic lupus erythematous (SLE), fever, weight loss, arthritis, and arthralgias occur most often. Butterfly rash of the face and lymphadenopathy occur in less than half the cases. Pulmonaryeffusion, hepatomegaly, splenomegaly, and Raynaud syndrome occur in less than one-third of patients with SLE.

38. Answer: 3

Rationale: The massive release of mediators triggers a series of events in target organs. Prior sensitization to the antigen must have occurred to trigger an anaphylactic reaction. Anaphylaxis may result from injection of an antigen, ingestion of food or drugs, or inhalation of antigens.

39. Answer: 1

Rationale: The release of histamine results in bronchospasm, vasodilation, and vascular permeability, leading to wheezing, increased mucus production in the lung, and edema of the airway.

40. Answer: 2, 3

Rationale: The onset of acute graft-versus-host disease (GVHD) occurs less than 100 days after bone marrow transplant (BMT). It results from immunocompetent donor T lymphocytes attacking the host tissues. The most common sites involved in acute GVHD include the skin, GI tract, and liver, with symptoms being dependent on the organ involved. Additional sites of involvement in chronic GVHD include the mouth, eyes, lungs, and neuromuscular system. Acute GVHD is graded from I to IV, with IV being most severe. Chronic GVHD is graded from 0 to 3, with 3 being most severe. The prevention strategy includes prophylactic immunosuppressive medication (i.e., calcineurin inhibitor and a short course of methotrexate, mycophenolate, or sirolimus).

41. Answer: 3

Rationale: The signs and symptoms of graft-versus-host disease (GVHD) include maculopapular rash; generalized erythroderma with desquamation; increased bilirubin; increased AST and SGOT; and/or increased alkaline phosphatase, abdominal cramping, and diarrhea. Infection is characterized by fever, mental status changes, and headaches. Decreased RBCs, hematocrit, and hemoglobin and the presence of petechiae are signs of anemia. Fever, chills, and urticaria are indications of a reaction to white blood cells (WBCs) in the bone marrow.

42. Answer: 4

Rationale: T lymphocytes are the white blood cells (WBCs) responsible for control of the immune response. In systemic lupus erythematous (SLE), T-suppressor cells are decreased and cellular activity is inhibited, leading to hypergammaglobulinemia and B-cell proliferation. Patients with SLE often present with lymphopenia but a higher proportion of B cells to T cells. The overall count of B cells is decreased compared with that in a healthy individual.

43. Answer: 2

Rationale: The T4 lymphocyte is known as the T-helper cell. These cells are responsible for the proliferation of lymphocytes and macrophages, causing activation of the cells in response to an antigen. The B lymphocytes are effector cells that mediate humoral responses by production of antibodies. The band neutrophil and segmented neutrophil are slightly mature and fully mature neutrophils, respectively. Neutrophils are the most abundant cells in the bone marrow and blood.

44. Answer: 3

Rationale: Based on the history of an HIV-positive test and the symptoms presented, the patient is at risk for *P. jirovecii* pneumonia. Further examination would include chest radiography and pulse oximetry (for oxygen saturation). The lack of purplish lesions is considered in ruling out Kaposi sarcoma. *Klebsiella pneumoniae* is a nosocomial infection, not community acquired. *Mycoplasma pneumoniae* infection is typically seen in teenagers and older adult patients with an insidious onset of symptoms.

45. Answer: 4

Rationale: HBIG alone has been demonstrated to be effective in preventing HBV transmission. There is no IgC antibody. IgA is the secretory immunoglobulin found in tears, saliva, and mucous secretions of the lung and gastrointestinal tract. IgE mediates allergic reactions. Pegylated-interferon (PEG-IFN) is used for chronic HBV infection.

46. Answer: 2

Rationale: Type I hypersensitivity reaction causes an immediate wheal and flare reaction. Contact dermatitis is

seen in type IV (delayed) reaction. Hematuria is seen in type II reaction that is caused by preformed circulating cytotoxic antibodies, such as in a blood transfusion reaction or autoimmune hemolytic anemia. High fever may be seen in type III hypersensitivity reaction when large quantities of antigen-antibody complexes are released in the body.

47. Answer: 2

Rationale: Sexually active teenagers are the fastest-growing group of HIV-positive patients because of unprotected sexual activity. Immunocompromised patients and elderly adults are at no greater risk for developing HIV than any other group. However, an increasing number of middle-aged males are becoming HIV positive from their association with prostitutes after the loss of their partners. Risk factors for HIV include unprotected sexual contact with persons of unknown HIV status, multiple sexual partners, intravenous drug use, hemophilia, and blood transfusions received before 1985.

48. Answer: 1

Rationale: Changes in the electrocardiogram (ECG) are associated with coronary and myocardial ischemia. Although ECG changes suggest myocardial injury, there is no change in the serum enzyme levels. Other signs and symptoms include hypotension and tachycardia.

49. Answer: 3

Rationale: Cotton-wool spots are the most common ophthalmologic problem associated with systemic lupus erythematous (SLE), are signs of vascular insufficiency, and are described as edematous and ischemic neuronal tissues that appear as fluffy areas on a funduscopic exam. They are also a common symptom of amaurosis fugax (retinal artery occlusion). Retinal hemorrhages and arteriovenous (AV) nicking may be seen in patients with hypertension. Conjunctivitis is an infection of the conjunctiva.

50. Answer: 1

Rationale: Patients with allergic rhinitis should monitor the air quality and allergy index in their area and understand their allergy triggers. A surgical-type mask will not filter out small allergens. Remaining inside during allergy season is an unrealistic expectation and can lead to decreased socialization and increased depression for the patient. Patients can enjoy a summer garden if they are careful about the choice of plants and flowers. For example, the patient with an allergy to ragweed should avoid daisies, dahlias, and chrysanthemums.

51. Answer: 3

Rationale: The operating room (OR) nurse likely has a latex allergy. The incidence of latex allergies has increased dramatically since the onset of standard precautions and increased use of latex gloves. In an effort to meet the increased demand for gloves, changes in the manufacturing process have resulted in a higher protein count in the gloves. The increased exposure to the protein has led to a proliferation of health care workers being diagnosed with a latex allergy.

52. Answer: 2

Rationale: Latex allergy is a progressive disorder that worsens with continual exposure. The symptoms range from contact dermatitis to anaphylaxis. Currently, latex allergy affects 17% of health care workers and 39% of dental professionals. Latex allergy is an acquired immune response to the latex protein allergen. No vaccine is available; the only defense is to avoid contact with latex.

53. Answer: 2

Rationale: The typical allergic facies consist of allergic "shiners" (black eyes), Dennie-Morgan lines (extra crease below the lower eyelids), and mouth breathing. Pale, boggy, blue-gray nasal mucosa and sneezing are common symptoms. "Skier's nose" is a watery rhinorrhea in response to cold air. The nasal discharge with allergies is usually clear, not thick, which often is associated with a bacterial infection.

54. Answer: 3

Rationale: Type IV hypersensitivity reactions are delayed hypersensitivity disorders with symptoms that start after 1 day of exposure, such as with poison ivy contact; symptoms are not immediate. Flowering plants are nonallergenic because their pollen is heavy and spread by insects, not the wind as in grass, tree, and weed pollens. Tree and grass pollens result in a type I hypersensitivity reaction that is immediate on exposure, resulting in atopic dermatitis, allergic rhinitis, asthma, or urticaria.

Pharmacology

55. Answer: 2

Rationale: The laboratory tests ordered would be complete blood count (CBC) with differential, lipase, lactic acid, electrolytes, BUN, creatinine, and liver function tests (LFTs). Assessment of immune function (CD4 count, viral load) is unnecessary at this point and would not change the management of the acute illness. Having the amylase, lipase, lactic acid, and LFTs would assist in

the diagnosis of pancreatitis, but it would not provide information on the patient's hydration status, the status of the biliary system, or the presence of acute infection.

56. Answer: 4

Rationale: Procainamide, hydralazine, and isoniazid have been shown to induce a lupus-like syndrome. Discontinuation of the medication results in the disappearance of the clinical signs and symptoms. Antibiotics (e.g., sulfonamides, penicillin) have been associated with anaphylactic reactions in some patients. Oral contraceptives may increase blood pressure and the risk for thromboembolism. Nonsteroidal antiinflammatory drugs (NSAIDs) (e.g., ibuprofen) have been associated with gastrointestinal upset and gastric pain, especially when taken on an empty stomach, and are contraindicated in patients with renal disease.

57. Answer: 2, 4

Rationale: The approach to the patient with asplenia should include ensuring that all vaccinations are up-to-date as well as administration of HBV, meningococcal, and pneumococcal vaccinations along with a yearly influenza immunization and Td booster every 10 years. The patient is over the recommended age for the HPV vaccination. The HAV vaccination was approved for use in 1995, so this patient could not have received it. Penicillin prophylaxis is not routinely recommended in adults, unless an asplenic patient has experienced previous sepsis or is immunocompromised.

58. Answer: 1

Rationale: Giant cell (temporal) arteritis, seen primarily in elderly patients, can lead to blindness if not treated immediately with corticosteroids. The usual daily dose of prednisone is 60 mg in divided doses initially and then in a single morning dose (every-other-day steroids are not used). A slow taper is initiated after 4 weeks if the patient is asymptomatic and the ESR is decreased. Tapering of the dose is individualized, and the patient may be on drug therapy for several months to years. The average time for disease remission is 3–4 years (range, 1–10 years).

59. Answer: 3

Rationale: Drug allergies are common in many patients, especially to antibiotics. The goal of initial therapy should be to understand the type of reaction the patient had to the initial medication therapy. The best and safest option is to avoid any medications that cause allergies and choose a related medication. In many cases, bacterial sensitivities restrict the ability to choose different classes of antibiotics. When a medication causes an allergy in a patient and it is the only medication available, desensitization therapy should be initiated starting with the lowest possible dose along with close monitoring. Desensitization therapy should never be used in patients who experienced reactions such as Stevens-Johnson syndrome or erythema multiforme.

60. Answer: 2, 4, 5, 6

Rationale: Chloroquine phosphate, doxycycline, mefloquine, and primaquine are medications used for malaria prophylaxis. Ceftriaxone is used for bacterial septicemia and respiratory and urinary tract infections caused by gram-negative bacilli. Ampicillin is used to treat infections with a variety of organisms and as prophylaxis for bacterial endocarditis.

61. Answer: 1

Rationale: Unless there is a secondary bacterial infection, antibiotics are contraindicated. Antihistamines and reduction of exposure to the allergen will help reduce the symptoms. For continued control and stabilization of the mast cells, corticosteroids are indicated.

62. Answer: 1

Rationale: Adults are at greater risk for the development of adverse drug reactions, probably because of the increased number of medications used and the amount of exposure and effects of aging on the immune system. Patients with prior drug reactions are more likely to develop reactions to new drugs. The risk of an adverse drug reaction occurs in the first 2–3 weeks of therapy. Prolonged course of therapy, high dosage, and intermittent therapy increase the risk of an adverse reaction. Genetic factors may increase mediator and metabolic pathway activity. The patient's gender has no effect, except with muscle relaxants and chymopapain, where female patients are at greater risk of an adverse drug reaction. The route of drug administration contributes to the risk, with IV, IM, SC, PO, and topical ranked in the order of greatest to least risk.

63. Answer: 3

Rationale: Treatment of chronic urticaria involves initial treatment with second-generation antihistamines and leukotriene receptor antagonists (montelukast), followed by first-generation antihistamines and doxepin (Silenor). Patients for whom these therapies fail require stronger systemic immunosuppressants, such as omalizumab, cyclosporine, or tacrolimus. Omalizumab is an IgG monoclonal antibody that inhibits IgE receptors. Adalimumab is contraindicated in this patient due to a risk of reactivation of tuberculosis. Corticosteroids are indicated only for short-term control of symptoms and are avoided for long-term use.

64. Answer: 3

Rationale: Trimethoprim-sulfamethoxazole (TMP-SMX) is used to treat as well as prevent *P. jirovecii* pneumonia,

usually with a 21-day course, with up to 7–10 days for a clinical response. Fluconazole and amphotericin B are antifungal drugs. Acyclovir is an antiviral used primarily to treat herpes simplex virus types 1 and 2 and herpes zoster (shingles).

65. Answer: 1

Rationale: NSAIDs that inhibit cyclooxygenase 1 (COX-1), such as aspirin and ibuprofen, often exacerbate symptoms in patients with urticaria and should be avoided. Selective COX-1 inhibitors such as celecoxib are generally well tolerated. Antibiotics and other medications should be restricted only for patients with known allergies to those medications.

66. Answer: 2

Rationale: The chronic use of nasal decongestants for more than 3 days can result in a rebound effect when discontinued, leading to increased nasal congestion from reflex vasodilation. The condition may take as long as 2–3 weeks to resolve. Allergic rhinitis is not a self-limiting illness associated only with spring and fall. Even though therapy is initiated, the patient should be instructed to avoid exposure to the allergen as much as possible.

67. Answer: 4

Rationale: Azathioprine is an immunosuppressant that acts as a prodrug to 6-mercaptopurine. This blocks DNA synthesis by preventing purine metabolism of proliferating T and B cells. This medication has many side effects, including a high risk of myelosuppression; increased risk of malignancy; as well as many gastrointestinal effects, including nausea, vomiting, and diarrhea. Because of the metabolism of xanthine oxidase, dosages of allopurinol must be reduced or entirely avoided due to risk of toxic myelosuppressive effects.

68. Answer: 4

Rationale: The major advantage of the second-generation antihistamines is that they do not cross the blood-brain barrier and therefore do not cause sedation and psychomotor dysfunction. There is little anticholinergic activity and less dry mouth and constipation. The cost of these antihistamines is 15–30 times greater than for the first-generation antihistamines. The medications are rapidly absorbed within 1–2 hours of PO administration on an empty stomach.

69. Answer: 1

Rationale: Sympathomimetics (adrenergics) cause vasoconstriction, thereby reducing edema and secretions. Inhaled corticosteroids stabilize mast cells and block degranulation.

70. Answer: 1

Rationale: The use of H_1 blockers can cause paradoxical central nervous system (CNS) stimulation, resulting in ataxia in older adult patients. Antihistamines can cause many simultaneous side effects in older adults, such as impaired vision and gait, which can lead to falls, and impaired thinking, which can interfere with functional skills (cognition) and could necessitate an unnecessary hospitalization or nursing home stay. Antihistamines also may interact with the older adult patient's numerous medications and exacerbate the side effects (e.g., dry mouth, constipation).

71. Answer: 2

Rationale: The patient should be instructed not to use over-the-counter (OTC) medications without consulting the adult-gerontology primary care NP or pharmacist. The nurse should explain that OTC drugs and herbal supplements are considered medications and that they may interact with prescribed medications. To avoid possible interactions, the patient should inform the adult-gerontology primary care NP of all the OTC drugs and herbals the patient is taking. The patient should be cautioned on the extended use of topical antihistamines. Antihistamines do not affect circulating histamine, so the patient must avoid exposure to a known allergen. Constipation and urinary retention are adverse effects that should be reported to the adult-gerontology primary care NP.

72. Answer: 2

Rationale: An advantage of using loratadine is that the once-daily dosing helps with patient compliance. The cost is greater than for some first-generation antihistamines. Loratadine with pseudoephedrine (Claritin D) is an antihistamine/decongestant with twice-daily or extended-release (daily) dosing.

73. Answer: 4

Rationale: Medications such as antihistamines and corticosteroids are used to counter mediator release and block release of additional mediators. NSAIDs, antibiotics, and decongestants are contraindicated in the treatment of anaphylactic reaction.

74. Answer: 2

Rationale: Treatment for Raynaud phenomenon (RP) includes avoiding triggers, especially exposure to cold temperatures. Pharmacologic treatments for RP include the initial use of dihydropyridine calcium channel blockers, amlodipine, and nifedipine.

75. Answer: 2

Rationale: Of patients receiving procainamide, 20% develop clinical drug-induced systemic lupus erythematous (SLE). The other drugs listed have not been associated with an SLE-like syndrome.

76. Answer: 2

Rationale: Severe malaise, pallor, stridor, and dyspnea are signs and symptoms associated with a severe anaphylactic reaction. Symptoms may occur immediately or up to 2 hours after exposure to the allergen. Severe reactions require immediate intervention.

77. Answer: 3

Rationale: Hydroxychloroquine (HCQ) is an aminoquinoline derivative used to treat malaria, but it can also be used as an immunosuppressant for autoimmune disorders, such as rheumatoid arthritis, primary Sjögren syndrome, porphyria cutanea tarda, and systemic lupus erythematosus. The most common and severe side effect of taking this medication is ocular toxicity, which can occur in the form of a retinopathy or as corneal damage. Other side effects can include muscular damage to the heart, causing restrictive cardiomyopathy, renal failure, myelosuppression and hypoglycemia. HCQ can exacerbate conditions such as G6PD deficiency, psoriasis, and porphyrias. Patients who begin HCQ should have a baseline eye examination and reexamination no less than every 5 years.

78. Answer: 2

Rationale: Epinephrine would be the first-line drug to be injected for the treatment of the respiratory distress associated with an anaphylactic reaction. The dose for epinephrine (SC) is 0.3–0.5 mL/kg using the 1 mg/mL solution for an adult. The onset of action of Benadryl is not fast enough. Lidocaine would only topically treat the pain and not the respiratory problem. Anti-inflammatory drugs would not be given initially but may be given later, if needed, for generalized discomfort or pain at the sting site.

79. Answer: 4

Rationale: Although diphenhydramine, brompheniramine, and chlorpheniramine are antihistamines and could be prescribed, loratadine would have less central nervous system-sedating effects.

Head, Eyes, Ears, Nose, & Throat (HEENT)

7

Physical Examination & Diagnostic Tests

Head

1. The adult-gerontology primary care NP is examining lymph nodes in the neck. Which nodes are palpated in the anterior triangle of the neck?
   1. Posterior cervical chain.
   2. Anterior superficial chain.
   3. Periauricular lymph nodes.
   4. Supraclavicular lymph nodes.

Eyes

2. When using an ophthalmoscope, the adult-gerontology primary care NP:
   1. Holds the ophthalmoscope in the right hand (uses right eye) while examining the patient's left eye.
   2. Starts the examination with the ophthalmic lens set at zero.
   3. Begins in a position 1 inch from the eye to check the red light reflex.
   4. Examines the anterior chamber in a well-lighted room and asks the patient to focus on an object.

3. The adult-gerontology primary care NP checking for strabismus would use which test?
   1. Cover-uncover test.
   2. Vertical prism test.
   3. Ishihara plates test.
   4. Snellen eye chart test.

4. The adult-gerontology primary care NP observes lid lag in a patient with:
   1. Myasthenia gravis.
   2. Hyperthyroidism.
   3. Hordeolum.
   4. Chalazion.

5. The adult-gerontology primary care NP is examining an older adult patient. There is a glossy white circle around the pupils of the eyes with yellowing of the sclera, and the pupils have a decreased reaction to the direct light reflex. The patient has a history of presbyopia. What is the correct interpretation of these findings?
   1. Beginning development of cataracts with a significant decrease in visual acuity.
   2. Expected changes in the eyes as a result of the aging process.
   3. Decrease in depth perception and early eye changes associated with glaucoma.
   4. Visual changes secondary to long-term treatment with digoxin and corticosteroids.

6. The adult-gerontology primary care NP is preparing to examine the eyes of an adult patient. To examine the retinal vessels and assess for hemorrhages, the adult-gerontology primary care NP uses which aperture on the ophthalmoscope?
   1. Small aperture.
   2. Red-free filter.
   3. Slit.
   4. Grid.

7. When testing the eyes for the presence of a normal consensual response, the adult-gerontology primary care NP:
   1. Shines the light into the patient's pupil and observes the rate of pupillary constriction.
   2. Directs the light into one pupil and observes for the constriction or response of the other pupil.
   3. Holds a card in front of one eye and has the patient focus on a fixed object, removes the card, and observes movement of the newly uncovered eye.
   4. Asks the patient to focus on an object, and then directs a light source to the bridge of the nose while observing for symmetric reflection in both eyes.

8. On ophthalmic examination, there appears to be a narrowing or blocking of the vein at the point where an arteriole crosses over it. The significance of this finding is:
   1. The need to evaluate the patient for chronic hypertension.
   2. The possibility of increased ocular pressure associated with glaucoma.
   3. Its association with papilledema, causing decreased venous drainage.
   4. It may represent a small embolus in the retinal vessels.

9. When examining the eyes, the adult-gerontology primary care NP determines that the pupils constrict when a patient shifts their gaze from a far object to a near one. This is interpreted as:
   1. Accommodation.
   2. Intact extraocular motor nerves.
   3. Appropriate consensual response.
   4. Visual acuity within normal limits.

10. During a physical exam, the adult-gerontology primary care NP notes xanthelasma. What laboratory test will the nurse order?
    1. ESR.
    2. CBC.
    3. Thyroid profile.
    4. Lipid profile.

Ears

11. When examining the ears of an adult patient, the adult-gerontology primary care NP determines that the tympanic membrane (TM) is pearl gray, shiny, and translucent. This is interpreted as:
    1. Scarring from previous infections.
    2. Decreased circulation to the membrane.
    3. Presence of serous fluid behind the membrane.
    4. Normal characteristics of the adult ear.

12. The Rinne test is performed to compare bone conduction (when the tuning fork is placed on the mastoid bone) with air conduction (when the tuning fork is held near the ear). A normal Rinne test is described as:
    1. Equal conduction through the mastoid bone and ear canal.
    2. Air conduction is greater than bone conduction.
    3. Bone conduction is twice as long as air conduction.
    4. Sound is clearer with bone conduction than with air conduction.

13. When assessing the tympanic membrane (TM), specific landmarks are determined and described according to the face of a clock. Where are the normal landmarks for the right TM located?
    1. Direct light reflex located at 5- to 6-o'clock position and malleus at 1- to 2-o'clock position, with the umbo in the center.
    2. Manubrium slanted to the left, with malleus at 10-o'clock position.
    3. Direct light reflex in center of membrane, with malleus at 9-o'clock position.
    4. Umbo is to the left of the center, with anterior malleolar folds at the 10-o'clock position.

Nose

14. During a routine physical examination, an adult-gerontology primary care NP notes three horizontal creases across the lower bridge of the nose in an adolescent patient. What should be the next appropriate response?
    1. Refer the patient to the dermatologist for further evaluation.
    2. Assume that the finding is normal and continue with the examination.
    3. Prescribe fexofenadine (Allegra) for the patient.
    4. Ask the patient about symptoms of sneezing, rhinorrhea, congestion, tearing, and itching of the nose/eyes/ears.

15. The adult-gerontology primary care NP understands that the nasal mucosa:
    1. Is dark pink, smooth, and moist.
    2. Is pale and translucent in appearance.
    3. Is pale and boggy.
    4. Is red and swollen.

Throat

16. A throat culture is indicated for the following suspected cause of pharyngitis:
    1. Rhinovirus and coronavirus infection.
    2. Group A β-hemolytic streptococci (GABHS).
    3. Mononucleosis.
    4. *Candida albicans.*

17. An adolescent arrives at the clinic with a complaint of low-grade fever, sore throat, slight headache, and fatigue for the past week. On physical examination, the adult-gerontology primary care NP finds exudative tonsils bilaterally, erythematous pharynx with white patches, and enlarged posterior cervical neck nodes. The adult-gerontology primary care NP would expect which laboratory test result?
    1. Positive rapid strep test.
    2. Positive monospot test.
    3. Increased neutrophil count.
    4. Positive viral throat cultures.

Disorders

Head

18. The adult-gerontology primary care NP sees a 60-year-old white woman of Norwegian descent in her office for a 2-day complaint of pain in her right frontotemporal region and jaw claudication that is worse at night. She has had a low-grade fever of 100.1°F (38.3°C) and has felt tired for the past 2–3 days. She guards the area and asks you not to touch it, as it hurts. The most likely differential diagnosis for this patient is:
    1. Temporomandibular joint dysfunction.
    2. Trigeminal neuralgia.
    3. Giant cell (temporal) arteritis.
    4. Preherpetic neuralgia.

19. An adult patient presents to the office with a white plaque near the base of the tongue. The adult-gerontology primary care NP notes that the plaque does not wipe off and assesses it as:
    1. Hemangioma.
    2. Leukoplakia.
    3. Papilloma.
    4. Erythroplasia.

20. Which of the following are predominant risk factors for oral carcinoma?
    1. History of dental infections and age younger than 40 years.
    2. Tobacco use and alcohol use.
    3. Infection with human papillomavirus and tobacco use.
    4. Alcohol use and history of dental abscess.

21. The hallmark of early oral cancer is:
    1. Tissue retraction.
    2. Thickening oral tissues.
    3. Persistent red and/or white patch and nonhealing ulcer.
    4. Halitosis and cough.

22. An adult male patient is being evaluated for a complaint of a sore throat. He states that he has difficulty swallowing and has mild oral pain. On examination, the adult-gerontology primary care NP finds that the patient's mouth, tongue, and pharynx are coated with white, curdlike plaques that are difficult to remove and leave a red surface when scraped with a tongue blade. What would be the best next action for the adult-gerontology primary care NP to take at this time?
    1. Refer the patient to an ear, nose, and throat specialist for evaluation.
    2. Prescribe amoxicillin 500 mg PO tid for 10 days.
    3. Encourage the patient to have HIV screening.
    4. Recommend only clear liquids for the next few days.

23. The adult-gerontology primary care NP knows that the most common site for head and neck cancer is the:
    1. Sinuses.
    2. Oral cavity.
    3. Larynx.
    4. Nasal cavity.

Eyes

24. A patient presents to an office of an adult-gerontology primary care NP complaining of acute-onset severe right eye pain with no precipitating injury. The patient has blurred vision and reports seeing halos around lights. On exam, the pupil is dilated and fixed. The adult-gerontology primary care NP recognizes that this is a condition that requires immediate evaluation by an ophthalmologist, and the patient is sent to the emergency department for further care. The most likely cause of patient's symptoms is:
    1. Open-angle glaucoma.
    2. Closed-angle glaucoma.
    3. Corneal abrasion.
    4. Iritis/uveitis.

25. A patient is being prepared for cataract surgery. What information is important for the adult-gerontology primary care NP to explain to the patient?
    1. The procedure is short, and the patient usually goes home the morning after the surgery.
    2. Both eyes will be patched for the first 24 hours, and it is important for the patient to stay in bed.
    3. The patient may have problems with headache and eye pain for the first 24 hours and should take the pain medication provided.
    4. Patients usually go home 2–3 hours after the surgery; the patient will have increased tearing, but it should not be painful.

26. A patient who is a sheet metal worker reports a foreign body sensation in his right eye that began shortly after working this morning. The initial assessment would most likely be to:
    1. Instill a topical anesthetic.
    2. Assess visual acuity.
    3. Examine the eye using a penlight.
    4. Examine the eye using fluorescein.

27. A patient works as a welder. He finished work about 8 hours ago and discovered that the protective glass on his welding hood was cracked. He is complaining of severe left eye pain and photophobia. The most likely diagnosis and next best action are:
    1. Chemical keratitis; dilate with atropine twice daily.
    2. Viral conjunctivitis; supportive treatment with artificial tears.
    3. Corneal abrasion; oral analgesics and an ophthalmic antibiotic ointment.
    4. Ultraviolet keratitis; ophthalmic antibiotic.

28. An older adult patient presents to the clinic with complaints of bilateral blurred vision that has increasingly worsened over the past 2 years. The patient also has a problem with night driving but denies eye pain. The adult-gerontology primary care NP would first evaluate for the presence of:
    1. Glaucoma.
    2. Retinal detachment.
    3. Degeneration of the macula.
    4. Cataracts.

29. An adult patient presents to the adult-gerontology primary care NP for evaluation of a "red" right eye for 24 hours. The patient states that when he awoke, the eye was matted shut. The patient denies trauma to the eye, eye pain, and any changes in vision. During the exam, it is noted that the pupils are equal and reactive, and there is mild conjunctival hyperemia bilaterally and a significant amount of yellowish discharge. The adult-gerontology primary care NP treats this patient for:
    1. Allergic conjunctivitis.
    2. Corneal abrasion.
    3. Viral conjunctivitis.
    4. Bacterial conjunctivitis.

30. Which assessment of the eye is a deviation from common age-related physiologic changes?
    1. Arcus senilis.
    2. Presbyopia.
    3. Sensitivity to glare.
    4. Sustained nystagmus.

31. During a routine physical examination of a 30-year-old patient, the adult-gerontology primary care NP identifies arcus senilis. What is the significance of this disorder?
    1. High potential for future blindness.
    2. None because this is a normal variant of the aging process.
    3. Abnormal lipid metabolism requiring further evaluation.
    4. Hereditary variant of no consequence.

32. A 70-year-old patient comes to the clinic complaining of an increased sensitivity to glare, difficulty adapting to darkness, and altered depth perception. The adult-gerontology primary care NP should suspect:
    1. Cataract.
    2. Macular degeneration.
    3. Glaucoma.
    4. Normal age-related physiologic changes.

33. An adolescent reports that he awoke this morning with eyelid redness and a swelling after being on a camping trip with friends. The adult-gerontology primary care NP notes that the adolescent is afebrile and the eyelid is non-tender and uniformly swollen. The most likely diagnosis is:

1. Blepharitis.
2. Hordeolum.
3. Insect bite.
4. Dacryocystitis.

34. In assessing an adult with bacterial conjunctivitis, the adult-gerontology primary care NP finds:
    1. Minimal tearing, moderate itching, and profuse exudate.
    2. Severe itching, moderate tearing, and minimal discharge.
    3. Minimal itching, moderate tearing, and mucoid exudate.
    4. Minimal itching, moderate tearing, and profuse exudate.

Ears

35. In teaching patients how to avoid acoustic trauma because of noise in the very loud range, the adult-gerontology primary care NP knows that noise is loudest from a:
    1. Vacuum cleaner.
    2. Power lawn mower.
    3. Clothes washer.
    4. Food blender.

36. A geriatric patient is complaining of difficulty hearing in both ears and states that the problem seems to have steadily worsened over the past few years. What finding would support a diagnosis of presbycusis?
    1. Complaint that they can hear voices but that everyone mumbles.
    2. Rinne test indicating air conduction greater than bone conduction.
    3. History of long-term tetracycline therapy for chronic infections.
    4. Weber test localizing increased tone in left ear versus right ear.

37. Which of the following organisms is *least likely* to cause otitis media?
    1. *Moraxella catarrhalis.*
    2. *Streptococcus pneumoniae.*
    3. *Staphylococcus aureus.*
    4. *Haemophilus influenzae.*

38. Which assessment finding of the ear would indicate a deviation from the normal aging process?
    1. A dull, retracted, and white tympanic membrane.
    2. An elongated lobule.
    3. A sensorineural hearing loss.
    4. A bulging tympanic membrane with a distorted cone of light.

39. Which statement by the adult-gerontology primary care NP indicates an understanding of conductive hearing loss in the older patient?
    1. "This has occurred because of damage of the eighth cranial nerve from gentamicin."

2. "This is a result of an inner ear infection."
3. "This is a normal part of aging and is referred to as presbycusis."
4. "This may be reversible after the cerumen is removed from the ear canal."

40. Sensorineural hearing loss is common in industrial settings and preventable with the use of adequate hearing protection. This type of hearing loss is usually first noted with changes at what level?
    1. 500 Hz.
    2. 200 Hz.
    3. 1000–2000 Hz.
    4. 3000–6000 Hz.

41. An adolescent is diagnosed by the adult-gerontology primary care NP with acute otitis media (AOM). During a pneumatic otoscopy, the adult-gerontology primary care NP expects the tympanic membrane (TM) to be:
    1. Immobile and painful, with absent or decreased landmarks.
    2. Mobile and painful, with absent or decreased landmarks.
    3. Immobile and not painful, with landmarks visualized.
    4. Mobile, not painful, full, and bulging.

42. A 16-year-old is on the school swim team and is seen by the adult-gerontology primary care NP for ear pain. The patient is afebrile. The left ear canal is extremely edematous and moderately inflamed, with thick, yellowish drainage at the external meatus. The most likely diagnosis is:
    1. Acute otitis media.
    2. Serous otitis media.
    3. Sinusitis.
    4. Otitis externa.

Nose

43. An adult-gerontology primary care NP sees an older adult and diagnoses the patient with an idiopathic anterior epistaxis. The bleeding site was visualized and chemical cautery was successful at stopping the bleeding. Which of the following discharge instructions should be provided to the patient?
    1. Avoid touching or placing any lubricants, such as petroleum jelly or antibiotic ointment into the nostrils.
    2. If the patient has the urge to sneeze, the patient should do so with the mouth closed.
    3. If bleeding recurs, the patient should perform digital compression of the nose with the patient's cervical spine hyperextended in a "sniffing" position for 5 minutes.
    4. Encourage the patient to use a humidifier at home and squirt nasal saline liberally.

44. An adult patient presents to the adult-gerontology primary care NP's office with the following complaints for the past 10 days: fever and complaints of right facial pain, copious yellow nasal discharge, and acute pain and headache, primarily when bending over. The physical examination is significant for right maxillary sinus tenderness upon palpation. The most likely diagnosis is:
    1. Chronic sinusitis.
    2. Acute sinusitis.
    3. Dental abscess.
    4. Giant cell (temporal) arteritis.

45. The adult-gerontology primary care NP notes a nasal septal perforation on a young adult. What does the adult-gerontology primary care NP suspect as the cause?
    1. Deviated nasal septum.
    2. Chronic epistaxis.
    3. Nose picking.
    4. Cocaine use.

46. An adult patient presents to the clinic complaining of sinus infection and states that symptoms started 3 days ago. The patient is complaining of rhinorrhea/congestion with green/yellow discharge from the nose. The patient reports a slight cough and postnasal drip. The patient denies fever, facial pain, or tooth pain. The patient requests an antibiotic to help him clear up this sinus infection. An appropriate response to this patient's request would be:
    1. "I agree, this is a sinus infection requiring an antibiotic. Here is a prescription for amoxicillin/clavulanate (Augmentin)."
    2. "Before we proceed with any treatment options, we should do some tests first. I will order a CT scan of your sinuses before prescribing any medication."
    3. "A viral infection associated with common cold causes 98% of sinus infections that clear up on their own. An antibiotic will not be helpful in clearing a viral infection and can actually do harm if taken for nonbacterial sinusitis. Let's talk about other treatment options that will help you feel better."
    4. "I am going to order some blood work. A white blood cell count lab test can help us distinguish between viral and bacterial infections. I will call you with results and treat you accordingly. In the meantime, use a saline nose spray twice a day."

47. The adult-gerontology primary care NP is teaching a public education program about the most effective preventive measure against the common cold, which is:
    1. Judicious use of vitamin C during cold season.
    2. Ensuring adequate sleep and fluids.
    3. Meticulous handwashing, preferably with an antibacterial soap and warm water.
    4. Avoiding contact with children and adults who have a runny nose, cough, and sore throat.

Throat

48. A rare complication of streptococcal pharyngitis that leads to contralateral uvular deviation, asymmetric tonsillar hypertrophy, muffled voice on exam but no stridor, drooling, or difficulty breathing or swallowing is recognized by adult-gerontology primary care NP as:
    1. Peritonsillar abscess.
    2. Peritonsillar cellulitis.
    3. Retropharyngeal abscess.
    4. Epiglottitis.

49. A 20-year-old patient presents to the adult-gerontology primary care NP's office with a chief complaint of "severe sore throat" for 3 days. The patient states that he also "ran a fever, but does not know how high it got," and has been very fatigued. Physical examination reveals enlarged tonsils with large, patchy exudate; erythematous pharynx; and nontender posterior cervical lymphadenopathy. The remainder of the examination is unremarkable. The adult-gerontology primary care NP would most likely make a diagnosis of:
    1. Infectious mononucleosis.
    2. Leukemia.
    3. Scarlet fever.
    4. Oral candidiasis.

50. Which of the following clinical findings is most likely associated with bacterial streptococcal pharyngitis?
    1. Rhinorrhea.
    2. Cough.
    3. Enlarged erythematous tonsils with exudate.
    4. Small oral vesicles.

Pharmacology

51. An adult patient returns to the office of an adult-gerontology primary care NP 1 week after he was diagnosed with acute otitis externa and was started on otic ciprofloxacin/dexamethasone (Ciprodex). He explains that his symptoms of pain and itching of his left ear have worsened with the use of the medication. In addition, he now notes a white discharge from his left ear. Examination reveals a mildly edematous erythematous ear canal with white discharge and a normal tympanic membrane. An appropriate treatment for this patient would include:
    1. Continue the current medication and prescribe antipyrine/benzocaine (Auralgan).
    2. Discontinue Ciprodex and prescribe carbamide peroxide (Debrox).
    3. Discontinue Ciprodex, and irrigate the ear canal, and prescribe clotrimazole 1% (Canesten) solution.
    4. Continue the current medication and prescribe oral amoxicillin twice daily.

52. Mild circumoral swelling of the lips without airway obstruction in a 65-year-old male who is allergic to shellfish that started 2 days ago after eating at a seafood restaurant should be treated with which of the following?
    1. Epinephrine (EpiPen), 0.3 mg injected subcutaneously.
    2. Diphenhydramine (Benadryl) 25 mg PO tid.
    3. Lisinopril (Zestril) 10 mg once daily.
    4. Montelukast sodium (Singulair) 10 mg daily at nighttime.

53. An adolescent who has a history of severe allergic rhinitis asks for a recommendation of a medication to try. The first-line agent for this condition is:
    1. Fluticasone (Flonase) nasal spray, 2 sprays in each nostril daily.
    2. Azelastine (Astelin) nasal spray, 2 sprays in each nostril bid.
    3. Pseudoephedrine (Sudafed) 120 mg orally bid.
    4. Fexofenadine (Allegra) 180 mg orally daily.

54. When the adult-gerontology primary care NP decides to prescribe an antibiotic for the treatment of acute sinusitis, which antibiotic is recommended as first-line empiric therapy for non–penicillin-allergic adults:
    1. Amoxicillin (Amoxil).
    2. Doxycycline (Vibramycin).
    3. Azithromycin (Zithromax).
    4. Amoxicillin-clavulanate (Augmentin).

55. A geriatric patient is diagnosed with chronic open-angle glaucoma. She has a past history of bradycardia and first-degree atrioventricular block. In consideration of her treatment, what medication is to be avoided?
    1. Pilocarpine (Isopto Carpine).
    2. Timolol (Timoptic).
    3. Hydrochlorothiazide (HydroDIURIL).
    4. Acetazolamide (Diamox).

56. The treatment plan for a patient diagnosed with infectious mononucleosis includes which of the following?
    1. Resting during the acute phase.
    2. Avoiding exercise during the acute phase.
    3. Corticosteroids during the acute phase.
    4. Ampicillin orally for 10 days.

57. Which antibiotic would be appropriate for the adult-gerontology primary care NP to prescribe for beta-lactamase production by strains of *Haemophilus influenzae* and *Moraxella catarrhalis* in an adolescent with acute otitis media?
    1. Amoxicillin (Amoxil).
    2. Erythromycin-sulfisoxazole (Pediazole).

3. Penicillin V potassium (Pen-Vee K).
4. Amoxicillin with clavulanic acid (Augmentin).

58. A patient arrives at the clinic having an acute attack of Ménière disease. Which three medications would the adult-gerontology primary care NP to prescribe?

1. Lorazepam (Ativan).
2. Meclizine (Antivert).
3. Atropine.
4. Furosemide (Lasix).
5. Nortriptyline (Pamelor).
6. Penicillin.

Physical Examination & Diagnostic Tests

Head

1. Answer: 2

Rationale: The conceptualization of triangles is useful in determining the location of palpable lymph nodes in the neck. The sternocleidomastoid muscle is the division between the anterior (containing the anterior superficial cervical chain) and the posterior (containing the posterior cervical chain) triangles. The trapezius muscle marks the posterior border of the posterior triangle. The supraclavicular nodes are palpated in the angle formed by the clavicle and the sternocleidomastoid muscle.

Eyes

2. Answer: 2

Rationale: The correct use of the ophthalmoscope involves using the right hand and right eye to examine the patient's right eye. The room should be semidarkened for best visualization. The examiner initially inspects the lens and vitreous body from a distance of about 12 inches (at zero setting) and moves closer to the eye, usually rotating the lenses to the positive numbers (+15 to +20), which assists in focusing on near objects.

3. Answer: 1

Rationale: The cover-uncover test is used to detect latent strabismus. The vertical prism test is performed to assess for amblyopia. The Ishihara test is used to examine color perception. The Snellen test is done to assess visual acuity.

4. Answer: 2

Rationale: Lid lag occurs in patients with hyperthyroidism and is evaluated by having the patient follow the examiner's finger as it is slowly moved up and down. The patient has lid lag if sclera can be seen above the iris as the patient looks downward. Ptosis is a drooping lid margin that falls at the pupil or below and may indicate an oculomotor lesion or myasthenia gravis. A chalazion is a chronic, sterile, lipogranulomatous inflammatory lesion of the meibomian gland, whereas a hordeolum is an acute inflammation of one of the glands in the eyelid.

5. Answer: 2

Rationale: Yellowing of the sclera and arcus senilis (also known as corneal arcus) is a benign, yellow-whitish ring

around the limbus and is seen in the older adult due to age-related physiologic changes. Cataracts occur as a result of opacity of the lens of the eye that causes partial or total blindness. The visual acuity and depth perception of the patient cannot be determined from the information provided.

6. Answer: 2

Rationale: The red-free filter is used to visualize the vessels and hemorrhages in better detail by improving contrast. This setting will make the retina look black and white. The small aperture is used when the pupil is very constricted; the slit is used to examine contour abnormalities of the cornea, lens, and retina; and the grid is used for estimating the size of lesions found in the fundal area.

7. Answer: 2

Rationale: A light beam shining onto one retina causes pupillary constriction in both that eye, termed the *direct reaction* to light, and in the opposite eye, referred to as the *consensual reaction.*

8. Answer: 1

Rationale: Chronic hypertension stiffens and thickens arteries, resulting in arteriovenous nicking. Intraocular pressure cannot be determined from an ophthalmic examination. Papilledema is associated with swelling around the optic disc with blurred margins. Small emboli are represented by an abrupt impediment or severe narrowing of an arteriole not associated with where the retinal veins and arteries cross.

9. Answer: 1

Rationale: Accommodation is the ability of the lens to change shape. Changes in pupil size when focusing from near to distant objects (and vice versa) tests for accommodation. Extraocular movements refer to the ability to move the eye in six cardinal directions. Consensual response is constriction of the eye in response to light being shined in the opposite eye. The Snellen eye chart is used to determine visual acuity.

10. Answer: 4

Rationale: Xanthelasma is a soft or hard yellow plaque on the inside corners of the eyelids (near the inner canthus). It is made up of cholesterol and is found more often on the upper lid than the lower lid. Xanthelasma is a type of xanthoma and is associated with hyperlipidemias, so a lipid profile would be an appropriate test to order.

Ears

11. Answer: 4

Rationale: The normal tympanic membrane (TM) is thin, translucent, shiny, and slightly concave with a pearl gray or pale pink appearance. This describes the normal characteristics of the TM. There is no evidence indicating scarring, presence of fluid, or decreased circulation to the membrane.

12. Answer: 2

Rationale: The Rinne test is positive (or normal) when air conduction is greater than bone conduction (AC > BC). If the patient hears the tuning fork better by bone conduction, the Rinne test is negative, which suggests a conductive hearing loss.

13. Answer: 1

Rationale: Direct light reflex located at 5- to 6-o'clock position and malleus at 1- to 2-o'clock position, with the umbo in the center, describes the correct position for the landmarks on the right ear. The manubrium slants to the right with the malleus at the 1- to 2-o'clock position for the right ear. The direct light reflex in the center of the membrane with the malleus at the 9-o'clock position describes the correct position for the left ear. The umbo is in the center with the anterior malleolar folds at the 1- to 2-o'clock position for the right ear.

Nose

14. Answer: 4

Rationale: The adult-gerontology primary care NP recognizes the nasal crease to be a result of uncontrolled allergic rhinitis, which may be seasonal or perennial as the patient repeatedly wipes the nose with palm. Dermatologic evaluation is not necessary. The finding is not normal. Before treatment is prescribed, a thorough history on allergic rhinitis should be obtained.

15. Answer: 1

Rationale: The nasal mucosa is normally dark pink, smooth, and moist. A pale, boggy mucosa suggests chronic allergy. A red and swollen mucosa suggests acute allergic rhinitis. The normal secretion is mucoid. Purulent, crusty, or bloody secretions are abnormal.

Throat

16. Answer: 2

Rationale: Diagnostic studies used to detect group A [beta]-hemolytic streptococci (GABHS or GAS) infection include a throat culture and a rapid antigen detection test (RADT). Throat culture has been considered the gold standard method to establish the microbial cause of acute pharyngitis. RADT is often used because it is rapid and convenient; however, RADT is less sensitive (true positive) than a throat culture. A positive monospot test result reveals heterophile antibodies. The monospot test is highly specific and sensitive. *Candida albicans* and rhinovirus are not diagnosed by bacterial cultures. Rhinovirus is one of the most common viral causes of pharyngitis. Oral candidiasis, a fungal infection, can be diagnosed with a potassium hydroxide smear showing mycelia (hyphae) or pseudo-mycelia (pseudohyphae) yeast forms.

17. Answer: 2

Rationale: The patient in this situation had risk factors (age) and symptoms of mononucleosis, so the monospot or heterophile antibody test should be conducted. The classic triad of mononucleosis symptoms includes sore throat, fever, and posterior cervical lymphadenopathy with or without mild tenderness. Rapid screening for streptococcal infection can be done using a throat swab with antigen agglutination kits and would be obtained first, but the result would probably be negative. WBC count would be ordered for bacterial pharyngitis; an increased neutrophil count is found with bacterial infection, and lymphocytosis is found with mononucleosis.

Disorders

Head

18. Answer: 3

Rationale: Giant cell (temporal) arteritis is most commonly seen in women of Scandinavian descent and presents with pain in the frontotemporal region that is exquisitely tender. Trigeminal neuralgia typically presents as a sharp, shooting, momentary pain with radiation to the jaw or cheek. Preherpetic neuralgia is a preeruption phase of shingles that can present 2–3 days prior to the vesicular rash. It is a diagnosis of exclusion that is confirmed by a rash appearing 2–3 days after the onset of the discomfort. Temporomandibular joint (TMJ) dysfunction presents as pain and tenderness over the TMJ joint, frequently associated with chewing and jaw movement.

19. Answer: 2

Rationale: Oral leukoplakia is a precancerous lesion that presents as white patches or plaques of the oral mucosa that cannot be rubbed off. Hemangiomas are usually benign tumors made up of blood vessels that typically appear as a purplish or reddish, slightly elevated area of skin that can include the lips, tongue, and buccal mucosa. Erythroplasia is an asymptomatic, red, velvety lesion on the oral or genital mucosa that is considered a precancerous lesion. Papillomas are benign verrucous lesions that are manifestations of human papillomavirus (HPV) infection.

20. Answer: 2

Rationale: Tobacco use and alcohol use are among the greatest risk factors for oral cavity and oropharyngeal cancers. Smokers are many times more likely than non-smokers to develop these cancers. Tobacco smoke from cigarettes, cigars, or pipes can cause cancers anywhere in the mouth or throat. Drinking alcohol increases the risk of developing oral cavity and oropharyngeal cancers, as about 7 of 10 patients with oral cancer are heavy drinkers. The disease is age related, occurring in those over 40 years of age and increasing with age. Infection with cancer-causing types of human papillomavirus (HPV), especially HPV-16, is a risk factor for some types of head and neck cancers, particularly oropharyngeal cancers that involve the tonsils or the base of the tongue.

21. Answer: 3

Rationale: Erythroplasia is accompanied by an inflammatory reaction in a patient with suspected oral cancer. Lesions persisting over 14 days strongly suggest early oral cancer. Tissue retraction and thickening of the oral tissues are later signs of oral cancer. Halitosis (odor) may be associated with dysfunction within the oral cavity (dental caries), nasal cavity, sinuses, or esophageal disorders. Cough is the primary symptom of respiratory disorders such as acute bronchitis or pneumonia.

22. Answer: 3

Rationale: Adults who present with thrush (oral candidiasis) may be immunologically impaired. It is important to screen these adults for HIV and diabetes mellitus as frequency of oral candidiasis increases with both of those illnesses. Treatment with amoxicillin is not the appropriate action, because the presenting disorder describes a fungal infection.

23. Answer: 2

Rationale: The adult-gerontology primary care NP knows that the risk factors for head and neck cancer include tobacco and alcohol use, poor oral hygiene, and occupational exposure to asbestos, nickel, wood, or leather. The most common site is in the oral cavity, accounting for 48% of head and neck cancer diagnoses.

Eyes

24. Answer: 2

Rationale: Closed-angle (acute) glaucoma is a medical emergency that requires immediate ophthalmological evaluation. Corneal abrasion is commonly seen with contact lens wear or in the presence of ocular trauma. Open-angle glaucoma is most often an asymptomatic chronic condition. Iritis/uveitis is an infection/inflammation of the deeper structures of the eye and is most often associated with trauma or infection. Dilated, fixed pupils are not seen with iritis/uveitis.

25. Answer: 4

Rationale: Patients go home almost immediately after the procedure. The eye may be patched, depending whether anesthesia was local or topical. The patient may experience some discomfort, but pain should not be a problem. The patient can be mobile and active as tolerated.

26. Answer: 2

Rationale: Initial assessment of visual acuity would provide the basis for comparison in the event of complications. Visual acuity should be measured before the instillation of a topical anesthetic or fluorescein. Following visual acuity assessment, an examination of the eye using a penlight is performed to evaluate for a penetrating foreign body.

27. Answer: 4

Rationale: Photokeratitis, also known as *ultraviolet keratitis* or *UV keratitis*, is an acute syndrome that occurs after ultraviolet irradiation of the eyes and can be intensely painful. Although the exposure may not initially be apparent to the patient, there is a latency period of approximately 6–12 hours between exposure and onset of symptoms. Photokeratitis is generally a self-limited condition with complete resolution. Initial treatment consists of oral analgesics and lubricant antibiotic ointments. An eye injury resulting from a welder's arc is commonly known as *flash burn, welder's flash,* or *arc eye.*

28. Answer: 4

Rationale: A cataract is an opacity of the lens of the eye that causes partial or total blindness. Cataracts are characterized by painless loss of visual acuity over time. Retinal detachment most often occurs suddenly, with partial loss of the field of vision. Glaucoma results in the loss of peripheral vision, and macular degeneration involves primarily the central vision field.

29. Answer: 4

Rationale: Bacterial conjunctivitis presents with injection of the conjunctiva, no pain, and with a history of purulent discharge. Bacterial conjunctivitis is usually in one eye, and viral conjunctivitis is more common in both eyes. Viral conjunctivitis will usually present with acute onset of a red eye with itching, photophobia, and excessive watery discharge. Unlike conjunctivitis with infectious causes, allergic conjunctivitis typically presents simultaneously in both eyes with the predominant feature of itching. The chief complaint of a corneal abrasion is pain.

30. Answer: 4

Rationale: Sustained nystagmus is indicative of a neurologic complication. The other options include normal age-related changes.

31. Answer: 3

Rationale: Arcus senilis is the deposit of lipids at the junction of the cornea and sclera that is present in many people over age 50 years. When identified in younger individuals, it may be related to a disorder of lipid metabolism. High cholesterol is more likely associated with a similar gray or white arc visible around the entire cornea (circumferential arcus) in younger adults.

32. Answer: 4

Rationale: These findings are normal age-related physiologic changes. Signs and symptoms of cataracts include reduced visual acuity; painless progressive loss of vision; and sensitivity to light, especially at night (night driving). Reduced color discrimination and presbyopia may also develop. Macular degeneration presents with a loss of central vision. Primary open-angle glaucoma presents with occasional headaches and seeing halos around lights but may be asymptomatic in its early stages. Primary angle-closure glaucoma can present with decreased vision, seeing halos around lights at night, and conjunctival redness.

33. Answer: 3

Rationale: Generalized, diffuse swelling and erythema of the eyelid is associated with an insect bite. Blepharitis is a chronic inflammatory condition characterized by erythema and scaling of the lid margins. Hordeolum, or stye, is an acute, purulent inflammation of the sebaceous glands (usually the glands of Zeis or the meibomian tear glands) of the eyelids and usually does not involve the entire eyelid. It may be painful, especially over the gland. Dacryocystitis is an inflammation of the lacrimal sac that is characterized by erythema and swelling over the lacrimal duct.

34. Answer: 4

Rationale: Classic signs of bacterial conjunctivitis include those symptoms listed along with complaints of eyelids being "glued shut" on awakening. Severe itching, moderate tearing, and minimal discharge symptoms are indicative of allergic conjunctivitis. Minimal itching, moderate tearing, and mucoid exudate symptoms are indicative of viral conjunctivitis.

Ears

35. Answer: 2

Rationale: Although all identified household appliances are noisy, the patient should wear a protective ear device when using a power lawn mower regularly for long periods.

36. Answer: 1

Rationale: In presbycusis, the ability to hear high-frequency sounds is diminished. These patients have difficulty distinguishing consonant sounds, so words such as *shoe* and *true* are heard as "oo." The Rinne test indicates that bone conduction is greater than air conduction. Tetracyclines are not ototoxic. The patient's family history may or may not contribute to the problem. If the hearing loss is sensorineural, the sound will be heard best in the normal ear when performing a Weber test. Normally, sound should be of equal intensity in both ears.

37. Answer: 3

Rationale: The key factor that contributes to acute otitis media (AOM) is a dysfunctional eustachian tube. The actual cause is unknown, but it may be sequelae of upper respiratory tract infections or allergies that result in edema of the eustachian tube, or it may result from reflux of nasopharynx bacteria into the eustachian tube. The most frequent bacterial organisms that infect the middle ear, especially in children, are similar to those of the nasopharynx: *S. pneumoniae, H. influenzae,* and *M. catarrhalis. Staphylococcus aureus* is one of the most common causative organisms in otitis externa.

38. Answer: 4

Rationale: A bulging tympanic membrane with a distorted cone of light would be indicative of an inflammation of the middle ear (AOM). The other options indicate age-related physiologic changes.

39. Answer: 4

Rationale: Conductive hearing loss may result from acute otitis media (AOM), perforation of the eardrum, and obstruction of the ear canal, as by cerumen. The other options result in sensorineural hearing loss.

40. Answer: 4

Rationale: Noise-induced hearing loss is a sensorineural hearing deficit that begins at the higher frequencies (3000–6000 Hz) and develops gradually as a result of chronic exposure to excessive sound levels.

41. Answer: 1

Rationale: The diagnosis of acute otitis media (AOM) is clinical, made by otoscopy, and based on the appearance of the tympanic membrane (TM). The bony landmarks are absent or decreased. The TM may be full, bulging, or retracted, with pus, and the light reflex is distorted. Pneumatic otoscopy reveals decreased or absent TM mobility.

42. Answer: 4

Rationale: The patient has the clinical findings of otitis externa, an inflammation and infection of the external ear canal predisposed by excessive wetness, such as swimming. Common organisms responsible for otitis externa include *Pseudomonas aeruginosa*, *Proteus mirabilis*, and *Enterobacter aerogenes* or fungal organisms of the *Aspergillus or Candida* species. Sinusitis clinical findings focus on sinus pain and a purulent nasal discharge. Clinical findings of otitis media include ear pain, full or bulging tympanic membrane, decreased or negative mobility, and possible erythema. Findings associated with serous otitis media include opaque or translucent tympanic membrane with air bubbles; landmarks may be absent, and the light reflex may be diffuse or absent.

Nose

43. Answer: 4

Rationale: Idiopathic epistaxis is most common and majority of epistaxis occurs in the anterior aspect. Although it is possible to eliminate bleeding with nasoconstricting agents and digital compression for at least 10–15 minutes with the cervical spine flexed "chin to the chest," some patients require chemical cauterization. Following a successful cauterization, the patient should be instructed to use a humidifier at home; squirt nasal saline liberally; and apply lubricants with a cotton swab, such as petroleum jelly or antibiotic ointment intranasally as dry air contributes to bleeding and re-bleeding. The patient should not sneeze with the mouth closed, as that increases intranasal pressure.

44. Answer: 2

Rationale: The patient is experiencing the classic characteristics of acute sinusitis. Viral causes of sinusitis show improvement by day 10, and bacterial sinus infections persist longer. A dental abscess can cause pain that radiates to the sinuses but more often causes constant, severe, tooth-associated pain and jaw tenderness. Giant cell (temporal) arteritis causes pain in the jaw and face but no nasal discharge.

45. Answer: 4

Rationale: Nasal snorting of cocaine results in nasal congestion and discharge. Because cocaine is a potent sympathomimetic, the nasal passages appear similar to what is found on physical exam of patients who abuse nasal decongestants (e.g., oxymetazoline [Afrin]). Chronic use of cocaine causes the nasal septal mucosa to become ischemic, which leads to tissue atrophy and eventual septal perforation, which is noted on physical exam and should be followed up with questions about snorting cocaine.

46. Answer: 3

Rationale: Because overwhelmingly most sinus infections are viral, it is recommended to avoid antibiotics during the first 7–10 days unless there is strong supporting evidence of bacterial infection, which this patient does not have. A CT scan is not typically taken at the initial visit, unless there is treatment failure. All patients with chronic sinusitis should have a CT scan. A white blood cell count is also not helpful initially in most mild to moderate cases. Initial treatment is focused on pain relief, nasal irrigation, and nasal decongestants.

47. Answer: 3

Rationale: Transmission of cold viruses is indirect (e.g., self-inoculation from virus on surfaces of inanimate objects to mucous membranes of the nose and mouth). Viruses are less likely to be spread by the aerosol route. Thus, the patient should avoid touching the nose and mouth unless the hands have been thoroughly washed. It is impractical to avoid contact because cold viruses are found everywhere. Although many individuals believe vitamin C prevents colds, research to support this claim is minimal.

Throat

48. Answer: 1

Rationale: Asymmetrical tonsillar hypertrophy with contralateral uvular deviation are hallmark signs of peritonsillar abscess, whereas peritonsillar cellulitis is associated with deep erythema that extends beyond the tonsils and pharynx without structural changes. Retropharyngeal abscess is a deep soft tissue infection that is difficult to diagnose on exam but is frequently accompanied by stridor. Drooling, tripoding, and dysphagia are a classic clinical triad indicating epiglottitis.

49. Answer: 1

Rationale: Mononucleosis is often seen in adolescents and young adults. It often presents with sore throat, fever, tonsillar exudate, lymphadenopathy, and malaise. Leukemia presents with symptoms of fever, fatigue, and weight loss, as well as lymphadenopathy and bone pain. Scarlet fever, a complication of streptococcal pharyngitis, presents with sore throat, fever, abdominal pain, headache, erythematous fine rash, and strawberry tongue. Oral candidiasis presents with white, curdlike plaques on erythematous mucosa. The tongue is red with a white coat.

50. Answer: 3

Rationale: The clinical presentation of pharyngitis varies and depends on the causative agent. Characteristics of bacterial pharyngitis include sore throat, headache, erythema of the tonsils with white or yellow exudate, dysphagia, tender anterior cervical adenopathy, and fever. Small oral vesicles are seen with herpangina, an infection caused by the coxsackie virus. Cough is typically the primary symptom of acute bronchitis; the presence of cough decreases likelihood of streptococcal pharyngitis. Rhinorrhea is associated with allergic rhinitis.

Pharmacology

51. Answer: 3

Rationale: The adult-gerontology primary care NP recognizes that the patient's condition is a result of otomycosis, a fungal infection of the external auditory canal that occurs either as a solitary infection or as a subsequent infection associated with use of antibiotic and steroidal otic therapy. The mainstay of treatment is meticulous cleaning of the ear canal and antifungal therapy. Otic antibiotics must be discontinued, as they may be a causative agent and have no clinical benefit at this time. Carbamide peroxide (Debrox) is used to treat partial or complete earwax obstructions.

52. Answer: 2

Rationale: Mild allergic angioedema without airway obstruction should be treated with oral antihistamines and glucocorticoids. Lisinopril can be a causative agent of ACE inhibitor–induced angioedema. An EpiPen is reserved for patients who are having anaphylaxis and should always be given intramuscularly.

53. Answer: 1

Rationale: Intranasal steroids (e.g., fluticasone) are most effective for moderate to severe allergic rhinitis, and they do not have any systemic side effects. Fexofenadine (Allegra) is a second-line choice for allergic rhinitis. The other medications listed are reasonable alternatives as they are effective, but they are not without side effects. Oral decongestants such as pseudoephedrine can cause insomnia, nervousness, or urinary retention. Azelastine (Astelin) can cause sedation and is expensive.

54. Answer: 4

Rationale: Amoxicillin has been recommended as a first-line agent in the past because of its narrow spectrum and relatively low cost. However, there is increasing emergence of antimicrobial resistance among respiratory pathogens, including pneumococci and *H. influenzae*. Amoxicillin-clavulanate rather than amoxicillin is recommended as empiric first line therapy for non-penicillin-allergic adults.

Doxycycline is a reasonable alternative for first-line therapy and can be used in patients with a penicillin allergy. Azithromycin is not recommended for empiric therapy, because of its high rate of resistance of *S. pneumoniae*.

55. Answer: 2

Rationale: Topical beta blockers such as timolol lower intraocular pressure but can be absorbed systemically. The major side effects are similar to those associated with systemic beta-blocker therapy, which can include a worsening of heart failure, bradycardia, and heart block. Topical beta blockers are contraindicated in some patients with cardiac or pulmonary disease.

56. Answer: 1

Rationale: Treatment of mononucleosis includes bed rest while the patient has fever and myalgia (10–14 days), supportive acetaminophen or ibuprofen, warm saline gargles, and throat lozenges or analgesic spray. The patient must avoid strenuous exercise and contact sports for 2 months because of the risk of splenic rupture. Splenomegaly is seen in 50% to 60% of all patients with infectious mononucleosis. Corticosteroids are recommended only for patients with impending airway obstruction, and an immediate referral to an otolaryngologist is warranted. Ampicillin is not recommended, because of the viral etiology of this disease. Additionally, rashes are common in patients with infectious mononucleosis and are treated with amoxicillin or ampicillin. About 95% of patients with mononucleosis recover uneventfully with supportive treatment.

57. Answer: 4

Rationale: Amoxicillin with clavulanic acid (Augmentin) is effective against beta-lactamase production. Erythromycin-sulfisoxazole has recently been reported as less effective. Amoxicillin is ineffective against beta-lactamase production, as is penicillin V.

58. Answer: 1, 2, 3

Rationale: For symptom relief during an acute attack, benzodiazepines (diazepam or lorazepam) decrease vertigo and anxiety; antihistamines (meclizine/dimenhydrinate) decrease vertigo and nausea; anticholinergics (atropine) lessen abnormal sensations; and antiemetics (prochlorperazine) reduce nausea and motion sickness. Diuretics as a maintenance medication may assist in reducing acute attacks by decreasing endolymphatic pressure and volume; however, there is insufficient evidence to recommend routine use. Tricyclic antidepressants and antibiotics are not first-line medications for an acute attack.

Integumentary

Physical Examination & Diagnostic Tests

1. The adult-gerontology primary care NP is performing a physical examination on a female patient as part of a scheduled office visit. Which finding, if noted, would represent a normal process associated with aging?
   1. Yellow-colored nails.
   2. Thinning of hair.
   3. Brittle nails.
   4. Absence of lesions.

2. The adult-gerontology primary care NP identifies clubbing on a male patient during an examination. Based on this finding, which three diagnostic tests/assessment techniques would be ordered?
   1. Imaging studies of the hands.
   2. Orthostatic blood pressures.
   3. Pulse oximetry reading.
   4. ECG.
   5. Chest x-ray.

3. The adult-gerontology primary care NP describes an annular skin lesion as usually arranged in:
   1. Groups of vesicles erupting unilaterally.
   2. A line.
   3. A pattern of merging together, not discrete.
   4. A circle, or ring shaped.

4. A patient has pitting of the nails. The adult-gerontology primary care NP understands this is associated with:
   1. Psoriasis.
   2. Iron-deficiency anemia.
   3. Malnutrition.
   4. Hyperthyroidism.

5. What diagnostic test would be appropriate to order for a patient who has acanthosis nigricans?
   1. Skin biopsy.
   2. Liver function tests (LFTs).
   3. Fasting blood glucose (FBS).
   4. IgE electrophoresis.

6. The adult-gerontology primary care NP is inspecting a dark-skinned individual for signs of jaundice. The best place to observe jaundice in dark-skinned individuals is:
   1. Sclera of the opened eye.
   2. Palms and soles of the hands and feet.
   3. Oral mucosa.
   4. Nail beds.

7. When assessing an adult's hydration status, the best place to evaluate skin turgor on an adult is:
   1. Just below the clavicle.
   2. Below the scapula on the back.
   3. On the inside of the forearm.
   4. On the back of the hand.

8. The Wood lamp may be used to evaluate skin lesions. When the light is shone on the patient's skin, a green-yellow fluorescence indicates:
   1. Presence of fungi.
   2. Lichenification.
   3. Keratinized cells.
   4. Bacterial colonies.

9. On exam of a patient's skin, the adult-gerontology primary care NP finds a lesion that is about 0.75 cm in diameter, brown, circumscribed, flat, and nonpalpable. What is the correct term for this lesion?
   1. Macule.
   2. Papule.
   3. Nodule.
   4. Wheal.

10. The history and physical of a patient indicates past occurrences of lichenification. The adult-gerontology primary care NP identifies the characteristics of this lesion as:
    1. Dried, crusty exudate, slightly elevated.
    2. Rough, thickened epidermis, accentuated skin markings.
    3. Keratinized cells shaped in an irregular pattern with exfoliation.
    4. Loss of epidermis with hollowed-out area and dermis exposed.

11. Clubbing of the nails commonly occurs in patients with chronic respiratory conditions. The adult-gerontology primary care NP assesses for this condition by:
    1. Evaluating the nail for transverse depressions and ridges.
    2. Placing the patient's hands together with palms inward and index fingers aligned.
    3. Placing nail beds of each index finger together to determine angle of nail plate.
    4. Determining if there is diffuse discoloration of the nail bed from decreased oxygenation.

12. A circumscribed, elevated lesion >1 cm in diameter and containing clear serous fluid is best described as a:
    1. Papule.
    2. Vesicle.
    3. Bulla.
    4. Pustule.

13. In performing a skin assessment, the adult-gerontology primary care NP understands that the following characteristic of a mole would necessitate immediate intervention:
    1. A 5-mm, symmetric, uniformly brown mole on the thigh that has not changed in appearance for more than 5 years.
    2. Multiple small (1–3 mm) flat moles across the upper back that are dark brown in color, round, and have smooth edges.
    3. A 3-cm, waxy papule with a "stuck-on" appearance, noted on the face.
    4. A new, 5–6-mm brown mole with an irregular red border that is occasionally pruritic.

14. Dermatophyte skin infections can be diagnosed from skin scrapings and prepared with which solution for microscopic exam?
    1. Hydrochloric acid.
    2. 10% or 20% potassium hydroxide (KOH) solution.
    3. Crystal violet.
    4. Distilled water.

15. When administering skin tests to an immunocompromised patient, the adult-gerontology primary care NP must consider:
    1. The importance of not applying more than one skin test at a time.
    2. That the skin test may react more aggressively than expected.
    3. The practice of using positive and negative control solutions.
    4. That an immunocompromised patient should not have skin testing.

Skin Disorders

16. A 65-year-old presents to the clinic for evaluation of small rough areas on his face that have increased in size over the past year. He states that he had several similar lesions on his neck removed a few years ago. Physical examination reveals 1 cm × 1 cm areas of erythematous, sandpaper-like lesions that are yellow to light brown in color above his brow. No discharge is noted. Which of the following should the adult-gerontology primary care NP educate the patient regarding lesions of this type?
    1. Risk of squamous cell carcinoma.
    2. Risk of melanoma.
    3. Risk of infection.
    4. The lesions are benign.

17. A 64-year-old female patient presents with an erythematous area of skin on her left buttock. She states that it is painful because it is located along her bikini line. She is worried she may not be able to continue to relax in the hot tub at her apartment community in the evenings. She denies any recent injuries to the area. Which of the following should the adult-gerontology primary care NP suspect as the most likely cause?
    1. *Pseudomonas aeruginosa.*
    2. *Staphylococcus aureus.*
    3. *Staphylococcus epidermidis.*
    4. Contact dermatitis.

18. A patient complains of intolerable itching in the pubic hair. On exam, the adult-gerontology primary care NP notes erythematous papules and tiny white specks in the pubic hair. The differential diagnosis includes all except:
    1. Pediculosis pubis.
    2. Scabies.
    3. Impetigo.
    4. Atopic dermatitis.

19. What finding would indicate to the adult-gerontology primary care NP that an immunoglobulin E–mediated potential trigger was suspected in the presence of an adult patient who had acute urticaria?
    1. Increase in fluid intake in the past 24 hours.
    2. Body temperature of 101°F.
    3. Patient had eaten seafood salad that day.
    4. Patient also presented with flulike symptoms.

20. A 70-year-old female presents to the clinic complaining of pain on her left arm. Inspection of the extremity reveals no erythema. Her skin is intact with no evidence of lesions. The patient's past medical history includes herpes zoster. Which clinical diagnosis would the adult-gerontology primary care NP make as supported by this patient's presentation and past medical history?
    1. Phantom pain.
    2. Postherpetic neuralgia.
    3. Urinary tract infection.
    4. Tinea infection.

21. An older adult woman has an area of vesicles in clusters with an erythematous base that extend from her spine, around and under her arm and breast, to the sternum on her left side. She states that the area was very tender last week and that the vesicles started erupting yesterday. She is complaining of severe pain in the area. What is the probable diagnosis for this condition?
    1. Psoriasis.
    2. Herpes zoster.
    3. Contact dermatitis.
    4. Cellulitis.

22. What is a chronic skin condition that is sometimes associated with arthritis?
    1. Eczema.
    2. Psoriasis.
    3. Neurodermatitis.
    4. Pityriasis rosea.

23. Which is a true statement about psoriasis?
    1. It is usually worse in the summer.
    2. It is highly contagious.
    3. It can be aggravated by stress.
    4. All patients have accompanying pruritus.

24. What information should be provided to a patient with actinic keratosis?
    1. The affected areas are a normal part of aging and are benign.
    2. These lesions can develop into squamous cell carcinomas.
    3. This is part of an allergic reaction, and the offending allergen needs to be identified.
    4. This skin condition responds well to sunlight, which will help alleviate the symptoms.

25. The following are all true statements regarding urticaria except:
    1. Most cases of acute urticaria involve IgE-mediated mast cell degranulation.
    2. Chronic urticaria may be related to occult infections.
    3. Urticaria is characterized by red, itchy wheals a few millimeters to a few centimeters in size.
    4. Laboratory studies are necessary to identify the causative agent.

26. A patient known to be positive for HIV presents with several painless, persistent, raised purple lesions on the lower arm. What is the most likely diagnosis of the lesions?
    1. Seborrheic dermatitis.
    2. Molluscum contagiosum.
    3. Kaposi sarcoma.
    4. Fungal infection.

27. In making a differential diagnosis between nummular eczema (dermatitis) and dyshidrotic eczematous dermatitis, the adult-gerontology primary care NP knows:

    1. Nummular eczema is characterized by flushing and clusters of papulopustules on the cheek and forehead.
    2. Dyshidrotic eczematous dermatitis is a chronic vesicular type of hand-and-foot eczema characterized by vesicles (tapioca-like), scaling, lichenification, and pruritus.
    3. Nummular eczema is a hereditary disorder characterized by chronic, usually bilateral scaly plaques on exposed areas (knees, elbows).
    4. Dyshidrotic eczematous dermatitis affects primarily young adults, is contagious, and is characterized by firm papules with a cleft surface and multiple conical vegetations.

28. A middle-aged male patient presents to the clinic with a complaint of being bitten last night by another individual during a fight. He has a bite mark on his forearm, and the skin has been broken. He reports he does not remember any recent vaccinations for tetanus. Recommended treatment by the adult-gerontology primary care NP should include all the following except:
    1. Administer Tdap (Adacel).
    2. Instruct patient to watch for signs of infection.
    3. Initiate treatment with a beta-lactam penicillin.
    4. Close the wound with sutures or Nexcare Steri-Strips.

29. Nail involvement secondary to primary foot-and-hand tinea, characterized by accumulation of subungual keratin that produces thickened, distorted, crumbling nails, is termed:
    1. Hippocratic nails.
    2. Onychomycosis.
    3. Koilonychia.
    4. Anonychia.

30. A middle-aged patient presents for an office visit with a complaint of a measles-like rash on his trunk and spreading to his extremities. He was seen several days ago for bronchitis and started on trimethoprim-sulfamethoxazole (TMP-SMX; Septra) ds 1 tab PO bid. What is the recommended action for the adult-gerontology primary care NP?
    1. Instruct the patient to continue the medication and see if any change occurs in the rash.
    2. Discontinue TMP-SMX.
    3. Take the patient off medication for 3 days, then restart the drug.
    4. Decrease TMP-SMX to half-dose.

31. A patient complaining of hyperhidrosis should be counseled that:
    1. This is a normal occurrence.
    2. There are no therapies for this complaint.
    3. Bathing in 20% alcohol solution of aluminum chloride hexahydrate (Drysol) may be beneficial.
    4. A history and physical exam need to be completed to rule out any medical etiologies.

32. During the physical exam, the adult-gerontology primary care NP assesses a maculopapular skin lesion on a patient's back that is warty, scaly, greasy in appearance, and light tan in color. What would be the probable diagnosis?
    1. Actinic keratosis.
    2. Basal cell carcinoma.
    3. Seborrheic keratosis.
    4. Senile lentigines.

33. The adult-gerontology primary care NP is assessing an older patient diagnosed with herpes zoster (shingles) in the prodromal stage. What would the practitioner expect to find on the assessment of this patient?
    1. Erythematous lesions present over four different parts of the body.
    2. Red, pinpoint, painless rash.
    3. Linear burning pain in a line on only half the patient's chest that does not cross the midline.
    4. Painless purulent lesions for 2 days followed by complaints of itching, burning, and nausea.

34. A retired farmer presents with a dome-shaped, pearly, firm nodule with telangiectasia on his nose. In making a diagnosis, the adult-gerontology primary care NP recognizes this to be:
    1. Compound nevus.
    2. Melanoma.
    3. Bullous pemphigoid.
    4. Basal cell carcinoma.

35. An adult female presents with an irregular, variegated nevus on her lower left back that has doubled in size in the past 3 months. What would be an appropriate action for the adult-gerontology primary care NP?
    1. Do a punch biopsy to confirm the diagnosis.
    2. Take a photograph of the lesion and recheck it in 1 month.
    3. Refer immediately to a dermatologist.
    4. Reassure the patient that these are normal changes related to hormone variations.

36. An older adult patient presents with pain in the right chest wall for the past 48 hours. On exam, the adult-gerontology primary care NP notices a vesicular eruption along the dermatome and identifies this as herpes zoster. The adult-gerontology primary care NP informs the patient that:
    1. All symptoms will disappear in 3 days.
    2. Oral medication can dramatically reduce the duration and intensity of symptoms.
    3. The patient has chickenpox, which may be contagious to grandchildren until the lesions are completely gone.
    4. The eruptions will recur at regular intervals.

37. A young adult female presents to the adult-gerontology primary care NP's office stating that she has had a red rash over her trunk for 2 weeks that does not itch. She has tried over-the-counter lotions and creams, but the rash is still there. The rash started as a small, round, red patch on her chest and has since spread across her chest, back, arms, and legs. A physical exam reveals a generalized distribution of erythematous and scaly macular lesions that run parallel to each other, creating a "Christmas tree" pattern. The adult-gerontology primary care NP should:
    1. Do a thorough medication history, investigate any potential allergens, and send the patient to an allergy specialist.
    2. Prescribe triamcinolone 0.025% cream (Aristocort A) bid for 2 weeks.
    3. Teach the patient that this viral disease is self-limiting, lasting 6–8 weeks, and to avoid prolonged or excessive exposure to sunlight.
    4. Refer the patient to a dermatologist for a biopsy.

38. An adult male patient presents to the adult-gerontology primary care NP's office complaining of flulike symptoms, a large red spot in the right groin, headaches, and generalized muscle pain. These symptoms have persisted for about 4–5 weeks. In taking the history, it would be most important to determine whether the patient:
    1. Was using new skin care products.
    2. Was taking any new medications, such as vitamins or herbal therapies.
    3. Has had a recent insect bite or was potentially exposed to insects such as ticks.
    4. Has been exposed to a person with tuberculosis.

39. When do bites from insects, spiders, snakes, and bees most often occur?
    1. High humidity months.
    2. Spring to early fall.
    3. Winter.
    4. Any time of the year.

40. Medical management for a brown recluse spider bite includes:
    1. Warm moist soaks to the affected area.
    2. Ice pack and elevation and immobilization of the area.
    3. Active and passive range of motion (ROM) to the area.
    4. Avoidance of antihistamines.

41. A scout leader is explaining about snakes and snake bites, and says to his group about the coral snake, "Red on yellow, kill a fellow; red on black, venom lack." Later, one of the boys is bitten by a snake described as having broad rings of red and black, separated by narrow rings of yel-

low. The adult-gerontology primary care NP understands that this patient will probably experience all the following except:

1. Numbness and change in sensation.
2. Local swelling at the fang mark site.
3. Dizziness and diplopia.
4. No symptoms, as the snake was not venomous.

42. The adult-gerontology primary care NP is examining a patient with a diagnosis of pityriasis rosea. Which three statements are correct about the condition?
    1. Pruritus is not present.
    2. Vesicles progressing to pustules occur within 2–3 days of eruption.
    3. Salmon-colored patch with fine scales is commonly noted on face, hands, and feet.
    4. Typical Christmas tree pattern of lesion distribution is observed.
    5. Presence of a herald patch before onset of generalized rash.

43. A young adult reports itching that seems to be worse at night. On examination, the adult-gerontology primary care NP notes a rash on the sides of the fingers and inner aspect of the elbows. The rash causes little bumps that often form a line that is approximately 2–3 mm long and the width of a hair. What does the adult-gerontology primary care NP suspect?
    1. Scabies.
    2. Hives.
    3. Fleas.
    4. Ticks.

44. What are common sites for atopic dermatitis in adults?
    1. Cheeks, forehead, and scalp.
    2. Wrists, ankles, and antecubital fossae.
    3. Antecubital fossae, face, neck, and back.
    4. Appears in the creases of the elbows or knees and nape of neck.

45. An older adult presents with complaints of a red, greasy scaly rash on his scalp, forehead, and eyebrow. What is the most likely diagnosis?
    1. Seborrheic dermatitis.
    2. Atopic dermatitis.
    3. Psoriasis.
    4. Rosacea.

46. What presenting symptom would be associated with the bite of a brown recluse spider?
    1. Paresthesias in all extremities.
    2. Edematous, erythematous area with coalescing macules.
    3. Tissue sloughing in the bite area within 8–10 hours.

4. Development of a central black eschar of "sinking infarct" within 24–48 hours.

47. An 84-year-old female patient presents to the office with bilateral varicosities on her lower extremities noted in the calf area. Varicosities appear to be superficial, but the patient wants to know if there is any therapeutic option that may reduce their appearance. Detection of pulses is within normal limits. Based on the patient's stated concern, the adult-gerontology primary care NP would suggest which of the following therapies?
    1. Laser therapy.
    2. Debridement of varicosities.
    3. Use of supportive compression stockings.
    4. Hydrotherapy.

48. What is a recommended treatment option for actinic keratoses?
    1. Hydrotherapy.
    2. Observation, as this is not considered to be a premalignant lesion.
    3. Topical chemotherapy.
    4. Systemic chemotherapy.

49. The adult-gerontology primary care NP understands that cat bites become infected more often than dog bites because:
    1. Dogs have a "cleaner mouth" than cats.
    2. Cat bites are often deep puncture wounds.
    3. Dog bites are usually on the face, which makes them less susceptible to infection.
    4. Cat bites are usually associated with clawing and spreading of microorganisms.

50. An adult was bitten by a neighbor's dog 3 days ago. He has developed an infection in a large wound on his lower leg. What would be an appropriate management strategy for the patient?
    1. Prescribe amoxicillin-clavulanate (Augmentin).
    2. Approximate the edges of the wound together with suture.
    3. Prescribe cephalexin (Keflex).
    4. Have the patient return to the clinic for follow-up in 2 weeks.

51. An adult has been bitten by a black widow spider while doing yard work. He is having a severe reaction; the adult-gerontology primary care NP expects:
    1. Hypotension and shock.
    2. Rash with bump or boil.
    3. Black eschar of sloughing tissue within 4 hours of the bite.
    4. Abdominal cramping, nausea, and headache.

Pharmacology

52. An adult male patient presents for removal of a tick on his abdomen that he noticed 6 hours ago after he returned from hunting. He is sure it was not there this morning when he showered. He complains of no symptoms. A physical exam reveals an adult *Ixodes* tick attached just inferior to the left navel. No erythema or discoloration of the skin is noted. The patient inquires about prophylaxis for Lyme disease. Which of the following should the adult-gerontology primary care NP recommend?
    1. Doxycycline 200 mg PO bid for 7 days.
    2. Doxycycline 200 mg PO once.
    3. Reassurance.
    4. Serologic testing for Lyme disease.

53. What would be the appropriate management for a patient with herpes zoster (shingles)?
    1. Acyclovir (Zovirax).
    2. Miconazole (Monistat-Derm).
    3. Clotrimazole (Lotrimin).
    4. Corticosteroid (prednisone).

54. An adult male patient is diagnosed with seborrheic dermatitis of the face. Which of the following treatments should the adult-gerontology primary care NP choose as initial therapy? Select three therapeutic treatments.
    1. Ketoconazole 2% topical.
    2. Chlorhexidine gluconate 4% topical.
    3. Betamethasone topical 0.1%.
    4. Hydrocortisone 2.5%.
    5. Clobetasol ointment 0.5% topical.

55. An obese woman presents to the clinic with complaints of tenderness and irritation under both of her breasts. An exam reveals a very irritated, moist, inflamed area with macules and papules present. What is the best treatment for the woman?
    1. Nystatin cream bid/tid for 10 days, with thorough drying of the area and exposure to light and air.
    2. Systemic antistaphylococcal antibiotics (dicloxacillin) and soaking with moist pads of normal saline three times daily.
    3. Gentle washing of the area and removal of crusts, then application of antibiotic ointment.
    4. Antiviral treatment (acyclovir) and topical ointment to prevent secondary infection.

56. Which three treatment options would the adult-gerontology primary care NP include in a plan of care for a patient presenting with scalp lesions attributable to psoriasis?
    1. Vigorous scalp massage every other day to facilitate plaque removal.
    2. Coal tar–based ointment.
    3. Topical vitamin D analogue.
    4. Topical emollients.
    5. Fluid replacement.

57. Which classification of drugs has the potential to aggravate psoriasis?
    1. Beta blockers.
    2. Thiazide diuretics.
    3. Vasodilators.
    4. Tricyclic antidepressants.

58. An adult female presents with cellulitis along the right side of her face extending near her orbit. Upon physical examination, pain is noted with ocular movements, right-sided blepharitis, and low-grade fever. Which of the following treatments should the adult-gerontology primary care NP anticipate as initial treatment?
    1. Trimethoprim-sulfamethoxazole.
    2. Clindamycin.
    3. Vancomycin plus ceftriaxone.
    4. Vancomycin plus metronidazole.

59. All the following are true of postherpetic neuralgia, except:
    1. Capsaicin cream (Zostrix) may alleviate some of the discomfort.
    2. In most patients, the postherpetic pain gradually subsides over several weeks.
    3. Acyclovir (Zovirax) 200 mg 5 caps daily PO in divided doses is an effective therapy.
    4. It is more common in patients over age 60 years.

60. An older adult male patient presents to the outpatient health clinic with complaints of pruritus of both hands and axillae. Upon examination, multiple papules are visualized between the fingers and in both axilla. Small burrows can be appreciated proximal to the papules. Which of the following should the adult-gerontology primary care NP choose as treatment?
    1. Hydrocortisone.
    2. Permethrin.
    3. Diphenhydramine.
    4. Ketoconazole.

61. An adult-gerontology primary care NP is examining multiple geriatric patients with pediculosis in an assisted living facility. Which of the following treatments should be initiated first?
    1. Lindane shampoo.
    2. Ivermectin oral.
    3. Crisaborole oral.
    4. Pyrethrin shampoo.

62. When treating infections suspicious of MRSA, the adult-gerontology primary care NP should be aware that which of the following is true regarding use of bacitracin or mupirocin (Bactroban)?
    1. Both medications are equally effective against MRSA.
    2. Mupirocin is more effective against MRSA.
    3. Bacitracin is more effective against MRSA.
    4. Neither is effective against MRSA.

63. An 82-year-old male presents as a new patient to the health clinic. During his initial visit, he requests a refill of prednisone that his previous primary care provider prescribed. He states that he has taken 20 mg by mouth daily for more than 10 years due to a single outbreak episode of pemphigus vulgaris. He states that he has been asymptomatic for 9 years and reports no other medical conditions. The adult-gerontology primary care NP should take which of the following next steps?
    1. Taper prednisone and prescribe tacrolimus.
    2. Discuss tapering the prednisone dose.
    3. Refill the patient's prednisone.
    4. Discontinue prednisone immediately.

64. When treating genital warts with topical podophyllin, it is important for the adult-gerontology primary care NP to:
    1. Apply the preparation directly to the wart and approximately 5 mm around the base.
    2. Cover with a dressing so that the solution remains moist, and caution the patient not to remove the dressing for 24 hours.
    3. Instruct the patient to wash off the medication in 4–6 hours.
    4. Treat with liquid nitrogen before applying podophyllin.

65. An adult patient who is being treated for acne rosacea presents to the office complaining of continued facial redness despite topical treatments. Which four medications would the adult-gerontology primary care NP consider including in the treatment regimen that may also provide reduced facial flushing?
    1. Furosemide (Lasix).
    2. Clonidine (Catapres).
    3. Niacin.
    4. Ondansetron (Zofran).
    5. Propranolol (Inderal).

66. A 70-year-old male patient presents to the clinic with complaints of intense itching. Examination of the skin reveals several areas of erythema with no observable lesions. The patient relates that this redness is due to his scratching to obtain relief. Which medication noted in the patient's medication profile could possibly contribute to his reported pruritus?
    1. Topical emollient.
    2. Corticosteroids.

3. Diuretic therapy.
4. Antihistamines.

67. What is the recommended treatment of rosacea?
    1. Oral hydrocortisone.
    2. Oral ketoconazole.
    3. Low-dose tetracycline.
    4. Topical 5-fluorouracil.

68. An adult female patient presents to the health clinic complaining of a pruritic and uncomfortable area under her left arm for 2 days. She states that she has been unable to shave under her arms. Examination of the left axilla reveals multiple follicular pustules. The area is mildly erythematous and painful to touch. Which of the following interventions should the adult-gerontology primary care NP choose?
    1. Reassurance.
    2. Topical clindamycin.
    3. Penicillin PO.
    4. Trimethoprim/sulfamethoxazole PO.

69. An adult female patient presents with a pruritic rash on the extensor areas of her arms and legs for several months that is debilitating. She also complains of diarrhea and bloating for several years and is subsequently diagnosed with celiac disease. Which of the following medications would best be indicated for the cutaneous eruption of this syndrome?
    1. Corticosteroids PO.
    2. Tazarotene topical.
    3. 5-Fluorouracil topical.
    4. Dapsone PO.

70. When using lidocaine with epinephrine 1%–2% as a local anesthetic in the repair of an injury, it is essential to remember that the maximum allowable dose is:
    1. 4.5 mg/kg.
    2. 2.5 mg/kg.
    3. 10 mg/kg.
    4. 15 mg/kg.

71. What therapeutic treatment option would be prescribed by the adult-gerontology primary care NP for a frail female patient who presents with several skin tears with no other contributory findings in a physical examination?
    1. Diuretic therapy to prevent fluid accumulation.
    2. Use of topical emollients to hydrate skin.
    3. Baby aspirin to prevent cardiovascular disease.
    4. Antibiotic to prevent infection.

72. An older adult patient presents to the adult-gerontology primary care NP complaining of a painful, tingling rash across the right side of the abdomen. An exam reveals vesicles with erythematous bases; some of the vesicles are draining cloudy fluid, whereas others are crusted. The adult-gerontology primary care NP makes the diagnosis of herpes zoster infection, and the patient is prescribed antiviral therapy. The patient states that the painful rash has caused difficulty sleeping for the past 4 nights. What would be appropriate therapy for this patient's pain?
    1. Amitriptyline (Elavil) 10 mg PO hs and nonsteroidal antiinflammatory drugs (NSAIDs) prn as directed.
    2. High-dose corticosteroid therapy.
    3. Application of heat directly to the area involved.
    4. No appropriate therapy is currently available to treat neuropathic pain.

73. An adult female patient presents to the health clinic complaining of excessive armpit sweating. She states that she has been "excessively sweaty" for as long as she can recall, but she inquires about treatment due to a new job that requires her to present publicly. She denies nervousness or anxiety and has no medical problems. Her only medication is oral contraceptives. She is prescribed aluminum chloride hexahydrate (Drysol) 20% to be applied to the underarms. Which three considerations should the adult-gerontology primary care NP educate the patient about regarding this medication?
    1. Avoid sunlight.
    2. Stinging sensation of affected area.
    3. Apply to wet skin.
    4. Avoid contact with broken or recently shaved skin.
    5. Use at bedtime.

74. A young adult female patient presents several days after being examined and treated for a localized skin infection for which she was prescribed oral antibiotics. Today she complains of a new-onset systemic maculopapular rash. She complains of intense pruritus but is in no acute distress. Her vital signs are within normal limits. A physical exam reveals diffuse small macules and papules. Which

of the following should be the priority treatment in this patient?
1. Prednisone 40 mg IV once, now.
2. Topical corticosteroid cream.
3. Diphenhydramine 50 mg IV once, now.
4. Immediate cessation of antibiotic treatment.

75. The adult-gerontology primary care NP knows development of which of the following is possible regarding use of tacrolimus (Protopic) topically for treatment of recurrent psoriasis or atopic dermatitis?
    1. Lymphoma.
    2. Staphylococcal scalded skin syndrome.
    3. Seborrheic dermatitis.
    4. Bullous pemphigoid.

76. On a return visit to the clinic, a patient receiving sulfonamide therapy exhibits generalized rash, mucous membrane lesions, skin sloughing on the palms and feet, high fever, and generalized malaise. These findings would alert the adult-gerontology primary care NP to consider:
    1. Hepatitis B.
    2. Stevens-Johnson syndrome.
    3. HIV infection/AIDS.
    4. *Pneumocystis carinii* pneumonia.

77. Which three treatments can be used for treatment of tinea versicolor?
    1. Selenium sulfide.
    2. Ciclopirox.
    3. Zinc pyrithione.
    4. Prednisone.
    5. Tretinoin.

78. While attending a rural public high school, an adolescent was bitten on the hand by a raccoon. At the rural clinic, the adult-gerontology primary care NP cleansed the wound. What would be the next action?
    1. Administer tetanus antitoxin.
    2. Contact local animal control authorities.
    3. Administer rabies immune globulin (RIG) and human diploid cell vaccine (HDCV).
    4. Teach the patient how to do hourly soaks to the hand using normal saline and peroxide.

8 Integumentary Answers & Rationales

Physical Exam & Diagnostic Tests

1. Answer: 2

    Rationale: Thinning of hair would be associated with normal age progression. Appearance of yellow nails would indicate a pathological process, notably a fungal infection. Brittle nails would also indicate a pathological process, notably related to vascular deficits. Absence of lesions does not correlate with the normal aging process. It is more likely that as a patient ages, lesions may become more prominent based on a combination of genetics, lifestyle, and environment.

2. Answer: 3, 4, 5

    Rationale: The presence of clubbing is an abnormal finding indicating compromise in perfusion that can originate from the pulmonary or cardiovascular system. Therefore, obtaining a pulse oximetry reading would provide evidence of a patient's current perfusion. An ECG could provide evidence of cardiac status in terms of rate and rhythm. A chest x-ray would provide evidence of the cardiac silhouette as well as lung fields, thus allowing for an overview of the patient's cardiac and respiratory status. Imaging studies of the hands would not necessarily reveal pathology, unless the practitioner suspected structural deformities. There is no evidence to support ordering orthostatic blood pressures in a patient who presents with clubbing, unless there is evidence of dizziness or fainting episodes.

3. Answer: 4

    Rationale: The term "annular" stems from the Latin word "annulus," meaning ringed. Lesions are circular or ovoid patches with a red periphery and central clearing (e.g., tinea corporis). Multiple groups of vesicles erupting unilaterally following the course of cutaneous nerves are described as herpetiform or zosteriform (herpes zoster). Linear lesions are arranged in a line (allergic contact dermatitis to poison ivy). Confluent lesions merge and are not discrete (scarlet fever rash).

4. Answer: 1

    Rationale: Psoriasis, peripheral vascular disease, diabetes, tuberculosis, and other infectious diseases, such as syphilis, are associated with pitting deformities of the nail that may vary from pinpoint to pinhead size and may be linear or irregular in distribution. Iron-deficiency anemia, eczema, malnutrition, and pellagra are associated

    with koilonychia (spoon nails). Hyperthyroidism and hypothyroidism are associated with onycholysis, which is a separation of the nail from the nail bed starting at the free edge and progressing proximally.

5. Answer: 3

    Rationale: Acanthosis nigricans (AN) typically occurs in patients who are obese or have diabetes and is a benign dermatosis characterized by velvety, hyperpigmented, hyperkeratotic plaques in body folds and creases (armpits, groin, and neck), which is associated with hyperinsulinemia and insulin resistance. A fasting blood glucose would be an appropriate diagnostic test to order.

6. Answer: 1

    Rationale: The place to inspect for jaundice is in that portion of the sclera that is observed when the eye is open. If jaundice is suspected, the posterior portion of the hard palate should be examined for a yellowish cast. Pallor and cyanosis can be noted in the nail beds, palms, and soles. Oral mucosa may be affected by surface stains.

7. Answer: 1

    Rationale: On an adult, the best place is just below the clavicle or on the abdomen.

8. Answer: 1

    Rationale: Fungal lesions will be visualized as a green-yellow fluorescence when viewed with the Wood lamp in a dimly lit room.

9. Answer: 1

    Rationale: A macule is less than 1 cm in diameter, nonpalpable, flat, and brown, red, purple, or tan (freckles, flat moles, rubella). A papule is elevated and palpable (warts, pigmented nevi). A nodule is 1–2 cm in diameter, solid, elevated, and deeper (lipoma). A wheal is elevated and irregular and has a variable diameter (insect bites, urticaria).

10. Answer: 2

    Rationale: Lichenification occurs with chronic irritation, often of an exposed extremity (chronic dermatitis). Crusts are dried exudate; scales are heaps of keratinized cells from exfoliation (psoriasis); and loss of epidermis is excoriation, as seen in an abrasion.

11. Answer: 3

    Rationale: The angle between the nail plate and the proximal nail fold when viewed from the side is >180 degrees and should form a diamond in clubbed nails. Normal nails form a 160-degree angle and should form a diamond shape between them when the nail beds of the index fingers are placed together. Transverse ridges and grooves may occur from trauma. Placing the palms together provides no assessment data. Diffuse discoloration may result from a fungal infection or an injury.

12. Answer: 3

    Rationale: Bulla is the correct term. A papule is solid. A vesicle is <1 cm in diameter, and a pustule contains a purulent exudate.

13. Answer: 4

    Rationale: The appearance of a new mole with high-risk features, including irregular border, color changes, and changes in sensation (e.g., pruritus), would necessitate immediate biopsy and/or referral to a dermatologist. Uniform moles, those that are symmetric and have smooth borders, and those not showing signs of change can be followed with annual skin assessments. Seborrheic keratosis is a benign skin growth, usually on sun-exposed areas, and appearing as waxy or "stuck-on" that requires no treatment.

14. Answer: 2

    Rationale: Under microscopic exam, fungal scrapings in 10% or 20% potassium hydroxide (KOH) solution will appear as threadlike hyphae crossing cell walls. The other solutions are not indicated to identify dermatophytes.

15. Answer: 3

    Rationale: It is important to remember to apply controls when skin testing the immunocompromised patient. A positive control test (histamine dichloride solution) is used to determine whether the patient reacts to histamine. If there is not an immediate reaction to histamine, the results of allergy skin tests can be difficult to interpret. A negative control test contains a solution (glycerinated saline) that does not contain histamine or allergen. If a reaction occurs, the skin is too sensitive to allow for correct interpretation of allergy skin tests.

Skin Disorders

16. Answer: 1

    Rationale: These lesions are most likely actinic keratosis. Actinic keratosis is a premalignant lesion at high risk of developing into squamous cell carcinoma of the skin. Actinic keratosis is most likely seen in sun-exposed areas and is described as a sandpaper-like lesion of a yellow to light brown coloration that may be erythematous. The patient should be referred to a dermatologist for further evaluation and removal of the lesion.

17. Answer: 1

    Rationale: Hot tub folliculitis caused by *Pseudomonas aeruginosa* should be suspected in any patient presenting with folliculitis and recent exposure to hot tubs. The infected area is most often in an area where wet clothing causes extended close contact with infected water. *Staphylococcus* should be suspected in patients without a known exposure or risk factor because it is the most common cause of folliculitis overall.

18. Answer: 3

    Rationale: Intense itching is characteristic of pediculosis pubis, scabies, and atopic dermatitis. Impetigo starts out as a tender erythematous papule and progresses through a vesicular to a honey-crusted stage with no itching.

19. Answer: 3

    Rationale: Urticaria arising from immunoglobulin E–mediated potential trigger could occur from food sensitivity/allergen exposure. Water intake and temperature elevations would be associated with nonimmunologically mediated causes. Flulike symptoms would be associated with non–immunoglobulin E–mediated causes due to presence of viral infection.

20. Answer: 2

    Rationale: A potential complication that can occur following activation of herpes zoster virus with an acute episode is the chronic progression to that of postherpetic neuralgia. Unlike with acute presentations, there is no evidence of customary lesions associated with shingles leading patients to present with pain presentations classified as allodynia. Phantom pain presents in patients with an amputation. Although most elderly patients present with atypical symptoms in the presence of urinary tract infections, on the basis of this patient's past medical history, it is more likely that she is experiencing a complication of herpes zoster. Tinea infection would present with a skin lesion finding.

21. Answer: 2

    Rationale: Herpes zoster typically presents with a history of tenderness followed by eruptions and vesicles that follow a dermatome on one side of the body. The condition is very painful. Other symptoms may include fever, headaches, and malaise. Psoriasis is characterized by thick, white, silvery, or red patches of skin. Contact dermatitis is a rash caused by touching something. Cellulitis is a skin infection characterized as red, hot, swollen, and tender skin.

22. Answer: 2

Rationale: Approximately 10%–30% of people with psoriasis develop an accompanying form of arthritis called psoriatic arthritis. The other options are dermatologic conditions that are not directly associated with arthritis.

23. Answer: 3

Rationale: Stress can aggravate psoriasis. Sunlight helps psoriasis, so it is usually better in the summer. It is not contagious, and only about 30% of patients with psoriasis have pruritus.

24. Answer: 2

Rationale: Actinic keratoses are potentially precancerous lesions that are commonly found in areas of skin exposed to sunlight.

25. Answer: 4

Rationale: Laboratory studies are not likely to be helpful in evaluation of urticaria. Identification of causes is usually based on history and physical findings. The other statements are true of urticaria.

26. Answer: 3

Rationale: Although any of these conditions can affect the skin, particularly of a patient who is HIV-positive, the description relates most closely to Kaposi sarcoma and warrants a biopsy.

27. Answer: 2

Rationale: Despite the name "dyshidrotic" eczematous dermatitis (bullous form called pompholyx), there is no evidence of sweating. Most patients have an atopic history, and emotional stress is often a precipitating factor in the appearance of the vesicles. Nummular (discoid) eczema is a chronic, pruritic, inflammatory dermatitis that occurs as coin-shaped plaques composed of papules and vesicles on an erythematous base. Rosacea is characterized by flushing and clusters of papulopustules on the cheek and forehead. Psoriasis is a hereditary disorder characterized by chronic, usually bilateral scaly plaques on exposed areas (knees, elbows). A verruca or common wart affects primarily young adults, is contagious, and is characterized by firm papules with a cleft surface and multiple conical vegetations.

28. Answer: 4

Rationale: Delay wound closure until determination of no infection in approximately 24–48 hours. Mouth flora of humans is abundant, and a bite carries the risk of heavy bacterial inoculum and severe infection. Antibiotics are indicated. A Td booster should be given every 10 years. Tdap may be given as one of these boosters if the patient has never received Tdap before. Typically, one dose of Tdap is routinely given at age 11 or 12 years. People who did not get Tdap at that age should get it as soon as possible. Tdap may also be given after a severe cut or burn to prevent tetanus infection.

29. Answer: 2

Rationale: Onychomycosis is the correct term. Hippocratic nails are clubbed nails and fingers associated with chronic heart and lung disorders. Koilonychia is a concavity of the nail plate often associated with iron-deficiency anemia. Anonychia is a total congenital absence of the nail.

30. Answer: 2

Rationale: In case of suspected drug reactions, it is recommended that the drug be eliminated and documented in the patient's record so that it is not reintroduced.

31. Answer: 4

Rationale: Excessive sweating may be normal, but a history and physical exam are needed to rule out underlying causes. Therapies can be offered. Drysol is for use only on the feet and axilla.

32. Answer: 3

Rationale: The assessment describes a seborrheic keratosis. The actinic keratosis is an irregular, rough, scaly, white-to-erythematous macular lesion found most often on sun-exposed areas, such as on the dorsal surface of the hands, arms, neck, and face. It has malignant potential. The basal cell carcinoma is a smooth, round nodule with a pearly gray border and central induration. Senile lentigines are gray-brown, irregular, macular lesions on sun-exposed areas of the face, arms, and hands.

33. Answer: 3

Rationale: Herpes zoster (shingles) is a vesicular dermatomal eruption related to a reactivation of latent varicella virus. It increases with advanced age and is characterized by burning pain and paresthesia along one or two dermatomes, not crossing the midline, and may be accompanied by fever, malaise, or headache. The vesicular stage lasts 2–3 weeks. The vesicles are initially clear or blood filled and become purulent. The area along the dermatome is erythematous, and the vesicles crust and then scab, which may leave hypopigmented scars. The other options discuss painless lesions and are not specific to this prodromal stage.

34. Answer: 4

    Rationale: These are classic signs of a basal cell carcinoma, also supported by the patient's employment history. Melanoma would be pigmented; compound nevus would not be firm or have telangiectasia; and bullous pemphigoid results in bullous lesions.

35. Answer: 3

    Rationale: Refer this patient immediately to a dermatologist because the findings are highly suspicious for a melanoma. A punch biopsy should never be done on a suspected melanoma, and any delay could be detrimental to the outcome.

36. Answer: 2

    Rationale: Oral acyclovir is very effective in reducing the intensity and duration of the symptoms if started early in the course of the disease. Herpes zoster does not usually recur at regular intervals but frequently lasts for several weeks. Once the rash has developed crusts, the person is no longer contagious. Shingles is less contagious than chickenpox, and the risk of a person with shingles spreading the virus is low if the rash is covered.

37. Answer: 3

    Rationale: The patient presents with a classic case of pityriasis rosea, a benign, self-limiting skin eruption of unknown etiology. Although a medication/allergen history would be warranted, referral to an allergy specialist or dermatologist would not be necessary. Triamcinolone would not be indicated, because the treatment is mainly symptomatic. Sunlight in moderate amounts has been shown to hasten healing in some patients.

38. Answer: 3

    Rationale: The signs and symptoms presented are classic for Lyme disease, which is transmitted by ticks. Therefore, it would be important to inquire about potential exposure to ticks before the signs and symptoms developed. Exposure to new skin care products would be important if the practitioner suspected an allergic reaction, which is not consistent with the signs and symptoms. Although always important, a thorough medication history probably will not reveal the cause of the signs and symptoms in this case. Tuberculosis does not present in this manner.

39. Answer: 2

    Rationale: Insects reproduce, are more active, and are present in greater numbers in the warm months of spring to early fall.

40. Answer: 2

    Rationale: Heat application is contraindicated; ice packs are preferred, as is elevation, to decrease the edema. The area should be immobilized. Tdap or Td may be given along with antihistamines to reduce swelling and relieve itching.

41. Answer: 4

    Rationale: This was a venomous coral snake bite. The typical symptoms are those listed, as well as nausea, vomiting, and muscle fasciculations.

42. Answer: 3, 4, 5

    Rationale: A "herald patch" usually appears on the skin first. This is usually an oval- or round-shaped patch which can vary from 2 to 5 cm in diameter and is salmon-colored with fine scales. It is followed within days by a regional outbreak of numerous smaller erythematous patches, thus providing a key diagnostic clue with smaller lesions oriented along skin cleavage areas (Langer lines) in a "Christmas tree" pattern. It most commonly appears on the chest or upper back, although it can sometimes appear on the abdomen, neck, back, thigh, or upper arms. Mild pruritus occurs, which typically causes the patient to seek medical assistance.

43. Answer: 1

    Rationale: The location and appearance of the lesions are typical of scabies. A rash causes little bumps that often form a line that are approximately 2- to 3 mm long and the width of a hair. The inflammatory lesions are erythematous and pruritic papules most commonly located in the finger webs, flexor surfaces of the wrists, elbows, axillae, buttocks, genitalia, feet, and ankles. The older adult may itch more severely with fewer cutaneous lesions and is at risk for extensive infestations, probably related to a decline in cell-mediated immunity. In addition, there may be back involvement in those who are bedridden.

44. Answer: 4

    Rationale: Atopic dermatitis in adults may be generalized; however, it frequently appears in the creases of the elbows or knees, dorsa of the feet, and nape of the neck in adults, who may have late-onset dermatitis or experience a relapse of a childhood condition. Localized eczema (e.g., chronic hand or foot dermatitis, eyelid dermatitis, or lichen simplex chronicus) may continue throughout adulthood; typically, atopic dermatitis declines with increasing age.

45. Answer: 1

    Rationale: Seborrheic dermatitis is usually salmon in color and has a red, greasy appearance with thick adherent crusts and indistinct margins. There is minimal pruritus. In adults, it is most commonly located in hairy skin areas: scalp and scalp margins, eyebrows and eyelid margins, nasolabial folds, ears and retroauricular folds, presternal area, middle to upper back, buttock crease, inguinal area, genitals, and armpits. Rashes in atopic dermatitis and eczema are pink, or red if inflamed, and have a whiter, nongreasy appearance. Scalp psoriasis is more sharply demarcated than seborrheic dermatitis and has crusted, infiltrated plaques rather than mild scaling and erythema. Rosacea is characterized by facial flushing, erythema, papules, pustules, and telangiectasia in a symmetric, central facial distribution and is uncommon in older adults (over 60 years of age).

46. Answer: 4

Rationale: Brown recluse spiders produce sharp pain at the instant of the bite, with subsequent minor swelling and erythema. Tissue necrosis may occur within the next 24–96 hours. A blue-gray to black macular halo may surround the bite, with eventual widening and sinking of the center of the lesion, leading to a "sinking infarct." This leaves a deep ulcer that requires weeks or months to heal.

47. Answer: 1

Rationale: With regard to appearance, use of laser or sclerotherapy is the best practice option to decrease the appearance of varicosities. Debridement is not recommended, because there is no indication of vascular compromise. The patient reports no clinical symptoms related to the varicosities, so the use of supportive compression stockings would not be indicated, as they would not reduce the patient's cosmetic concerns. Hydrotherapy is not an acceptable treatment for varicosities.

48. Answer: 3

Rationale: Actinic keratosis is considered to be a precancerous lesion, and topical chemotherapy is indicated for the affected areas. Hydrotherapy is not suggested as a treatment option. Cryotherapy can be used as a treatment option along with photodynamic therapy, scraping, or curettage.

49. Answer: 2

Rationale: Deep puncture wounds are more likely to become infected with anaerobic organisms. The narrow, sharp feline incisors deeply puncture tissue and may easily penetrate a bone or joint. Bites on the hand have the highest infection rate, whereas bites on the face have the lowest rate.

50. Answer: 1

Rationale: Amoxicillin-clavulanate is an excellent choice for the empiric treatment of animal bites. Cephalexin is not indicated, because of resistant strains of *Pasteurella multocida,* an organism present in 25% of dog bites and 50% of cat bites. Avoid first-generation cephalosporins (e.g., ce-

phalexin), penicillinase-resistant penicillins (e.g., dicloxacillin), macrolides (e.g., erythromycin), and clindamycin when it is not administered with another medication, as these medications are not effective against *Pasteurella multocida.* An infected bite should be followed daily until the infection clears. Open wound management is indicated, not suturing.

51. Answer: 4

Rationale: In addition to these symptoms, bronchospasm, hypertension, seizures, and altered mental status may occur. Black eschar is associated with a brown recluse spider bite. Rash with bump or boil is typical of a bug bite.

Pharmacology

52. Answer: 3

Rationale: Lyme disease is caused by the spirochete *Borrelia* species and is transmitted by the *Ixodes* tick, endemic to the eastern United States. Nymphal (young) ticks more commonly transmit the disease than adults and are unlikely to transmit the bacteria until after 48–72 hours of attachment. Prophylactic one-time treatment with doxycycline 200 mg PO is indicated only if the tick is positively identified as an *Ixodes* tick, the tick has been attached for 36 hours or longer (or a known exposure within the same time), and the patient resides in an endemic area. Endemic areas include the eastern United States but specifically the northeastern states and Great Lakes areas, including portions of Minnesota and Wisconsin. Serologic testing is not indicated, as early diagnostic indicators such as IgM antibodies to *Borrelia* will not begin appearing until 1–2 weeks after infection.

53. Answer: 1

Rationale: Antiviral therapy with acyclovir 800 mg 5 times daily for 7 days may expedite healing if started within 2–3 days of onset, especially in immunocompromised individuals. Miconazole and clotrimazole are antifungal creams. Prednisone would only be used to decrease the incidence of postherpetic neuralgia and may increase the incidence of disseminated infection, so it is not recommended during the acute phase.

54. Answer: 1, 3, 4

Rationale: Initial therapy in treatment of seborrheic dermatitis of the face includes topical low-potency corticosteroids, including hydrocortisone, as well as topical antifungals, including ketoconazole and ciclopirox. Systemic medications and higher-potency topical corticosteroids, such as clobetasol, are not indicated for initial therapy or uncomplicated disease.

55. Answer: 1

   Rationale: The description is consistent with intertriginous candidiasis, which is treated with an antifungal ointment or oral medication. It is not a staphylococcal infection; the area needs to be kept dry, not moist. An antibiotic ointment will not relieve the problem. Herpes zoster is treated with antiviral medications; this case is not described as particularly painful, and it is bilateral.

56. Answer: 2, 3, 4

   Rationale: The presence of psoriasis on the scalp can be extensive, leading to scaling of the entire scalp. Included in the plan of care to treat scaling, one should use topical therapies such as coal tar ointment, emollients, and/or topical vitamin D analogues. Vigorous scalp massage would be contraindicated because that could lead to more discomfort and irritation. The process of removal of scales is done gently to facilitate response of medication to the surface area. Fluid replacement is not indicated in the treatment of psoriasis.

57. Answer: 1

   Rationale: Beta blockers can exacerbate psoriasis. They are believed to decrease cAMP-dependent protein kinase, an inhibitor of cell proliferation. Drugs in the other classifications have no known effect on psoriasis.

58. Answer: 3

   Rationale: The patient most likely has orbital cellulitis due to low-grade fever and pain with ocular movements compared with preseptal cellulitis. Orbital cellulitis should be treated more aggressively, including vancomycin plus ceftriaxone, cefotaxime, ampicillin-sulbactam, or piperacillin-tazobactam. Immediate treatment is indicated due to the risk of possible intracranial invasion. The other answer choices are for secondary treatment or for treatment of preseptal (periorbital) cellulitis.

59. Answer: 3

   Rationale: Acyclovir treats the acute phase during initial eruption of vesicular lesions and offers no benefit for postherpetic pain.

60. Answer: 2

   Rationale: The patient in this scenario likely has scabies, caused by the *Sarcoptes scabiei* mite. Treatment is aimed at both symptom relief and prevention of transmission. Treatment should include either permethrin 5% cream or oral ivermectin. For severe cases, combination treatment may be used. Other treatment choices include crotamiton, malathion, or lindane. Lindane is indicated only as an alternative therapy due to risk of serious side effects.

61. Answer: 4

   Rationale: Pediculosis is more common in children but can regularly be seen in long-term care facilities and older adults living in close quarters. Pediculosis is caused by the head louse (*Pediculus humanus capitis*). Initial treatments include over-the-counter pyrethrins, such as pyrethrin shampoo and permethrin lotion. Prescription medications include ivermectin lotion, benzyl alcohol lotion, malathion lotion, and spinosad topical suspension. The medication lindane has been restricted to use as a second-line agent due to the risk of serious side effects and should be limited to one use. Additional care, including washing linens and clothing, should be instituted. Crisaborole (Eucrisa) is a new medication approved in December 2016 for the treatment of atopic dermatitis and would not be indicated.

62. Answer: 2

   Rationale: It is important to note that mupirocin (Bactroban) is a more effective treatment of MRSA infections. Mupirocin is indicated for use for topical skin infections, as surgical skin prophylaxis, or intranasally to eliminate MRSA colonization. Bacitracin is indicated for skin infections but has been shown to have decreased effectiveness against MRSA infections. Other topical anti-infectious agents include retapamulin (Altabax) and combinations of bacitracin with neomycin and polymyxin B.

63. Answer: 2

   Rationale: Pemphigus vulgaris is an autoimmune disease in which antibodies are formed against dystonin in hemidesmosomes in the skin. This results in painful and sometimes fatal blistering of the skin. Pemphigus vulgaris has a variable course, and the goal of therapy should be to minimize further blister formation as well as to promote healing. High-potency topical glucocorticoids, such as clobetasol, as well as systemic glucocorticoids are first-line treatments. Patients who achieve remission for more than 2 months should be evaluated for discontinuation of therapy or ongoing therapy at the lowest dose to prevent relapse. It is important to always taper long-term glucocorticoids. Additional immunosuppressive agents (tacrolimus) would not be indicated for this patient, because he has been asymptomatic for 9 years and has been tolerating glucocorticoids.

64. Answer: 3

   Rationale: Patients need to be instructed to wash off podophyllin. It should be applied sparingly, only to the wart and avoiding normal skin, and allowed to dry thoroughly before the patient dresses. No rationale exists to treat with both liquid nitrogen and podophyllin.

65. Answer: 1, 2, 4, 5

Rationale: Certain medications, such as clonidine (Catapres), ondansetron (Zofran), and propranolol (Inderal), can help to decrease facial flushing. Furosemide (Lasix) does not have any reported effect on facial flushing. Niacin or vitamin B_3 can cause facial flushing due to vasodilation effects.

66. Answer: 3

Rationale: Diuretic agents may cause elderly patients to experience systemic pruritus. Topical emollients would not cause pruritus, but rather would be used to decrease symptomatic complaints. Corticosteroids and antihistamines also would be effective in decreasing symptomatic complaints.

67. Answer: 3

Rationale: Systemic treatment with low-dose tetracycline is very effective for rosacea; topical treatment with metronidazole or low-dose hydrocortisone may also be useful. Oral cortisone and antifungal agents are not known to be effective. Topical 5-fluorouracil is used in the treatment of actinic keratosis, a precancerous skin condition.

68. Answer: 2

Rationale: Folliculitis of the axilla without other risk factors or exposures is most likely caused by *Staphylococcus aureus*. Medical treatment is not usually indicated in singular eruptions of folliculitis. Patients with multiple sites or moderate skin involvement should first be treated with topical mupirocin and clindamycin. Oral antimicrobials are indicated for refractory or severe cases, including beta-lactam antibiotics, TMP/SMX, clindamycin, or doxycycline for 7–10 days.

69. Answer: 4

Rationale: The mainstay of treatment of celiac disease is removal of gluten-containing products from the diet and oral dapsone (Aczone) for the treatment of dermatitis herpetiformis. Some patients may also be treated with topical corticosteroids as a secondary treatment or if intolerant to dapsone. Dapsone may cause hemolysis in patients with G6PD deficiency. Tazarotene is a topical retinoid indicated for treatment of acne and psoriasis.

70. Answer: 1

Rationale: The maximum allowable dose for adults is 4.5 mg/kg of lidocaine with epinephrine and 5 mg/kg of lidocaine without epinephrine. Although local anesthetics are often used, the maximum allowable doses are rarely emphasized, and overdose can result in anaphylactic shock.

71. Answer: 2

Rationale: Skin tears are seen in the frail elderly population, and therapeutic treatment should be focused on maintaining hydration of the skin. Diuretic therapy could lead to dehydration. Baby aspirin therapy is unrelated to the appearance of skin tears. Antibiotic therapy would be used only if infection was suspected or identified upon examination.

72. Answer: 1

Rationale: Amitriptyline in low doses is effective in treating neuropathic pain. Nonsteroidal antiinflammatory drugs (NSAIDs) may also be effective in treating the inflammatory component of herpes zoster pain. The most effective nonpharmacologic method of treating pain from shingles is the application of cool compresses. Heat may exacerbate neuropathic pain in some patients. Antidepressants and anticonvulsants are effective adjuvant therapies in the treatment of neuropathic pain.

73. Answer: 2, 4, 5

Rationale: Aluminum chloride hexahydrate (Drysol, Hypercare) is a common topical treatment for hyperhidrosis. It should be applied directly to the affected area at bedtime on only clean, dry skin and may be held in place with a snug-fitting shirt or plastic wrap for maximum effectiveness. This medication should not be applied to broken or recently shaved skin due to the risk of irritation. Common side effects include discomfort or a stinging sensation of the skin that may subside over time. Patients with skin irritation should discontinue treatment.

74. Answer: 4

Rationale: The patient most likely has experienced morbilliform (drug-induced) drug eruption, also commonly called an exanthematous drug eruption, which is a type IV hypersensitivity reaction that typically occurs 5–14 days after treatment. Many medications can cause reactions, but antibiotics like penicillin, cephalosporins, macrolides, quinolones, and TMP/SMX are some of the most commonly implicated. Treatment priorities involve first stopping the offending agent followed by symptomatic treatment with corticosteroids and/or antihistamines. Immediate treatment with diphenhydramine or systemic corticosteroids would not be indicated, because this patient is clearly not experiencing an acute reaction.

75. Answer: 1

   Rationale: Tacrolimus is a calcineurin inhibitor that inhibits T-cell activation. Calcineurin inhibitors are second-line agents used as treatment for refractory psoriasis and atopic dermatitis. A black box warning was added in 2006 due to a possible risk of cutaneous malignancy development. For this reason, tacrolimus should be limited in treatment and used as a second-line agent. Systemic tacrolimus administration should be given only under the care of a provider familiar with immunosuppressive therapies due to significant risk of side effects, including neurotoxicity, renal toxicity, and increased infection risk.

76. Answer: 2

   Rationale: Stevens-Johnson syndrome is a severe form of erythema multiforme that can be fatal. The clinical picture is mucous membrane lesions, conjunctival and corneal lesions, fever, malaise, arthralgia, and sloughing of the skin of the hands and feet. Distinguishing characteristics of the syndrome are eruption of vesicles, mucosal ulcerations, and sloughing skin.

77. Answer: 1, 2, 3

   Rationale: Tinea versicolor (pityriasis versicolor) is a common skin infection caused by the fungal organism *Malassezia furfur*. Treatment involves topical antifungals (azoles, ciclopirox, terbinafine), selenium sulfide, and zinc pyrithione. Systemic antifungals are reserved for recurrent or extensive presentations. Patients should be educated that treatment may take several months to resolve symptoms. Treatment with corticosteroids or a retinoid would be ineffective.

78. Answer: 3

   Rationale: Any bite potentially associated with an animal that may harbor rabies (skunks, bats, raccoons, foxes, coyotes, and rats) should be treated with both active and passive rabies immunization. Tetanus antitoxin would be indicated if the patient was not current on the immunization. Animal authorities would be called after the initial treatment to locate the animal and euthanize it so that the brain could be examined for rabies, but this should not delay prophylactic treatment.

Endocrine

9

Physical Examination & Diagnostic Tests

1. With nearly 70% of the adult population being overweight, including obesity, it is important to distinguish a bulge of subcutaneous fat at the base of the neck from a goiter. Which of the following statements is true regarding how to differentiate them?
   1. Swallowing cannot be relied upon, as both tissues move up and down when drinking fluid.
   2. Fat layers remain in a fixed position, but a thyroid gland moves up and down while drinking.
   3. Goiters are typically visibly defined from the lateral position of observation.
   4. Fatty tissue appears to be less prominent when observed from the side compared with an enlarged thyroid.

2. What is the correct procedure for palpation of a patient's thyroid gland?
   1. Stand behind the patient, hyperextend the head, and palpate both sides simultaneously.
   2. Have the patient lower the chin and tilt the head slightly toward the side being evaluated.
   3. Hyperextend the head and have the patient lean away from the side being evaluated.
   4. Have the patient lean away from the side being examined and take a swallow of water.

3. A 16-year-old adolescent with diabetes is noncompliant with consuming a healthy diet. In addition, the adult-gerontology primary care NP notes that he seems unconcerned about any consequences of his activities, such as riding a motorcycle without a helmet. Which factor is typical of adolescence and pertinent to this adolescent's overall health?
   1. Less involvement with parents.
   2. Less dominant role with peer group.
   3. Secure sense of self and high self-esteem.
   4. Experimenting with risky behaviors.

4. When a patient sips water and swallows, the thyroid gland:
   1. Moves downward and slightly posterior, and feels smooth on palpation.
   2. Elongates and enlarges during the swallow and immediately returns to a resting position.
   3. Moves slightly out during the sipping and backward during the swallowing.
   4. Moves upward during the swallow and feels symmetric and smooth to palpation.

5. Which characteristics of skin, hair, and nails are correctly listed for the thyroid condition?
   1. Thin nails and coarse and dry but warm skin are associated with hyperthyroidism.
   2. Thicker nails, coarse skin, and hair that breaks off easily are linked with hypothyroidism.
   3. Fine hair, coarse skin, and onycholysis of the nails are found with hyperthyroidism.
   4. Puffy facies, brittle nails, and hyperpigmented skin are associated with hypothyroidism.

6. Select the facial feature description linked with the correct endocrine pathology:
   1. Coarse facial features, heavier brow line, and prominent jaw: acromegaly.
   2. "Moon face," extra hair growth on the upper lip and chin with acne on the back and chest: acromegaly.
   3. Wide-eyed look with nervous tic and bulging eyes: hypothyroidism.
   4. Lid lag, moist skin, periorbital puffiness: hypothyroidism.

7. The laboratory value that points most directly to parathyroid abnormality is:
   1. Low TSH.
   2. Elevated calcium.
   3. Elevated magnesium.
   4. Depressed phosphate.

8. While conducting the interview for a physical exam, the adult-gerontology primary care NP identifies which finding in the patient's history as being commonly associated with thyroid carcinoma?
   1. Family history of thyroid cancer.
   2. History of hyperthyroidism.
   3. Irradiation of the neck.
   4. Smoking for 15 years.

9. When doing a physical exam on a patient with hyperthyroidism, a common neurologic finding is:
   1. Memory, attention, and problem-solving deficits.
   2. Diminished deep tendon reflexes.
   3. Severe cognitive impairment.
   4. Delusions and psychosis.

10. The treatment goal for glycemic control in a person with type 2 diabetes is to achieve and maintain hemoglobin A1C level (HgbA1C) of:
    1. <10%.
    2. 6%–9%.
    3. <7%.
    4. >8%.

11. Which finding would alert the adult-gerontology primary care NP that a patient might be experiencing a problem with the endocrine system?
    1. Coagulation abnormalities and fatigue.
    2. Growth abnormalities and glucose intolerance.
    3. Hypoxia and jaundice.
    4. Steatorrhea and abdominal distention.

12. The adult-gerontology primary care NP notes a solitary thyroid nodule on a patient during a routine physical exam. The next step for diagnostic testing is:
    1. Thyroid scan and antibody level.
    2. TSH level and ultrasound.
    3. X-ray film of the thyroid.
    4. Fine-needle aspiration (FNA) biopsy.

13. An adult female patient presents to the adult-gerontology primary care NP's office complaining of fatigue, weakness, and weight gain over the past 4 months. Physical exam reveals elevated blood pressure (BP), facial and supraclavicular fullness, hirsutism noted on the face, proximal muscle weakness, and facial and truncal distribution of acne. Appropriate laboratory tests the adult-gerontology primary care NP should order include:
    1. Antinuclear antibody (ANA) and rheumatoid factor (RF).
    2. Three-hour glucose tolerance test and lipid profile.
    3. RBC count and a calcium level.
    4. Dexamethasone suppression test, urinary-free cortisol level, and TSH and T_4.

14. The adult-gerontology primary care NP would anticipate which laboratory values in the patient with Graves disease?
    1. TSH levels to be increased.
    2. TSH levels to be decreased.
    3. TSH levels to be within normal limits (WNL).
    4. T_4 levels to be decreased.

15. Which information is correct regarding foot screening using a nylon filament (5.07-gauge Semmes-Weinstein)?
    1. Use a 25-g filament and apply along the perimeter of any scar or ulcer tissue.
    2. Apply the filament at a 45-degree angle to the skin surface.
    3. Apply sufficient force for approximately 1.5 seconds to cause the filament to bend.
    4. Slide the filament across the skin and make repetitive contact with each of the 10 sites.

16. What two abnormal imaging studies should prompt the adult-gerontology primary care NP to perform an assessment for primary parathyroid dysfunction?
    1. Improving DEXA (bone density) scores in conjunction with bisphosphonate therapy.
    2. Early poor bone density scores in premenopausal women.
    3. Thyroid nodule scan that shows the nodule is not "hot" (is not actively producing thyroid hormone).
    4. Kidney stone noted on KUB film (kidneys, ureter, bladder).
    5. X-ray of the pelvis showing "Brim sign."

17. To make the diagnosis of diabetes, the patient must have two fasting plasma glucose levels documented on two occasions greater than or equal to:
    1. 200 mg/dL.
    2. 140 mg/dL.
    3. 126 mg/dL.
    4. 110 mg/dL.

Disorders

18. The adult-gerontology primary care NP is planning to teach a client with newly diagnosed diabetes about his condition. Before the adult-gerontology primary care NP provides instruction, what is most important to evaluate? The patient's:
    1. Required dietary modifications.
    2. Understanding of the exchange list.
    3. Ability to administer insulin.
    4. Present understanding of diabetes.

19. The etiology of type 1 diabetes can be best described as:
    1. An autosomal dominant genetic disorder.
    2. Autoimmune destruction of the beta cells.
    3. Overnutrition and resulting obesity as the major risk factor.
    4. Prevented by exercise, which increases the concentration of insulin receptors.

20. Dehydration during hot outdoor temperatures is accelerated by interruption of ADH (antidiuretic hormone) by the ingestion of:
    1. Sugar.
    2. Salt.
    3. Alcohol.
    4. Grilled meats.

21. The adult-gerontology primary care NP understands that acromegaly is typically caused by:
    1. Hypersecretion of benign pituitary tumors.
    2. Hyposecretion of pituitary hormones.
    3. Hypersecretion of adrenal cortex hormones.
    4. Metastatic tumors within the pituitary.

22. A patient has been diagnosed with diabetes for more than 5 years. To whom should the adult-gerontology primary care NP maintain an annual referral for this patient?
    1. Cardiologist.
    2. Dietitian.
    3. Vascular surgeon.
    4. Ophthalmologist.

23. Hirsutism presenting in a female with normal menstruation and normal plasma androgens is most likely:
    1. An ovarian tumor.
    2. Cushing syndrome.
    3. Idiopathic.
    4. Polycystic ovary disease.

24. Pathophysiologic causes of decreased testosterone levels develop in the:
    1. Hypothalamus.
    2. Anterior pituitary.
    3. Testes.
    4. All the above.

25. **QSEN** When counseling a patient with diabetes on foot care, it is important to emphasize:
    1. Daily foot soaks in warm, soapy water.
    2. Careful daily foot inspections.
    3. Trimming corns and calluses regularly.
    4. Trimming toenails close to the nail bed.

26. An adult patient presents to the adult-gerontology primary care NP for evaluation of polyuria, polydipsia, and weight loss. Which laboratory result would require immediate intervention by the adult-gerontology primary care NP?
    1. A1C of 14%.
    2. Serum glucose of 150 mg/dL.
    3. A1C of 6.0%.
    4. Serum glucose of 65 mg/dL.

27. An adult patient is being evaluated for hypoglycemia because of a blood sugar level of 58 mg/dL. The adult-gerontology primary care NP would begin the differential diagnosis by:
    1. Deciding if the hypoglycemia is fasting or postprandial.
    2. Ascertaining if it is related to alcohol use.
    3. Deciding if the patient has other medical problems.
    4. Reassuring the patient that it is a benign problem.

28. An older adult male patient complains of lethargy, cold intolerance, weight gain, and yellowing of the palms. The most important laboratory study ordered by the adult-gerontology primary care NP in diagnosing this condition is:
    1. Complete blood count.
    2. Liver enzymes.
    3. Thyroid panel.
    4. Cardiac enzymes.

29. A middle-aged, normally healthy female presents for evaluation of intermittent palpitations. She also reports mood variability, tremulousness, difficulty falling asleep, and a 10-lb weight loss despite a normal appetite. She feels warm most of the time and wonders if she is perimenopausal. She has no history of heart disease. The objective data that would yield the most useful information would be:
    1. Electrocardiogram (ECG).
    2. TSH, free T_4.
    3. Electrolytes.
    4. Serum hormone level.

30. An adult woman presents to the clinic complaining of fatigue, weakness, weight gain despite lack of appetite, and feelings of depression. Physical exam reveals an obese, alert patient with thinning hair, bilateral chest puffiness, increased facial hair, supraclavicular fat pad, thin arms and legs, purple striae on the abdomen, and multiple ecchymotic areas on the extremities. Her vital signs are BP of 158/96 mm Hg, pulse of 88 beats/min, and respiration of 22 breaths/min. Laboratory results show FBS of 200 mg/dL and an electrolyte panel within normal limits (WNL), except for potassium of 3.0 mEq/L, hemoglobin of 11.8 g, and hematocrit of 34%. This assessment information would support the adult-gerontology primary care NP's diagnosis of:
    1. Addison disease.
    2. Pheochromocytoma.
    3. Cushing syndrome.
    4. Hypoaldosteronism.

31. Due to its position in the base of the brain and its impact on the optic structures, tumors of the pituitary gland frequently manifest as:
    1. Exophthalmos.
    2. Loss of vision in half of the visual field.
    3. Ocular muscle disturbances.
    4. Loss of central vision.

32. Clinical findings in a patient with hypothyroidism include:
    1. Hyperactive bowel sounds.
    2. Oily skin and acne.
    3. Postural tremors of the hands.
    4. Edema of the face and eyelids.

33. A young adult male reports anxiety, tremulousness, headaches, palpitations, and sweating 2–4 hours after eating. Physical exam is normal. No lab results are currently available. No medical conditions are noted in the history. What is the most likely diagnosis?
    1. Dumping syndrome.
    2. Hypoglycemia.
    3. Alcohol abuse.
    4. Hyperthyroidism.

34. A woman comes to your office complaining about adrenal fatigue because she has had continuous stress in the past year. What do you know about this condition?
    1. It is an "Internet diagnosis" not recognized by the scientific community as a formal syndrome.
    2. It is another term for laboratory-confirmed subclinical adrenal insufficiency.
    3. It is a constellation of symptoms commonly found in individuals who have adrenal gland secretion higher than usual levels.
    4. It is the most common complaint in persons seeking opiate drugs.

35. Which of the following is the most likely etiology for hypercalcemia in the medically well asymptomatic adult?
    1. Hyperthyroidism.
    2. Hyperparathyroidism.
    3. Hyperpituitarism.
    4. Hypothyroidism.

36. A middle-aged male with no previous medical history presents with a 30-lb weight gain in 2.5 months. He denies any medication use or allergies. He was recently laid off from a very active job and has been sedentary. Physical exam reveals BP of 172/111 mm Hg, central obesity, and FBS of 200 mg/dL. What is the most likely cause of the patient's weight gain?
    1. Cushing syndrome.
    2. Hypothyroidism.
    3. Depression.
    4. Diabetes.

37. A middle-aged woman presents with agitation, confusion, fever, tachycardia, and diaphoresis. Her daughter states that nausea, vomiting, and abdominal pain preceded these symptoms. The patient has no history of cardiac disease, diabetes, or substance abuse. She was started on some "antidrug" 2 weeks ago and is scheduled for some form of throat surgery next week (per her daughter). Based on this history, the adult-gerontology primary care NP immediately orders:
    1. TSH, T_4.
    2. Urinalysis.
    3. Spinal tap.
    4. Computed tomography of the head.

38. A 45-year-old female patient presents to the office complaining of a 6-month history of fatigue, 15-lb weight gain, lethargy, an inability to tolerate cold temperatures, forgetfulness, hair loss, and constipation. Physical exam findings include dry, coarse skin; periorbital edema and puffy facies; bradycardia; hyporeflexia and muscle weakness; and a smooth, goitrous thyroid. The adult-gerontology primary care NP would make the diagnosis of:
    1. Heart failure.
    2. Diabetes mellitus.
    3. Hypothyroidism.
    4. Thyroid cancer.

39. A patient with diabetes has been taking 6 U of regular insulin and 12 U of NPH insulin in the morning. In the evening, she has been taking 3 U of regular insulin and 8 U of NPH insulin. The patient has been monitoring her blood glucose levels (mg/dL) and shows the adult-gerontology primary care NP the following chart:

	7:00 AM	Noon	5:00 PM	Bedtime
Monday	100	76	98	109
Tuesday	119	75	88	110
Wednesday	119	66	86	100
Thursday	123	70	111	122
Friday	128	60	99	110

The adult-gerontology primary care NP adjusts the patient's insulin by:
    1. Increasing the regular insulin.
    2. Decreasing the regular insulin.
    3. Decreasing the NPH insulin.
    4. Increasing both insulins.

40. The role of the adult-gerontology primary care NP in the initial management of a patient with a thyroid nodule involves:
    1. Referring the patient to an endocrinologist for further evaluation.
    2. Obtaining fine-needle aspiration (FNA) biopsy of the nodule and sending it to cytology.
    3. Ordering an ultrasound and a thyroid panel.
    4. Ordering levothyroxine (Synthroid) to reduce the size of the nodule.

41. Once considered a "rare occurrence" or cause of hypertension, it is now recognized that what percentage of hypertensive patients have a component of adrenal gland disease?
    1. 5%.
    2. 10%–20%.
    3. 30%–50%.
    4. >50%.

42. When teaching a patient with diabetes about "sick day" guidelines, the adult-gerontology primary care NP explains that the patient should:
    1. Stop measuring blood glucose and only check urine for ketones.
    2. Not take the usual dose of insulin at the usual time.
    3. Be sure to take metformin (Glucophage) and acarbose (Precose), even if nausea and vomiting are present.
    4. Administer extra doses of regular insulin according to instructions for blood glucose levels above 240 mg/dL.

43. A young adult female patient presents to the clinic with complaints of nervousness, tremulousness, palpitations, heat intolerance, fatigue, weight loss, and polyphagia. After a complete history and physical, along with thyroid function tests, the adult-gerontology primary care NP makes the diagnosis of hyperthyroidism, recognizing that the most common cause of this condition is:
    1. Thyroid cancer.
    2. Graves disease.
    3. Pituitary adenoma.
    4. Postpartum thyroiditis.

44. A young adult male patient presents to the office stating that he found a lump in his neck while shaving. Physical exam reveals a firm, 2-cm nodule that is fixed, nontender, and located on the right lobe of the thyroid gland. Right posterior cervical lymphadenopathy is also noted. The adult-gerontology primary care NP should:
    1. Order a TSH level and ultrasound and refer the patient to a surgeon for a possible fine-needle aspiration (FNA) biopsy of the nodule.
    2. No intervention is necessary at this time; schedule a follow-up visit in 6 months.
    3. Prescribe levothyroxine (Synthroid) 0.1 mg PO daily and schedule a 6-week follow-up visit.
    4. Immediately ablate the patient's thyroid with radioactive iodine and refer him to an endocrinologist.

45. A patient with Graves disease is to have radioactive iodine (I^{131}) therapy. Which information is important for the adult-gerontology primary care NP to include when teaching about this treatment?
    1. Patients are highly radioactive for approximately 7 days after treatment and need to be isolated.

2. Patients should not become pregnant during or after receiving this therapy because of the teratogenic effects to the fetus that occur due to chromosomal abnormalities.
    3. Patients may become hypothyroid after this treatment and therefore need to have regular TSH and T_4 levels drawn, with the potential for thyroid hormone replacement therapy.
    4. This therapy is contraindicated in patients with cardiac disease.

46. During an evaluation of a patient with prediabetes (glucose intolerance), the adult-gerontology primary care NP identifies what finding in the patient's objective data as being associated with the increasing insulin resistance?
    1. Triglycerides >150 mg/dL.
    2. High-density lipoprotein >40 mg/dL in men and >50 mg/dL in women.
    3. Blood pressure <130/85 mm Hg.
    4. Fasting blood sugar <110 mg/dL.

47. While taking a history on a patient, the adult-gerontology primary care NP identifies what finding that may be associated with osteopenia/osteoporosis?
    1. High calcium intake.
    2. Minimal alcohol intake.
    3. Smoking 1 pack/day for 20 years.
    4. Walking 30 minutes 4 days a week.

48. Of the following risk factors for osteoporosis, which would the adult-gerontology primary care NP see primarily with men?
    1. Smoking 2 packs of cigarettes a day.
    2. Excessive use of alcohol.
    3. Low testosterone level.
    4. Minimal exercise.

49. When prescribing a meal plan for a patient with type 2 diabetes, the adult-gerontology primary care NP tells the patient that the macronutrient with the most influence on postprandial glucose levels is:
    1. Fiber.
    2. Fat.
    3. Protein.
    4. Carbohydrate.

50. A common cause of poor control of type 1 diabetes during the adolescent period is:
    1. Too frequent evaluation of blood sugar.
    2. Increased intake of protein.
    3. Too much exercise.
    4. Denial of the severity of the condition.

51. On physical examination of a 14-year-old girl complaining of amenorrhea, the adult-gerontology primary care NP notes BP 138/90 mm Hg, pulse of 98 beats/min, broad chest with widely spaced nipples, Tanner stage I, webbing of neck, low hairline, and prominent, anomalous ears. The adult-gerontology primary care NP suspects:
    1. Klinefelter syndrome.
    2. Marfan syndrome.
    3. Fragile X syndrome.
    4. Turner syndrome.

52. When does the adult-gerontology primary care NP suspect that undiagnosed primary hyperaldosteronism is at play in hypertension management?
    1. When the average BP remains above 140/80 mm Hg despite being on two antihypertensive medications.
    2. When BP readings consistently remain above 160/100 mm Hg with three antihypertensive medications.
    3. When BP readings take more than 6 weeks to respond to initial treatment.
    4. When BP readings remain above 150/100 mm Hg and are associated with hyperkalemia.

53. An adolescent male patient presenting with recent-onset nocturia, polydipsia, polyphagia, weight loss, and blurred vision is most likely experiencing the symptoms of:
    1. Type 1 diabetes.
    2. Type 2 diabetes.
    3. Urinary tract infection (UTI).
    4. Mononucleosis.

Pharmacology

54. Adult-gerontology primary care NPs are very familiar with the precautions about tapering of steroid medications. Which of the following is a true statement about the actual need and/or process of doing so that the adult-gerontology primary care NP understands?
    1. All dosing regimens, no matter the dose and the duration of therapy, require tapering of doses.
    2. Patients who have had several steroid prescriptions in the past year are at lessened risk of sustaining a poor outcome if the doses are not tapered.
    3. Dosing regimens lasting longer than 2 weeks require consideration of a tapering schedule.
    4. Pulse doses of steroid (i.e., 3-day bursts) do not require tapering if they occur more than 6 months apart.

55. When prescribing oral medications for an overweight patient with type 2 diabetes who also has a voracious appetite, the adult-gerontology primary care NP is likely to prescribe which medication to encourage weight loss and reduce appetite, as an adjunct to improved diet and exercise?
    1. Exenatide (Byetta).
    2. Pioglitazone (Actos).
    3. Metformin (Glucophage).
    4. Glyburide (Micronase).

56. Timing of taking thyroid medication has traditionally been in the morning on an empty stomach. If the patient insists on taking thyroid medication with an evening meal, is this acceptable? What would be two appropriate responses?
    1. No, the circadian rhythm cycles are best supported with AM dosing.
    2. This is acceptable if there is a 2- to 4-hour separation from an ingested full evening meal.
    3. There is no difference between AM and PM dosing guidelines.
    4. This is a feasible option if there are no other medications taken at that time that would cause interactions or absorption issues.

57. Glargine (Lantus) is an insulin analogue that essentially has no peak and is *usually* administered:
    1. Before meals.
    2. With lispro insulin (Humalog) in one injection.
    3. Before breakfast and dinner.
    4. Once daily.

58. An adult male patient with type 2 diabetes has a creatinine level of 1.8 mg/dL. Which of the following drugs is contraindicated?
    1. Pioglitazone (Actos).
    2. Metformin (Glucophage).
    3. Rapaglinide (Prandin).
    4. Acarbose (Precose).

59. Patients started on metformin (Glucophage) need to be monitored closely for what potential side effect?
    1. Significant increase in weight.
    2. Elevation of LDL level.
    3. Lactic acidosis.
    4. Increase in insulin requirements.

60. A patient with type 2 diabetes is taking glipizide (Glucotrol) 10 mg PO bid. In evaluating the medication's effectiveness, the adult-gerontology primary care NP knows that glipizide reduces blood glucose by:
    1. Delaying the cellular uptake of potassium and insulin.
    2. Stimulating insulin release from the pancreas.
    3. Decreasing the body's need for and use of insulin at the cellular level.
    4. Interfering with the absorption and metabolism of fats and carbohydrates.

61. The adult-gerontology primary care NP would expect which symptom to be a side effect of metformin (Glucophage)?
    1. Gastrointestinal (GI) upset.
    2. Photophobia.
    3. Hypoglycemia.
    4. Skin eruptions.

62. The sodium-glucose cotransporter 2 (SGLT2) inhibitor medications are known to contribute to which of the two following outcomes in patients with type 2 diabetes:
    1. Reduced A1C level.
    2. Weight loss.
    3. Decreased issues of vaginal yeast infections.
    4. Decreased risk of breast and bladder cancers.
    5. Urinary retention.

63. A patient is receiving antithyroid medication. The adult-gerontology primary care NP understands that:
    1. Lifelong daily treatment is necessary to keep TSH levels within the normal range.
    2. Antithyroid medications do not cross the placenta.
    3. The drugs are somewhat expensive and have serious cardiac and hematologic side effects.
    4. Patients remain on drug therapy for 1–2 years, and then the medication is gradually withdrawn.

64. When prescribing an antihypertensive medication for a patient with type 2 diabetes, the drug classifications that would tend to reduce insulin sensitivity are:
    1. Diuretics and calcium channel blockers.
    2. Diuretics and beta blockers.
    3. Calcium channel blockers and ACE inhibitors.
    4. Alpha blockers and ACE inhibitors.

65. A 35-year-old female sees the adult-gerontology primary care NP with a complaint of cold intolerance, fatigue, dry skin, weight gain, and heavy menstrual periods. Physical exam reveals a pulse of 58 beats/min; a "waxy," sallow complexion; and a firm goiter. Her TSH level is 176 mU/L. What is the best treatment choice for this patient?
    1. Begin levothyroxine (Synthroid) at 25 mcg (0.025 mg) PO daily and repeat TSH in 2 weeks.
    2. Administer loading dose of PO levothyroxine and start full replacement dose.
    3. Administer loading dose of IV levothyroxine and start on half replacement dose.
    4. Begin levothyroxine at 100 mcg (0.1 mg) PO daily and recheck TSH in 6 weeks.

66. The adult-gerontology primary care NP is performing a preoperative evaluation of a man scheduled to undergo coronary artery bypass grafting. Physical exam reveals mild facial puffiness, hoarse voice, and dry skin. The results of thyroid function tests show that the patient has a TSH level of 34 mU/L. What is the recommended treatment for the patient?
    1. Give loading IV bolus of levothyroxine (Synthroid) 500 mcg (0.5 mg) and proceed with surgery.
    2. Cancel surgery and send him home to begin levothyroxine PO 100 mcg (0.1 mg), then reschedule surgery.
    3. Begin PO levothyroxine and monitor the patient in the hospital until he is euthyroid.
    4. Proceed with surgery and treat the patient's hypothyroidism postoperatively.

67. The adult-gerontology primary care NP is seeing an obese, middle-aged female patient for a follow-up visit. She was diagnosed with type 2 diabetes 3 months ago and started on a regimen of diet and exercise. Today, her fasting plasma glucose is 200 mg/dL and A1C is 10%. She has lost 2 lb. She reports her home glucose monitoring has ranged from 180–300 mg/dL. The rest of her chemistry profile is within normal limits (WNL). What is the best treatment choice for the patient?
    1. Review her diet and exercise plan, increase exercise regimen, and reduce caloric intake. Schedule her for another follow-up in 3 months.
    2. Start her on sliding-scale insulin and instruct her on recording glucose and insulin requirements. Schedule her to return in 1 week for reevaluation regarding long-acting insulin.
    3. Initiate treatment with metformin (Glucophage).
    4. Initiate treatment with an oral sulfonylurea agent (e.g., glyburide).

68. What is associated with chronic overtreatment with levothyroxine (Synthroid)?
    1. Tachycardia.
    2. Osteoporosis.
    3. Insomnia.
    4. Sweating.

69. A middle-aged male presents for a diabetes follow-up exam. He has been in good health without identified complications of diabetes. His FBS is 100 mg/dL, and his personal records indicate that he is taking insulin at the prescribed amounts and times. His vital signs are BP 142/98 mm Hg, pulse 80 beats/min, and respiration 20 breaths/min. What two actions would be included in today's plan?
    1. Begin diuretics and a beta blocker.
    2. Begin ACE inhibitor and consider a diuretic.
    3. Obtain ECG and chest x-ray.
    4. Return for BP check in 5–7 days.
    5. Order a serum creatinine and urine microalbuminuria test.

70. An adult male has recently been started on insulin. His regimen is two daily injections, with two-thirds of the total daily insulin in the morning and one-third in the evening. He is using the 70/30 mixture of intermediate- and short-acting insulin in both injections. He presents for a follow-up visit with his FBS log. The adult-gerontology primary care NP notes that his recorded glucose levels before the evening meal have been 60–70 mg/dL. Other checks during the day are 100–120 mg/dL. What adjustment needs to be made?
    1. Intermediate insulin: change 70/30 combination to self-mix and reduce AM dose.
    2. Regular insulin: reduce AM dose of 70/30.
    3. Intermediate insulin: reduce AM dose of 70/30.
    4. Regular insulin: change 70/30 combination to self-mix and reduce AM regular dose.

71. A patient on antithyroid drug therapy for hyperthyroidism presents with complaints of palpitations and dry mouth for the past 2 days. He has had a cough and cold symptoms for the past 3 days, which he has been treating with over-the-counter medications. Which medication would the adult-gerontology primary care NP encourage the patient to avoid?
    1. Benzocaine (Chloraseptic) lozenges.
    2. Guaifenesin (Robitussin).
    3. Ibuprofen (Advil).
    4. Pseudoephedrine (Sudafed).

72. What is the most frequent complaint of patients who use insulin pumps?
    1. Problems with elevated glucose after changing the catheter-type (non-needle) infusion set.
    2. Skin and site problems with dressing adhesive not sticking; redness and pain at infusion site.
    3. Mechanical problems with the pump's digital readout.
    4. Understanding "sick day" management modifications.

73. The adult-gerontology primary care NP understands that pioglitazone (Actos) or rosiglitazone (Avandia) is indicated for:
    1. Prenatal patients with gestational diabetes.
    2. "Brittle" patients with type 1 diabetes.
    3. Patients with type 2 diabetes requiring insulin who have poor glycemic control and insulin resistance.
    4. Patients with type 2 diabetes to prevent the rapid postprandial blood glucose surges by delaying carbohydrate absorption.

74. An older patient with a history of hypertension and coronary bypass surgery has been diagnosed with hypothyroidism. Appropriate medication management is:
    1. Levothyroxine (Synthroid) 100 mcg (0.1 mg) daily and return in 6 weeks for follow-up.
    2. Desiccated thyroid extract 2 grains daily and return in 6 weeks for follow-up.

3. Levothyroxine (Synthroid) 25 mcg (0.025 mg) daily for 6 weeks with a gradual increase in dosage every 4–6 weeks until a therapeutic level is obtained.
4. Methimazole (Tapazole) 15 mg daily in three divided doses, gradually increasing the dose every 4 weeks until a therapeutic level is obtained.

75. A patient is newly diagnosed as being hypothyroid and is placed on levothyroxine (Synthroid) 100 mcg (0.1 mg) PO daily. What should be the adult-gerontology primary care NP's approach to follow-up?
    1. No follow-up visits are necessary.
    2. The patient should return to the clinic in 4–6 weeks for TSH measurement and determination of any symptomatic improvement.
    3. The patient should have weekly levothyroxine levels measured.
    4. The patient should have monthly CBCs while on levothyroxine (Synthroid) because the medication has been found to be myelosuppressive.

76. Classes of medications typically used to treat hyperthyroid conditions include:
    1. Antibiotics and corticosteroids.
    2. ACE inhibitors, anxiolytics, and antithyroid medications.
    3. Beta blockers, NSAIDs, and antithyroid medications.
    4. Calcium channel blockers and corticosteroids.

77. A patient with hypothyroidism receiving daily levothyroxine (Synthroid) for 3 weeks presents to the clinic with complaints of intermittent chest pain. What is the appropriate therapeutic response?
    1. Discontinue levothyroxine because chest pain is a contraindication to its continuance.
    2. Schedule the patient for a stress test.
    3. Decrease dose of levothyroxine, order an electrocardiogram (ECG), and consult immediately with endocrine and/or cardiology health team members.
    4. Prescribe an anxiolytic agent for the patient.

78. The adult-gerontology primary care NP understands that lispro insulin (Humalog):
    1. Can be injected just before eating.
    2. Is less costly than regular insulin.
    3. Increases the likelihood of late postprandial hypoglycemia due to its length of action.
    4. Causes teratogenic effects.

79. When prescribing sulfonylureas, the adult-gerontology primary care NP educates the patient that the most common side effect of therapy is:
    1. Upset stomach.
    2. Diarrhea.
    3. Angina.
    4. Hypoglycemia.

80. The primary action of pioglitazone (Actos) and rosiglitazone (Avandia) is to:
    1. Decrease hepatic glucose output.
    2. Increase secretion of insulin from the pancreas.
    3. Increase glucose uptake into the muscle and fat.
    4. Increase postprandial uptake of glucose into the intestine.

81. A patient has been discharged to home on DDAVP (desmopressin acetate) for diabetes insipidus after removal of a pituitary tumor. On exam, the adult-gerontology primary care NP notes that the patient is lethargic but has 4+ deep tendon reflexes. The adult-gerontology primary care NP suspects:
    1. Noncompliance with therapy.
    2. Water intoxication.
    3. Increased vasopressor effect.
    4. Interaction with over-the-counter (OTC) cough medicine products.

82. During a retrospective review of an established patient, the adult-gerontology primary care NP notes that the photographs of the person show more than just typical aging. They include increased spacing of teeth without loss of dentition, a deep furrowing of the brow, enlarging jaw, and a widening of the nose. What would be the initial intervention the adult-gerontology primary care NP should consider?
    1. Treat without intervention until the symptoms become of symptomatic concern.
    2. Investigate with an oral glucose tolerance test (OGTT).
    3. Test first to rule out a thyroid disorder.
    4. Draw an insulin-like growth factor 1 (IGF-1) test.

83. Primary Cushing disease is linked to suppression of pituitary control over steroid homeostasis. Secondary Cushing syndrome must be considered in which of the following patient groups?
    1. Type 1 diabetes.
    2. Patients with chronic hypertension who respond to medications.
    3. Patients with cancers, especially of small cell variety.
    4. Any patient who is obese.

84. Some diabetic medication groups are being associated with a link to cancer. Which of the following drugs and links to possible cancer types is correct? Select two responses that identify the pairs of drugs and links to possible cancer.
    1. The thiazolidinediones (TZD group) and bladder cancer.
    2. The biguanides and pancreatic cancer.
    3. The glucagon-like peptide agonists (GLP-1) and thyroid cancer.
    4. The sulfonylureas and prostate cancer.
    5. The incretin mimetics and stomach cancer.

85. Which of the following osteoporosis medications does not carry the critical warning that the patient must take the medication with a full glass of water and remain upright 30–60 minutes after dosing?
    1. Alendronate (Fosamax).
    2. Ibandronate (Boniva).
    3. Risedronate (Actonel).
    4. Zoledronic acid (Zometa).

86. A young adult is taking DDAVP (desmopressin) nasally. The patient also has allergies to the local plants, which creates a good amount of nasal congestion. What medication education is important to emphasize?
    1. If the patient is taking an antihistamine, the patient cannot take the DDAVP.
    2. If the patient's nasal passages are full of mucus, the patient should blow the nose to clear it prior to taking the DDAVP.
    3. The congestion makes the use of inhaled DDAVP ineffective, so the dose will have to be taken orally until the allergies diminish.
    4. The patient needs to take the DDAVP at least 1 hour apart from any oral antihistamine.

87. Education concerning home blood sugar testing with a personal glucometer includes the following key point:
    1. Use the matching test strips designed for the particular glucometer because different brands are not interchangeable.
    2. When opening a new canister of test strips, recalibration or setting control codes is no longer needed.
    3. The values obtained from self-monitoring glucometers match serum blood values.
    4. Remember to cleanse the fingertip or alternative testing site with alcohol prior to using the lancing-type device.

88. What blood test can be drawn to help identify whether the patient has type 1 or type 2 diabetes?
    1. Hemoglobin A1C.
    2. Glycosylated fructose.
    3. C-peptide level.
    4. Apo A vs Apo B.

89. Which group of antihypertensive agents have some positive impact on the development of diabetic nephropathy?
    1. Alpha blockers.
    2. Beta blockers.
    3. Calcium channel blockers.
    4. ACE inhibitors.

90. Which two of the following diabetic medication groups is linked with higher risks for hypoglycemia when given as monotherapy?
    1. Biguanides.
    2. Insulins.
    3. Sulfonylureas.
    4. Incretin mimetics.
    5. DDP-4 inhibitors (gliptins).

9 Endocrine Answers & Rationales

Physical Exam & Diagnostic Tests

1. Answer: 2

   Rationale: Goiters are typically not visible from the lateral aspect in most patients without regard to weight. When examining, inspection from the side to identify any enlargement between the cricoid cartilage and the suprasternal notch is helpful. Any prominence noted in this area should be measured with a ruler and recorded. If the prominence is larger than 2 mm (0.08 inch), there is a high likelihood of goiter. A small goiter is one to two times the normal size of the thyroid, and a large goiter is more than twice normal size.

2. Answer: 2

   Rationale: When examining the thyroid, it is important that the patient relax the sternocleidomastoid muscles, which is done by having the patient tilt toward the side being evaluated.

3. Answer: 4

   Rationale: The peer group is important and influences the adolescent, which often manifests as experimentation with risky behaviors (riding a motorcycle without a helmet, not eating healthily to manage diabetes). Later on, as the adolescent approaches young adulthood, more thought is given to risky behaviors and the consequences, and a more secure sense of self develops.

4. Answer: 4

   Rationale: The thyroid gland is fixed to the cricoid cartilage and superior portion of the trachea and thus ascends during swallowing. This assists the adult-gerontology primary care NP to distinguish thyroid structures from other neck masses. The gland's size, degree of enlargement, consistency, surface characteristics, and the presence of nodules or bruits are noted during the exam.

5. Answer: 2

   Rationale: Puffiness of the face and the skin around the eyes (periorbital) as well as dry, thickened skin, with coarse, breakable hair are linked with chronic low thyroid states. Classic signs of hyperthyroidism are onycholysis (brittle nails, Plummer nails), warm, velvety skin, fine hair with hair loss, and pretibial edema. Onycholysis is the loosening or separation of a fingernail or toenail from its nail bed and is associated with fungal infections, trauma, and hyperthyroidism.

6. Answer: 1

   Rationale: Coarse facial features, heavier brow line, and prominent jaw are associated with acromegaly. Other findings include frontal skull bossing (prominent, protruding forehead), mandibular overgrowth, maxillary widening, teeth separation, malocclusion, overbite, and skin thickening on the face (tongue, lips, and nose). Moon face as well as extra hair growth on the upper lip and chin with acne on the back and chest are typical Cushing characteristics. A wide-eyed look with nervous tic, bulging eyes (exophthalmos), lid lag, and warm, moist skin are associated with hyperthyroidism. Periorbital puffiness is associated with hypothyroidism.

7. Answer: 2

   Rationale: The increased bone turnover related to abnormal parathyroid hormone levels is linked with increased calcium levels. Changes in other lab values can be associated with bone loss, but the link is stronger with calcium changes.

8. Answer: 3

   Rationale: Papillary carcinoma, the most common form of thyroid cancer, is associated with a history of exposure to radiation. Family history, history of hyperthyroidism, and smoking are not considered significant risk factors for this malignancy.

9. Answer: 1

   Rationale: Memory, attention, and problem-solving deficits are often-noted symptoms with hyperthyroidism. The high level of thyroid hormone affects the nervous system, causing sympathomimetic symptoms such as brisk deep tendon reflexes, fine rapid tremor of the hands, restlessness, irritability, insomnia, dreams, nightmares, and rarely severe cognitive impairment and psychosis.

10. Answer: 3

    Rationale: The American Diabetes Association recommends an A1C level of <7% as an important treatment goal to decrease the risk of long-term complications. A lab test result of >6.5% A1C is an indication that action needs to be taken, either by a change in medication or a reinforcement of education. Counseling should be provided for prediabetes patients with A1C >5.7%. In some older patients, those with multiple comorbidities, or limited life expectancy, a goal of <8% may be used.

11. Answer: 2

Rationale: Growth abnormalities are associated with anterior pituitary dysfunction and glucose intolerance with diabetes related to pancreatic dysfunction. Coagulation abnormalities and fatigue would be associated with hematologic dysfunction. Hypoxia would be associated with oxygenation problems and jaundice with liver or biliary problems. Steatorrhea is associated with malabsorption syndrome, cystic fibrosis, and other issues of the exocrine pancreas.

12. Answer: 2

Rationale: The primary care provider may obtain TSH, T_3, T_4, and T_7 levels as well as an ultrasound. Ordering antibody levels, thyroid scans, or fine-needle aspiration (FNA) biopsy should be done after coordination with the endocrine team. The FNA aspirate is sent for cytology and interpretation.

13. Answer: 4

Rationale: The low-dose dexamethasone suppression test is the best screening test, and the 24-hour urine test for free cortisol (UFC) is the best confirmatory test to use for Cushing disease. Late-night salivary cortisol is a screening test that would be elevated. Thyroid-stimulating hormone (TSH) and thyroxine (T_4) may also be appropriate to rule out a thyroid condition because some of the patient's signs and symptoms are consistent with thyroid dysfunction. Antinuclear antibody (ANA) and rheumatoid factor (RF) are ordered when rheumatoid arthritis or systemic lupus erythematosus (SLE) is suspected; however, the patient's clinical picture is not consistent with these conditions. The red blood cell (RBC) count would be done to rule out anemia, a potential problem for this patient based on the history of fatigue, but the rest of the clinical picture indicates more than anemia. No clinical findings support a calcium level being drawn.

14. Answer: 2

Rationale: Thyroid-stimulating hormone (TSH) levels should be decreased in a patient with Graves disease because thyroid-stimulating immunoglobulins bind to TSH receptors, which increase thyroxine (T_4) and triiodothyronine (T_3) synthesis and release, subsequently suppressing TSH levels.

15. Answer: 3

Rationale: The correct procedure is to use a 10-g (5.07-gauge Semmes-Weinstein) filament and apply it to 10 sites on the foot (1 on the top of the foot and 9 on the heel, sole, and toes). The filament is applied perpendicular (90-degree angle) to the skin surface with sufficient force for 1.5 seconds to cause the filament to bend. The filament should not be allowed to slide across the skin or make repetitive contact with each test site. Randomizing the selection of test sites (start with great toe → heel → instep area → 5th metatarsal) and the time between successive tests to reduce patient guessing and having the patient close the eyes are also helpful.

16. Answer: 2, 4

Rationale: Parathyroid dysfunction typically occurs in older age, but it is commonly the cause of unexplained osteoporosis in younger to middle-aged adults. The most frequent first presentation on imaging is kidney stones. "Brim sign" (thickened iliopectineal line or pelvic brim) is noted on an x-ray in patients who have Paget disease.

17. Answer: 3

Rationale: The American Diabetes Association has defined the diagnostic criteria for diabetes to include any one of the three following methods, which must be confirmed on a subsequent day:
- Random plasma glucose ≥200 mg/dL and acute symptoms (polyuria, polydipsia, polyphagia).
- Fasting plasma glucose ≥126 mg/dL.
- Plasma glucose ≥200 mg/dL during an oral glucose tolerance test (OGTT).
- Hemoglobin A1C >6.5%.

Disorders

18. Answer: 4

Rationale: Assessing diet and understanding of the exchange list and the administration of insulin are certainly important considerations in diabetes education. However, they cannot be initiated until the adult-gerontology primary care NP evaluates the patient's knowledge of his or her disease state, which is the reason that option 4 is correct. When two options appear to say the same thing, only in different words, then look for another answer; that is, eliminate the options that you know are incorrect. Options 1 and 2 both refer to the client's understanding of nutrition.

19. Answer: 2

Rationale: Type 1 diabetes is caused by destruction of the beta cells mediated through the immune system. The other three choices refer to type 2 diabetes.

20. Answer: 3

Rationale: During dehydration, an increased release of ADH (vasopressin) from the pituitary gland acts on the kidneys to increase reabsorption of water and provide protective functions. Alcohol ingestion, in contrast, inhibits the release of ADH, preventing water reabsorption in the kidneys causing free water loss.

21. Answer: 1

Rationale: Pituitary masses associated with acromegaly are usually benign tumors that create a disruption in normal feedback mechanisms. Symptoms noted on physical exam result from the effects of growth hormone (GH) excess or from the secreting tissue effect of the pituitary mass on surrounding brain structures. This is not typically an adrenal cortex dysfunction. Although tumors can cause acromegaly symptoms, pituitary masses associated with acromegaly are typically noncancerous lesions.

22. Answer: 4

Rationale: An annual eye exam with the pupils dilated should be done by a specialist who can recognize subtle abnormalities. Diabetic retinopathy is the most common eye disease among people with diabetes. Although the other referrals can offer important contributions to diabetes care, these would be done on an as-needed basis rather than annually.

23. Answer: 3

Rationale: Because of the normal menstrual periods and androgen plasma level, hirsutism would be considered in a premenopausal woman. There are iatrogenic causes (i.e., medications). Diseases related to the ovaries would cause changes in the menstrual cycle and, with Cushing syndrome, would be associated with adrenal androgen overproduction.

24. Answer: 4

Rationale: Testosterone production is regulated by the hypothalamic-pituitary-testicular (HPT) axis, so abnormalities in any of these areas can affect the production of testosterone.

25. Answer: 2

Rationale: It is important for patients with diabetes to have their feet inspected daily either by self-exam or by a family member. Feet should be washed daily but never soaked. Corns and calluses should receive a professional's care. Nails should be trimmed straight across to avoid injury to the nail beds.

26. Answer: 1

Rationale: An A1C of >8.0% indicates poor glucose control over the past few months. According to American Diabetes Association (ADA), an A1C of >8.0% is equal to an average daily blood glucose of 355 mg/dL. The normal serum glucose for adults ranges from 70 to 120 mg/dL. Diabetic acidosis is not of concern until the glucose level is >300 mg/dL.

27. Answer: 1

Rationale: True hypoglycemia can be organized around whether it is fasting or postprandial. Postprandial hypoglycemia may be caused by early adult-onset diabetes or postgastrectomy syndrome. Fasting hypoglycemia is most often caused by excessive doses of insulin, sulfonylureas alone, or with biguanides and thiazolidinediones.

28. Answer: 3

Rationale: The symptoms of lethargy, cold intolerance, weight gain, and yellowing of the palms suggest hypothyroidism, and thyroid studies (e.g., TSH) would be most useful. A complete physical would be performed, and liver etiology is still a differential. Xanthoderma (yellowing of palms) typically occurs only due to a coexisting carotinemia. Thyroid etiology is the "most likely" choice because cold intolerance is given.

29. Answer: 2

Rationale: This middle-aged female patient presents with many of the classic symptoms of early hyperthyroidism (e.g., tremulousness, racing pulse, difficulty falling asleep, weight loss despite a normal appetite, and feeling warm). A suppressed thyroid-stimulating hormone (TSH) with an elevated free T_4 establishes the diagnosis of hyperthyroidism.

30. Answer: 3

Rationale: The patient's physical findings and habitus, along with hypertension and hypokalemia, are associated with Cushing syndrome, which is a state of excessive cortisol production due to a pituitary tumor. A Cushing-like syndrome is often associated with prolonged glucocorticoid administration. Obesity is the primary finding in Cushing syndrome, along with the "moon face," lipoma growths on the upper back, truncal obesity, hirsutism in women, and impotence and loss of body hair in men. Addison disease is characterized by hyperkalemia, hyponatremia, hypoglycemia, anemia, and hypercalcemia. Patients with hypoaldosteronism (impaired renin secretion) have hyperkalemia. Pheochromocytoma would be included in the differential diagnosis of this patient because of the hypertension; the other findings are not consistent with this diagnosis.

31. Answer: 2

Rationale: Hemianopia (also called hemianopsia) is loss of vision in half of the visual field and is a classic sign of pituitary enlargement. It can be unilateral or bilateral (bitemporal hemianopsia), depending on the extent of the lesion. Exophthalmos is associated with thyroid hyperactivity. Ocular muscle control is less likely with pituitary lesions. Central vision loss is most associated with diabetes mellitus and age-related macular degeneration.

32. Answer: 4

Rationale: Accumulation of hyaluronic acid in interstitial tissues increases capillary permeability to albumin and causes the interstitial edema of the face and eyelids in patients with hypothyroidism.

33. Answer: 2

Rationale: Although alcohol abuse may be a cause of hypoglycemia, the patient is presenting with classic symptoms of postprandial hypoglycemia. Assessment for alcohol abuse as the etiology of the hypoglycemia would be advisable. Increased circulating thyroid hormones increase beta-cell sensitivity and increase insulin release. This does not typically manifest as hypoglycemia; instead, most patients with hyperthyroidism develop glucose intolerance due to an antagonism of the peripheral action of insulin on cells.

34. Answer: 1

Rationale: This "syndrome" of collective complaints has yet to be found to have a basis in actual physiologic laboratory values. It is not an established complaint in the endocrine community; however, patients presenting with these issues should have a laboratory workup done to establish other underlying causes with appropriate treatment plans.

35. Answer: 2

Rationale: Hyperparathyroidism accounts for more than 60% of patients with hypercalcemia and is likely to be the explanation for elevated serum calcium levels.

36. Answer: 1

Rationale: Although depression may explain the weight gain, Cushing syndrome is the correct diagnosis for the constellation of symptoms of rapid weight gain, hypertension, and elevated blood sugar. These symptoms suggest adrenal dysfunction. Serum cortisol and adrenocorticotropic hormone (ACTH) levels should be checked.

37. Answer: 1

Rationale: The woman is likely experiencing the life-threatening syndrome that can occur in decompensated hyperthyroidism. The clues are her symptom presentation and progression, the new "antidrug," and upcoming throat surgery, which suggest that the patient is likely on PTU or methimazole and has thyroid cancer. Although other possible causes of delirium are eventually considered, the adult-gerontology primary care NP needs to go with the probabilities of occurrence within the given context.

38. Answer: 3

Rationale: The symptoms (weight gain, lethargy, inability to tolerate cold temperatures, forgetfulness, hair loss, and constipation) describe the classic presentation of a patient with hypothyroidism. A patient with heart failure would have jugular venous distention, rales, and peripheral edema. The criteria for diagnosing diabetes mellitus are polydipsia, polyphagia, polyuria, and weight loss. Thyroid cancer typically presents without many physical symptoms other than hoarseness and dysphagia, and often the only physical finding is a hard, fixed nodule on the thyroid gland.

39. Answer: 2

Rationale: The patient's blood sugar levels are low around lunchtime, which is when the regular insulin is peaking (3–4 hours), so a reduction in the regular insulin would address this problem.

40. Answer: 3

Rationale: The adult-gerontology primary care NP's role in primary care for a patient with a thyroid nodule involves initially the early identification of the thyroid nodule on physical exam and ordering an ultrasound and thyroid panel, then referring the patient to an endocrinologist for further evaluation, and possibly obtaining some preliminary thyroid-stimulating hormone (TSH) and antibody testing. The endocrinologist performs the fine-needle aspiration (FNA) if the nodule is <1 cm with normal TSH level. Levothyroxine may or may not be used to diminish the size of the nodule, based on the findings derived from the FNA and the endocrinologist's chosen treatment plan.

41. Answer: 2

Rationale: Primary aldosteronism is considered the most common cause of secondary hypertension. Approximately 10%–15% of all patients with hypertension are now considered to have "inappropriate aldosterone secretion" for a variety of reasons. Primary aldosteronism is particularly common in patients with resistant hypertension, with a prevalence of approximately 20%.

42. Answer: 4

Rationale: Patients with diabetes must understand that when they are sick, blood glucose levels will probably increase, even when they are not eating. They need to monitor blood glucose levels every 2–4 hours. The medications metformin and acarbose should not be given until the patient's nausea and vomiting have subsided and the patient has resumed a normal diet; blood glucose monitoring is important during this time. Dehydration will increase the risk of metabolic acidosis for patients on metformin.

43. Answer: 2

Rationale: Graves disease, an autoimmune condition also known as "diffuse toxic goiter," is the most common cause of hyperthyroidism in this age group. Much less common causes include cancer of the thyroid, adenoma of the pituitary gland, and postpartum (or silent) thyroiditis.

44. Answer: 1

Rationale: The thyroid-stimulating hormone (TSH) level should be ordered to determine whether the patient is euthyroid, hypothyroid, or hyperthyroid, along with an ultrasound. The patient should also be sent to an endocrinologist or surgeon because all nodules of the thyroid should be biopsied to rule out malignancy. "Watching and waiting" is inappropriate without having a biopsy performed. Thyroid hormone replacement therapy would be indicated only for patients found to be hypothyroid and in whom thyroid cancer has been ruled out. Thyroid ablation may be indicated in patients whose fine-needle aspiration (FNA) biopsy results are positive for thyroid cancer, but this cannot be determined without an endocrinologist's intervention.

45. Answer: 3

Rationale: Hypothyroidism often follows this treatment, with 50% of patients requiring replacement therapy in the first year and almost 100% requiring therapy in 10 years. For this reason, regular monitoring of thyroid-stimulating hormone (TSH) and T_4 levels should be performed. Patients emit a small amount of radioactivity after receiving the dose used to treat this condition and do not require isolation for 7 days. Radioactive iodine is perceived to be safe, without an increased risk of chromosomal abnormalities; therefore no contraindication exists to becoming pregnant after therapy, although patients are counseled to avoid pregnancy during treatment and to avoid children and pregnant women after receiving the oral ablation dose. This therapy is recommended for patients who have cardiac disease associated with their thyroid condition.

46. Answer: 1

Rationale: Improper use of glucose increases the release of free fatty acids, which elevates triglycerides. The other values are still within normal limits.

47. Answer: 3

Rationale: Smoking causes thinning of the bones and can lead to osteopenia/osteoporosis. A diet high in calcium with minimal alcohol intake and walking are all self-care practices that may prevent or delay the onset of osteopenia/osteoporosis.

48. Answer: 3

Rationale: Low testosterone levels may result from prostate cancer treatment and long-standing liver disease. Smoking, excessive use of alcohol, and minimal exercise are risk factors of osteoporosis that can occur in both men and women.

49. Answer: 4

Rationale: Carbohydrate is the macronutrient with the greatest impact on the postprandial glucose levels. Ingested protein has minimal effect on the blood glucose levels. A diet high in fat may be associated with cardiovascular disease. Fiber has little effect on the plasma glucose response, but it may result in decreased low-density lipoprotein (LDL) cholesterol.

50. Answer: 4

Rationale: All these contribute significantly to difficulty controlling diabetes in the teenage years. Hormonal changes and the desire to become independent increase emotional conflicts. Teens have a great desire to be like their peers and do not want to be regimented in following a specific diet and adhering to a treatment plan.

51. Answer: 4

Rationale: These findings are consistent with Turner syndrome: short stature, gonadal dysgenesis, lymphedema (usually appearing in infancy), left-sided heart or aortic abnormalities, primary amenorrhea, and delayed onset of puberty. Fragile X syndrome is an inherited condition usually affecting males and characterized by a long, narrow face and prominent ears, mild to profound intellectual disability, hyperactivity and poor attention span, and autistic-type behavior. Marfan syndrome is a connective tissue disorder of tall and thin adolescents that is characterized by long limbs, narrow hands, long, slender fingers, and nearsightedness. Klinefelter syndrome is characterized by small testes, sterility, gynecomastia, and long legs.

52. Answer: 2

Rationale: Resistant hypertension needs a full workup to include adrenal impact, especially when BP readings remain above 160/100 mm Hg despite the patient being on three antihypertensive medications. Aldosterone excess results in renin suppression via feedback mechanism, hypertension due to volume expansion and sodium retention, and low potassium due to increased renal losses. The risk is highest in those with familial early stroke and hypertension incidence and in those with hypokalemia, adrenal incidentaloma, and sleep apnea.

53. Answer: 1

Rationale: Type 1 diabetes usually (but not always) appears before age 30 years and is heralded by the three "Ps": polydipsia, polyuria, and polyphagia.

Pharmacology

54. Answer: 3

Rationale: Continuous dosing of steroid medication conditions the adrenal feedback system to become less sensitive to discontinuation of the exogenous hormone supply, which normally would trigger a natural ramp-up of innate steroid production. Duration longer than 2 or 3 weeks and moderate to high doses trigger the need to evaluate current values and prepare for a gradual reduction in dosage before the patient stops taking the steroid medication.

55. Answer: 1

Rationale: Incretin mimetic medications, such as exenatide, are associated with weight loss. Metformin is associated with weight neutrality and appetite suppression. Glyburide is considered a second-generation sulfonylurea, which tends to stimulate insulin secretion from the pancreas, thus causing a slight weight gain. Pioglitazone is an insulin sensitizer and increases glucose uptake in the muscle and fat. Common side effects include fluid retention and an increase in central adiposity.

56. Answer: 3, 4

Rationale: There is no change in thyroid function and hormone levels in patients who take evening doses, as long as there is a separation of meals and the standard medication review to avoid drug-to-drug interactions. It is also recommended to take medications such as levothyroxine in the evening, typically due to side effect profiles such as insomnia rather than efficacy.

57. Answer: 4

Rationale: Glargine is a long-acting basal insulin usually given once daily and lasts almost 24 hours without a peak. This clear insulin must be given alone and not mixed with other insulins in the same syringe. Lispro insulin is a rapid-acting insulin usually given three times daily with meals. A basal insulin can be used at the same time with a different injection. In rare cases, basal insulins are given more than once per day, but this is not usual practice.

58. Answer: 2

Rationale: Metformin should not be given to men with a serum creatinine level ≥1.5 mg/dL or to women with a serum creatinine level ≥1.4 mg/dL, because it can predispose the patient to lactic acidosis. Pioglitazone and rapa-

glinide are metabolized primarily in the liver and require monitoring of liver function tests. Acarbose is metabolized mainly in the gastrointestinal tract.

59. Answer: 3

Rationale: Lactic acidosis is a potentially severe and fatal reaction to metformin. Metformin does not contribute to weight gain; it often helps with weight loss and decreases low-density lipoprotein (LDL), triglyceride levels, and insulin requirements.

60. Answer: 2

Rationale: Sulfonylureas reduce blood glucose by stimulating insulin release from the pancreas. Over time, these drugs also may actually increase insulin effects at the cellular level and decrease glucose production by the liver, which is why sulfonylureas are used in patients with type 2 diabetes who still have a functioning pancreas.

61. Answer: 1

Rationale: Anorexia, nausea, and a metallic taste in the mouth are common side effects. Over time, gastrointestinal (GI) symptoms subside and can be relieved by taking the medication with food or by starting at a lower dose. Metformin has a safety profile that does not include hypoglycemia unless mixed with other agents that trigger it.

62. Answer: 1, 2

Rationale: Positive outcomes include better glucose control over time and some potential weight loss. This SGLT2 medication class (e.g., canagliflozin, dapagliflozin) is linked to an increase in genital yeast infections, and some agents have been associated with increasing risks of cancer (though low on the basis of current information). A new black box warning was published May 2017 to state that canagliflozin increases the risk of foot and leg amputations and should be used with caution. There is also the side of effect of increased desire to urinate.

63. Answer: 4

Rationale: Antithyroid medications or thionamides (propylthiouracil; methimazole) are relatively inexpensive and do cross the placenta. The patient remains on the medications for 1–2 years with the hope of a permanent remission of symptoms when the medications are withdrawn.

64. Answer: 2

Rationale: Both of these drug classifications (diuretics and beta blockers) tend to reduce insulin sensitivity and can cause hyperglycemia. Angiotensin-converting enzyme (ACE) inhibitors, calcium channel blockers, and selective alpha blockers are metabolically neutral; some may actually have a beneficial effect.

65. Answer: 4

Rationale: The patient's symptoms indicate hypothyroidism, as does the elevated thyroid-stimulating hormone (TSH) level (normal levels are 0.5–4.7 mU/L). A full replacement dose of levothyroxine should be the goal for the patient with a standard starting dose of 100–125 mcg (0.1 to 0.125 mg) for a 70-kg person. The TSH level should be checked in 6 weeks, which is the time it may take for a given dose to become effective. Loading doses should never be given, except for coma, which is treated by IV medication in the hospital.

66. Answer: 4

Rationale: Patients with coronary disease found to be mildly to moderately hypothyroid can safely undergo urgent surgery (including bypass procedures) without prior replacement. The rate of complications is no greater than for nonhypothyroid patients, and the cardiac risks are less compared with initiating replacement therapy preoperatively.

67. Answer: 3

Rationale: Metformin is a better option in an obese patient because it is frequently associated with weight neutrality or even some weight loss, whereas sulfonylureas may actually cause weight gain. Insulin is now considered an option, but the use of a sliding scale is no longer current practice. Diet and exercise were unsuccessful, and the longer the patient's blood sugar remains elevated, the greater her risk for end-organ damage. An A1C level in this range (10%) requires aggressive treatment to decrease vascular complications.

68. Answer: 2

Rationale: Chronic overtreatment is associated with osteoporosis; the other options are related to acute overdose of levothyroxine and can be relieved by omitting the dose for 3 days and then starting on a lower dose.

69. Answer: 4, 5

Rationale: To initiate treatment for elevated blood pressure (BP), it is recommended that three elevated readings be recorded on three separate occasions. No evidence suggests that this patient had increased BP at prior visits. This patient should first be checked for microalbuminuria, which would indicate the immediate starting of an ACE inhibitor, especially because microalbuminuria is often the first sign of impending renal damage. The microalbuminuria test is typically performed in conjunction with a creatinine test to provide an albumin-to-creatinine ratio.

70. Answer: 1

Rationale: This is the best answer because the AM intermediate dose will affect the glucose level before din-

ner. Altering the regular insulin will affect levels before lunch and before bedtime; however, these levels are acceptable. To reduce the intermediate dose while maintaining the level of regular insulin, the patient will need to self-mix the intermediate and regular insulin, using less of the intermediate. A more modern approach is to use basal insulin (long-acting) plus mealtime rapid-acting insulins.

71. Answer: 4

Rationale: Pseudoephedrine and other decongestant medications that contain sympathomimetics lead to adverse reactions of central nervous system (CNS) overstimulation, palpitations, headache, hypertension, and nervousness. Guaifenesin in combination with dextromethorphan and phenylpropanolamine (Robitussin-CF) or pseudoephedrine (Robitussin-PE) can also cause palpitations and CNS overstimulation. Guaifenesin with dextromethorphan (Robitussin-DM) may cause gastrointestinal (GI) upset, drowsiness, headache, and rash. Many over-the-counter (OTC) medications also have an iodine component that may alter thyroid levels.

72. Answer: 2

Rationale: Infusion site problems and skin irritation are by far the most frequent complaints of patients who use an insulin pump and often are the reason why the pump is discontinued. Patients also find it is more time-consuming and costly. However, the Diabetes Control and Complications Trial (DCCT, 1993) researchers reported a reduced risk of microvascular complications when insulin pumps and multiple daily injections were used.

73. Answer: 3

Rationale: Pioglitazone and rosiglitazone act by decreasing peripheral insulin resistance in skeletal muscle and adipose tissue without enhancing insulin secretion and improving glucose tolerance in patients with type 2 diabetes. Prenatal patients are managed with insulin or metformin, not an insulin sensitizer. The action of alpha-glucosidase inhibitors, such as acarbose (Precose) and miglitol (Glyset), prevents the rapid postprandial blood glucose surges by delaying carbohydrate absorption (known as "starch blockers").

74. Answer: 3

Rationale: Older patients, especially those with heart disease, need to be started on the smallest amount of thyroid medication replacement (between 12.5 mcg and 25 mcg, not 100 mcg) followed by gradual increases until a therapeutic level is achieved. If thyroid replacement occurs too quickly, the heart may decompensate; 2 grains of thyroid extract is too much. Methimazole is an antithyroid medication used to treat hyperthyroidism.

75. Answer: 2

Rationale: The response to therapy is based on a clinical symptomatology and a thyroid-stimulating hormone (TSH) assay approximately 4–6 weeks after the initiation of therapy. This is continued until a stable dose is obtained. TSH and a free T_4 level are the two standard tests that can be used to monitor the status of the thyroid; a levothyroxine level cannot be measured. Levothyroxine is not a myelosuppressive.

76. Answer: 3

Rationale: Beta blockers are initially prescribed to reduce the signs and symptoms of the condition and to reduce the peripheral conversion of T_4 to triiodothyronine (T_3); nonsteroidal antiinflammatory drugs (NSAIDs) are indicated for reducing inflammation associated with thyroiditis; and antithyroid medications (propylthiouracil [PTU]; methimazole) are used to treat severe hyperthyroidism. Corticosteroids are sometimes used in the treatment of thyroiditis, but the remaining classes (antibiotics, angiotensin-converting enzyme [ACE] inhibitors, calcium channel blockers, and anxiolytics) are not routinely used in the management of hyperthyroidism.

77. Answer: 3

Rationale: Monitoring TSH is the most accurate way to assess thyroid function in a patient taking levothyroxine. Decreasing the dose of levothyroxine and evaluating the patient's cardiac status are the appropriate interventions in this situation, in addition to quickly involving the other health care team members. Discontinuing the thyroid replacement would be inappropriate because the patient remains hypothyroid and requires therapy for life. An anxiolytic may be a helpful adjunct, but it is not appropriate as the sole intervention, because it ignores the cardiac symptoms.

78. Answer: 1

Rationale: Lispro (Humalog) was the first analogue of human insulin and has several advantages over regular insulin, including more rapid onset and shorter duration of action. It reaches peak activity in 1–2 hours and has a 4-hour duration, versus 6–8 hours for regular insulin. It is convenient because it can be injected immediately before eating (10–15 minutes). It is also more expensive than regular insulin, and some third-party payers may not reimburse patients.

79. Answer: 4

Rationale: Hypoglycemia and weight gain are the most common side effects of sulfonylurea therapy.

80. Answer: 3

Rationale: Pioglitazone (Actos) and rosiglitazone (Avandia) decrease insulin resistance, which increases the glu-

cose uptake in the muscle and fat. Metformin decreases hepatic glucose output. Oral sulfonylureas increase insulin secretion in the pancreas. The alpha-glucosidase inhibitors increase postprandial glucose uptake in the intestine.

81. Answer: 2

Rationale: DDAVP (desmopressin acetate) promotes reabsorption of water in the renal tubules, which can lead to water intoxication. The signs of water intoxication are lethargy, behavioral changes, disorientation, and neuromuscular excitability.

82. Answer: 4

Rationale: The earlier the intervention, the better the outcome for the patient with acromegaly. Initially, the common practice and best single test is to measure insulin-like growth factor-1 (IGF-1), which, if normal, rules out acromegaly. Levels twice the upper limit suggest acromegaly. Although not a pancreas-centered disorder, the oral glucose tolerance test (OGTT) is performed as follow-up testing and is a sensitive diagnostic evaluation (done after checking the IGF-1 level), except in patients with known diabetes whose diabetes is uncontrolled. In normal patients, the values fall into normal ranges; in patients with acromegaly, growth hormone (GH) is suppressed by the blood sugar load. The GH level is measured before the OGTT is done and then again at 2 hours. GH levels may remain >2 ng/mL in patients with acromegaly. Although thyroid enlargement can be part of a general organomegaly presentation, it is not the typical cause of this clinical presentation.

83. Answer: 3

Rationale: Although abnormal glucose control is a hallmark of Cushing disease, it is typically in patients with diabetes who have a metabolic syndrome presentation, not in the type 1 diabetes group. Hypertension under good control is not linked to steroid overproduction; it is the patient who does not respond to medication who is evaluated for adrenal issues. Bronchogenic and other small cell types of cancers have been known to produce "ectopic" steroids. The "moon face" of Cushing syndrome is not the same as that of someone who is simply overweight.

84. Answer: 1, 3

Rationale: Bladder cancer, although rare, is linked with the selective sodium glucose cotransporters (SGLT2) and the thiazolidinediones (TZDs). Medullary cancer risk has prompted issuance of a black box warning for the glucagon-like peptide agonist (GLP-1) medications. The biguanides, incretin mimetics, and sulfonylureas do not have these black box warnings.

85. Answer 4

Rationale: Zoledronic acid (Zometa) is administered as an intravenous (IV) infusion. The others are all oral medications that carry the need to remain sitting upright to decrease the risk for esophageal irritation. The IV medication does require good hydration to decrease renal risks.

86. Answer: 2

Rationale: Nasally inhaled DDAVP (desmopressin) must have direct contact with the nasal mucosa for absorption. Secretions, especially those that are thicker, prevent this, so clearing the nasal passages with an effective nasal clearing blow will provide some additional time for "topical" absorption. There are no major problems with concurrent antihistamine use that would decrease the amount of secretions. The DDAVP is not taken orally, so the precaution about separation by 1 hour is not needed.

87. Answer: 1

Rationale: Test strips are proprietary to the specific monitor. Test strips are frequently not interchangeable, even in monitors from the same manufacturer. Similarly, lancets are specific to the device used to provide a skin puncture. Some newer monitors do not require frequent calibrations or a code number. Handwashing must be completed with soap and water. Alcohol is not used to cleanse the digits, unless medically indicated. Serum, capillary, and deeper puncture glucose values do vary, especially over time.

88. Answer: 3

Rationale: Naturally occurring insulin has a C-peptide bond, which is removed during the processing of exogenous insulin as a drug. The level of C-peptide in the blood can show how much insulin is being made by the pancreas. Classically, a patient with type 1 diabetes has no C-peptide bonds because all circulating insulin is from exogenous sources. In comparison, a patient with type 2 diabetes is expected to have some innate insulin production, so C-peptides should be present. The hemoglobin A1C or glycosylated fructose can be used for either patient group. The Apo A and B levels deal with lipid values, not sugars. It should be noted that newer research shows that some patients with type 1 diabetes actually produce a bit of natural insulin, especially after the initial period, so the C-peptide laboratory is not the absolute determinant of disease status.

89. Answer: 4

Rationale: Although the reduction of hypertension is important to renal health, the angiotensin-converting enzyme (ACE) inhibitors and some selected angiotensin II receptor blocker (ARB) agents have a "renal protective" effect apart from the vascular tension issue. This does not extend to their direct renin inhibitor "cousins." There may be some positive impact from the sodium glucose cotransporter (SGLT-2) group, but more research is needed.

90. Answer: 2, 3

Rationale: The risk of low blood sugar is greatest with the oldest of the diabetic remedies. This is especially true when insulins are mixed with sulfonylureas. The relative lack of hypoglycemic episodes with the other drug groups makes them a safer alternative.

10

Musculoskeletal

Physical Examination & Diagnostic Tests

1. The adult-gerontology primary care NP is performing a history and physical examination on a 72-year-old female patient who is complaining of slight pain in the left shoulder. Which observation would indicate that further testing should be initiated?
   1. Slight swelling is noted.
   2. Brisk capillary refill is noted in the fingers of the left hand.
   3. Bilateral comparison reveals similar pain in the right shoulder.
   4. Limited range of motion in the joint.

2. Which diagnostic test provides a general indicator that inflammation is occurring within the musculoskeletal system?
   1. C-reactive protein.
   2. Antinuclear antibodies.
   3. ESR.
   4. A1C.

3. A goniometer is a measurement device used in the musculoskeletal exam of a patient. The adult-gerontology primary care NP uses this tool to determine:
   1. Strength of the muscles in the extremities.
   2. Degree of joint flexion and extension.
   3. Range of motion of the extremities.
   4. Point of joint flexion that is painful.

4. The adult-gerontology primary care NP places a patient in the prone position with the knee flexed 90 degrees. The tibia is firmly opposed to the femur by exerting downward pressure on the foot. The leg is rotated externally and internally. If locking of the knee occurs, this is accurately called a positive:
   1. Drawer sign.
   2. McMurray test.
   3. Apley test.
   4. Bulge sign.

5. A patient has numbness and tingling in the thumb and first two fingers when pressing the backs of the hands together (flexes wrists at 90 degrees) for 60 seconds. This is a positive:
   1. Tinel sign.
   2. Drawer sign.
   3. McMurray test.
   4. Phalen maneuver.

6. What is the sign that occurs when compressing the suprapatellar pouch back against the femur and feeling for fluid entering the spaces?
   1. Drawer sign.
   2. Kernig sign.
   3. Balloon sign.
   4. Bulge sign.

7. De Quervain tenosynovitis can be diagnosed in part by a positive:
   1. Finkelstein test.
   2. Tinel sign.
   3. Phalen maneuver.
   4. Lachman test.

8. The primary exam techniques used for assessing the musculoskeletal system are:
   1. Inspection and percussion.
   2. Auscultation and palpation.
   3. Inspection and palpation.
   4. Palpation and percussion.

9. What criteria can the adult-gerontology primary care NP use to suggest a diagnosis of polymyalgia rheumatica (PMR)?
   1. Chest radiograph showing pulmonary hyperinflation, asymmetric joint pain, and an elevated serum C-reactive protein (CRP).
   2. Serum protein electrophoresis, clonal bone marrow plasma cells ≥10% or biopsy-proven bony or soft tissue plasmacytoma, and presence of related organ or tissue impairment.
   3. Corticosteroid challenge, erythrocyte sedimentation rate (ESR) >40 mm/h, proximally and bilaterally distributed aching, morning stiffness (lasting 30 minutes or more) persisting for at least 2 weeks, and age 50 years or older.
   4. ESR <40 mm/h, emitting seronegative symmetric synovitis with pitting edema and tremor with rigidity.

10. When performing an assessment, the adult-gerontology primary care NP understands that the metacarpophalangeal (MCP) joints are frequently involved with:
   1. Gout.
   2. Rheumatic fever.
   3. Rheumatoid arthritis (RA).
   4. Osteoarthritis (OA).

11. In the evaluation of polyneuropathy, which study would *not* be recommended?
   1. Erythrocyte sedimentation rate (ESR).
   2. Complete blood count (CBC).
   3. Glycosylated hemoglobin (A1C).
   4. Electromyography (EMG).

12. In accurately assessing a patient who reports a back injury, it is critical to question:
   1. Family history of back problems.
   2. Previous injury.
   3. Personal history of chronic illness.
   4. Mechanism of injury.

13. The Tinel sign and Phalen maneuver are used in identifying a common workplace condition that the adult-gerontology primary care NP recognizes as:
   1. Lateral epicondylitis.
   2. Carpel tunnel syndrome.
   3. Dupuytren disease.
   4. Thoracic outlet syndrome.

14. An older adult patient complains of fatigue, weakness, lightheadedness, and anorexia. He also complains of hot, swollen proximal interphalangeal (PIP) and metacarpophalangeal (MCP) joints. These symptoms occurred 5 months ago and recurred a few days ago. Which laboratory findings would be most conclusive of these assessments?
   1. High mean corpuscular volume (MCV), low serum ferritin.
   2. Normal mean corpuscular volume (MCV), high serum ferritin.

3. Elevation in uric acid level.
4. Elevation in white blood cell (WBC) count.

15. How is the talar tilt test conducted?
   1. The tibia is grasped with one hand, and backward pressure is applied to the heel.
   2. The ankle is gently inverted, and laxity of the ligament is graded.
   3. The examiner passively inverts, everts, dorsiflexes, and plantar-flexes the ankle.
   4. The patient actively inverts, everts, dorsiflexes, and plantar-flexes the ankle.

16. Varus pressure on a knee that is slightly flexed (30 degrees) tests:
   1. Medial collateral ligament stability.
   2. Lateral collateral ligament stability.
   3. Medial cruciate ligament stability.
   4. Lateral meniscus tear.

17. The adult-gerontology primary care NP is assessing an adolescent girl for scoliosis. How is this test conducted?
   1. Have the adolescent bend at the waist, and look for asymmetry in the back and hip area.
   2. Examine the adolescent fully clothed, paying particular attention to the hips and back.
   3. Have the adolescent walk heel-to-toe, and observe the gait and pelvis.
   4. Place the adolescent on her back, and flex the knees and observe for misalignment.

18. A 66-year-old male patient presents with lower back pain, fatigue, and weight loss for the past 4 months. Five months ago, he had a right humeral fracture. Lab analysis reveals serum calcium 12.2 mg/dL, hemoglobin 9.2 g/dL, hematocrit 27.1%. A lumbar x-ray is ordered and displays areas of hypodensity in the vertebral column as well as generalized osteopenia. Dipstick urinalysis reveals increased albumin. Which of the following tests would provide the most definitive diagnosis?
   1. CT of the lumbar spine.
   2. Bone marrow biopsy.
   3. Digital rectal exam.
   4. Prostate biopsy.

19. A young adult twisted his knee and comes to the clinic complaining of knee pain. He also states that in the past few weeks his knee has "locked up a couple of times." On examination, a positive McMurray test result is elicited. This is consistent with a diagnosis of:
   1. Anterior cruciate ligament tear.
   2. Dislocated patella.
   3. Medial meniscus tear.
   4. Chondromalacia patella.

Disorders

20. Which observation by the adult-gerontology primary care NP would lead to inclusion of a differential diagnosis of osteoporosis in a 78-year-old female patient who is complaining of bone and joint pain?
    1. Decrease in skin turgor.
    2. Low vitamin D level.
    3. Bilateral swelling of the feet.
    4. Temperature elevation.

21. The adult-gerontology primary care NP realizes that the most common cause of shoulder pain in adults is:
    1. Frozen shoulder.
    2. Thoracic outlet syndrome.
    3. Impingement syndrome.
    4. Osteoarthritis.

22. A 45-year-old female complains of knee pain when kneeling and a "clicking" noise when walking up steps. The adult-gerontology primary care NP notes slight knee effusion and tenderness when palpating the patella against the condyles. The diagnosis for this patient is:
    1. Anterior cruciate tear.
    2. Dislocated patella.
    3. Chondromalacia patella.
    4. Patellar tendonitis.

23. A patient has been diagnosed with a complete rotator cuff tear of the left shoulder. The nurse would expect the patient to have difficulty in:
    1. Abducting the left arm.
    2. Supinating the left forearm.
    3. Shrugging the shoulders.
    4. Touching the left hand to the right shoulder.

24. An adult-gerontology primary care NP is reviewing patient histories to determine whether there is increased risk for the development of osteoporosis in a group of elderly patients. Which three observations would confirm increased risk?
    1. Male gender.
    2. Female patient with body mass index (BMI) of 28 kg/m^2.
    3. Patient taking oral prednisone therapy prescribed for skin irritation.
    4. Female gender.
    5. Patient history of seizure disorders being managed with antiseizure medication.

25. A patient has been diagnosed with polymyalgia rheumatica (PMR). The adult-gerontology primary care NP understands that this disorder is:
    1. An autoimmune, multisystem problem in which the body makes antibodies to its own proteins.
    2. A degenerative disorder with no inflammatory changes in which joint cartilage wears away with age and eventually causes bone spurs.
    3. An inflammatory disorder involving the axial skeleton and large peripheral joints.
    4. A chronic inflammatory connective tissue disorder that affects primarily older women and is associated with giant cell (temporal) arteritis.

26. In teaching a patient about fibromyalgia, the adult-gerontology primary care NP includes what information?
    1. Diagnostic studies such as ESR and CBC are important tools to confirm disease progression.
    2. Avoid stretching exercises and daily low-impact aerobics.
    3. Take ibuprofen (Motrin) 200 mg q4–6h prn for pain and amitriptyline (Elavil) 10 mg 1–2 hours before bedtime.
    4. Apply heat or massage "trigger points" to reduce pain.

27. The adult-gerontology primary care NP understands that chronic synovitis with pannus formation is the basic pathophysiologic finding in patients with:
    1. Systemic lupus erythematosus (SLE).
    2. Ankylosing spondylitis (AS).
    3. Rheumatoid arthritis (RA).
    4. Osteoarthritis (OA).

28. The adult-gerontology primary care NP is examining a patient who is complaining of pain in her hips and knees. She has a history of osteoarthritis. On exam, the joints are painful to movement and are warm to touch. The best immediate therapy for this patient is:
    1. Physical therapy for range of motion of affected areas.
    2. Decreased physical activity and immobilizing splints for affected joints.
    3. Moist heat and/or cold therapy on painful joints.
    4. ESR to determine level of activity.

29. A 79-year-old female presents to the clinic for follow-up related to a recent fall (1 week ago) that took place in the home setting. No fractures were reported on the basis of prior imaging studies and/or physical examination. The patient had fallen on her right side, and there were several bruises noted on the right forearm that have resolved. Which physical finding, if noted by the adult-gerontology primary care NP, would warrant further inquiry?
    1. Brisk capillary refill of the fingers bilaterally.
    2. Palpable nodule located on the right forearm.
    3. Patient complains of feeling tired, but no more than usual.
    4. Patient has clear nasal discharge but no evidence of cough or respiratory compromise.

30. The history of a patient who may have contracted Lyme disease may include what characteristic?
    1. Erythematous rash on the bridge of the nose and on the cheeks with discoid patches on the trunk.
    2. Immediate development of arthritis symptoms, especially in the knees.
    3. Expanding rash with central clearing within 1 month of being bitten by a tick.
    4. Early symptoms of meningitis and myocarditis.

31. The adult-gerontology primary care NP understands that finding Heberden nodes in a physical exam of a patient is a cardinal sign of:
    1. Septic arthritis.
    2. Rheumatoid arthritis (RA).
    3. Gouty arthritis.
    4. Osteoarthritis.

32. Competing diagnoses for an adult male patient who presents with acute onset of unilateral inflammation, pain, and erythema of the first metatarsophalangeal (MTP) joint could be:
    1. Gout, cellulitis, and osteoporosis.
    2. Cellulitis, rheumatoid arthritis, and gout.
    3. Osteoporosis, fibromyalgia, and cellulitis.
    4. Septic arthritis, rheumatoid arthritis, and osteoarthritis.

33. Diseases that often present as polyarthritic disorders include:
    1. Lyme arthritis, rheumatic heart disease, ankylosing spondylitis, and psoriatic arthritis.
    2. Rheumatoid arthritis (RA), gout, Reiter syndrome, and osteoarthritis.
    3. Gonococcal arthritis, systemic lupus erythematosus (SLE), and septic arthritis.
    4. Polymyalgia rheumatica (PMR), Lyme arthritis, pseudogout, and psoriatic arthritis.

34. A common injury can most often cause a meniscus tear under which circumstances?
    1. The knee is almost completely extended, and the tibia is externally rotated.
    2. An applied external force is sufficiently strong to cause external rotation or hyperextension of the knee.
    3. Valgus or varus pressure on the knee occurs at full extension and at 30 degrees of flexion.
    4. The knee is simultaneously twisted and flexed during an injury.

35. Pain in a lumbosacral strain typically begins:
    1. Immediately with the injury.
    2. 1–2 hours after injury.
    3. 6–8 hours after injury.
    4. 12–36 hours after injury.

36. An acute onset of pain that descends down to the lower leg and foot of a 25-year-old obese adult is likely to be a symptom of:
    1. Lumbosacral strain.
    2. Herniated intervertebral disc injury.
    3. Osteomyelitis.
    4. Osteoporosis.

37. The adult-gerontology primary care NP sees a patient with trauma to the knee that caused it to "give out," followed by severe pain and effusion. Later, he had "locking" of the knee with pivoting or turning. This patient has probably suffered:
    1. Patellofemoral stress syndrome.
    2. Growing pains.
    3. Shin splints.
    4. Patellar subluxation.

38. A patient with patellofemoral syndrome has quadriceps setting as a recommended exercise. The adult-gerontology primary care NP would teach the patient to:
    1. Lie supine on the floor with legs extended, dorsiflex the foot, and push the thigh into the floor.
    2. Sit on the floor, lean back on the elbows, flex one knee to 90 degrees, and extend the other completely and hold for 5 seconds.
    3. Lie on the floor and flex both knees to about 20 degrees with a rolled towel underneath them, and extend one leg and hold for 5 seconds.
    4. Use resistive exercises with an elastic band.

39. Which risk factor is associated with gout?
    1. Female gender.
    2. Age 20 years.
    3. Ingestion of salicylate medications.
    4. Overuse of extremity.

40. A third-degree ankle sprain is associated with:
    1. Minimal ecchymosis, moderate edema, and a stable joint.
    2. Moderate ecchymosis, moderate edema, and an unstable joint.
    3. Marked ecchymosis, marked edema, and a stable joint.
    4. Marked ecchymosis, marked edema, and an unstable joint.

41. A patient with rheumatoid arthritis presents for follow-up. What is the best evaluative question the adult-gerontology primary care NP can ask that will help determine the severity of the disease?
    1. "Were you able to drive the car to your appointment today?"
    2. "Were you able to fix your dinner last night?"
    3. "How long does it take for your joints to loosen up after you get up in the morning?"
    4. "How many pounds can you carry?"

42. A 35-year-old woman is seen with a complaint of diffuse musculoskeletal pain, stiffness, and fatigue for the past 3 months. The pain is worse in the morning and also with changes in weather. She states that she wakes up in the morning feeling tired. The result of her physical exam is normal, except for pain on digital palpation in 12 tender points. Her laboratory results are unremarkable. The most likely diagnosis is:
    1. Fibromyalgia.
    2. Myofascial syndrome.
    3. Rheumatoid arthritis (RA).
    4. Depression.

43. When counseling a postmenopausal 60-year-old female patient on prevention of osteoporosis, all of the following are therapeutic recommendations *except*:
    1. Cessation of smoking.
    2. Daily intake of 200 mg of calcium and 40 IU of vitamin D.
    3. Continue hormone replacement therapy (HRT).
    4. Monitor bone loss by dual-energy x-ray absorptiometry (DEXA) every 1–2 years.

44. A patient tells the adult-gerontology primary care NP that she has "whiplash." The adult-gerontology primary care NP understands that this is:
    1. Cervical facet joint dysfunction.
    2. Cervical disc injury.
    3. Zygapophyseal joint injury.
    4. Cervical strain.

45. A patient presents with a complaint of sudden pain and swelling in the knee unrelated to an injury. He also has chills and fever. On exam, the knee is warm, tender, and swollen with evidence of effusion. What action would the adult-gerontology primary care NP take first?
    1. Splint the affected joint.
    2. Obtain aspiration of synovial fluid from the affected joint.
    3. Initiate treatment with nonsteroidal antiinflammatory drugs (NSAIDs).
    4. Recommend rest, ice, compression, and elevation of affected joint.

46. When determining the specific etiology of polyarticular complaints, which clinical clues are most helpful for diagnosis?
    1. Laboratory identification of antinuclear antibodies (ANA) and ESR.
    2. Radiograph of the affected joints.
    3. Affected joint pattern and presence or lack of inflammation.
    4. Sexual history of the patient.

47. A patient with ankylosing spondylitis (AS) is receiving education on managing her disease. The adult-gerontology primary care NP would teach the patient all of the following *except*:
    1. Regular exercise program.
    2. Maintenance systemic corticosteroid therapy.
    3. Use of indomethacin (Indocin) for discomfort.
    4. Observation for signs and symptoms of iritis.

48. An adult patient comes to the office complaining of foot pain. He can recall no specific injury, but he gives a history of being an occasional runner who drinks 6 to 10 beers on weekends. What physical findings would the adult-gerontology primary care NP expect to find?
    1. Redness, swelling, and warmth of first metatarsophalangeal joint.
    2. Swelling, ecchymosis, and decreased range of motion of ankle.
    3. Swelling of foot and decreased circulation.
    4. Decreased range of motion of ankle and obvious bone deformity.

49. Which of the diet selections indicate that the older patient understands health education regarding the prevention of osteoporosis?
    1. Chicken and baked potato.
    2. Glass of skim milk and toasted cheese sandwich.
    3. Hamburger and salad.
    4. Ice cream sundae with whipped cream.

50. During the history, which of the following questions would best assist the adult-gerontology primary care NP in diagnosing osteoarthritis (OA) versus rheumatoid arthritis (RA)?
    1. "Is your joint pain symmetric and localized?"
    2. "Does your morning stiffness usually last several hours?"
    3. "Have you experienced fatigue, weakness, and weight loss?"
    4. "Is your joint pain asymmetric and worse with movement and relieved by rest?"

51. The number one cause of disability in adults under age 45 is:
    1. Cancer.
    2. Fracture.
    3. Low back pain.
    4. Migraines.

52. Primary treatment of joint injury involves:
    1. Rest, ice, compression, and elevation.
    2. Narcotic pain control and radiograph.
    3. Specialist referral and magnetic resonance imaging.
    4. Nonsteroidal antiinflammatory drugs (NSAIDs) and exercise.

53. The most common complaint in a patient with back injury who has cauda equina syndrome, a surgical emergency, is:
    1. Urinary retention.
    2. Numbness below the level of injury.
    3. Weakness in the lower extremities.
    4. Leg pain.

54. Recognition of annular tears is important in the diagnosis of back pain because:
    1. They require immediate surgery.
    2. They are often misdiagnosed as strains or sprains, leading to herniation.
    3. They result in rapid paralysis.
    4. Radiography would reveal them, but x-rays are usually not ordered initially.

55. What chronic musculoskeletal problem may occur after an injury, is characterized by a 3-month history of pain on both sides of the body (above and below the waist), and tenderness in at least 11 of 18 specified points?
    1. Chronic osteoarthritis.
    2. Reflex sympathetic dystrophy.
    3. Tendinitis.
    4. Fibromyalgia.

56. Which patient is at highest risk for osteoporosis?
    1. A 55-year-old male smoker and retired athlete.
    2. A 60-year-old, 105-lb, postmenopausal white female switchboard operator.
    3. A 42-year-old black female intensive care unit nurse who is lactose intolerant.
    4. A 50-year-old obese white woman with three children living on a farm.

57. A 38-year-old secretary complains of pain in her hands at night. On exam, the adult-gerontology primary care NP notes wasting of the thenar eminence of both hands and dry skin on the thumb, index, and middle fingers. The adult-gerontology primary care NP suspects:
    1. Carpal tunnel syndrome.
    2. Transient ischemic attack.
    3. Osteoarthritis.
    4. Raynaud phenomenon.

58. A 53-year-old woman presents with complaints of morning stiffness in the neck and back. She has pain in her pelvis and shoulder as well as fatigue. Her laboratory studies reveal elevated ESR, normal rheumatoid factor, normal creatine phosphokinase, and normochromic normocytic anemia. Her physical exam reveals an elevated temperature, bilateral pain, and stiffness of the pectoral and pelvic muscles. Based on this information, the most appropriate diagnosis is:
    1. Polyarteritis nodosa.
    2. Wegener granulomatosis.
    3. Polymyalgia rheumatica (PMR).
    4. Rheumatoid arthritis.

59. A 55-year-old woman with a prior diagnosis of polymyalgia rheumatica (PMR) presents with headache, low-grade fever, aching, stiffness, fatigue, malaise, and anorexia. Based on the information, the adult-gerontology primary care NP would make a preliminary diagnosis of:
    1. Influenza.
    2. Pneumonia.
    3. Temporal arteritis.
    4. Rheumatoid arthritis.

60. A man comes into the clinic complaining of low back pain that radiates down the lateral thigh. The pain began suddenly on the job after lifting a heavy object. The adult-gerontology primary care NP would further evaluate the patient for which three conditions:
    1. Compression fracture of lower lumbar vertebrae.
    2. Piriformis syndrome.
    3. Spinal cord injury.
    4. Compression of a lumbar disc.
    5. History of spinal cord injury.

61. An 80-year-old resident of a long-term care facility with a history of multi-infarct dementia (MID) is alert but disoriented to person, place, and situation. His only health problems are MID and osteoarthritis. Over the past 2 weeks, he has become agitated and exit-seeking and is constantly rubbing his knees. The adult-gerontology primary care NP suspects that the patient is experiencing:
    1. Worsening dementia.
    2. Pain.
    3. Urinary tract infection (UTI).
    4. Acute cerebral infarct.

62. An adolescent complains of right knee pain immediately after running in track practice. On examination, the knee is warm to touch, and a tender, swollen tibial tuberosity is noted. The adult-gerontology primary care NP suspects:
    1. Osgood-Schlatter disease.
    2. Rheumatoid arthritis.
    3. Acute tendinitis.
    4. Posttraumatic knee effusion.

63. Nighttime extremity pain in school-age children that is deep but not present in the joints and that may be caused by inflammation of the muscle bodies in tight fascial sheaths and by periods of high activity is:
    1. Osgood-Schlatter disease.
    2. Patellofemoral stress syndrome.
    3. Growing pains.
    4. Shin splints.

64. The adult-gerontology primary care NP is teaching crutch walking to an adolescent with a lower-leg cast for a fractured tibia. Instructions for assisting the adolescent to walk up the stairs would include:
    1. Place both crutches on the upper step and step up with unaffected leg while balancing on crutches.
    2. Position the affected leg on the upper step and use the crutches to move up.
    3. Place the unaffected leg on the upper step and move affected leg and crutches up together.
    4. Position the affected leg and the crutch on the upper step and bring the unaffected leg up with the crutch.

65. An adolescent patient is being evaluated by the adult-gerontology primary care NP for knee pain. The patient is active in sports in his school but can recall no specific injury to the knee. On examination, the adult-gerontology primary care NP finds unilateral swelling of the anterior aspect of the tibial tubercle, which is tender. The most likely diagnosis is:
    1. Stress fracture.
    2. Patellar dislocation.
    3. Osgood-Schlatter disease.
    4. Neumann syndrome.

Pharmacology

66. A 65-year-old postmenopausal female has been treated with alendronate (Fosamax) for 6 years. Current screening indicates no increase in risk factors. Based on clinical guidelines, which treatment option would the adult-gerontology nurse primary care practitioner suggest to the patient?
    1. Discontinue medication at this time.
    2. Switch medication from oral to intravenous route in order to maintain adequate coverage.
    3. Add vitamin D 500 IU/day to the treatment regimen.
    4. Increase calcium supplementation to 1500 mg/day.

67. The adult-gerontology primary care NP is seeing a middle-aged, severely arthritic woman who has been receiving maintenance therapy of prednisone 10 mg/day for the past 6 weeks. She now presents as acutely ill with signs and symptoms of acute pneumonia. She is fatigued and weak with loss of appetite, and her blood pressure (BP) is lower than at previous visits. Which action should be taken in regard to prednisone?
    1. Immediately discontinue the medication.
    2. Increase the dosage to 60 mg/day, then taper back to 10 mg/day.
    3. Gradually taper from 10 to 1 mg/day.
    4. Maintain the dosage at 10 mg/day.

68. An elderly patient is being treated with colchicine for prophylaxis related to an acute gout attack. Based on this information, the adult-gerontology primary care NP will assess the patient for which of the following?
    1. Constipation.
    2. Fluid retention.
    3. Fever.
    4. Dehydration.

69. What is the initial drug of choice for a patient with rheumatoid arthritis (RA)?
    1. Tramadol.
    2. Aspirin.
    3. Methotrexate.
    4. Hydrocortisone.

70. A patient with rheumatoid arthritis (RA) is placed on prednisone 5 mg PO qd. In teaching the patient about her medication, it would be important for the adult-gerontology primary care NP to include what information?
    1. When the symptoms of arthritis subside, she will be able to quit taking her medication.
    2. It is important to take the medication as prescribed, even after the redness and swelling decrease.
    3. Increased fluid intake is important to prevent renal damage by the steroids.
    4. The medication should be taken about 30 minutes before eating.

71. What is the correct drug therapy for an adult with an acute episode of gout?
    1. Indomethacin (Indocin) 25 mg PO prn.
    2. Naproxen (Naprosyn) 100 mg PO bid.
    3. Colchicine 0.6 mg two tablets PO × 1, then repeat in 1 hour × 1.
    4. Indomethacin (Indocin) 50 mg q8h × 6–8 doses, then 25 mg q8h until resolution.

72. An adult-gerontology primary care NP is reviewing the medication profile of an older adult male patient with a history of renal failure who now presents with an acute exacerbation of gout. Which action should be taken by the adult-gerontology primary care NP at this time?
    1. Assess medications being taken for pain control.
    2. Monitor daily weights.
    3. Discontinue use of NSAIDS.
    4. Withhold dialysis treatments until gouty attack has subsided.

73. If a 24-hour urine test indicates that a patient is secreting too much uric acid (>900 mg/day), the adult-gerontology primary care NP would prescribe:
    1. Aspirin 325 mg PO daily.
    2. Tylenol 325 mg PO q4–6h prn.
    3. Indomethacin (Indocin) 25 mg PO q8h, then increase at weekly intervals by 25 mg daily.
    4. Allopurinol (Zyloprim) 100 mg PO qd × 1 week, then increase daily dose by 100 mg to a maximum of 300 mg/day.

74. Disease-modifying drugs for rheumatoid arthritis in adults include:
    1. Ibuprofen (Motrin, Advil), sulindac (Clinoril), and salicylates (aspirin, Disalcid).
    2. Corticosteroids (prednisone, methylprednisolone).
    3. Misoprostol (Cytotec).
    4. Hydroxychloroquine (Plaquenil), sulfasalazine (Azulfidine), methotrexate, and gold sodium thiomalate (Myochrysine).

75. What is the drug of choice for treatment of gout in the older adult patient?
    1. Xanthine oxidase inhibitors.
    2. Aromatase inhibitors.
    3. Angiotensin-converting enzyme inhibitors.
    4. Beta blockers.

76. Gold compounds are contraindicated in patients with all of the following conditions *except:*
    1. Renal disease.
    2. Hepatic disease.
    3. Rheumatoid arthritis.
    4. Blood dyscrasia.

77. The adult-gerontology primary care NP, in using best practice, would prescribe which dosage for vitamin D supplementation for the elderly patient to prevent osteoporosis?
    1. 1500 mg of vitamin D every other day.
    2. 400 IU on a daily basis.
    3. 800–1000 IU on a daily basis.
    4. 600 mg of vitamin D on a daily basis.

78. The most appropriate medication used to control pain for a patient with osteoarthritis would be:
    1. Acetaminophen.
    2. Systemic corticosteroids.
    3. Gold salts.
    4. Misoprostol.

79. What is a serious side effect of ibuprofen in the older adult patient?
    1. Rebound headaches.
    2. Impairment of renal function.
    3. Neuropathy.
    4. Pancreatic failure.

80. A patient has been on methotrexate (Rheumatrex) for 6 weeks. This was the medication of choice for her severe refractory rheumatoid arthritis (RA). What parameters should the adult-gerontology primary care NP monitor?
    1. Monthly platelet count and CBC with differential.
    2. Urinalysis, blood sugar, and ECG every 2 weeks.
    3. Monthly CBC, urinalysis, and electrolytes.
    4. Coagulation studies, electrolytes, and CBC every week.

81. A middle-aged male patient presents with a complaint of waking up yesterday morning with a swollen and painful big toe. The patient reports he has "never had anything like this before" and has not had previous health problems. On exam, the big toe is red, hot, and tender in the joint with inflammation extending into the surrounding tissue. His temperature is 99.8°F (37.7°C), and his WBC count is mildly elevated. Needle aspiration of joint fluid reveals urate crystals. What is the best treatment choice that the adult-gerontology primary care NP could recommend for the patient?
    1. Bed rest, very-low-calorie diet, and increased fluid intake.
    2. Allopurinol (Zyloprim) 200 mg PO daily, continuing dose for maintenance therapy once symptoms resolve.
    3. Naproxen (Naprosyn) 500 mg PO tid, continuing full dose until symptoms resolve, then tapering and discontinuing over 72 hours.
    4. Injection of intra-articular corticosteroid to the affected joint.

82. What is the preferred medication used to treat chronic pain symptoms in elderly patients as a first-line therapy?
    1. Acetaminophen.
    2. NSAIDs.
    3. Opioid analgesics.
    4. Anticonvulsants.

83. An older adult woman comes into the clinic complaining of "sores" in her mouth. The adult-gerontology primary care NP observes several inflamed ulcers on her gums and lips. Which medication would the nurse identify as most likely to cause this problem?
    1. Propranolol (Inderal).
    2. Spironolactone (Aldactone).
    3. Fexofenadine (Allegra).
    4. Alendronate (Fosamax).

10 | Musculoskeletal Answers & Rationales

Physical Exam & Diagnostic Tests

1. Answer: 4

   Rationale: With regard to musculoskeletal system, limitation of range of motion of the joint indicates that further testing should be initiated. Slight swelling in the context of related pain may be due to an injury, but unless swelling is pronounced, the area should just be monitored. Brisk capillary refill is a normal finding. The presence of pain in both shoulders may indicate osteoarthritic changes.

2. Answer: 3

   Rationale: ESR provides a general indicator that inflammation is occurring within the musculoskeletal system. C-reactive protein is a specific indicator relative to cardiac disease. Antinuclear antibodies provide specific information related to immunological diseases. A1C provides information related to glycemic control.

3. Answer: 2

   Rationale: The goniometer is used to determine the degree of joint flexion and extension or joint range of motion.

4. Answer: 3

   Rationale: A positive Apley test result, locking of the knee, or the sound of clicks and pain, may indicate a torn meniscus. The drawer sign tests the integrity of cruciate ligaments with the patient in a sitting and lying, not prone, position. The McMurray test assesses for medial meniscus injury when the knee is fully flexed and the tibia is externally rotated, with varus pressure applied to the knee while extended. For medial meniscus tears, the test is performed while applying valgus pressure to the knee.

5. Answer: 4

   Rationale: The Phalen maneuver, when present, suggests carpal tunnel syndrome. The Tinel sign also tests for carpal tunnel syndrome, but it is performed by lightly percussing over the median nerve on the volar (palmar) side of the wrist, with characteristic tingling or shocklike sensations across the palm, thumb, and first two fingers. The drawer sign and McMurray test are used to assess the knee.

6. Answer: 3

   Rationale: The balloon sign occurs when considerable fluid is in the suprapatellar pouch, with possible ballottement of the patella. The bulge sign is for testing fluid in the knee joint and is elicited with the knee extended by applying pressure to the medial aspect and watching for a bulge or fluid wave. A patellar tap suggests fluid in the knee as the patella clicks against the femur. The drawer sign tests the cruciate ligaments with the patient in a sitting and lying position. The Kernig sign for meningeal irritation is the inability to extend the lower leg when that leg is flexed at the hip, or there may be resistance or pain during elicitation of the sign.

7. Answer: 1

   Rationale: Pain with gentle deviation of a fist (thumb tucked under the other four fingers) to the ulnar side is a positive Finkelstein test result and an indication of de Quervain disease, which is swelling and tenderness over the volar portion of the "snuffbox" resulting from chronic tenosynovitis. A positive Tinel sign (tapping gently over carpal tunnel causing tingling in thumb, index finger, and middle and radial half of ring finger) and a positive Phalen maneuver (holding dorsum of hands flexed 90 degrees back to back with the same distribution of tingling) are indicative of carpel tunnel syndrome. A positive Lachman test result indicates stability of the cruciate ligament of the knee.

8. Answer: 3

   Rationale: The musculoskeletal system is examined by a visual inspection and palpation of the bones, joints, and surrounding musculoskeletal soft tissue. Percussion is generally not done, and auscultation is not appropriate to the system being examined.

9. Answer: 3

   Rationale: Patients with polymyalgia rheumatica (PMR) have a rapid, dramatic clinical response to corticosteroid therapy. Serum protein electrophoresis is used to rule out myeloma. The erythrocyte sedimentation rate (ESR) is elevated in a number of diseases and is not specific to PMR. The chest radiograph is used to diagnose diseases affecting the lungs and thorax. The serum C-reactive protein (CRP) would be elevated in PMR.

10. Answer: 3

    Rationale: The wrist, metacarpophalangeal (MCP) and proximal interphalangeal (PIP) joints, and other small joints of the hands and feet are involved with rheumatoid arthritis (RA). The great toe is most often involved with gout. The large joints of the hip, knee, and shoulder, along with the distal interphalangeal (DIP) joint and base of the thumb, are involved with degenerative joint disease (osteoarthritis).

11. Answer: 2

Rationale: It would not be necessary to obtain a complete blood count (CBC). The A1C measurement would be ordered to evaluate the relative control of diabetes. Electromyography (EMG) is most often performed to evaluate both nerve conduction and needle electrode exam. Many toxins and inflammatory processes are involved with polyneuropathy, so the erythrocyte sedimentation rate (ESR) would be a helpful diagnostic tool for identifying the inflammatory process, even though it is a nonspecific test for the condition.

12. Answer: 4

Rationale: A thorough history is very important in assessing any patient with an injury, but with a back injury, the mechanism will provide the best indication of the extent of the injury and the proper diagnostic and treatment approaches. Determining loss of bowel or bladder control could indicate an emergent condition, cauda equina syndrome.

13. Answer: 2

Rationale: Carpel tunnel syndrome, a compression neuropathy of the median nerve at the wrist, is commonly caused by repetitive finger and wrist motion and results in a positive Tinel sign and Phalen maneuver. The Tinel sign is considered positive when tapping over the nerve with a reflex hammer causes tingling in the distribution of the nerve. The Phalen maneuver is performed by fully flexing the wrist passively and noting tingling in the thumb or fingers.

14. Answer: 2

Rationale: The clinical assessments point to a chronic inflammatory process such as rheumatoid arthritis (RA). The dizziness, fatigue, lightheadedness, and weakness may be a problem with anemia. The anemia of chronic disease is either a microcytic or normocytic anemia. The value that differentiates the anemia of chronic disease from other anemias is the serum ferritin (iron stores). The value will be either normal or high. A mean corpuscular volume (MCV) of 104 indicates a macrocytic anemia, which would not include the anemia of chronic disease. Low serum ferritin would not be considered a possibility with this disorder. The uric acid level would be elevated in gout. The white blood cell (WBC) count does not address the signs of anemia.

15. Answer: 2

Rationale: The talar tilt test is a ligamentous stress test that detects excessive ankle inversion by examining the integrity of the lateral ankle ligaments, particularly the calcaneofibular ligament. Anterior ankle stability is tested in the anterior drawer test, in which the tibia is grasped by the examiner's one hand while the heel is firmly grasped, and backward pressure is applied to the tibia with the examiner's other hand. In passive range of motion, the examiner inverts, everts, dorsiflexes, and plantar-flexes the foot and ankle. The patient puts the foot and ankle through the complete range in active range of motion.

16. Answer: 2

Rationale: Varus pressure on a slightly flexed knee tests lateral collateral ligament stability. Valgus pressure tests medial collateral ligament stability. Cruciate ligaments are tested with the anterior drawer test. The McMurray test assesses medial meniscus injury when the knee is fully flexed and the tibia is externally rotated, with varus pressure applied to the knee while extended.

17. Answer: 1

Rationale: The adolescent should remove her shirt (leave on bra or swimsuit top) and bend at the waist. The adult-gerontology primary care NP should examine for uneven hips and shoulders.

18. Answer: 2

Rationale: The patient most likely has multiple myeloma. This is best evidenced in this question as bone pain, hypercalcemia, and x-rays that show lytic bone lesions and osteopenia. In the absence of osteopenia or lytic bone lesions, an MRI scan may be ordered. Diagnosis of multiple myeloma requires greater than or equal to 10% clonal plasma cells found via bone marrow biopsy combined with related organ damage or tissue impairment. End-organ damage often presents as renal insufficiency due to excess light chains and presents as albuminuria. Electrophoresis will reveal M proteins.

19. Answer: 3

Rationale: A positive McMurray test result (palpable click and pain when rotating the foot laterally and extending the leg) along with the symptoms is indicative of a medial meniscus tear. The drawer test is done to evaluate anterior cruciate ligament tears (knee flexed with foot on table; sit on foot and grasp both sides of tibia at knee; pull tibia forward; abnormal if movement of tibia is away from the joint).

Disorders

20. Answer: 2

Rationale: Low vitamin D level may be associated with a clinical diagnosis of osteoporosis. A decrease in skin turgor is a normal consequence of the aging process.

Bilateral swelling of the feet may be due to vascular insufficiency and/or a consequence of standing. An elevation in temperature is typically not associated with osteoporosis.

21. Answer: 3

Rationale: Impingement syndrome is usually caused by rotator cuff tendinitis, which occurs when internal/external rotation is impaired. Frozen shoulder can occur after a rotator cuff injury, especially if a sling is used for a prolonged period. With the Adson or Wright maneuver, thoracic outlet syndrome would indicate a decrease or loss of the radial pulse when the patient abducts the arm and holds a deep breath while hyperextending the neck and turning the chin toward the raised arm.

22. Answer: 3

Rationale: These are common symptoms of chondromalacia patella. With anterior cruciate tears, the patient generally cannot bear weight on the extremity without it buckling or giving way. With a dislocated patella, the patient would have severe pain associated with considerable effusion (loss of normal knee hollow on sides of patella) and possible patellofemoral compartment. Patellar tendonitis, or jumper's knee, causes pain, weakness, and swelling of the knee joint, but no "clicking" noises.

23. Answer: 1

Rationale: With a complete rotator cuff tear (most commonly a rupture of supraspinatus tendon), the patient would have difficulty abducting the arm and impaired internal/external rotation. Touching the hand to the opposite shoulder is adduction.

24. Answer: 3, 4, 5

Rationale: Increased risk for the development of osteoporosis in the elderly patient is seen in females as opposed to their male counterparts, as well as in individuals who are on prednisone and/or antiseizure therapy. In terms of body mass index (BMI) or weight, individuals who are small framed are at greater risk of developing osteoporosis than those who are considered to be of normal weight or in the slightly overweight range.

25. Answer: 4

Rationale: Polymyalgia rheumatica (PMR) is a chronic inflammatory connective tissue disorder that affects primarily older women and is associated with giant cell (temporal) arteritis. Anemia is common in PMR, along with an elevated erythrocyte sedimentation rate (ESR). There is a common complaint of morning stiffness; rheumatoid factor is negative. An autoimmune, multisystem disorder is characteristic of systemic lupus erythematosus (SLE). A degenerative joint disorder is characteristic of osteoarthritis. An inflammatory disorder involving the axial skeleton and large peripheral joints is characteristic of ankylosing spondylitis.

26. Answer: 3

Rationale: Diagnostic studies are of little value and benefit, except to rule out other causes, such as polymyalgia rheumatica (PMR) or hypothyroidism. Treatment is symptomatic; the usual drugs are amitriptyline (Elavil), nonsteroidal antiinflammatory drugs (NSAIDs), tramadol (Ultram), cyclobenzaprine (Flexeril), temazepam (Restoril), zolpidem (Ambien), pregabalin (Lyrica), duloxetine (Cymbalta), and triazolam (Halcion). Engaging in daily, slow, low-impact aerobics, preferably done in the late afternoon or early evening, is encouraged. Heat and massage are helpful, but not on the "trigger points."

27. Answer: 3

Rationale: The chronic inflammatory disorder of rheumatoid arthritis (RA) involves synovial hypertrophy caused by chronic synovitis and pannus formation that results in progressive destruction of the cartilage, ligament, tendons, and bone. Ankylosing spondylitis (AS) usually involves the large peripheral joints (e.g., sacroiliac) and is characterized by extreme kyphosis. There is no inflammation with osteoarthritis (OA). Systemic lupus erythematosus (SLE) has a distribution of symptoms similar to that of RA, but no pannus formation.

28. Answer: 3

Rationale: Moist heat or cold, whichever relieves the pain more effectively, is appropriate to use on acutely affected joints. Physical therapy is recommended after the acute involvement of the joint; care must be taken to decrease repetitive movements. Immobilization is avoided because it tends to increase the stiffness of the joint. The erythrocyte sedimentation rate (ESR) is not an appropriate indicator to determine the level of activity in patients with osteoarthritis.

29. Answer: 2

Rationale: The patient has had a recent fall, so the appearance of a palpable nodule requires further inquiry as this can be indicative of further vascular damage. Brisk capillary refill is a normal finding. The fact that the patient complains of feeling tired but that this has not changed from previous reporting is unremarkable. The fact that the patient has clear nasal discharge with no other contributory cold or flulike symptoms is unremarkable.

30. Answer: 3

Rationale: Expanding rash with central clearing may also be described as the "bull's-eye rash," which is associated with Lyme disease. An erythematous rash on the bridge of the nose and on the cheeks describes the malar or "butterfly" rash of systemic lupus erythematosus. The arthritis symptoms and other complications (meningitis and myocarditis) occur later in the disease process, especially if the patient is not treated with antibiotics, usually tetracycline, doxycycline, or amoxicillin.

31. Answer: 4

Rationale: Deformities (bony protuberances) of the distal interphalangeal (DIP) joints are called Heberden nodes and are cardinal signs of osteoarthritis. The DIP joints are seldom involved with rheumatoid arthritis (RA). Gouty arthritis most often affects the great toe. Joints are warm, red, tender, and swollen with septic arthritis.

32. Answer: 2

Rationale: Cellulitis usually presents with warm, erythematous, painful areas of the skin. Symptoms of erythema, edema, and pain of the first metatarsophalageal (MTP) joint are a common presentation for gout. Symptoms present in rheumatoid arthritis (RA) are similar: red, swollen, and painful joints. The inflammation of RA is usually symmetric but can present as erythematous, swollen joints. Systemic symptoms may also be present. Osteoporosis most often occurs in postmenopausal women because of bone loss that occurs with the decline of estrogen in the blood. Bone thinning leads to fractures, not inflammation of joints or skin. Osteoarthritis presents as pain and stiffness with decreased range of motion, stiffness in the morning for a few minutes that relieves with movement, and occasionally joint effusions. Point tenderness in 11 of 18 sites with digital palpation is present in fibromyalgia. Joint swelling and erythema are not present. In septic arthritis, joint pain, inflammation, and erythema would be accompanied by systemic symptoms of fever and chills. It would be considered in the differential diagnosis for this patient.

33. Answer: 1

Rationale: Lyme arthritis, rheumatic heart disease, ankylosing spondylitis, psoriatic arthritis, rheumatoid arthritis (RA), Reiter syndrome, osteoarthritis, gonococcal arthritis, systemic lupus erythematosus (SLE), and polymyalgia rheumatica (PMR) typically occur as polyarthritic disease. Gout, septic arthritis, and pseudogout most often occur as monoarthritis.

34. Answer: 4

Rationale: A patient who sustains a meniscal tear can usually recall a twisting injury of the knee followed by pain and effusion over the joint line. A strong force or injury that causes

external rotation or hyperextension of the knee is a common mechanism of injury for collateral or cruciate ligament injuries. Valgus and varus are tests for stability of the knee joint, which involve applying medial and lateral pressure to the knee during full extension and flexion of 30 degrees.

35. Answer: 4

Rationale: As the soft tissue swells, pain onset occurs usually about 12–36 hours after injury.

36. Answer: 2

Rationale: Herniated intervertebral disc pain typically descends to the lower leg and foot. Lumbosacral strain causes pain in the back, buttock, and sometimes thigh. Osteomyelitis must be preceded by an event that permits an infectious agent to enter the bone. Osteoporosis occurs most often in postmenopausal women.

37. Answer: 4

Rationale: At the time a patellar subluxation occurs, a traumatic event causes the knee to "give out," and the patella is usually laterally displaced; severe pain and an effusion result. Subsequent to the injury, the patient will notice a locking sensation in the knee with pivoting or turning. Patellofemoral stress syndrome is a form of overuse syndrome. Pain of a dull, aching quality is present in the knee, sometimes with clicking. Long periods of sitting or activities that involve knee flexion as well as compression of the patella in the groove cause increased pain. Growing pains usually occur at night and resolve by morning. The pain is deep and does not involve the joints. In shin splints, inflammation of muscles along the medial shaft of the tibia due to overuse causes aching pain. Rest improves the pain.

38. Answer: 1

Rationale: In quadriceps setting, with the foot dorsiflexed, the thigh is pressed downward against the floor and held for 5 seconds. The straight leg raise involves lifting an extended leg while sitting on the floor and leaning back on the elbows with the opposite leg flexed to 90 degrees. A terminal arc extension requires that the patient lie on the floor supine with extended legs flexed to 20 degrees over a rolled towel. The patient then extends one leg and holds for 5 seconds. The exercise is repeated with the opposite leg. All of these exercises can be used to stretch and strengthen the quadriceps muscles in those with patellofemoral stress syndrome. Resistive exercises with an elastic band are general exercises that can be done with the extremities.

39. Answer: 3

Rationale: Gout generally affects men over age 30 and is associated with obesity; lead intoxication; starvation; and use of some medications, including salicylates, diuretics, pyrazinamide, and alcohol.

40. Answer: 4

Rationale: A third-degree sprain is a complete tear of a ligament resulting in marked edema, ecchymosis, pain, and an unstable joint.

41. Answer: 3

Rationale: Morning stiffness or activity and the length of time required for maximal improvement are American Rheumatism Association Classification criteria for rheumatoid arthritis (RA) and useful, measurable tools for effects of treatment. The other questions are good indicators of quality of activities of daily living but do not give a full, overall, measurable picture of the patient's joint discomfort.

42. Answer: 1

Rationale: This patient meets the classification criteria for fibromyalgia based on history of widespread pain and pain in 11 of 18 tender points. Myofascial syndrome symptoms are more focal, with no associated fatigue or sleep disorder. A patient with rheumatoid arthritis (RA) would have abnormal serologic study results. Depression may cause musculoskeletal pain and fatigue but would not include reproducible tender points.

43. Answer: 2

Rationale: This is a subtherapeutic amount of calcium and vitamin D. Recommended calcium for women ages 51 and older is 1200 mg daily and 800–1000 IU daily of vitamin D. The other choices are recommendations for prevention of osteoporosis.

44. Answer: 4

Rationale: Most whiplash injuries are associated with a cervical neck strain related to spasm of the cervical and upper back muscles from injury.

45. Answer: 2

Rationale: The patient's symptoms are indicative of septic arthritis, which is a medical emergency; if not treated promptly, the joint may be severely damaged or destroyed. Exam of the joint fluid is the most important diagnostic test. The other choices may provide some symptomatic relief, but the first goal of treatment is to determine whether the joint is septic.

46. Answer: 3

Rationale: When developing a differential diagnosis, the history and physical exam will help narrow the differen-

tiation. Other procedures are important in completing the evaluation, but the most important information is the pattern of joints affected and whether it is inflammatory or noninflammatory disease.

47. Answer: 2

Rationale: Corticosteroids have limited value in treating ankylosing spondylitis (AS), and long-term use is associated with many serious side effects. Important treatment includes regular exercise to strengthen supporting muscles and use of nonsteroidal antiinflammatory drugs (NSAIDs) for pain. Approximately one-third of patients have recurrent attacks of acute iritis.

48. Answer: 1

Rationale: Trauma, increased alcohol intake on weekends, and physical stress have all been implicated in acute gout. Gout occurs primarily in adult men. Decreased circulation, ecchymosis, and bone deformity are not likely with acute gout.

49. Answer: 2

Rationale: Calcium intake is important in minimizing the development of osteoporosis. Both these foods contain calcium. The other options are not focused on calcium intake.

50. Answer: 4

Rationale: Signs and symptoms of osteoarthritis include asymmetric joint pain exacerbated by movement and relieved by rest. Stiffness is of short duration (<15 minutes) after inactivity or in the morning. Pain may be described as aching and poorly localized. The other questions are indicative of rheumatoid arthritis (RA).

51. Answer: 3

Rationale: Low back pain is the number one cause of disability and accounts for 25% of young adults aged 20–44 years reporting disabling work-related injuries.

52. Answer: 1

Rationale: The RICE principle is used for initial treatment: **R**est, **I**ce, **C**ompression, and **E**levation. All other treatments mentioned may be appropriate, but not as the primary treatment.

53. Answer: 1

Rationale: Although all symptoms may be associated with cauda equina syndrome, urinary retention and loss of bowel or bladder control are important clues to the immediate need for surgery.

54. Answer: 2

Rationale: Annular tears are tears of the annulus fibrosus of the intervertebral disc and are the first step toward herniation. Early recognition can help avoid the need for surgical repair of a subsequent herniation.

55. Answer: 4

Rationale: Fibromyalgia is a poorly understood condition that can prolong the normal treatment course of an injury considerably and is very difficult to treat. Osteoarthritis may follow an injury, as can reflex sympathetic dystrophy and tendinitis, but they do not have specified tender points.

56. Answer: 2

Rationale: The five risk factors for osteoporosis include being of female gender, white or Asian, over age 45, low body weight, postmenopausal, sedentary lifestyle, low calcium intake, and a smoker.

57. Answer: 1

Rationale: The patient's occupation and symptoms both suggest carpal tunnel syndrome. Initial treatment would involve night splinting, ice, and antiinflammatory medication.

58. Answer: 3

Rationale: Polymyalgia rheumatica (PMR) is an inflammatory disorder of the proximal muscles presenting as described. Polyarteritis nodosa, an inflammatory disorder affecting the small arteries, presents with muscle weakness, myalgias, headache, and subcutaneous nodules along leg and arm arteries. Wegener disease presents with mild anemia, dyspnea, cough, chest pain, hemoptysis, and abnormal urinalysis.

59. Answer: 3

Rationale: Up to 40% of patients with temporal arteritis have a previous history of polymyalgia rheumatica (PMR). Presenting complaints include headache, low-grade fever, muscle aching and stiffness, fatigue, malaise, and anorexia.

60. Answer: 1, 2, 4

Rationale: The patient is presenting with the classic symptoms of nerve root compression secondary to pressure from a protruding lumbar disc. The sciatic stretch test (straight leg raise) maneuver will increase the radiation of pain down the hip. In piriformis syndrome, the piriformis muscle (a narrow muscle located in the buttocks) compresses or irritates the sciatic nerve. Spinal cord injury will result in focal pain or tenderness, bruising, hematoma, and palpable step-offs along the spine.

61. Answer: 2

Rationale: This patient is likely experiencing an acute exacerbation of his osteoarthritis because he is constantly rubbing his knees. Because 85% of the residents of long-term care facilities have uncontrolled pain, he probably has uncontrolled pain. Starting him on routine acetaminophen (Tylenol) would be an excellent start to pain management. It is unlikely that the patient's dementia is worsening, because this is an acute problem. Although a urinary tract infection (UTI) is a good choice, the cues of rubbing the major joints would likely rule out a UTI as the problem. The patient is not exhibiting any neurologic symptoms, which would rule out an acute cerebral infarct.

62. Answer: 1

Rationale: Osgood-Schlatter disease (tibial tubercle apophysitis) is characterized by a painful, self-limiting tibial tubercle swelling that leads to knee pain, especially during periods of rapid growth. Extension of the knee against resistance or application of pressure over the tibial tubercle aggravates the pain. Pain worsens with activity and subsides with rest.

63. Answer: 3

Rationale: Growing pains usually occur at night and resolve by morning. The pain is deep and does not involve the joints. Osgood-Schlatter disease results from degeneration of the tibial tubercle because of overuse and a rapid growth spurt. Pain and swelling occur over the tibial tubercle. Symptoms are exacerbated by activities that involve the quadriceps muscle. Another form of overuse syndrome is patellofemoral stress syndrome. Pain of a dull, aching quality is present in the knee, sometimes with clicking. Long periods of sitting or activities that involve knee flexion as well as compression of the patella in the groove cause increased pain. In shin splints, inflammation of muscles along the medial shaft of the tibia results from overuse and causes aching pain. Rest improves the pain. Improper warm-up exercises or extended exercise by an unconditioned person, especially in unsuitable shoes, can lead to this pain.

64. Answer: 3

Rationale: The unaffected leg goes up the step first, and then the crutches, followed by the affected leg. This allows for stability and weight bearing on the unaffected leg, with the crutches supporting the affected leg.

65. Answer: 3

Rationale: Osgood-Schlatter disease is common in late childhood and adolescence. The risk for disease increases in patients who are involved in strenuous activity, especially involving the quadriceps muscle. The usual treatment is NSAIDs and rest.

Pharmacology

66. Answer: 1

Rationale: Patients who have low fracture risk after being treated with alendronate (Fosamax) for at least 5 years qualify for a drug holiday because the effects of the medication are still present. There is no need to switch the route of medication. Vitamin D supplementation should be within 800 to 1000 IU/day. Calcium supplementation greater than 1200 mg/day may be associated with an increased risk of complications ranging from kidney stones to cardiac events.

67. Answer: 2

Rationale: Patients on chronic steroid therapy should be evaluated for adrenal insufficiency during an acute illness, which increases stress. Signs and symptoms indicate subtle clinical manifestations of adrenal insufficiency. Recommended treatment is to treat the patient empirically with stress-dose corticosteroid during acute illness. Stopping the medication or maintaining the same dose may precipitate acute adrenal insufficiency.

68. Answer: 4

Rationale: The use of colchicine in the elderly patient can lead to the presence of nausea, vomiting, diarrhea, and dehydration. Constipation, fluid retention, and fever are not associated findings.

69. Answer: 2

Rationale: Aspirin is the first choice. Nonsteroidal antiinflammatory drugs (NSAIDs) can be used, but the antiinflammatory and antipyretic effects of aspirin, plus its low cost, make it the initial drug of choice. Methotrexate is used for severe cases that do not respond to aspirin or NSAIDs. Steroids may be given but are not the drug of choice. Tramadol is effective in RA pain but is not a first-line therapy.

70. Answer: 2

Rationale: The patient needs to understand the importance of maintaining the prescribed steroid dose. When symptoms decrease, the medication is effective. It is not influenced by fluids and should be taken with food.

71. Answer: 3

Rationale: This is the only effective dose listed for the treatment of an acute episode of gout. The other doses are incorrect and insufficient as dosed. The maximum dose of colchicine for an acute gout attack is 1.8 mg.

72. Answer: 3

Rationale: Patients with chronic renal disease should not be on NSAID therapy, as it relates to control of gout. The adult-gerontology primary care NP should be assessing pain medications for their effectiveness and monitoring the patient's weight as critical assessments. Withholding dialysis treatment would be against the standard of care.

73. Answer: 4

Rationale: Allopurinol works to keep the serum uric acid level lower. The goal of therapy is a serum uric acid level <6.5 mg/dL. The other medications listed do not help lower serum uric acid levels, and aspirin can precipitate a gout attack.

74. Answer: 4

Rationale: These drugs modify rheumatoid arthritis (RA) when nonsteroidal antiinflammatory drugs (NSAIDs), such as ibuprofen, sulindac, and salicylates, have not worked. Corticosteroids can be used until the disease-modifying agents begin to work. Misoprostol is used to prevent ulcer development related to long-term medication use.

75. Answer: 1

Rationale: Xanthine oxidase inhibitors are the drug of choice for the treatment of gout in the older adult patient. Aromatase inhibitors are used in the treatment of certain cancers. Angiotensin-converting enzyme inhibitors are used in the treatment of cardiac disease and hypertension. Beta blockers are used in the treatment of cardiac disease and migraine headaches.

76. Answer: 3

Rationale: Gold is indicated for treatment of rheumatoid arthritis (RA) and is contraindicated in the presence of the other listed diseases.

77. Answer: 3

Rationale: Recommendations for vitamin D for patients ages 50 and older are 800–1000 IU on a daily basis. Vitamin D is measured in international units as opposed to the metric system of weights. For individuals who are below age 50, the recommendation is between 400 and 800 IU.

78. Answer: 1

Rationale: Acetaminophen or nonsteroidal antiinflammatory drugs (NSAIDs) are generally used for pain relief in patients with osteoarthritis. Systemic corticosteroids are not indicated in osteoarthritis. Gold salts may be one of several pharmacologic approaches to the treatment of rheumatoid arthritis. Misoprostol is used to minimize the development of NSAID-induced gastric ulcers.

79. Answer: 2

Rationale: Renal function may already be reduced in older adults, and ibuprofen can further impair renal function, which, in turn, can result in nephrosis, cirrhosis, and congestive heart failure.

80. Answer: 1

Rationale: The patient should be monitored for blood dyscrasias on a monthly basis, which would be a CBC with differential and platelet count. Women of childbearing age should avoid pregnancy.

81. Answer: 3

Rationale: Nonsteroidal antiinflammatory drugs (NSAIDs) (naproxen) are the recommended treatment for an acute gout attack in patients able to tolerate NSAID therapy. Allopurinol is contraindicated in an acute attack and can even precipitate an attack in the early stages of treatment. Low-calorie diets increase risks of gouty attacks. Joint injection would not be a first-line treatment choice, but for refractory cases in patients unable to take oral medication, it may be an option.

82. Answer: 1

Rationale: Acetaminophen is the preferred first-line therapy in treating pain in elderly patients due to its low profile for side effects if dosing regimens are followed according to therapeutic guidelines. The other medications can be used if acetaminophen dosing does not provide adequate relief, but these other drugs have a higher profile for side effects and as such should be used cautiously in the elderly patient.

83. Answer: 4

Rationale: Gastritis and oral ulcers are common complications of alendronate (Fosamax). Alendronate is used to increase calcium absorption in patients with osteoporosis. If these effects occur, the medication should be discontinued. The medications in the other options do not cause this problem.

Neurology

11

Physical Examination & Diagnostic Tests

1. The adult-gerontology primary care NP is evaluating the mobility status of an older adult patient with the Timed "Up and Go" (TUG) test. The expected time frame for the patient to complete this test is:
   1. 10 seconds.
   2. 30 seconds.
   3. 45 seconds.
   4. 60 seconds.

2. An 80-year-old presents to the office with new-onset syncope. Which five of the following diagnostic strategies should the adult gerontology primary care NP request?
   1. Carotid Doppler.
   2. CBC.
   3. ECG.
   4. Hemoccult.
   5. Orthostatic vital signs.
   6. Parathyroid hormone level.

3. To evaluate the neurologic system for appropriate sensory system functioning in the geriatric patient, it is appropriate to determine the presence of stereognosis. This is done by having the patient:
   1. Rapidly touch the index finger and then the nose.
   2. Distinguish between a coin and a key by touch.
   3. Stand with heels together and eyes closed.
   4. Close eyes and identify familiar odors.

4. To determine cerebellar functioning in the geriatric patient, the adult-gerontology primary care NP would perform:
   1. "Get Up and Go" test.
   2. The Romberg test.
   3. Kinesthesia assessments.
   4. SPICES assessment.

5. When assessing the neurologic status of an elder, the adult-gerontology primary care NP expects:
   1. Alcohol abuse is a rare cause of peripheral neuropathy in elders.
   2. It is a national recommendation to screen all elderly for dementia.
   3. Physical illness should be a differential with any cognitive change.
   4. Sensory testing is recommended in the lower extremities only.

6. What is considered a "soft" (or equivocal) neurologic sign?
   1. Positive Babinski reflex in an adult.
   2. Mirroring hand movements of the extremities.
   3. Brudzinski sign.
   4. Kernig sign.

7. A 60-year-old patient presents with new-onset seizures and his wife reports "he's just been different from himself" for the past 2 weeks. The patient is stable and sitting comfortably in the exam room. As the patient moves to the exam table you note slight ataxia. On neurologic assessment, he has a diminished pupillary response on the right. What imaging modality will you recommend?
   1. A CT scan without contrast.
   2. A PET scan.
   3. An angiogram of the brain.
   4. An MRI with contrast.

8. A patient is having difficulty controlling seizures and is referred for an electroencephalogram (EEG). The adult-gerontology primary care NP explains:
   1. This test will cause some discomfort and a sedative will be provided before the test.
   2. It will be important for her to take her regular dosages of paroxetine (Paxil) and phenytoin (Dilantin) before the test.
   3. The procedure is painless and she will not experience discomfort or electrical shock.
   4. After the test, she will be on bed rest for 8 hours and will be given clear liquids for 12 hours.

9. Which cranial nerve is being tested when the adult-gerontology primary care NP asks the patient to raise the eyebrows, smile, frown, or puff out the cheeks?
   1. Hypoglossal nerve.
   2. Acoustic nerve.
   3. Glossopharyngeal nerve.
   4. Facial nerve.

10. The adult-gerontology primary care NP notes an absent patellar reflex in a healthy patient. What might the practitioner ask the patient to do?
    1. Lift both arms above the head and count to five slowly as the reflex is tested.
    2. Raise both legs slowly and then lower and immediately test for the reflex.
    3. Clench both hands together and pull while the reflex is tested.
    4. Close eyes and hold breath while examiner tests for the reflex.

11. The adult-gerontology primary care NP is performing a vaginal examination on a patient with a history of spina bifida. With the insertion of the metal speculum, the patient suddenly feels nauseated and is sweating, and her skin turns blotchy. What is your most immediate reaction to this situation?
    1. Provide reassurance.
    2. Put a blanket over the patient's legs.
    3. Assess blood pressure.
    4. Remove the speculum.

12. With the patient in the supine position, the adult-gerontology primary care NP gently flexes the patient's neck in the direction of the chin touching the chest. If there is pain and resistance to the flexion, and if the hips and knees flex at the same time, the nurse accurately describes this finding as:
    1. Phalen sign.
    2. Romberg sign.
    3. Kernig sign.
    4. Brudzinski sign.

13. **QSEN** The adult-gerontology primary care NP is seeing an 82-year-old patient who lives in a townhome and routinely needs to climb two sets of stairs to get to the bedroom. Which two instruments would be appropriate to assess the patient's fall risk?
    1. The Tinetti Balance and Gait Assessment.
    2. The Timed Get Up and Go Test.
    3. The SPICES Questionnaire.
    4. The Strength and Timing Instrument.
    5. Trendelenburg Test.
    6. Phalen Test.

14. Which of the following differentials would be priority in a patient with new-onset syncope?
    1. Cardiac dysrhythmias.
    2. Postural hypotension.
    3. Symptomatic hypoglycemia.
    4. Vasovagal syncope.

15. Which statement about the diagnosis of essential tremor is correct?
    1. The tremor is noticed most often at rest.
    2. The tremor occurs more often in upper extremities.
    3. The tremor does not cause functional impairment.
    4. The tremor will not affect voice quality.

16. The adult-gerontology primary care NP understands that dysdiadochokinesia refers to:
    1. Trouble with speech.
    2. Memory impairment.
    3. Impaired rapid alternating movements.
    4. Neurologic triad of gait, memory, and speech dysfunction.

Disorders

17. Which statement regarding meningitis in the elderly is correct?
    1. Symptoms are more pronounced in elderly.
    2. *Neisseria meningitidis* is the most common bacterial cause.
    3. Outcomes are improved with use of systemic steroids.
    4. Neurosurgery does not affect risk of meningitis.

18. The adult-gerontology primary care NP is seeing a 65-year-old patient with a presenting concern of headache. Which question would be most valuable in developing differentials for this patient?
    1. Do you have a family history of headaches?
    2. How old were you when the headaches began?
    3. When did this headache begin?
    4. Where is your headache located?

19. Which statement about Parkinson disease is correct?
    1. Symptom onset typically begins in the fifth decade of life.
    2. Women are affected more often than men.
    3. There is no genetic risk in the development.
    4. Hallucinations are a common comorbidity.

20. The adult-gerontology primary care NP understands that the most common form of facial paralysis in the adult patient is:
    1. Facial nerve fasciitis.
    2. Trigeminal neuralgia.
    3. Bell's palsy.
    4. Herpes zoster.

21. A patient has a history of injury at the fifth thoracic vertebra (T5), and his condition has stabilized. The adult-gerontology primary care NP understands that, with this level of injury, the patient most likely will not be able to:
    1. Perform coordinated movements with his hands, such as writing.
    2. Achieve lower body strength and coordination for walking.
    3. Have adequate upper body strength to drive a car.
    4. Maintain the upper body coordination required for eating.

22. An older patient is diagnosed with postpolio syndrome. The most common symptom is:
    1. Gastrointestinal upset, headache, and malaise.
    2. New onset of weakness, fatigue, and pain.
    3. Sudden onset of lower limb paralysis after an acute infection.
    4. Headache, fever, and elevated blood pressure and pulse.

23. The adult-gerontology primary care NP is discussing safety measures for the home environment of a patient with Parkinson disease. It would be important for the adult-gerontology primary care NP to include what information?
    1. Sleep on a firm mattress that is high off the floor to facilitate getting into and out of bed.
    2. Pour hot liquids with the cup or container placed on the table to avoid spilling.
    3. Place a sheepskin pad on the bed to decrease the development of decubiti.
    4. Perform passive and active range of motion twice daily to prevent contracture.

24. A patient presents to a rural clinic after a diving accident. The adult-gerontology primary care NP suspects a spinal cord injury at the fifth cervical vertebra (C5). While awaiting emergency transport services, which assessment would be a priority in this level of injury?
    1. Checking for voluntary movement of extremities and sensation below the level of injury.
    2. Assessing breath sounds and evaluating movement of diaphragm with respiration.
    3. Maintaining cervical flexion to facilitate airway until cervical traction is initiated.
    4. Beginning neurologic checks with careful documentation of location of pain sensations.

25. Many patients who suffer from recurrent headaches have similar symptoms with each episode. Which is a sign that a headache may be from a more serious cause?
    1. It occurs on the right side.
    2. Rhinorrhea occurs with the headache.
    3. It becomes more and more painful.
    4. It increases when the patient bends over.

26. Epidemic meningococcal meningitis occurs rarely. This control is a result of:
    1. Live immunization recommendations on a national level.
    2. Lower community carrier rates.
    3. Improved socioeconomic conditions.
    4. Earlier detection and recognition of outbreaks.

27. Which of the following are considered three risk factors for the development of Parkinson disease?
    1. Exposure to pesticides.
    2. History of concussion.
    3. Farming.
    4. Occupational exposure to rubber.
    5. Limited tobacco and caffeine use.

28. The adult-gerontology primary care NP understands that benign paroxysmal positional vertigo:
    1. Is described as vertigo and nystagmus with positional change and occurs most often in older adults.
    2. Is more common in young persons and occurs suddenly and in episodes that include vertigo, tinnitus, hearing loss, feeling of fullness in the ears, and nausea and vomiting.
    3. Follows a viral syndrome (upper respiratory or gastrointestinal) with exacerbation of the vertigo with position change without hearing loss or tinnitus.
    4. Involves gradual hearing loss and tinnitus along with vertigo, eventually with facial numbness and weakness.

29. A 52-year-old patient presents with a "funny feeling in my feet and calves, like I can't feel them." The sensation has been continuous over the past 2 days and seems to be worsening. The patient is otherwise healthy except for a recent upper respiratory infection. Your primary differential based on the history above is:
    1. Amyotrophic lateral sclerosis.
    2. Guillain-Barré syndrome.
    3. Multiple sclerosis.
    4. Muscular dystrophy.

30. Which three of the following conditions are included in the differential diagnosis of a patient with facial paralysis?
    1. Herpes zoster.
    2. Bell palsy.
    3. Trigeminal neuralgia.
    4. Otitis media.
    5. Myasthenia gravis.

31. What would be appropriate to include in the health promotion plan for a patient with a diagnosis of multiple sclerosis?
    1. Avoid aerobic exercise, due to muscle weakness.
    2. Keep warm (especially extremities) to improve neurologic function.
    3. Avoid antioxidants (vitamins C and E, beta-carotene); they contribute to loss of myelin sheath.
    4. Consume a low-fat, high-fiber diet with daily cranberry juice and calcium supplement.

32. A patient has had a stroke and is incontinent of urine. The family should be taught to:
    1. Restrict fluid intake.
    2. Insert a Foley catheter.
    3. Establish a scheduled voiding pattern.
    4. Reposition the patient often to reduce the discomfort of urgency.

33. What is the best approach to test the hearing of a patient with Bell's palsy?
    1. Stand out of sight of the patient and ask the patient to move or do something.
    2. Use a tuning fork to test for lateralization of sound.
    3. Stand in front of the patient and whisper "Raise your hand."
    4. Snap your fingers next to the patient's ear and ask if the sound was heard.

34. Physical findings in a 50-year-old female patient who wears a left lower leg brace are weight of 100 pounds, height of 65 inches, and vital signs within normal limits. She has developed postpolio symptoms. The adult-gerontology primary care NP suggests that the patient:
    1. Gain weight to prevent further disability.
    2. Exercise all muscle groups vigorously to prevent disuse syndrome.
    3. Avoid exposure to cold or chilling, which may cause a loss of strength in the affected muscle.
    4. Reduce the amount of time using the brace for joint support to prevent further loss of strength.

35. A patient presents to the clinic with symptoms of unilateral tremor, rigidity, flexed posture, bradykinesia, loss of postural reflexes, and freezing. The adult gerontology primary care NP recognizes these symptoms as:
    1. Multiple sclerosis.
    2. Myasthenia gravis.
    3. Parkinson disease.
    4. Brain tumor.

36. Inflammation and swelling of the seventh cranial nerve with resultant unilateral facial muscle paralysis is called:
    1. Bell's palsy.
    2. Temporal (giant cell) arteritis.
    3. Facial droop.
    4. Trigeminal neuralgia.

37. The adult-gerontology primary care NP understands that the following trigger helps differentiate a migraine from a tension headache:
    1. Alcohol.
    2. Bright lighting and noxious stimuli.
    3. Stressful situations.
    4. Sleep pattern disturbances.

38. The adult-gerontology primary care NP is teaching a patient about migraine headaches. Select three statements that are true about migraine headaches.
    1. Migraine is likely related to both vascular and chemical changes in the brain.
    2. Migraine and related headaches are disorders of an infectious response in the neurons.
    3. Genetic and environmental factors are influential in migraine.
    4. During migraine, the pain is described as pounding or throbbing and is aggravated by physical activity.
    5. Migraine headache feels like a tight band around the head.
    6. Migraine headache is unilateral, reaches maximum intensity in 15 minutes, and lasts 90 minutes.

39. Which symptom(s) can occur in a patient who has experienced a transient ischemic attack (TIA) in the anterior cerebral circulation?
    1. Bilateral vision disturbance and diplopia.
    2. Dysarthria (speech disturbance).
    3. Disorders of behavior and cognition.
    4. Bilateral motor and sensory dysfunction.

40. Many visits to emergency departments by adults are prompted by headaches. Which symptom may help the adult-gerontology primary care NP differentiate a migraine headache from a headache that may indicate severe problems?
    1. It is preceded by an "aura."
    2. It occurs mainly behind one eye and tends to be grouped.
    3. Onset is sudden and accompanied by nuchal rigidity.
    4. It occurs mainly on awakening.

41. An adult patient presents with a complaint of facial paralysis that started suddenly. In making a diagnosis, the adult-gerontology primary care NP considers which of the following symptoms of Bell's palsy?
    1. Concurrent paralysis of the opposite arm and leg.
    2. Pain in the (ipsilateral) ear that accompanied or preceded the paralysis.
    3. Loss of bowel control.
    4. Loss of hearing on the opposite side.

42. An older adult woman is present when her husband is admitted for a myocardial infarction. She complains that she is having numbness and tingling in her hands and face. Her heart rate is 98 beats/min and her respiratory rate is 32 breaths/min. What is the best action for the adult-gerontology primary care NP to take?
    1. Administer oxygen per nasal cannula at 3 L/min.
    2. Schedule a magnetic resonance imaging (MRI) appointment.
    3. Provide calming interventions by explaining the probable reason for the symptoms.
    4. Administer amitriptyline (Elavil) 25 mg PO.

43. The adult-gerontology primary care NP is evaluating an older adult's tremor. Which assessment finding would be characteristic of an essential tremor rather than a parkinsonian tremor?
    1. The handwriting is not affected.
    2. The tremor occurs with purposeful movements.
    3. The tremor occurs at rest.
    4. The tremor worsens with beta blockers or alcohol.

44. Which assessment may be evaluated in a patient with Parkinson disease?
    1. Macrographia.
    2. Micrographia.
    3. Exaggeration of rapid successive movements.
    4. Increased swinging of arms while walking.

45. A patient recently diagnosed with multiple sclerosis asks the adult-gerontology primary care NP about the disease process. The adult-gerontology primary care NP knows that:
    1. 90% of patients have a quickly progressive form of the disease.
    2. 90% of patients, after the first onset of symptoms, have relapses and remissions.
    3. 10% of patients will respond to corticosteroids.
    4. 10% of patients have problems with optic neuritis and sensory loss.

46. A 30-year-old female patient has had several episodes of incontinence, weakness, visual loss, and some ataxia. Physical exam reveals slight swelling of the optic disc on funduscopy, difficulty with heel-to-toe walking, lower extremity weakness, and 2+ deep tendon reflexes. Which condition does the adult-gerontology primary care NP suspect?
    1. Multiple sclerosis.
    2. Parkinson disease.
    3. Amyotrophic lateral sclerosis.
    4. Myasthenia gravis

47. A patient has a 3-year history of recurrent headaches once or twice a month lasting 12–18 hours. When the patient presents at the clinic, she has taken 6 g of acetaminophen in the past 12 hours with no relief. The adult-gerontology primary care NP would:
    1. Recommend a parenteral narcotic analgesic as well as prescribe opioids for prn use.
    2. Consider an analgesic rebound relative to the dose of acetaminophen taken.
    3. Order naproxen (Anaprox) for prophylactic treatment of the headaches.
    4. Order an EEG and MRI to rule out pathology.

48. A patient presents to the emergency department, stating it is the "worst headache of my life." The patient reports that the headaches have not responded to the usual over-the-counter headache remedies. What is a priority differential?
    1. Brain tumor.
    2. Migraine.

3. Onset of newly diagnosed seizure disorder.
4. Subarachnoid hemorrhage.

49. A patient with a recent history of a left hemisphere stroke returns to the clinic for a checkup. What symptoms would the adult-gerontology primary care NP anticipate the patient to exhibit?
    1. Left-sided weakness.
    2. Bilateral weakness of lower extremities.
    3. Difficulty with speech.
    4. Left visual field deficit.

50. The adult-gerontology primary care NP is evaluating a group of older adult patients for risk factors of an embolic stroke. Which condition would be least likely to precipitate this type of stroke?
    1. Mitral valve disease.
    2. Atrial fibrillation.
    3. Endocarditis.
    4. Diabetes mellitus.

51. A patient returns to the clinic for a follow-up visit. She has a history of simple partial seizures. When questioning the patient, the adult-gerontology primary care NP would identify recurrence of this seizure activity if the patient reported:
    1. Short episodes when she loses consciousness, but does not fall.
    2. No loss of consciousness, but jerking and tingling of her right leg, and then right hand.
    3. Auditory hallucinations, unconsciousness, and urinary incontinence.
    4. Short period of unconsciousness, followed by period of confusion.

52. An older adult woman comes to the clinic complaining of having difficulty when she tries to do her needlework. She walks straight, although somewhat slowly, and no rigidity is noted on movement. She states the shaking in her hands stops when she holds her hands in her lap. What tentative diagnosis would the adult-gerontology primary care NP make?
    1. Parkinson disease.
    2. Transient ischemic attack.
    3. Benign essential tremor.
    4. Resting tremor.

53. A patient with a history of myasthenia gravis presents with ptosis, facial weakness, dysphagia, and generalized weakness. What is important for the adult-gerontology primary care NP to ask and establish initially?
    1. When did the symptoms first begin, and have they increased in severity?
    2. What medications is the patient taking, and when did he last take them?
    3. What activity was the patient participating in when the symptoms began?
    4. Has the patient experienced any seizure activity with the increase in symptoms?

54. A patient presents with miosis and ptosis with anhidrosis of the ipsilateral face and neck. The initial diagnosis would be:
    1. Horner syndrome.
    2. Damage to cranial nerves III and IV.
    3. Ménière syndrome.
    4. Mycotic aneurysm.

55. The adult-gerontology primary care NP is talking with a well-appearing, 42-year-old patient who mentions a concern over the past 3 months with swallowing. Which four differentials should be considered?
    1. Cranial nerve XI (glossopharyngeal nerve) dysfunction.
    2. Cranial nerve X (vagus nerve) dysfunction.
    3. Thyromegaly.
    4. Esophageal cancer.
    5. Epiglottitis.
    6. Multiple sclerosis.

56. The initial symptoms of amyotrophic lateral sclerosis are:
    1. Weakness in the lower extremities and urinary incontinence.
    2. Weakness in the upper extremities and dysfunction in fine motor skills.
    3. Spasticity and hyperreflexia.
    4. Loss of continence and drooling.

57. Which four findings below are associated with Guillain-Barré syndrome?
    1. A recent viral illness.
    2. Weakness more profound in the upper extremities.
    3. Headache and nuchal rigidity.
    4. Visual changes.
    5. Respiratory distress or failure.
    6. Protein in cerebral spinal fluid analysis.

58. The adult-gerontology primary care NP is seeing a patient for new-onset headaches. Which statement by the patient would cause the most concern?
    1. "This headache makes me sick to my stomach."
    2. "This headache is behind my right eye and is giving me stabbing pain."
    3. "This headache has awakened me from sleep for the past week."
    4. "I have needed to wear dark glasses for the past 3 days in a row."

59. The adult-gerontology primary care NP is treating a patient with Parkinson disease. What finding should the adult-gerontology primary care NP anticipate?
    1. Visual hallucinations and paranoia.
    2. Bowel and bladder dysfunction.

3. Disorders in extraocular movements.
4. Pulmonary hypertension associated with left ventricular failure.

60. Which of the following statements is correct concerning brain tumors?
    1. Meningiomas are the most frequent type of primary malignant tumors.
    2. A history of breast cancer has no associated risk for brain tumor.
    3. Seizures are a common clinical finding.
    4. Increased intracranial pressure is a classic early finding in meningioma.

61. The adult-gerontology primary care NP recognizes that cerebral edema usually presents within what time frame following a head trauma?
    1. 24 hours.
    2. 48 hours.
    3. 72 hours.
    4. 1 week.

62. Which four symptoms are findings associated with post-concussion syndrome?
    1. Anxiety.
    2. Behavioral disturbances.
    3. Headaches.
    4. Fine tremors.
    5. Hallucinations.
    6. Sleep disturbances.

63. The adult-gerontology primary care NP recognizes which of the following two criteria as correct concerning multiple sclerosis (MS)?
    1. The onset is most likely between the ages of 20 to 50 years.
    2. It affects males and females equally.
    3. It is more commonly diagnosed in northern climates.
    4. Native Americans, Eskimos, and Asians are affected more than other ethnicities.
    5. MS is a result of exclusively an autoimmune disorder.

64. The adult-gerontology primary care NP is reviewing the records of a patient who is recovering from a stroke. The records indicate the patient is experiencing homonymous hemianopia. This is interpreted as:
    1. Partial loss of visual acuity in the peripheral area of the visual field.
    2. Diplopia in the eye contralateral to the cerebral lesion.
    3. Nystagmus in both eyes, but movements are dissimilar.
    4. Loss of vision in both eyes in either the right or the left half of the visual field.

65. An adolescent girl is accompanied to the clinic by her mother, who states the school reports that she "stares off into space a lot" and does not seem to pay attention during these brief periods, which typically last 1–3 minutes. The neurologic exam is within normal limits. What should the adult-gerontology primary care NP suspect in the patient?
    1. Grand mal seizure.
    2. Complex partial seizure.
    3. Absence seizure.
    4. Simple partial seizure.

66. A child is admitted to the rural clinic after a car accident in which she sustained a closed head injury and fractured femur. The child is lethargic and follows commands slowly, and her pupils are equal and reactive. The child is to be transferred to a hospital by air ambulance. In assessing the child, what would the adult-gerontology primary care NP consider as a significant change in her condition?
    1. Urine output is less than 500 mL in 24 hours.
    2. She complains of a headache in the frontal area.
    3. She is able to move her lower extremities to command.
    4. Vital signs are BP of 130/50 mm Hg and pulse of 70 beats/min.

67. Which is considered a likely cause of seizures in adolescents and young adults?
    1. Congenital abnormalities and metabolic disturbances.
    2. Metabolic disorders, CNS infection, and fever.
    3. Idiopathic disease, trauma, and substance abuse.
    4. Trauma, malignant tumor, and cerebrovascular accident.

Pharmacology

68. Which product would be the safest choice for an 81-year-old patient with insomnia?
    1. Diphenhydramine (Benadryl).
    2. Doxepin (Silenor).
    3. Oxazepam (Serax).
    4. Ramelteon (Rozerem).

69. Which product would cause the adult-gerontology primary care NP the greatest concern based on review of a medication list belonging to a 68-year-old who fell from a ladder hitting his right parietal region on asphalt?
    1. Metaxalone (Skelaxin).
    2. Ginseng (over-the-counter).
    3. Omeprazole (Prilosec).
    4. Acetaminophen (Tylenol).

70. A patient is taking an antiepileptic medication. The adult-gerontology primary care NP understands that the antiepileptic medication:
    1. Must be taken indefinitely.
    2. Is usually discontinued after 4 years of no seizure activity, and EEG confirms lack of seizure activity.
    3. Is usually given in combination with other antiepileptics or sedatives to reduce the seizure threshold.
    4. Must be given to all patients who experience a seizure.

71. A 67-year-old patient presents with the concern of right-sided facial pain. She describes the pain as burning and sharp. The pain has not awakened her from sleep. She explains she has to "press on it" when it starts and she does not talk or move her mouth because it worsens the pain. The adult-gerontology primary care NP will consider what management based on the symptoms above:
    1. Carbamazepine (Tegretol).
    2. Indomethacin (Indocin).
    3. Prednisone.
    4. Valaciclovir (Valtrex).

72. Pharmacologic management of patients with peripheral vestibulopathy includes:
    1. Meclizine (Antivert) 100 mg PO qid.
    2. Dimenhydrinate (Dramamine) 5 mg PO tid to qid.
    3. Scopolamine transdermal patch, 1 disc applied behind ear and left in place for 3 days.
    4. Prochlorperazine (Compazine) 25–50 mg PO q4h prn.

73. Which product would reduce essential tremors?
    1. Alcohol.
    2. Caffeine (over-the-counter).
    3. Pseudoephedrine (Sudafed).
    4. Enalapril (Vasotec).

74. The family of a patient with Parkinson disease brings him to the clinic because he is experiencing increasing difficulty with ambulation. The adult-gerontology primary care NP increases the patient's dose of carbidopa (25 mg)/levodopa (100 mg) (Sinemet 25–100 mg) from three to four times daily. What is important for the adult-gerontology primary care NP to teach the family regarding the increase in the dose of this medication?
    1. Sleep disorders are common side effects of carbidopa/levodopa.
    2. Carbidopa/levodopa has shown efficacy in slowing disease progression.
    3. Orthostatic hypotension can be problematic at higher dosing ranges.
    4. The medication should be given on an empty stomach.

75. The adult-gerontology primary care NP is seeing a 56-year-old patient with a history of hypertension, dyslipidemia, and Barrett esophagitis. The patient has experienced headaches since playing football in high school. Which product would you discourage the patient from continuing based on his chronic illnesses?
    1. Acetaminophen (Tylenol).
    2. Amlodipine (Norvasc).
    3. Sumatriptan (Imitrex).
    4. Prochlorperazine (Compazine).

76. Which medication class is recognized for the treatment of moderate to severe dementia?
    1. Cholinesterase inhibitors.
    2. NMDA receptor antagonists.
    3. SSRIs.
    4. Central alpha$_2$ agonists.

77. Before prescribing an abortive agent for migraines, a priority question to ask the patient would be:
    1. "Do you have a history of gastric colic?"
    2. "Do you have a history of panic episodes?"
    3. "Do you have a history of cardiac disease?"
    4. "Do you have a history of seizure disorder?"

78. **QSEN** What would be a priority teaching in a newly diagnosed patient initially using an anticonvulsant?
    1. Contact sports pose no risk to persons with epilepsy.
    2. The anticonvulsant medication will cause drowsiness.
    3. Avoid solitary activities.
    4. Medical alert bracelets are unhelpful.

79. Which factor is the greatest positive intervention for ischemic stroke?
    1. Cardiac rhythm control.
    2. Blood pressure control.
    3. Timely use of thrombolytics.
    4. Renal protection, including fluid support.

80. The adult gerontology primary care NP recognizes that which antibiotic class can interfere with the metabolism of first-generation antiepilepsy drugs, such as carbamazepine?
    1. Cephalosporins.
    2. Quinolones.
    3. Sulfonamides.
    4. Macrolides.

81. The adult-gerontology primary care NP is discussing the worth of the herpes zoster vaccination with a 62-year-old patient. What would be an accurate statement in promoting the vaccine?
    1. Postherpetic neuralgia is not a reason to accept the vaccine.
    2. A severe case of zoster increases the risk of postherpetic neuralgia.
    3. Age is not correlated with risk for postherpetic neuralgia.
    4. Herpes zoster cannot affect the central or peripheral nervous systems.

82. What information is important for the adult-gerontology primary care NP to teach the patient regarding the use of medications to treat trigeminal neuralgia?
    1. Medications may cause seizure-like activity.
    2. Therapeutic levels of the drug may take up to a month to be reached.
    3. Relief of the symptoms should occur within 24 hours of starting the medication.
    4. Permanent side effects are not a concern of this condition.

11 Neurology Answers & Rationales

Physical Exam & Diagnostic Tests

1. Answer: 1

Rationale: To complete the TUG test (also referred to as the "get up and go" test), the patient is asked to stand up from a chair with arms, walk 10 feet, then turn around and return immediately to the chair. The complete test should be performed within 10 seconds or less and correlates with functional dependence. Gait, balance, position change, and turning are evaluated. Additional testing is recommended if longer than 20 seconds are required to complete the test.

2. Answer: 1, 2, 3, 4, 5

Rationale: A carotid Doppler should be considered to recognize compromise in cerebral perfusion. A complete blood count to detect anemias and an ECG to investigate persistent or new-onset cardiac dysfunction are diagnostic strategies. A hemoccult will assist in detection of GI bleeding. Orthostatic vital signs will detect changes in cardiac output due to hypovolemia or medications.

3. Answer: 2

Rationale: Stereognosis is the ability to determine familiar objects by shape rather than visual identification. Rapidly touching the index finger and then the nose determines fine motor skills and coordination, standing with heels together and eyes closed determines proprioception (balance; posture), and closing the eyes and identifying familiar odors determines the functioning of the first cranial (olfactory) nerve.

4. Answer: 2

Rationale: The Romberg test assesses cerebellar function so it would be a reasonable method to evaluate an elder's balance. The "Get Up and Go" test assesses gait, balance, and position change and turning (also referred to as the "timed up and go" test [TUG]). Kinesthesia assessments determine proprioception ability. The SPICES assessment is an acronym of common older adult syndromes: **S** is for sleep disorders, **P** is for problems with eating or feeding, **I** is for incontinence, **C** is for confusion, **E** is for evidence of falls, **S** is for skin breakdown.

5. Answer: 3

Rationale: Urinary tract infection, pneumonia, and other infections are common causes of confusion. There is no national recommendation to screen an elderly patient for dementia unless there are signs of dementia. Alcohol abuse, diabetes, and vitamin B_{12} deficiency are common causes of peripheral neuropathy in elders. Sensory testing using light touch and pain is recommended in the distal upper and lower extremities.

6. Answer: 2

Rationale: Soft neurologic signs involve slight deviations of the central nervous system (CNS) that are present occasionally or inconsistently. Examples are short attention span; clumsiness; frequent falling (disturbances of gait); hyperkinesis; left-handed, but right-footed; language disturbances; anisocoria; and mirroring movements of the extremities (when one hand performs a movement, the other is also in motion). The other three options indicate a CNS problem that occurs consistently; Brudzinski and Kernig signs indicate meningeal irritation, and a positive Babinski reflex in an adult may indicate an upper motor lesion in the corticospinal tract.

7. Answer: 4

Rationale: The MRI will provide the clearest image and higher sensitivity to smaller lesions. Contrast will assist in visualizing blood vessels. The patient is stable at this time, or a CT scan without contrast would be the image of choice for immediate diagnosis of a bleeding vessel. A PET scan will provide information about highly active metabolic activity. This would be a secondary consideration following MRI findings. An angiogram of the brain will limit findings to vascular structures only.

8. Answer: 3

Rationale: The procedure is painless with no danger of electrical shock. All anticonvulsants, antidepressants, stimulants (caffeine, tobacco), and alcohol should be stopped. It would be concerning to see a selective serotonin reuptake inhibitor (SSRI) prescribed in a patient with seizures because SSRIs lower seizure threshold. There is no restriction on movement or diet after the procedure.

9. Answer: 4

Rationale: The facial nerve is tested by facial movement, taste, sensation, and corneal reflex. The hypoglossal nerve is tested by the patient sticking out the tongue. The acoustic nerve is tested by a hearing test. The glossopharyngeal nerve is tested by taste, gag reflex, and having the patient drink and swallow.

10. Answer: 3

Rationale: Augmentation of the patellar reflex can be obtained by having the patient isometrically tense muscles not directly involved with the reflex arc being tested, called the Jendrassik maneuver.

11. Answer: 4

Rationale: Patients with spina bifida can experience autonomic hyperreflexia as characterized by elevated blood pressure, sweating, blotchy skin, nausea, or goose bumps due to stimulation of the bowel, bladder, or skin below the spinal lesion area. During a physical exam, the following can be causes of hyperreflexia, which include reactions to a cold, hard examination table or cold stirrups; insertion and manipulation of a vaginal speculum; pressure during the bimanual or rectal examination; or tactile contact with hypersensitive areas. The vaginal speculum should be removed and the hyperreflexia ceases, the adult-gerontology primary care NP and the patient should mutually decide whether to continue the examination.

12. Answer: 4

Rationale: This describes Brudzinski sign. Phalen sign (maneuver) is elicited in carpal tunnel syndrome. The Romberg sign test is done to assess gross swaying by asking the patient to stand with feet together and eyes closed for 5 seconds. Kernig sign (inability to extend lower leg when leg is flexed at hip or when there is resistance or pain) along with Brudzinski sign indicate meningeal irritation and should be evaluated further.

13. Answer: 1, 2

Rationale: Both the Tinetti and the Timed Get Up and Go tests assess functional ability and fall risk. The SPICES Questionnaire assesses various geriatric syndromes. The Strength and Timing Instrument is not a valid assessment tool. The Trendelenburg test measures competency of the leg vein valves in patients with varicosities. The Phalen test is used to assess for carpal tunnel syndrome.

14. Answer: 1

Rationale: Cardiac dysrhythmias or alterations in cardiac output are priority due to risk of sudden death from cardiac or cerebral ischemia. Syncope can be associated with metabolic concerns due to electrolyte imbalance or alterations in glucose, as well as vagal sources from standing in one place or from straining/bearing down with bowel movement. Postural hypotension due to medications, nausea, vomiting, dehydration, or anemia are differentials as well.

15. Answer: 2

Rationale: Essential tremor is associated with action and is found more commonly in the upper extremities, head/neck, or voice. Essential tremor worsens with activity, causing impairment in fine motor activities, including dressing, sewing, writing, playing an instrument, or other hobbies a patient may enjoy.

16. Answer: 3

Rationale: Dysdiadochokinesia is difficulty with attempts at rapidly alternating movements (e.g., finger to nose).

Disorders

17. Answer: 3

Rationale: Corticosteroids improve outcomes in all adults, reducing long-term mortality. *Listeria monocytogenes* is more commonly associated with meningitis in the elderly. Atypical presentation is common in elderly, and expected physical exam findings are not as pronounced. Basilar skull fracture, sickle cell disease, immunosuppression, alcoholism, and neurosurgery all increase risk for infections of the central nervous system.

18. Answer: 2

Rationale: Headaches should decrease in frequency and severity with age. New onset of headaches after age 50 is considered a dangerous sign. Other dangerous signs include asymmetric responses to light in pupils, change in the patient's level of consciousness, headache described as "worst pain in my life," a "different" type of headache, headaches awakening the patient during sleep, painful temporal arteries, or behavioral changes.

19. Answer: 4

Rationale: Psychosis, including paranoia, hallucinations, and delusions are common in Parkinson disease, with up to 40% of patients experiencing hallucinations in end stage disease. The mean age of diagnosis of Parkinson disease is 70 years. There is a male prevalence and patients having a first-degree relative have twice the risk for Parkinson disease than the general population.

20. Answer: 3

Rationale: The most common form of facial paralysis is Bell's palsy, a disorder affecting the facial nerve characterized by muscle flaccidity of the affected side of the face. Trigeminal neuralgia is a disorder of cranial nerve V that is characterized by an abrupt onset of pain in the lower and upper jaw, cheek, and lips. Herpes zoster affects the dermatomes and does not cause a paralysis, but rather pain, herpetic grouped skin vesicles, and possibly postherpetic neuralgia.

21. Answer: 2

Rationale: Fifth thoracic vertebra (T5) injuries do not affect the coordination or capacity of the upper body, arms, and hands; the lower body is paralyzed. The patient should be able to do all activities listed except walk.

22. Answer: 2

Rationale: The cardinal signs of postpolio syndrome include onset of new weakness; fatigue; and pain along with hot or cold intolerance; and swallowing, speech, breathing, and sleep disturbances.

23. Answer: 2

Rationale: Pouring liquids is frequently a complicated task for this patient due to the tremors. If the cup or container to be filled is placed on the table, there is less chance of spilling the contents.

24. Answer: 2

Rationale: At this level of injury (C5), the intercostal muscles and diaphragm can be affected, and the patient may have respiratory compromise. Airway maintenance and avoiding flexion of the neck are critical.

25. Answer: 3

Rationale: If a headache becomes more and more severe, if there is new onset of severe headache in a patient over 35 years old, if the headache's character or progression is different from other headaches, or if there is vomiting, but no nausea, there could be a new and serious cause for the headache. The side on which the headache occurs, and accompanying rhinorrhea, may or may not be significant. Increasing pain when bending over is characteristic of sinus pressure or infection.

26. Answer: 3

Rationale: Improved sanitary and socioeconomic conditions have led to the marked reduction in the number of cases of epidemic meningitis. There is no research to support increased cases in communities with higher carrier numbers. Meningitis vaccine is not a live vaccination.

27. Answer: 1, 2, 3

Rationale: Pesticide exposure, concussion, and farming/agricultural work are all risk factors to developing Parkinson disease. Rubber is an occupational concern to the development of cancers, but is not associated with Parkinson disease. History of smoking as well as coffee and caffeine intake may reduce risk.

28. Answer: 1

Rationale: Benign paroxysmal positional vertigo usually occurs in older patients. Younger persons who experience a sudden episode of vertigo, tinnitus, hearing loss, sensation of fullness, and nausea and vomiting typically have Ménière disease. Peripheral vestibulopathy usually follows upper respiratory or gastrointestinal viral illness and involves nearly incapacitating vertigo that increases with positional changes, but not hearing loss or tinnitus. The adult-gerontology primary care NP should suspect acoustic neuroma if gradual hearing loss, tinnitus, and vertigo occur before the development of facial numbness and weakness.

29. Answer: 2

Rationale: Guillain-Barré syndrome presents with progressive paresthesias and weakness most commonly in the lower extremities. It can occur following a recent illness. The symptoms are bilateral. Amyotrophic lateral sclerosis typically presents with unilateral paresthesias in one of the upper extremities, as does multiple sclerosis in a lower extremity. Muscular dystrophy commonly presents in younger patients and with pain and stiffness.

30. Answer: 1, 2, 4

Rationale: The differential diagnosis for facial paralysis includes bacterial ear infections, Lyme disease, herpes zoster, Bell's palsy, mumps, temporal bone fracture, acoustic neuroma, other tumors, and demyelinating diseases. Trigeminal neuralgia is associated with intense facial pain, not paralysis. Myasthenia gravis is characterized by fluctuating weakness and fatigability, often subtle, that worsens during the day and after prolonged use of affected muscles; may improve with rest; ptosis may be observed.

31. Answer: 4

Rationale: In addition to the factors listed, keeping cool, not warm, is associated with improvement of neurologic function. A regular exercise program is encouraged, along with daily intake of a multivitamin, antioxidants, and low-dose aspirin (81 mg). Maintaining ideal body weight, having rest periods or naps daily, and becoming informed about the disease process are important aspects of promoting health.

32. Answer: 3

Rationale: Reestablishing regularity will assist in maintaining bladder control. A catheter exposes the patient to infection. Fluids should not be restricted.

33. Answer: 1

Rationale: Bell's palsy involves a sensorineural hearing loss. In contrast to being able to read lips, this patient must be able to hear the direction of sound without any visual prompting. The tuning fork assists in differentiating between air and bone conduction of sound.

34. Answer: 3

Rationale: In addition to regular health maintenance visits, the patient should be advised to avoid gaining weight and exercising to the point of muscle pain. Cold temperatures can cause a loss of muscle strength in the affected muscle groups and should be avoided. Assistive or orthotic devices (canes, walkers, braces) should be used, along with periodic evaluation of muscle strength and function.

35. Answer: 3

Rationale: The clinical presentation of Parkinson disease is asymmetric or unilateral tremor, rigidity, bradykinesia with freezing, and flexed posture with loss of postural reflexes. The classic finding of myasthenia gravis is fatigability, which is also characterized by fluctuating weakness, often subtle, that worsens during the day and after prolonged use of affected muscles, and may improve with rest with ptosis of the eye that may shift from eye-to-eye. Patients with multiple sclerosis can present with a number of neurologic signs and symptoms depending on the locations of the lesions within the CNS. Typical symptoms include fatigue, depression, emotional instability, epilepsy, memory loss, diplopia, sudden vision loss, facial palsy, dysarthria, dysphagia, muscle weakness or spasms, ataxia, vertigo, falls, hyperesthesia or paresthesia, pain, bowel or bladder incontinence, urinary frequency or retention, or impotence. Brain tumor signs and symptoms may include new onset or change in pattern of headaches with the headache gradually becoming more frequent and more severe, unexplained nausea or vomiting, vision problems, such as blurred vision, double vision or loss of peripheral vision, gradual loss of sensation or movement in an arm or a leg, changes in personality and other sensory issues.

36. Answer: 1

Rationale: The symptoms describe Bell's palsy, which is thought to be caused by a virus. This sudden onset of unilateral facial paralysis usually resolves within 2 weeks, but can endure for months. A few patients may have residual problems. Temporal or giant cell arteritis is a generalized, large-vessel vasculitis commonly affecting the branches of the proximal aorta that supply the neck and the extracranial structures of the head. Facial droop occurs with Bell palsy because of paralysis of the muscles innervated by the facial (seventh cranial) nerve. Trigeminal neuralgia is sudden pain along the fifth cranial nerve.

37. Answer: 4

Rationale: Sleep pattern disturbances, either too little or too much, may trigger a migraine headache. Lighting and noxious stimuli, along with alcohol use and stress, may trigger both tension and migraine headaches.

38. Answer: 1, 3, 4

Rationale: Headache disorders, including migraine, are disorders of neurovascular regulation and chemical changes in the brain, and are not associated with an infectious response. Migraine headache pain is described as pounding or throbbing and is aggravated by physical activity. A tension headache is described as a feeling of a tight band around the head with no nausea and vomiting. A cluster headache is severe, unilateral, retro-orbital pain reaching intensity within 15 minutes and lasting 90 minutes.

39. Answer: 3

Rationale: A wide variety of changes can occur in behavior and cognition after a transient ischemic attack (TIA). Bilateral vision disturbance, diplopia, dysarthria (speech disturbance), and motor/sensory problems on both sides of the body are problems associated with TIA in the posterior cerebral circulation.

40. Answer: 3

Rationale: A sudden onset headache and nuchal rigidity may indicate a subarachnoid hemorrhage. Migraine headache without aura is the most common; however, migraine with aura occurs before the onset of pain. Cluster headaches occur behind one eye and are grouped. Headaches associated with hypertension occur mainly on awakening.

41. Answer: 2

Rationale: Bell's palsy is typically preceded or accompanied by pain in the ear on the paralyzed side often 1–2 days before the onset of facial paralysis. The paralysis is confined to the face, and there is no bowel involvement. Postauricular pain, tinnitus, and a mild hearing deficit may occur on the affected side.

42. Answer: 3

Rationale: Patients who are under stress have periods of hyperventilation in which they "blow off" more carbon dioxide (CO_2) than necessary. They experience numbness and tingling in their hands and faces and may experience syncope. Reassurance and calming intervention techniques by explaining the voluntary component of the rapid breathing will often have dramatic results of correcting the symptoms. In the past, breathing into a paper bag was recommended because it was supposed to increase CO_2 level and relieve the symptoms of respiratory alkalosis; however, this is not supported in evidenced-based literature and may be dangerous in patients with hypoxia or other physiologic/pathologic causes for the hyperventilation.

43. Answer: 2

Rationale: The differentiating feature between the two tremors is that the essential tremor occurs with purposeful movements. Handwriting may be affected with both tremors. The tremor with Parkinson disease occurs at rest. Essential tremors improve with beta blockers as well as with alcohol.

44. Answer: 2

Rationale: Micrographia (small, cramped handwriting) is a classic manifestation of Parkinson disease. The patient has impairment of rapid successive movements and loss of automatic movements, such as swinging the arms while walking.

45. Answer: 2

Rationale: Multiple sclerosis (MS) is characterized by exacerbations and remissions of the symptoms. Only 10% of MS patients have a progressive form of the disease from the onset. Many patients (35%–40%) have problems of optic neuritis, sensory loss, and weakness, and do respond to corticosteroids.

46. Answer: 1

Rationale: Involvement of more than one CNS area, age 15–60 years, two or more separate episodes of symptoms involving different sites, or gradual progression over at least 6 months meet the criteria for multiple sclerosis.

47. Answer: 2

Rationale: The recommended dose for acetaminophen is no more than 4 g/day. This patient may be experiencing an analgesic rebound headache. Appropriate prophylactic medications for migraine include beta blockers (propranolol), tricyclic antidepressants (amitriptyline), selective serotonin reuptake inhibitors (paroxetine), anticonvulsants (topiramate), and calcium channel blockers (verapamil). It is not necessary to order expensive tests for patients with migraine or tension headache. Usually a careful, thorough history is sufficient.

48. Answer: 4

Rationale: This is a common patient complaint ("worst headache of my life") with a subarachnoid hemorrhage. This patient should have an emergent noncontrast CT scan of the brain and lumbar puncture with immediate referral to a neurologic surgeon, if either is positive.

49. Answer: 3

Rationale: The speech center (Broca area) is most often located in the left cerebral hemisphere. The patient would experience weakness of the right side of the body and a right-sided visual deficit as well.

50. Answer: 4

Rationale: Mitral valve disease, atrial fibrillation, and endocarditis all precipitate the development of an embolus that can result in an embolic stroke. Diabetes will precipitate occlusive disease of the cerebral arteries and the possible development of a thrombotic stroke, not an embolic stroke.

51. Answer: 2

Rationale: A simple partial seizure is characterized by unilateral paresthesia, numbness and tingling, and spastic movement of the extremities. The patient has no loss of consciousness or incontinence of the bowel or bladder.

52. Answer: 3

Rationale: The characteristics of a benign essential tremor are fine-to-coarse rhythmic tremors of the hands and feet that increase with activity and may be absent at rest. Frequently, the voice is also involved. An ingestion of a small amount of alcohol may decrease symptoms.

53. Answer: 2

Rationale: It is important to determine first whether the patient has stayed on the medication schedule. The symptoms may be the result of missed medication or overmedication, especially with pyridostigmine (Mestinon). The symptoms may also be exacerbated by exercise and heat.

54. Answer: 1

Rationale: The clinical presentation is classic for Horner syndrome, especially the lack of sweating (anhidrosis) on the ipsilateral (same) side of the face and neck as the eye symptoms. The patient needs to be referred for further neurologic workup.

55. Answer: 1, 3, 4, 6

Rationale: The glossopharyngeal nerve's motor function assists in swallowing. Thyromegaly can produce a feeling of fullness in the throat that is accompanied by dysphagia. Swallowing dysfunction is a late sign of esophageal cancers. Neuromuscular disorders, including multiple sclerosis, may be associated with dysphagia. Cranial nerve X (vagus) provides parasympathetic stimulation to secrete digestive enzymes in the gut, aid in peristalsis, as well as to provide the carotid reflex, involuntary actions of the heart, lung, and digestive systems. Its sensory innervation affects the area behind the ear and part of the external ear canal. Epiglottis is an airway-threatening, acute bacterial infection that is most commonly associated with *Haemophilus influenzae* type B. Patients with epiglottitis would not appear well.

56. Answer: 2

Rationale: The upper extremities are affected initially in 40%–60% of cases. A frequent sign is low-amplitude fasciculations. Lower extremity weakness occurs in 20% of cases initially. Spasticity and hyperreflexia are other symptoms as the disorder progresses. Loss of continence is not a common concern. Drooling is one of the bulbar symptoms that can be present early in the disease. Additional bulbar symptoms include dysarthria and dysphagia.

57. Answer: 1, 4, 5, 6

Rationale: Recent viral illnesses, visual changes, respiratory dysfunction, and protein in cerebral fluid analysis are all findings in Guillain-Barré syndrome. Weakness is most profound in the lower extremities, progressing upward, leading to the risk of respiratory dysfunction. Headache and nuchal rigidity are associated with meningitis. Visual changes are associated with multiple sclerosis.

58. Answer: 3

Rationale: Headaches that awaken the patient from sleep are associated with intracranial tumors. While nausea can also be present with increased intracranial pressure, intracranial tumors are associated with vomiting. Headache behind one eye is associated with cluster headaches, and photosensitivity is a common finding in migraine headaches.

59. Answer: 1

Rationale: Psychosis is a common comorbidity of Parkinson disease, with up to 40% of patients experiencing hallucinations. Bowel/bladder dysfunction, extraocular movement disorders, and cardiac complications, including left-ventricular pathology are not associated with Parkinson disease.

60. Answer: 3

Rationale: Approximately one half of patients with brain tumors have a seizure. A history of breast, lung, melanoma, renal, and colon cancer increases risk for brain metastases. Gliomas are the most common type of primary malignant brain tumors. Increased intracranial pressure is a late finding in slow-growing tumors.

61. Answer: 3

Rationale: Peak occurrence for cerebral edema usually is up to 72 hours after a neurologic insult. It gradually resolves over a 2- to 3-week period. Cerebral edema may be caused by either the initial injury to the neuronal tissue or secondarily in response to the biochemical cellular injury cascade, hypoxia, hypercarbia, or cerebral ischemia.

62. Answer: 1, 2, 3, 6

Rationale: Anxiety, behavioral changes, headaches, and sleep disturbances are associated with postconcussion syndrome. Hallucinations/psychosis and fine tremors are not associated with postconcussion syndrome.

63. Answer: 1, 3

Rationale: Multiple sclerosis (MS) is most commonly diagnosed in northern Europe, North America, and Australia. It is uncommon around the equator. It affects whites more than other ethnicities, and females three times more often than males. MS is not a result of any one disorder, but is felt to be due to environmental, genetic, and autoimmune interactions.

64. Answer: 4

Rationale: Homonymous hemianopia is the loss of the vision in one half of the visual field. Either the right or left field of vision may be affected. It is most often caused by a lesion or pathology in the optic tract or occipital lobe.

65. Answer: 3

Rationale: This accurately fits the description of a petit mal or absence seizure, which is a type of generalized seizure that begins in childhood and usually ends in early adulthood (30s). There is usually impairment of consciousness, automatic symptoms, and mild tonic-clonic symptoms. Classically, "staring off into space" is the reporting symptom.

66. Answer: 4

Rationale: An increase in the pulse pressure and decrease in pulse rate are indications of increasing cerebral edema and intracranial pressure, which would necessitate immediate intervention. A child's urine output should be 20–30 mL/h.

67. Answer: 3

Rationale: The most likely causes of seizures in adolescents and young adults are idiopathic disease, trauma, and substance abuse. Congenital abnormalities are the likely cause of seizures in newborns. In children under 6 years old, metabolic causes, CNS infection, and fever can cause seizures. Trauma, malignant tumor, and stroke are likely causes for seizures in elderly patients.

Pharmacology

68. Answer: 3

Rationale: Ramelteon (Rozerem) is a melatonin-receptor agonist which has the lowest side effect profile for elderly. Ramelteon should be avoided in severe hepatic impairment.

Diphenhydramine (first-generation antihistamine), doxepin (tricyclic antidepressant), and oxazepam (benzodiazepine) have anticholinergic properties including risk for sedation, confusion, falls, and urinary retention in the elderly patient.

69. Answer: 2

Rationale: Herbal products beginning with "G" are associated with anticoagulation. *Ginkgo biloba*, ginger, and garlic also contain similar properties. The patient's use of ginseng places him at higher risk for cerebral bleeding. Knowing prescribed medications, as well as over-the-counter and herbal products is critical when developing differentials following an injury. Metaxalone, omeprazole, and acetaminophen are not recognized for antico-agulants/antiplatelet properties.

70. Answer: 2

Rationale: Although most medication is discontinued after 4 years of no seizure activity, a confirmatory EEG should be obtained. Not all seizure patients require medication; referral to and monitoring by a neurologist are appropriate.

71. Answer: 1

Rationale: The patient's symptoms are diagnostic of trigeminal neuralgia. This disorder responds well to anticonvulsant therapy (carbamazepine). Indomethacin and prednisone reduce inflammation, but are not considered first-line therapy in trigeminal neuralgia. Valaciclovir is an antiviral used to treat herpes zoster. This patient's pain has several similarities with herpes zoster, but herpes zoster is more continuous pain, including while trying to sleep.

72. Answer: 3

Rationale: Scopolamine patches are placed behind the ear and provide medication for 3 days. The correct dose for meclizine (Antivert) is 12.5–25 mg PO tid to qid; for dimenhydrinate (Dramamine) 50 mg PO tid or qid; and for prochlorperazine (Compazine) 5–10 mg PO q4h prn.

73. Answer: 1

Rationale: Patients with essential tremors are at higher risk for alcohol abuse as alcohol reduces the tremor. Caffeine products (tea, soda, coffee, chocolate) and over-the-counter cold/cough medications worsen tremor. Beta blockers are used to reduce tremors, not ACE-inhibitors.

74. Answer: 3

Rationale: Carbidopa/levodopa (Sinemet) induces a number of adverse reactions, including hypotension, gastrointestinal (GI) upset, psychosis, and motor complications. For best absorption, it should not be given around meals, despite GI side effects. It exerts no known effect on slowing disease progression.

75. Answer: 3

Rationale: Sumatriptan targets 5-hydroxytryptamine (5-HT) receptors in the brain that are associated with headaches. Triptans cause vasoconstriction, which can place patients at risk for cardiac and cerebral ischemia, especially with a medical history of preexisting cardiac and vascular disease. Acetaminophen, amlodipine, and prochlorperazine do not place the patient at risk for vasoconstriction.

76. Answer: 2

Rationale: NMDA receptor antagonists (e.g., memantine) are recognized as the class for management of moderate-to-severe Alzheimer dementia. This group of medications control the effects of glutamate (the major excitatory transmitter in the CNS) at NMDA receptors, which are believed to play a critical role in learning and memory. The NMDA receptor regulates calcium entry into the neuron. Selective serotonin reuptake inhibitors (SSRIs) are antidepressants used in the treatment of depression and anxiety. Central alpha$_2$ agonists are used in the treatment of hypertension.

77. Answer: 3

Rationale: Abortive medications for migraines cause cranial vasoconstriction, which will be generalized to all vessels, including cardiac. A history of cardiac disease, especially ischemia, increases risk for cardiac event.

78. Answer: 2

Rationale: Patients should be aware that all antiseizure medications can cause drowsiness, so driving, bathing, swimming, using machinery, climbing, etc., are all risky behaviors, especially when starting new medications. Contact sports would not be encouraged because the patient would be at risk of worsening seizure control should a head injury occur. Avoiding solitary activities is not discouraged, providing machinery and high areas are not involved. Medical alert bracelets or necklaces allow expedient information should the patient be injured and unconscious following a seizure.

79. Answer: 3

Rationale: Timely intervention with thrombolytics has the best evidence for patient outcomes. The goal from onset of symptoms to thrombolytics is 180 minutes. The risk of disability is greatly reduced with thrombolytic use, and the benefits outweigh the risk of a bleed.

80. Answer: 4

Rationale: Macrolide antibiotics, such as erythromycin and clarithromycin, can increase the plasma concentration of carbamazepine; therefore, when these medications are used together, carbamazepine levels must be closely monitored.

81. Answer: 2

Rationale: The risk for postherpetic neuralgia increases with age as well as zoster severity. Postherpetic neuralgia can be a chronic, life-altering condition and is associated with increased risks of suicide. Zoster targets the peripheral nervous system (individual dermatomes), but can also infect the central nervous system, causing myelitis and encephalitis.

82. Answer: 3

Rationale: Onset of drug action and relief of trigeminal neuralgia symptoms occur in 24 hours, usually in 4–6 hours. Laboratory tests are usually monitored based on the specific medication, not a peak and trough. These medications may be given to treat seizures.

12

Gastrointestinal & Liver

Physical Examination & Diagnostic Tests

1. The adult-gerontology primary care NP is preparing to examine the abdomen of a patient. What is the correct sequence in which to conduct the exam?
   1. Inspection, palpation, percussion, auscultation.
   2. Palpation, percussion, auscultation, inspection.
   3. Percussion, palpation, auscultation, inspection.
   4. Inspection, auscultation, percussion, palpation.

2. The adult-gerontology primary care NP is seeing a 22-year-old male who recently returned from Thailand on a 2-month mission trip. He had a sudden onset of 5–7 loose, watery stools a day for the past month. He has had abdominal cramping, nausea, and stool urgency. The best course of action would be:
   1. Stool testing for culture and sensitivity, treatment with loperamide and rifaximin.
   2. Stool testing for ova and parasites, treatment with bismuth subsalicylate and levofloxacin.
   3. Stool testing for fecal leukocytes, treatment with probiotics.
   4. Stool testing for culture and sensitivity, treatment with loperamide and azithromycin.

3. When obtaining a history from a 21-year-old female adult patient with abdominal pain, which of the following should initially be assessed?
   1. Food effects on the pain.
   2. Location and onset of the pain.
   3. Change of pain with bowel movements.
   4. First day of last menstrual period.

4. To test for a positive obturator sign in a patient with abdominal pain, the adult-gerontology primary care NP:
   1. Passively flexes the right thigh at the hip, and medially rotates the leg from the 90-degree hip/knee flexion position.
   2. Asks the patient to take a deep breath while palpating in the abdominal right upper quadrant.
   3. Places his/her right hand above the patient's knee and has the patient raise the leg.
   4. Palpates the right abdomen one third the distance from the anterior superior iliac spine to the umbilicus.

5. The adult-gerontology primary care NP is performing the initial physical exam on a 51-year-old man. The history reveals that the patient's father died of colon cancer, but the patient is asymptomatic and has not had any screening for colon cancer. What is the best test to use to screen the patient?
   1. Barium enema and flexible sigmoidoscopy.
   2. CT colonography.
   3. Colonoscopy.
   4. Fecal occult blood, fecal immune testing, and stool DNA testing.

6. A 76-year-old male patient has end-stage liver disease. Which of the following lab abnormalities is most likely to be seen?
   1. Sodium 145 mEq/L.
   2. Bilirubin, total serum 0.9 mg/dL.
   3. Albumin 5.0 g/dL.
   4. INR 2.5.

7. The adult-gerontology primary care NP is obtaining recommended testing on patients born between 1945 and 1965 per the Center for Disease Control (CDC). Once a positive HCV Ab (hepatitis C antibody) test is found, the next step would be to:
   1. Call the patient and explain that hepatitis C is active and treatment is needed.
   2. Repeat the HCV Ab test to assure it is positive.
   3. Test with a hepatitis B panel.
   4. Test for HCV RNA.

8. A 25-year-old male patient comes in complaining that his girlfriend has been diagnosed with acute hepatitis B and he is afraid he may have it also. When testing the patient, the adult-gerontology primary care NP would determine a diagnosis of acute hepatitis B (HB) infection from the following blood test results:
    1. Negative HB surface antigen (HBsAg) and positive HB core antibody (HBcAb).
    2. Negative HB surface antigen (HBsAg) and positive HB surface antibody (HBsAb).
    3. Positive HB surface antigen (HBsAg) and positive HB core antibody (HBcAb).
    4. Negative HB core antibody (HBcAb) and negative HB surface antibody (HBsAb).

9. The diagnosis of early acute pancreatitis would be considered by the adult-gerontology primary care NP based on a history of severe constant acute upper abdominal pain that radiates to the back and which of the following laboratory results?
    1. White blood cell (WBC) count of 10,300/mm³.
    2. Serum alanine aminotransferase of 60 IU/L.
    3. Serum amylase of 100 U/L.
    4. Serum lipase of 850 U/L.

10. A 74-year-old male complains of rectal bleeding for the past year. He has no change in bowel habits and denies abdominal pain, weight loss, and rectal pain. He has seen blood in the toilet water and when wiping approximately once every few weeks, but lately the bleeding has increased. He had a colonoscopy for colon cancer screening 5 years ago. The adult-gerontology primary care NP should:
    1. Send the patient home with a fecal occult blood test.
    2. Schedule colonoscopy.
    3. Schedule a flexible sigmoidoscopy.
    4. Schedule a double contrast barium enema.

11. An overweight, middle-aged woman has right upper quadrant pain that radiates to her right subscapular area and is severe and persistent. She is also experiencing anorexia, nausea, and a fever. Her most recent meal was a double quarter-pound hamburger with cheese, French fries, and a vanilla milkshake. Based on this information, the adult-gerontology primary care NP examines the abdomen and percusses for costovertebral angle tenderness. The abdomen is tender in the right upper quadrant. Which of the following signs, if positive, corresponds to the correct diagnosis?
    1. Obturator sign; patient has appendicitis.
    2. Costovertebral angle tenderness; patient has a urinary tract infection.
    3. Murphy sign; patient has cholecystitis.
    4. McBurney point sign; patient has acute appendicitis.

12. A 47-year-old male presents with severe epigastric pain radiating into his back that began 1 day ago. He is taking lisinopril and metformin and was last seen 1 year ago in the office. He smokes one pack per day and drinks 4–5 beers a day. Lately he has had more beer on the weekends while watching football. The adult-gerontology primary care NP suspects acute pancreatitis due to alcohol. What would be the appropriate test to confirm the diagnosis?
    1. Amylase and lipase.
    2. Liver function tests.
    3. Abdominal ultrasound.
    4. Abdominal CT scan.

13. The adult-gerontology primary care NP reviews laboratory results for a patient that reveal a positive *Helicobacter pylori* stool antigen test. The adult-gerontology primary care NP would want to treat this if the patient complained of:
    1. Upper abdominal pain.
    2. Altered bowel habits.
    3. Dysphagia.
    4. Nausea.

Disorders

14. A 20-year-old female patient in her third year of college presents with altered stool consistency and frequency for the past 6 months. She notes there is no pattern and she cannot predict when she will have diarrhea. She notes increased stress as she prepares for final exams. The adult-gerontology primary care NP suspects irritable bowel syndrome (IBS). What other history would assist in a diagnosis of IBS?
    1. Weight loss of 15 lbs.
    2. Lower abdominal cramping that is associated with a bowel movement.
    3. Symptoms occur frequently after she has cereal with milk in the morning.
    4. Stomach upsets in high school.

15. A sudden onset of diarrhea that consists of 5–6 loose stools a day and awakens the patient at night with cramping, but without blood in the stools, would most likely be caused by:
    1. Infection.
    2. Irritable bowel syndrome.
    3. Ischemic colitis.
    4. Lactose intolerance.

16. The adult-gerontology primary care NP is discussing *Clostridium difficile* (CD) infection with the family of a 68-year-old female who lives with them and was recently diagnosed with CD infection. Which of the following statements would be the most important for the family to understand?
    1. CD infection has been reported to recur after an initial occurrence 50% of the time within 8 weeks.
    2. CD infection is the leading cause of health care–associated infections in hospitalized patients.

3. Hand-washing with alcohol-based hand sanitizer should be used in the home.
4. Have the patient use a separate bathroom from the rest of the family.

17. An adult male presents with midsternal chest pain with radiation to the neck and left arm. He denies other symptoms. He was seen in the emergency room and had a negative cardiac workup. What might be the diagnosis?
    1. Pneumonia.
    2. Costochondritis.
    3. Gastroesophageal reflux.
    4. Esophageal spasm.

18. The adult-gerontology primary care NP suspects peritonitis in a patient. What assessment finding is most indicative of peritonitis?
    1. Palpate and watch for a positive Murphy sign.
    2. Perform a rectal exam and test the stool for blood.
    3. Auscultate the abdomen for increased bowel sounds.
    4. Palpate for rebound tenderness.

19. An older adult woman is noted to have iron-deficiency anemia. She has no pain or rectal bleeding. What history would raise the suspicion of a gastric ulcer?
    1. Symptoms of acid reflux for the past 2 years, occurring at least 3 times a week.
    2. Postmenopausal with no recent history of vaginal bleeding.
    3. Weight loss of 10 lbs in the past 2 months.
    4. An ankle sprain requiring 800 mg of ibuprofen three times a day for the past 6 weeks.

20. A 45-year-old male is seen for anal itching and a rash. Symptoms have been present for 3 months and are worse after a bowel movement and at night. He uses medicated wipes to clean his perianal area several times a day. He notes intense itching, burning, and pain around the anus. He has no comorbidities and is otherwise healthy. He has tried hemorrhoid cream with no relief. The adult-gerontology primary care NP suspects pruritus ani. What would be the best treatment for him?
    1. Topical hydrocortisone cream applied to the perianal area 3 times a day for 6 weeks.
    2. Antifungal cream applied twice a day for 2 weeks.
    3. Keep the perianal skin dry and clean with water and avoid severe rubbing.
    4. Sitz baths 4 times a day and apply a moisture barrier cream such as zinc oxide daily for 3 weeks.

21. A patient with a chief complaint of diarrhea alternating with constipation, intermittent cramping, and bloating and relieved by a bowel movement is most likely:
    1. Antibiotic-induced diarrhea.
    2. Inflammatory bowel disease.
    3. Gastroenteritis.
    4. Irritable bowel syndrome (IBS).

22. Which patient presentation would most likely suggest dysphagia caused by esophageal spasm?
    1. They usually have more difficulty swallowing solids than liquids.
    2. There is a long history of gastroesophageal reflux.
    3. They have difficulty swallowing both solids and liquids.
    4. They have marked weight loss.

23. Which problem would most likely worsen the symptoms of gastroesophageal reflux disease (GERD)?
    1. Small sliding hiatal hernia.
    2. An empty stomach when lying down.
    3. Gaining 10 lbs over a period of months.
    4. Gastroparesis.

24. A patient comes to the emergency department concerned about pain and swelling in his groin. He tells the adult-gerontology primary care NP that his doctor said he has an incarcerated hernia. Which assessment finding correlates with an incarcerated hernia?
    1. Hernia that easily moves back and forth across the abdominal wall.
    2. Hernia that protrudes from the groin area and cannot be reduced into the abdomen.
    3. Hernia that is very painful to palpation with significant abdominal swelling.
    4. Hernia that decreases in size when the patient increases intra-abdominal pressure.

25. Which finding most likely indicates a need for an endoscopy in patients with heartburn?
    1. Any new onset of heartburn.
    2. Symptoms persisting after 8–12 weeks of empiric therapy.
    3. Negative *Helicobacter pylori (H. pylori)* test.
    4. Good response to empiric treatment after 7–10 days.

26. The adult-gerontology primary care NP has received a right upper quadrant ultrasound report that states: moderate hepatic steatosis, also known as nonalcoholic fatty liver disease (NAFLD). The 60-year-old male patient had elevated liver enzymes with an alanine transaminase (ALT) of 74 U/L and aspartate transaminase (AST) of 82 U/L. He has type 2 diabetes, hypertension, and a BMI of 36. Which statement below is most accurate concerning NAFLD?
    1. The most common cause of death in NAFLD is cardiovascular disease.
    2. He needs to consider bariatric surgery to improve his liver function.
    3. The most common cause of death in NAFLD is hepatocellular cancer.
    4. He has a 50% risk of developing cirrhosis.

27. The adult-gerontology primary care NP knows that the following principle is most important in understanding the pathophysiology of gastroesophageal reflux disease (GERD):
    1. A hiatal hernia is always a coexisting and major contributing factor.
    2. The lower esophageal sphincter (LES) has become a poor antireflux barrier.
    3. The amount of acid reflux depends on a familial tendency for GERD.
    4. Overeating, use of caffeine, and alcohol cause GERD.

28. Irritable bowel syndrome (IBS) affects:
    1. Men more than women.
    2. Children more than young adults.
    3. Women more than men.
    4. Elderly persons more than young adults.

29. The adult-gerontology primary care NP understands that hepatitis B can be transmitted through blood and blood products. Another mode of transmission of hepatitis B is:
    1. Respiratory contact.
    2. Arthropod vectors.
    3. Fecal-oral route.
    4. Perinatal exposure.

30. A rare but emergent potential complication of a hernia includes:
    1. Infection.
    2. Incarceration.
    3. Bowel obstruction.
    4. Testicular torsion.

31. Which form of viral hepatitis is transmitted by the fecal-oral route?
    1. Hepatitis A.
    2. Hepatitis B.
    3. Hepatitis C.
    4. Hepatitis D.

32. A 54-year-old female complains of intermittent crampy abdominal pain over the past 18 hours, loss of appetite, vomiting, abdominal bloating, and inability to have a bowel movement. She has a history of hysterectomy 20 years ago, cholecystectomy 5 years ago, and two laparoscopies for abdominal pain over the past 4 years. The adult-gerontology primary care NP sends her to the emergency room because the NP suspects:
    1. Appendicitis.
    2. Small bowel obstruction.
    3. Biliary ductal obstruction.
    4. Gastroenteritis.

33. An exam of the male genitalia that consists of inserting a finger into the lower scrotum and into the inguinal canal, and asking the patient to cough causes the adult-gerontology primary care NP to feel a sudden presence of a viscus that lies within the inguinal canal and comes through the external canal passing into the scrotum. This is most likely called:
    1. An indirect inguinal hernia.
    2. A direct inguinal hernia.
    3. A strangulated inguinal hernia.
    4. A femoral hernia.

34. The adult-gerontology primary care NP sees a 65-year-old female with constipation. She reports a history of "slow bowels" for most of her life and has taken laxatives on a regular basis. She has had worsening symptoms requiring her to increase bisacodyl (Correctol) from every other day to daily over the past 3 months. She still has a stool every 3–4 days and can have no stool for 7 days or more at times. She has no abdominal pain and never feels that she has a "good bowel movement." What is her most likely diagnosis?
    1. Loss of bowel function related to chronic stimulant laxative use.
    2. Pelvic floor dyssynergia.
    3. Colonic inertia.
    4. Irritable bowel syndrome—constipation predominant.

35. Which is true about enterobiasis (pinworm infection)?
    1. The parasite is in the soil and enters the body through the feet. It can cause anemia.
    2. The parasite causes pruritus around the anus because the gravid females exit through the anus at night and lay eggs on the skin. The human is the only host of this parasite.
    3. The eggs of this parasite enter the body by ingestion of dirt (pica) or dirt on unwashed vegetables that contain the eggs, or through water containing the eggs.
    4. This parasite is a protozoan. The source is usually contaminated water, but it is spread from person to person by fecal-oral contamination.

36. Nonpharmacologic management of GERD includes which of the following?
    1. Weight reduction and sleep with head of bed elevated 4–6 inches with blocks.
    2. Lying down and resting after meals and weight reduction.
    3. Drinking large amounts of fluids with meals and avoiding alcohol.
    4. Avoiding mint, orange juice, and milk.

37. When a patient complains of chronic constipation with no alarm symptoms, what should be the first step?
    1. Colonoscopy to rule out blockage from colon cancer.
    2. Defecography to rule out rectocele.

3. Increasing fiber intake to 30–35g a day.
4. Physical therapy to strengthen pelvic floor muscles.

38. An organism associated with etiology of peptic ulcer disease (PUD) is:
    1. *Streptococcus pneumoniae.*
    2. *Helicobacter pylori.*
    3. *Moraxella catarrhalis.*
    4. *Staphylococcus aureus.*

39. A common cause of cirrhosis and need for liver transplantation in the United States is:
    1. Hepatitis A.
    2. Nonalcoholic fatty liver disease.
    3. Chronic hepatitis B.
    4. Alcohol ingestion.

40. Prolapse of the anal cushion, made up of vascular, connective, and muscular tissue, through the anal canal below the dentate line describes:
    1. Rectal prolapse.
    2. External hemorrhoid.
    3. Rectocele.
    4. Internal hemorrhoid.

41. An acute illness with jaundice, anorexia, malaise, arthralgias, an incubation period of 2–6 months, a chronic and acute form, and that is transmitted by parenteral, sexual, and perinatal routes describes:
    1. Hepatitis A.
    2. Hepatitis B.
    3. Hepatitis C.
    4. Hepatitis E.

42. A patient with a history of cholelithiasis presents to the office complaining of increased right upper quadrant abdominal pain. The adult-gerontology primary care NP would arrange immediate hospital admission for possible, prompt intervention if the history also showed that the patient is:
    1. 40 years old and having diarrhea.
    2. 75 years old and diabetic.
    3. 5 weeks pregnant.
    4. 23 years old and obese.

43. An older adult male presents to the adult-gerontology primary care NP for evaluation of years of "heartburn" and recent significant weight loss (30 lbs in 1 month). He has been taking antacids and an oral histamine receptor antagonist (H_2 RA) for "years off and on," and has had some relief of his symptoms. He has a 60-pack-year history of cigarette smoking and drinks alcohol daily. What differential diagnosis must the adult-gerontology primary care NP consider first?
    1. Gastric ulcer.
    2. Gastroesophageal reflux disease (GERD).

3. Esophageal cancer.
4. Lung cancer.

44. A 70-year-old female complains of increased gas and bloating over the past 6 months. She has difficulty controlling the gas and expels it frequently. She also notes intermittent diarrhea after eating. The adult-gerontology primary care NP had seen the patient 6 months ago for bronchitis, but had not treated her with antibiotics. She notes symptoms are worse when she has cheese and ice cream. She denies lactose intolerance. The following lab tests were normal: complete blood count (CBC), comprehensive metabolic panel (CMP), and urinalysis (UA). Her thyroid stimulating hormone (TSH) was 5.2, with upper limit of normal 4.5 and a *Helicobacter pylori* IgG antibody was elevated. What is the most likely cause of her symptoms?
    1. Lactose intolerance.
    2. Celiac disease.
    3. Hyperthyroidism.
    4. *Helicobacter pylori* infection.

45. An adult patient presents to the adult-gerontology primary care NP complaining of weakness and vomiting. He gives a history of "several" drinks per day for the past 22 years and cirrhosis, diagnosed 6 months ago. The adult-gerontology primary care NP questions the patient about excessive bleeding. The patient reports two episodes of hematemesis. What emergent condition is the adult-gerontology primary care NP most concerned about?
    1. Bleeding peptic ulcer.
    2. Excessive nosebleed.
    3. Hemoptysis.
    4. Esophageal varices.

46. A 66-year-old male was sent to the adult-gerontology primary care NP after an evaluation for a cough by pulmonary function test. His pulmonary function test was normal and he is not responding to fluticasone propionate HFA or albuterol (Proventil HFA). He has had a dry cough for the past year that is worse after eating. Occasionally he wakens at night coughing. He denies chest pain, dyspnea, fever, or signs of an upper respiratory illness. He has type 2 diabetes and hyperlipidemia and is taking metformin and atorvastatin. He has no history of heart disease and had a negative ECG. He had gained 20 lbs but his weight has been stable for the past year. What is the likely cause of his cough?
    1. Environmental allergies including pollen.
    2. Exposure to fumes at his job where he is an auto mechanic.
    3. Sinusitis and postnasal drainage.
    4. Gastroesophageal reflux disease (GERD).

47. A young adult female presents to the adult-gerontology primary care NP for evaluation of 2 days of increasing crampy abdominal pain. She states that she also has some mild nausea, anorexia, and a low-grade fever. The patient states that the pain is periumbilical. Her STAT complete blood count reveals a slightly elevated white blood count, but is otherwise normal. What is the adult-gerontology primary care NP's next step in the care of this patient?
    1. Refer to a gynecologist for evaluation of possible ectopic pregnancy.
    2. Order a CT of the abdomen and refer to surgeon for evaluation of possible appendicitis.
    3. Observe overnight and reassess the next day.
    4. Place on a clear liquid diet and have patient watch for increasing symptoms.

48. An adult patient has early alcoholic cirrhosis diagnosed by a liver biopsy. While teaching the patient to manage her symptoms, the adult-gerontology primary care NP instructs that it is most important that the patient:
    1. Take daily vitamin E supplement.
    2. Decrease her alcohol intake to less than two drinks a day.
    3. Abstain from alcohol.
    4. Maintain a nutritious diet.

49. An older adult female patient age 72 years presents with fever, leukocytosis, and a sudden onset of lower left quadrant pain for the past 12 hours. She has not had a bowel movement since the pain began. The adult-gerontology primary care NP's top differential diagnosis would be:
    1. Appendicitis.
    2. Diverticulitis.
    3. Irritable bowel syndrome.
    4. Ruptured ovarian cyst.

50. Which patient would be at **lowest** risk for developing diverticular disease?
    1. A vegetarian on a high-fiber diet.
    2. A patient with chronic constipation for 10 years.
    3. An older patient on a six small meals a day diet.
    4. A patient on a low carbohydrate diabetic diet.

51. The adult-gerontology primary care NP knows that colon cancer screening with colonoscopy is recommended in which of these patients?
    1. A 35-year-old healthy Hispanic male.
    2. A 45-year-old healthy black male.
    3. An 85-year-old female with no symptoms.
    4. A 50-year-old female who had a negative colonoscopy for rectal bleeding 2 years ago.

52. The adult-gerontology primary care NP knows that in patients with ulcerative colitis that involves the entire colon (universal or pancolitis), careful surveillance of the colon is required because of an increased risk of:
    1. Colon cancer.
    2. Diverticulosis.
    3. Ischemic colitis.
    4. Irritable bowel syndrome.

53. Which is true of peptic ulcer disease (PUD) in older adult patients over the age of 65 years?
    1. Smoking does not increase the risk of PUD.
    2. Duodenal ulcers are more common in older adults.
    3. Perforation is a common complication.
    4. Weight loss and anorexia are often the only symptoms.

54. Which is true of early cancer of the esophagus in the older adult patient?
    1. Heavy alcohol intake and smoking increase the risk for adenocarcinoma of the esophagus.
    2. Esophageal cancer is associated with high caffeine use.
    3. Dysphagia for solids and cough may be the first symptoms.
    4. Boring-type mid-chest pain indicates mediastinal involvement and requires immediate surgery.

55. A patient has a history of colon polyps. The adult-gerontology primary care NP knows:
    1. A history of polyps increases the risk of colon cancer and more frequent screening is required.
    2. Hyperplastic polyps are a concern for malignancy.
    3. Small polyps <1 cm are not a concern.
    4. A colonoscopy is 100% accurate for finding colon polyps and cancer.

56. A young adult patient presents with a complaint of intermittent diarrhea and cramping for the past 2 years. Screening blood tests reveal iron-deficiency anemia and elevated liver transaminases. The adult-gerontology primary care NP suspects:
    1. Hepatitis B.
    2. Celiac sprue.
    3. Salmonella infection.
    4. Bleeding peptic ulcer.

57. A middle-aged male patient with elevated liver enzymes and no other symptoms has a history of type 2 diabetes and hypercholesterolemia. The adult-gerontology primary care NP would first consider:
    1. Nonalcoholic fatty liver disease (NAFLD).
    2. Autoimmune hepatitis.
    3. Celiac sprue.
    4. Drug-induced liver disease.

58. In patients suspected of having celiac sprue with elevated tissue transglutaminase antibodies (tTG),

but negative duodenal biopsy for villi blunting and celiac sprue, the adult-gerontology primary care NP knows:
1. The patient may have a negative biopsy because of being on a gluten-free diet for 3 weeks.
2. The positive antibodies are likely a false positive result.
3. The patient may have celiac disease.
4. The biopsy may be a false negative result.

59. A young female adult reports that she had the flu and recovered 2 weeks ago. She reports resolution of her symptoms, except she continues to have nausea, decreased appetite, and early satiety. The adult-gerontology primary care NP suspects:
1. A relapse of the influenza infection.
2. Postviral gastroparesis.
3. Vertigo, causing nausea related to a possible ear infection.
4. Peptic ulcer from taking ibuprofen.

60. Irritable bowel syndrome (IBS) can produce which of the following symptoms?
1. Abdominal cramping, rectal bleeding, and diarrhea.
2. Diarrhea alternating with constipation, but no pain.
3. Abdominal cramping, diarrhea, and fecal incontinence.
4. Abdominal cramping, diarrhea, and bloating.

61. When discussing diet with a patient with irritable bowel syndrome (IBS), the adult-gerontology primary care NP tells the patient to avoid:
1. Simple sugars.
2. Dairy products.
3. Red meat.
4. Vegetables.

62. Patient education for a patient with nonalcoholic fatty liver disease (NAFLD) should include:
1. Working on lowering cholesterol intake.
2. Discontinuing any statin medication.
3. Beginning exercise and working on weight loss with diet.
4. Taking vitamin A 15,000 IU daily.

63. This viral strain that can cause gastroenteritis is seen in adolescents and adults. It has a short incubation period (18–72 hours) and short duration of symptoms (24–48 hours). It is characterized by an abrupt onset of nausea and abdominal cramps, followed by vomiting and diarrhea, and is often accompanied by headache and myalgia. What is the most likely cause?
1. *Campylobacter.*
2. *Norovirus (Norwalk).*
3. *Rotavirus.*
4. *Cytomegalovirus.*

64. A 57-year-old female complains of fecal leakage intermittently and one episode of incontinence over the past 2 months. The adult-gerontology primary care NP elicits the following history: 3 vaginal childbirths, 8-lb babies, 1 forceps delivery, 1985–1990. Why was this history important?
1. It is routine aspect of past medical history that is elicited at each female patient visit.
2. It may provide a clue to possible etiology of fecal leakage and incontinence.
3. It indicates that the patient now has adult children and may be dealing with stress of the "empty nest."
4. Vaginal deliveries with large babies can cause a rectocele which would contribute to her incontinence.

65. An older adolescent is being seen for evaluation after a dirt-bike accident. The patient states that the bike flipped over and struck him on the abdomen. He has a hematoma just below the left anterior rib area. The adult-gerontology primary care NP must be particularly aware of which possibility?
1. Ruptured bowel due to blunt trauma.
2. Bladder trauma due to blunt trauma.
3. Hypovolemia due to ruptured spleen.
4. Arrhythmias.

Pharmacology

66. A 60-year-old male was referred by the adult-gerontology primary care NP to Gastroenterology for upper endoscopy because of a complaint of dysphagia. The patient was diagnosed with eosinophilic esophagitis. What treatment can the adult-gerontology primary care NP anticipate he will be taking?
1. Corticosteroids.
2. Sucralfate (Carafate).
3. Ranitidine (Zantac).
4. Omeprazole (Prilosec).

67. The adult-gerontology primary care NP is examining a 30-year-old obese man with a body mass index (BMI) of 35 who complains of almost daily indigestion and heartburn for the past year with a strong acid taste in the mouth about an hour after meals, and frequent belching and awakening at night with choking. The history is negative for chronic illnesses and alarm symptoms. A diagnosis of gastroesophageal reflux disease (GERD) is made. What is the best initial treatment for the patient?
1. Lansoprazole (Prevacid) 15 mg with breakfast daily.
2. Hyoscyamine (Levsin) 0.125 mg tid 15 minutes before eating.
3. Ranitidine (Zantac) 150 mg bid.
4. Omeprazole (Prilosec) 20 mg every morning 30–60 minutes before breakfast.

68. A 42-year-old female complains of rectal pain after a bowel movement that persists for an hour. This began 10 weeks ago, after a particularly hard, large stool. Since then she has had pain with every stool and has noted a slight amount of bleeding on the tissue paper. The adult-gerontology primary care NP suspects an anal fissure. What would be the most appropriate treatment for a chronic anal fissure?
   1. Sitz baths, psyllium fiber, and bulking agents.
   2. Topical lidocaine gel.
   3. Pramoxine-hydrocortisone cream (Analpram-HC singles rectal).
   4. Topical nitrate ointment 0.2%.

69. Which of the following would be prescribed by the adult-gerontology NP as initial treatment for a 72-year-old female with uncomplicated peptic ulcer disease (PUD) and negative *Helicobacter pylori* by stool antigen?
   1. Clarithromycin.
   2. Tetracycline and metronidazole and a histamine 2 receptor antagonist (H$_2$ RA).
   3. Pantoprazole (Protonix).
   4. Bismuth (Pepto-Bismol).

70. The adult-gerontology primary care NP is considering prescribing a nonsteroidal anti-inflammatory drug (NSAID) for an older adult male patient with a history of a coronary angioplasty and stent placement for osteoarthritis pain of the knee and hip. Which would be the best choice in order to prevent ulcers?
   1. Sucralfate qid (Carafate) along with celexicoxib (Celebrex) bid.
   2. Ranitidine bid (Zantac) along with naproxen bid (Naprosyn).
   3. Misoprostol (Cytotec) along with meloxicam 15 mg daily (Mobic.)
   4. Dexlansoprazole (Dexilant) along with celexicoxib (Celebrex).
   5. Sucralfate (Carafate) qid on an empty stomach and ibuprofen bid (Motrin).

71. After percutaneous or permucosal exposure to a hepatitis B source, what is the appropriate treatment for the patient?
   1. In an unvaccinated patient, begin the hepatitis B series.
   2. In a person with a positive hepatitis B surface antibody, no treatment is necessary.
   3. In a vaccinated person with a negative antihepatitis B surface antigen, give hepatitis B immune globulin (HBIG), and initiate a new hepatitis B vaccine series.
   4. In a patient with a positive antihepatitis B surface antibody who completed the entire hepatitis B vaccine series, give a hepatitis B booster.

72. Successful treatment for an adult patient with *Helicobacter pylori (H. pylori)*–induced peptic ulcer disease requires therapy with which regimen?
   1. Clarithromycin, amoxicillin, and omeprazole (Prilosec) for 14 days.
   2. Bismuth (Pepto-Bismol), cephalexin (Keflex), and metronidazole (Flagyl) for 10 days.
   3. Amoxicillin, bismuth (Pepto-Bismol), metronidazole (Flagyl), and cimetidine (Tagamet) for 10 days.
   4. Clarithromycin, tetracycline, cephalexin (Keflex), and lansoprazole for 14 days.

73. A primary therapy for patients with mild ulcerative colitis is:
   1. Metronidazole (Flagyl).
   2. Mesalamine (Delzicol).
   3. Ciprofloxacin (Cipro).
   4. Prednisone (Deltasone).

74. For a patient exposed to household or sexual contacts with hepatitis A, the adult-gerontology primary care NP would:
   1. Give immunoglobulin 0.02 mL/kg as soon as possible but no later than 2 weeks after exposure.
   2. Give one dose of HBIG and immunoglobulin 0.02 mL/kg as soon as possible.
   3. Give immunoglobulin 0.02 mL/kg and two doses of HBIG.
   4. Understand that no injections are needed.

75. A young woman presents with a history of recent unprotected sexual activity (in the past 2 weeks) with a partner now diagnosed with hepatitis B. She is currently asymptomatic and does not recall having a vaccine in the past. What is the best action for the adult-gerontology primary care NP?
   1. Obtain a hepatitis B envelope antibody test (anti-HBe).
   2. Administer one dose of HBIG.
   3. Obtain a viral load for hepatitis B.
   4. Administer one dose of HBIG and initiate vaccination.

76. What condition is a contraindication for the administration of the hepatitis B vaccine?
   1. Pregnancy.
   2. Lactation.
   3. Severe hypersensitivity.
   4. Age >60 years.

77. A 78-year-old patient was treated for community-acquired pneumonia with azithromycin and developed diarrhea 1 week after completing treatment. He is having 6–7 loose watery stools a day. He is afebrile and his white blood cell count was 10.1 K/μL. He has tested positive for

Clostridium difficile (CD) toxins A and B by stool enzyme immunoassay. The adult-gerontology NP knows the first-line treatment should be:

1. Probiotics (*Lactobacillus acidophilus* and *Lactobacillus casei*) once a day for 4 weeks.
2. Vancomycin (Vancocin) 125 mg PO qid for 10 days.
3. Metronidazole 500 mg PO tid for 10 days.
4. Vancomycin 500 mg PO qid for 4 days and metronidazole 500 mg IV tid for 3 days.

78. A patient takes bismuth subsalicylate (Pepto-Bismol). The patient calls the adult-gerontology primary care NP to report that his stools are unusually dark. He is not experiencing any gastric discomfort, orthostatic hypotension, or increased lethargy. How would the adult-gerontology primary care NP interpret the information?
    1. He is probably bleeding and should come in immediately.
    2. He ate something to affect the color of his stool.
    3. His stools are dark, secondary to Pepto-Bismol.
    4. The stool discoloration is caused by metronidazole.

12 | Gastrointestinal & Liver Answers & Rationales

Physical Exam & Diagnostic Tests

1. Answer: 4

   Rationale: Inspection and auscultation should be conducted first to prevent eliciting pain and undue guarding. The adult-gerontology primary care NP should auscultate and listen to the abdomen before percussing and palpating it, because palpation may alter the frequency of bowel sounds. If the exam is painful initially, the patient will be uncomfortable, which will not allow the examiner to continue.

2. Answer: 4

   Rationale: Acute diarrheal infections are common with travelers to developing countries. Diarrhea that lasts 14 to 30 days is classified as persistent and chronic if more than 30 days' duration. Guidelines recommend that stool be tested for culture and sensitivity. It is important to know the most common organisms seen in the travel location to test appropriately. In Thailand, *Campylobacter* and *Salmonella* are two of the most common causes of infectious diarrhea. These organisms cause invasive diarrhea and would not be treated with rifaximin as that is an antibiotic that is not absorbed, working only in the intestines. Quinolone-resistant *Campylobacter* is common in Southeast Asia, but is sensitive to macrolides, such as azithromycin. Concurrent treatment with loperamide may be used to provide symptom relief. Loperamide is an antiperistaltic, antidiarrheal medication that acts on opioid receptors in the gastrointestinal tract and does not enter the central nervous system. Bismuth subsalicylate (Pepto-Bismol) can be used for mild diarrheal illnesses but not concurrently with antibiotics. Bismuth has anti-inflammatory, antacid, and antidiarrheal effects though the action is not well understood. Probiotics are not recommended for treatment of acute diarrhea.

3. Answer: 4

   Rationale: Although all the information is important in determining the cause of abdominal pain, for a young female patient of childbearing age, ascertaining whether the patient is pregnant is a priority. A possibility of pregnancy would alter the testing that might need to be ordered, so a pregnancy test should be ordered. Additionally, abdominal pain may be from pelvic inflammatory disease or related gynecologic disorders. The adult-gerontology primary care NP should obtain a gynecologic, pregnancy, and recent sexual history, including dates of last two normal menstrual periods, condom use and other birth control use, and timing of last sexual intercourse. Food effects are important to ascertain because it may lead to a diagnosis of dietary intolerances. Location and associated symptoms are valuable to narrow down the differential diagnoses of the pain. Abrupt onset of pain has differential diagnoses that are different from pain that is recurrent/chronic, having occurred at least for 3 weeks. Acute pain can be visceral, parietal, or referred. Visceral pain originates in the hollow abdominal organs, due to contraction, distention or stretching of the organ and is usually felt along the midline of the abdomen. Parietal pain results from inflammation of the peritoneum, is usually severe and noted at the site of the originating disorder. Referred pain is usually noted distal to the site and is caused by innervation along the spinal level of the site. Referred pain may feel superficial or deep sensation. Change in bowel habits may indicate an intestinal origin if there is relief, even if only temporary. Pain not affected by a bowel movement or passing gas is not likely intestinal/colonic pain and may be related to other sources, such as kidney/bladder or the musculoskeletal system.

4. Answer: 1

   Rationale: Passive flexion and medial rotation of the right leg causes right hypogastric pain, a positive obturator sign, which suggests an inflamed appendix. A positive Murphy sign, severe pain and a brief inspiratory arrest, results when a patient takes a deep breath while the examiner applies pressure over the right upper quadrant suggestive of cholecystitis. The Psoas sign is positive with pain on pushing against the hand or with the patient on the left side extending and elevating of the right. When contraction or extension of the psoas muscle causes pain, is a sign of inflammation of the psoas muscle and a sign of appendicitis. McBurney point tenderness is in the right lower quadrant 2 inches from the anterior superior spinous process of ilium and is associated with acute appendicitis.

5. Answer: 3

   Rationale: A colonoscopy is the most accurate and sensitive test to screen for colon cancer. Additionally, when polyps or cancers are found they usually can be completely removed at the time. The improved equipment, medication for sedation and colon preparation has made this test safe and effective. Studies have found it to be the most effective screening in terms of cost, lives saved, and colon cancers prevented. Finding and removing colon polyps increase the prevention of colon cancer. A barium enema has poor sensitivity and specificity for locating polyps and cancer and is not recommended. The test requires a bowel preparation and is uncomfortable for the patient. A flexible sigmoidoscopy is a limited exam of the lower portion of the colon. The CT colonography performed by a CT scan, which adds the risk of radiation. It requires a bowel preparation and can be uncomfortable. It does not examine the rectum and can miss smaller polyps. Fecal occult blood testing has low sensitivity and specificity, and has limited use for screening. Fecal immunochemical testing and stool DNA testing are available and can detect polyps and cancers in the colon, but the sensitivity is lower than a colonoscopy.

6. Answer: 4

Rationale: Patients with end-stage liver disease are unable to form proteins, clotting factors and synthesize certain toxins. While no single serologic test can diagnose liver disease, hyponatremia, hyperbilirubinemia, hypoalbuminemia are often seen and used along with increased PT/PTT times and increased INR to monitor severity of end-stage liver disease.

7. Answer: 4

Rationale: Hepatitis C exposure will produce a positive HCV Ab; however, it is not necessarily indicative of active infection. Twenty percent of patients exposed to hepatitis C will clear the virus without treatment but will continue to have a positive antibody. Per guidelines from the American Association for the Study of Liver Diseases (AASLD), to determine current infection with hepatitis C virus, testing with the sensitive HCV RNA test is recommended after a positive HCV Ab. This will show presence of the virus. Repeating the antibody is not useful. Without confirmation, it is not appropriate to inform the patient of an active infection, but it should be explained that it is possible there is active infection. Testing for hepatitis B would be important since the risk factors are the same as for HCV, but is not the initial action to take.

8. Answer: 3

Rationale: Positive Hepatitis B surface antigen indicates active infection present. A positive core antibody can indicate infection, immunity, or an unclear interpretation, depending on other results. Negative surface antigen and positive core or surface antibody indicates immunity. Negative core and surface antibodies together indicate there is no immunity.

9. Answer: 4

Rationale: Serum lipase is thought to be more specific and remains elevated longer than amylase in acute pancreatitis. It is the preferred marker but it can be elevated in other conditions as well. An upper limit of 3–5 times normal may be needed to consider pancreatitis as diabetics tend to have higher than normal lipase levels, normally. Serum amylase and/or lipase elevated to three times normal or higher is one of the diagnostic criteria for acute pancreatitis. Amylase will elevate first, within 3–6 hours of onset and normalize in 3–5 days. Lower sensitivity and specificity make it less reliable than lipase and amylase can remain normal in up to one-fifth of patients with acute pancreatitis. In adults, the normal level for serum amylase is 30–110 IU/L and for serum lipase 13–141 IU/L. A mildly elevated serum transaminase may indicate chronic liver disease and if markedly elevated may be due to biliary ductal dilation. A mildly elevated WBC is nonspecific.

10. Answer: 2

Rationale: Colonoscopy, which examines the entire 6 feet of the colon, should be performed to rule out colon polyps and cancer. Rectal bleeding should always be evaluated. Though the cause of bleeding may be hemorrhoids, colon polyps, cancer, and inflammation need to be considered. During a colonoscopy, any polyps seen can be removed at that time. A flexible sigmoidoscopy examines the lower 40–50 cm of the colon, needs a bowel cleansing, and is done without sedation. Polyps or cancer seen would warrant a more thorough exam with a colonoscopy. A barium enema is not a reliable test for colon polyps and cancer. It is uncomfortable for the patient and has a low yield. It is not recommended. A fecal occult blood test would not be warranted as the patient is having rectal bleeding and results would not change the course of action.

11. Answer: 3

Rationale: The history, right upper quadrant pain that radiates to the right subscapular area, especially after a fatty meal, and positive Murphy sign are all associated with cholecystitis. A positive Murphy sign is noted with severe pain with inspiratory arrest on palpation of the right upper quadrant.

12. Answer: 4

Rationale: An abdominal CT scan will definitively identify pancreatic inflammation. Amylase and lipase will usually elevate during pancreatitis, but these are not definitive for diagnosis. Liver function tests may be elevated but are nonspecific. An abdominal ultrasound is a very poor test to examine the pancreas and most of the time the pancreas can be obscured by bowel gas.

13. Answer: 1

Rationale: *Helicobacter pylori* (*H. pylori*) is a bacterium that is common worldwide and is responsible for most gastric and duodenal ulcers (peptic ulcer disease) and gastric cancers. The most accurate noninvasive tests for active infection are the urea breath test and stool antigen test. Serum IgG and IgM antibody testing may not indicate a current infection as the antibodies will be present even after the infection is eradicated. *H. pylori* causes gastric inflammation, which can present as upper abdominal pain. Altered bowel habits may be indicative of irritable bowel syndrome, which is not known to have an association to the bacterium. Dysphagia, or difficulty swallowing, is an esophageal disorder and is common with gastroesophageal reflux disease. Nausea is a nonspecific symptom with no strong correlation to the bacterial infection.

Disorders

14. Answer: 2

Rationale: IBS is the most common disorder of gut-brain interaction, formerly known as a functional GI disorder. Newly revised diagnostic criteria include abdominal pain at least 1 day a week for the past 3 months with onset at least 6 months prior, and/or associated with a change in stool frequency and/or stool appearance. An unexplained weight loss is an alarm symptom that requires further investigation and is not associated with IBS. Symptoms with dairy intake may be lactose intolerance whereby the lack of the enzyme lactase inhibits the breakdown of mild sugar. A history of stomach upsets is nonspecific and could be related to gastroesophageal reflux, IBS, or other conditions.

15. Answer: 1

Rationale: Diarrhea is a common symptom with a wide differential. Clues include awakening at night and cramping without blood. A sudden onset that awakens a patient suggests pathology, which could be inflammation or infection. Obtaining a travel history, exposure to infection, and medication history may suggest infection. Irritable bowel syndrome is a functional disorder that does not awaken the patient. Ischemic colitis presents with rectal bleeding, as well as pain and diarrhea. Lactose intolerance and other dietary triggers cause functional diarrhea and cramping.

16. Answer: 4

Rationale: *Clostridium difficile* (CD) infection is highly transmissible and precautions need to be taken to prevent spread to other household contacts. The patient should use a separate bathroom because of the possibility of contamination of CD spores on surfaces. Hand

hygiene is extremely important to prevent transmission to others, but alcohol-based hand sanitizers are not effective against CD. These are nonsporicidal and do not remove CD from contaminated hands. Soap and water hand washing is necessary. CD infection can recur, but is reported at 10%–20%, not 50%. CD infection is the leading cause of health care–associated infections worldwide, elderly and hospitalized patients being particularly susceptible. However, CD infection can occur in the community as well. For the 2%–3% of healthy individuals that carry CD, the normal microbiome of the gut suppresses it. When antibiotics are taken, the balance of the microbiome is altered and CD can overgrow and produce toxins A, an enterotoxin and B, a cytotoxin. While CD infection usually is mild to moderate, it can be severe and develop into fulminant and life-threatening colitis.

17. Answer: 3

Rationale: A negative workup for cardiac disease leads to other considerations for chest pain. Gastroesophageal reflux can cause noncardiac chest pain and patients do not always have classic symptoms of reflux. This would be the most likely diagnosis to consider. Pneumonia is very unlikely without any respiratory symptoms. Costochondritis is a common musculoskeletal symptom of chest wall inflammation that is noted on palpation of the ribcage. Esophageal spasm can cause pain, but is usually accompanied by dysphagia and occurs during eating or drinking.

18. Answer: 4

Rationale: Rebound tenderness is found with placing pressure on the abdomen and quickly lifting the hand. Patients will complain of more pain with release of the pressure on the abdomen rather than the pressure itself. This suggests parietal peritoneal irritation and inflammation. Other signs include a positive cough test, guarding, and rigidity. Murphy sign is indicative of gallbladder inflammation and occurs with complaints of right upper quadrant pain and tenderness. Stool for occult blood is not a test for peritonitis as it would indicate gastrointestinal bleeding. Increased bowel sounds, also known as borborygmi, are more associated with the gastrocolic reflex and hyperactivity in intestines and would not be present with peritonitis. However, decreased bowel sounds may be present with peritonitis.

19. Answer: 4

Rationale: Nonsteroidal anti-inflammatory drugs (NSAIDs), such as ibuprofen, carry a high risk of gastrointestinal erosion and ulcers. There may be no symptoms until anemia is noted. Gastroesophageal reflux does not contribute to anemia, unless there is gastritis with erosions or other signs of bleeding. Postmenopausal history is significant because it rules out a cause of anemia, but not a concern for ulcer development. Weight loss of 5 lbs a month is a nonspecific symptom that needs further exploration.

20. Answer: 3

Rationale: Pruritus ani is an uncomfortable sensation around the anal orifice. It is common and may be associated with hemorrhoids. It affects men more than women and is more prevalent in ages 40–60 years. Idiopathic pruritus ani accounts for most of the cases, up to 75%, while secondary causes include proctitis, anal fistula, and psoriasis. The main symptom is intolerable impulse to scratch the perianal region, most often after a bowel movement and at bedtime. Hydrocortisone cream could relieve the symptoms but should be used for only a short period, 2 weeks or less. Long-term corticosteroid use can lead to atrophy, infections, and contact dermatitis. Antifungal cream would not be helpful unless there was secondary infection. The skin needs to be kept clean and dry and not vigorously rubbed. Moisture and creams are not helpful as the symptoms will continue. Some food and drink can exacerbate the symptoms and should be avoided, such as coffee, tea, cola, chocolate, and beer. Regular bowel habits are also important.

21. Answer: 4

Rationale: Irritable bowel syndrome (IBS) presents with abdominal pain and altered bowel habits that can be erratic and unpredictable. The symptoms can be aggravated by stress and food triggers. Diarrhea should not occur during sleep, but abdominal pain can occur at any time. Antibiotic-induced diarrhea occurs in association with a recent course of antibiotics, especially in the previous 3 months. Antibiotics may trigger *Clostridium difficile* colitis. Bacterial or viral gastroenteritis presents with a sudden onset of diarrhea and does not alternate with constipation. Inflammatory bowel disease (IBD) presents with more consistent symptoms of diarrhea and pain and possibly rectal bleeding. In fact, the symptoms of IBD can be present for months to years before diagnosis. Extraintestinal manifestations, such as arthritis and skin lesions, may be present and nocturnal diarrhea and fecal incontinence can be present if rectal inflammation is present.

22. Answer: 3

Rationale: Patients with dysphagia due to an esophageal spasm may report difficulty with both liquids and solids, as the spasm has closed the esophagus temporarily. Relaxation of the esophagus usually occurs within a minute and the food will pass down. This can cause choking with liquids as well. Spasm can occur for many reasons, one of which can be acid reflux. It is episodic, nonprogressive, and unpredictable. Difficulty swallowing solids and feeling that food is sticking is most likely because of an esophageal stricture or obstruction. Marked weight loss is not usually a symptom of dysphagia, unless is it related to esophageal cancer.

23. Answer: 4

Rationale: Gastroparesis can be a significant complication for patients with reflux. The lingering contents in the stomach contain acid and the frequency of reflux will be increased. Persons with a small sliding hiatal hernia are not likely to have a significant change in their symptoms. Reflux is less likely to occur after lying down with an empty stomach. Weight gain may worsen symptoms, but usually it is noted with a significant change in weight, not just 10 lbs.

24. Answer: 2

Rationale: The most common hernia is an inguinal hernia, protruding at the inguinal canal. Incarceration means the hernia cannot be reduced or returned to the abdominal cavity. A reducible hernia easily moves across the abdominal wall. There should be no abdominal swelling, and if the hernia is particularly painful and associated with nausea and vomiting, strangulation/incarceration should be considered as a surgical emergency, as there can be tissue necrosis.

25. Answer: 2

Rationale: An endoscopy is needed for patients with no/minimal response to therapy, indicated by persistent symptoms after 8–12 weeks of therapy. Heartburn may be characterized by burning substernal chest pain and may have gastroesophageal reflux. The factors that would raise a red flag would be long-term history of reflux, dysphagia, or weight loss. It is not recommended to test with endoscopy for all patients with heartburn. A negative *H. pylori* test lessens the chance of inflammation and ulceration. Response to treatment within 2 weeks is a positive indication that the patient has gastroesophageal reflux and can continue treatment and be followed in the office.

26. Answer: 1

Rationale: The most common cause of death with NAFLD is cardiovascular disease with hepatocellular carcinoma and liver disease as the second and third causes, respectively. Bariatric surgery for morbid obesity includes gastric bypass, sleeve gastrectomy, adjustable gastric band and biliopancreatic diversion with duodenal switch. These are done with the goal of weight loss to improve the patient's health, including improving diabetes and hypertension. Rapid weight loss which can occur after bariatric surgery may improve liver function tests but some studies demonstrate progression of liver disease and worsening liver fibrosis. The risk of cirrhosis is not 50%. Of patients with NAFLD, 30% will develop nonalcoholic steatohepatitis (NASH), which is characterized by inflammation, cell damage, and fibrosis. Cirrhosis develops in 15%–25% of patients with NASH.

27. Answer: 2

Rationale: The major factor contributing to reflux is an incompetent lower esophageal sphincter (LES), the antireflux barrier. A hiatal hernia is frequently present with reflux, but is not a significant factor in the pathophysiology, unless it is large, but may be associated with greater reflux and delayed esophageal acid clearance in patients with reflux. Gastroesophageal reflux disease (GERD) can be familial, but is not always a factor. Overeating, alcohol, and caffeine all relax the LES sphincter and increase stomach acid production, affecting symptoms, but are not the main causative factor.

28. Answer: 3

Rationale: Most epidemiologic studies demonstrate that IBS is up to 50% more common in females than in males, appears to be familial, and is estimated to affect 10% to 30% of the adult population in Western countries. A disease of young and middle-aged adults, IBS peak prevalence occurs in the third and fourth decades of life, and the condition is usually diagnosed before age 50.

29. Answer: 4

Rationale: A means of hepatitis B (HBV) transmission is from an infected mother to baby, perinatally. Before the hepatitis B vaccine, it was estimated that 30%–40% of chronic HBV infections were transmitted perinatally. Since the widespread use of the vaccine and guidelines of vaccinating newborns, this rate has dropped dramatically. The main routes of transmission are contact with an infected person including sexual, transfusions, sharing razors or toothbrushes, sharing needles, syringes, and other drug injecting equipment, blood and open sores, needle sticks or other sharp instruments. HBV is not spread by food, water, sharing eating utensils, breastfeeding, hugging, kissing, coughing, sneezing, or the fecal-oral route.

30. Answer: 2

Rationale: Symptoms of an incarcerated hernia that has strangulated include acute pain, redness, nausea, and vomiting and is considered a surgical emergency and requires immediate referral to a surgeon. Strangulated hernias should be surgically repaired as early as possible to prevent complications such as necrosis and viscus perforation. Bowel obstruction and testicular torsion are emergent conditions, but not associated with an incarcerated hernia.

31. Answer: 1

Rationale: Hepatitis A and E are transmitted by the fecal-oral route. Hepatitis A spreads rapidly in households and daycare centers for children. Risk is higher in daycare centers with young children who wear diapers. Outbreaks can also occur from contaminated food and water

infected with human sewage. Hepatitis B, C, and D are transmitted by blood. Hepatitis D only occurs as a coinfection with hepatitis B.

32. Answer: 2

Rationale: The patient's symptoms most likely represent a small bowel obstruction (SBO). The history of multiple abdominal surgeries provides a possible cause as adhesions commonly develop after surgery and are one of the most common causes of SBO. Appendicitis would be documented on a CT scan which would likely be done at the emergency room. Appendicitis can present with these symptoms, but the pain is usually progressive and not intermittent. Biliary ductal obstruction is unlikely as the patient's gallbladder has been removed and though stones can reform it takes many years, usually more than 5 years. Another cause of biliary obstruction is a neoplasm, but the patients usually do not have pain and bowels are not generally affected. Gastroenteritis usually is accompanied by diarrhea not constipation.

33. Answer: 1

Rationale: When there is a defect in the abdominal wall, a hernia can develop. The hernia is a protrusion of a peritoneal-lined sac (i.e., bowel or omentum) through the weakness in the abdominal wall. An indirect hernia protrusion occurs directly through the floor of the inguinal canal and exits through the external inguinal ring. A direct hernia is less common and occurs more in those over 40 years of age. It may be felt medial to the external canal, and rarely passes into the scrotum. A femoral hernia is noted when the femoral artery exits the abdomen and is the least common of pelvic hernias. It occurs more in females. A strangulated hernia is nonreducible and can be a surgical emergency.

34. Answer: 1

Rationale: Chronic long-term use of stimulant laxatives such as bisacodyl can worsen constipation as the bowels become dependent and develop a resistance to the stimulants. Pelvic floor dyssynergia can cause fecal incontinence, diarrhea, or constipation. But stimulant laxatives would cause diarrhea since the colon motility is not the problem. Colonic inertia is an infrequent cause of constipation and can be severe, it may be a differential diagnosis, but not the most likely. Irritable bowel syndrome has pain as a major symptom, which is not present with this patient's symptoms.

35. Answer: 2

Rationale: The pinworm parasites reside in the intestine. Females lay eggs on the skin outside the anus, resulting in extreme pruritus. The only host is humans and it is transmitted by the fecal-oral route, easily spreading among households, daycare centers, and schools. Hookworm larvae reside in the soil, enter the body through the feet, and can cause anemia. When dirt containing roundworm eggs are ingested through pica or unwashed vegetables, or if contaminated water is consumed, an intestinal infestation occurs. Giardiasis results from ingestion of the protozoan *Giardia lamblia* through contaminated water or oral-fecal transmission.

36. Answer: 1

Rationale: An important nonpharmacologic intervention for gastroesophageal reflux disease (GERD) is to advise the patient not to lie down within 2–3 hours after meals to allow the stomach to empty. Patients with GERD also should reduce weight, avoid large meals and exercise after meals, and elevate the head of the bed. Certain drinks (alcohol, mint, and orange juice) should be avoided because they can increase acid production and can relax the lower esophageal sphincter. Acidic foods (tomato products, spicy foods) may worsen symptoms of reflux and should be avoided. The patient should be taught to avoid bending after meals. Drinking large amounts of fluid with meals may affect GERD, depending on the volume of the fluids.

37. Answer: 3

Rationale: Lifestyle modifications should be the first step in managing constipation. Most patients do not have enough fiber in their diet. Thirty to thirty-five grams a day is recommended, most of which should come from the diet. Fiber supplements can help but do not add a significant amount of fiber. Patients need to read food labels to determine their fiber amount. Increasing fluids and exercise are also useful to maintain regular bowel function. In the absence of alarm symptoms such as weight loss, rectal bleeding, or significant abdominal pain, conservative therapy should be tried before considering testing. It is rare that colon cancer causes constipation and blockages as this would be an advanced cancer. Rectocele can be a cause of constipation, and should be considered if lifestyle modifications are not improving bowel function.

38. Answer: 2

Rationale: *Helicobacter pylori* has been shown to be responsible for most duodenal and gastric ulcers. The other common cause of ulcers is from use of nonsteroidal anti-inflammatory drugs (NSAIDs) at regular and/or high doses. The other organisms listed are implicated in other types of infections (e.g., acute otitis media; skin infections). *Streptococcus pneumoniae* and *Moraxella catarrhalis* have been implicated as causative agents in pneumonia.

39. Answer: 2

Rationale: Hepatitis A never becomes chronic and is not a cause of cirrhosis. Nonalcoholic fatty liver disease

(NAFLD) is common, affecting 15%–20% of the general population, and is related to the metabolic syndrome. Excess fat deposits, partially due to insulin resistance, can cause inflammation and scarring that lead to cirrhosis. NAFLD has been increasing in incidence and severity. Chronic hepatitis B is not a major of cirrhosis in the United States but is a world-wide epidemic and responsible for hepatocellular cancer. Alcohol in large and/or daily amounts can cause cirrhosis.

40. Answer: 2

Rationale: A hemorrhoid is a vascular anal cushion and can be internal (above the dentate line) or external (below the dentate line), which can enlarge and bleed. Everyone has internal hemorrhoids even though they may not have any symptoms. In a rectal mucosa prolapse, the wall of the rectum prolapses through the anal canal on straining. A rectocele is a herniation of the rectum into the vaginal wall and can cause constipation.

41. Answer: 2

Rationale: These characteristics describe hepatitis B. In 2014, it is estimated that there were 19,200 new cases in the United States. The incidence has declined by 82% since initiation of the vaccine in 1991. The incidence of chronicity is estimated to be between 850,000 and 2.2 million people. Hepatitis A has symptoms of fever and jaundice (up to 50%), but the incubation period is 15–50 days (average 30 days) and does not have a chronic form. Hepatitis C infection causes jaundice up to 25% of the time and can cause arthralgia, but there is no fever. The incubation period is 14–18 days (average 42–49 days). Up to 75% of those infected with hepatitis C will develop chronic infection. Hepatitis E is characterized by oral-fecal transmission that is associated with contaminated food and water, and has an incubation period of 14–60 days and no chronic disease state.

42. Answer: 2

Rationale: Although some patients need eventual intervention including a cholecystectomy, those who are older adults and diabetic are at increased risk for complications and should be hospitalized for prompt diagnosis, which could include a right upper quadrant (RUQ) abdominal ultrasound, and possibly a magnetic resonance cholangiopancreatography (MRCP). The MRCP is very sensitive at documenting a gallstone lodged in the bile duct. Abnormally elevated transaminases and possibly pancreatic enzymes would be present with bile duct blockage, and the patient may have secondary pancreatitis. Intravenous fluids, pain control, and surgical consultation would also be warranted. The other patients would need evaluations but could be started with outpatient testing.

43. Answer: 3

Rationale: Long-term GERD ("heartburn for years") without effective treatment (no complete relief of symptoms and no proton pump inhibitor) carries a risk of Barrett esophagus (a precursor to cancer) and esophageal adenocarcinoma, especially in a non-Hispanic white male smoker over the age of 50 years. Rapid weight loss is a concerning clinical finding that may indicate esophageal cancer or other cancer that had advanced to a hypermetabolic state. He also has a risk of squamous cell carcinoma of the esophagus as it is associated with cigarette smoking and alcohol use, but is less common than adenocarcinoma (ratio 1:2). Adenocarcinoma of the esophagus most commonly develops in men (men/women ratio 6:1) age 65 years and older. The symptoms of heartburn caused by either gastric ulcer or long-term GERD will not likely be controlled with an H_2 RA/antacid and would require a proton pump inhibitor daily. A patient with a gastric ulcer should be tested for *Helicobacter pylori* and would be questioned about a history of nonsteroidal anti-inflammatory drug (NSAID) use, and then treated appropriately. Clinical manifestations of lung cancer include cough, hemoptysis, dyspnea, chest pain, and weight loss, and the substantial pack-year history does place the patient at risk. This would be in the differential, but esophageal cancer would be the first diagnosis to rule out.

44. Answer: 1

Rationale: Intermittent diarrhea, gas, and bloating can occur after ingestion of dairy if the patient is lactose intolerant. This can occur at any time and can present after a viral illness. The decrease or loss of the enzyme lactase which breaks down lactose in dairy results in colonic bacteria breaking down the lactose and producing gas and diarrhea. Some patients can be extremely sensitive to all dairy, including butter. Patients with celiac disease are usually anemic and may have elevated liver enzymes. Hyperthyroidism can cause diarrhea, but the patient's TSH is high meaning she has hypothyroidism. *Helicobacter pylori* infection can cause abdominal pain and bloating, but would not necessarily cause diarrhea and the elevated antibody is not confirmatory of infection.

45. Answer: 4

Rationale: Esophageal varices are dilated submucosal veins that are a late sign and complication of cirrhosis because of scarring of the liver and portal hypertension. The cirrhosis would likely be advanced for varices to develop, usually in the esophagus, but can also occur in the stomach. As these varices are under high pressure, the patient can have anything from a slow leak of blood to a major, life-threatening bleed. The varices should be diagnosed by endoscopy and treated with beta blockers to lower the blood pressure. Of patients with cirrhosis, approximately 50% will develop gastroesophageal varices and will have a yearly rate of bleeding from 5% to 15%. A history of heavy alcohol intake may be the cause of this patient's cirrhosis. These patients can present clinically with bleeding, spontaneous "coffee grounds" or bright-red blood, hypotension, and eventual shock. The other choices could all be associated with this patient. A bleeding peptic ulcer is possible, but is not the first concern. An excessive nosebleed is possible because of thrombocytopenia from cirrhosis and would need to be explored. Hemoptysis implies lung disease.

46. Answer: 4

Rationale: Gastroesophageal reflux disease (GERD) can present with a variety of symptoms including atypical extraesophageal symptoms such as cough. Acid in the esophagus can trigger a bronchospasm resulting in a cough and other pulmonary symptoms. His weight gain coincides with the onset of the cough which can worsen reflux. The timing of the cough, after meals and at night, correlates with when reflux is likely to be occurring. Not everyone who has GERD is aware of it and has no classic heartburn on regurgitation. Environmental allergies can contribute but his symptoms would likely be more seasonal and not continuous the entire year, depending on his location. Exposure to fumes would trigger a cough, but pulmonary workup was negative and he did not respond to treatment. Sinusitis and postnasal drainage can cause a cough, but likely would be seasonal and not necessarily occurring after meals.

47. Answer: 2

Rationale: Increasing crampy abdominal pain that starts as periumbilical pain, anorexia, and fever are classic symptoms of appendicitis. A surgeon should evaluate the patient to decrease the risk of rupture. An abdominal CT scan has a high sensitivity to document appendicitis. Although ectopic pregnancy should always be a consideration in young females with abdominal pain, the characteristics of the pain and other symptoms are not typical of an ectopic pregnancy. However, a good gynecologic history would be needed. The patient should not be sent home unless the CT scan was negative, and then follow-up within 24 hours would be warranted.

48. Answer: 3

Rationale: Abstinence from alcohol, the most important treatment for cirrhosis, can halt progression of cirrhosis and reverse the damage, if the liver is minimally scarred. Continuing to drink even occasionally can be detrimental and rapidly increase the disease process. It is known that 1–2 drinks a day for a woman raises her risk of cirrhosis up to four times the risk of the general population. Recent research shows that current drinking may be more of a factor than a lifetime amount. The patient's diet should be nutritious and she should avoid herbal and other supplements because some have been known to cause liver toxicity. Vitamin E supplementation is being researched as treatment for nonalcoholic fatty liver disease. There is no standard recommendation for vitamin E treatment with cirrhosis.

49. Answer: 2

Rationale: Diverticulitis is defined as clinically evident macroscopic inflammation of a diverticulum or diverticula. It occurs in 4% of patients with diverticulosis. Patients usually present with a sudden onset of abdominal pain in the left lower quadrant. The patient may have a low-grade fever and leukocytosis. Patients with diverticulitis can have a range of mild to severe inflammation and 15% will develop complications. Nausea and vomiting may accompany severe pain. Appendicitis may present with pain in the periumbilical region that eventually travels to the right lower quadrant and may not be severe for several hours after onset. Other signs, including nausea and vomiting, leukocytosis, and fever, may or may not be present. Irritable bowel syndrome (IBS) may present with aching or cramping in the periumbilical or lower abdominal regions, often precipitated by meals and relieved by defecation. The pain can be severe occasionally, and there is an altered frequency and consistency of the stools. Fever, leukocytosis, and awakening at night are not indicative of IBS. A ruptured ovarian cyst would not be a differential in an older adult woman as the ovaries shrink and stop functioning with menopause.

50. Answer: 1

Rationale: A high-fiber diet is important for preventing and treating for diverticular disease, and vegetarians who eat increased amounts of fruits, vegetables, grains, and cereals with high fiber are in the lowest risk category. Chronic constipation causes chronic increased pressure in the sigmoid colon, which can increase the likelihood of bowel wall weakening and diverticula (out-pouches) developing. Small meals and low-fiber diets (low carbohydrate with low intake of grains) would also increase the risk of constipation.

51. Answer: 2

Rationale: The risk of colorectal cancer increases in patients over age 50 years for the general population, which is the age recommended to begin screening. However, patients who are black (African American, African) have a higher risk and do not respond well to treatment for colon cancer. It is recommended that patients who are black begin screening at 45 years of age. Colon cancer

is most frequently found in patients in their sixth and seventh decades of life. Almost all colon cancers begin as polyps, which can be slow growing, taking 8–15 years to begin to grow and eventually turn into cancer. Frequently, there are no symptoms, even with left-sided colon cancers and bright red rectal bleeding always should be explored. Although hemorrhoid bleeding would be the most common cause of rectal bleeding, without a colonoscopy, one cannot be definite. Screening recommendations change if there is a family history of colon polyps or cancer, especially first-degree relatives. Family members who were diagnosed before the age of 60 years greatly increases the risk for the patient and the screening is recommended for every 5 years, beginning at an age 10 years before the age of the family member at diagnosis. Colonoscopy is the most accurate and the only test where polyps can be removed at the time of testing. Symptoms such as weight loss, pain, and change in bowel habits are usually late signs. Patients over the age of 75 to 80 years are individually evaluated for continued screening. With no symptoms and no history of polyps, screening may be discontinued.

52. Answer: 1

Rationale: Colorectal cancer (CRC) risk in patients with left-sided and universal ulcerative colitis increases by 0.5%–1% per year after the 8th year of disease. Ulcerative colitis limited to the proctosigmoid region carries less of a risk. Crohn disease, which can affect any part of the gastrointestinal tract from the mouth to the rectum, carries a higher risk if the colon is involved. Colonoscopy with random biopsies every 1–2 years is recommended beginning 8–10 years after the inflammatory bowel disease began. Diverticulosis is common in the general population, but is less common in ulcerative colitis and is not a risk factor for CRC. Ischemic colitis occurs when a mesenteric artery is temporarily blocked and the colon at the splenic flexure develops ischemia from lack of blood flow. There is not a higher risk of ischemic colitis for patients with ulcerative colitis. Irritable bowel syndrome is common in the general population and in patients with ulcerative colitis, but it is a disorder of brain-gut interaction and does not increase risk of colon cancer.

53. Answer: 4

Rationale: Patients with a gastric ulcer may not have any symptoms, especially in the older adult. Weight loss and anorexia may be present, but the patient may attribute this to "getting older." The patient may not realize an ulcer is present until it bleeds and causes significant anemia. Smoking does increase the risk, and perforation can occur, but is not common. Gastric ulcers are thought to be more common than duodenal ulcers in older adult patients.

54. Answer: 3

Rationale: Dysphagia and cough with solid and liquid intake may be the first indication that the patient has cancer, but this is usually late in development. Alcoholism and smoking are the primary risk factors for squamous cell esophageal cancer, which is not as common as adenocarcinoma, which is usually associated with chronic GERD and Barrett esophagus. Caffeine intake in coffee of one or more cups a day, specifically, may be protective against esophageal, oral, and pharyngeal cancer. Midchest pain indicates late disease, which does not usually respond to treatment, including surgery.

55. Answer: 1

Rationale: A history of polyps does increase the risk of colon cancer and on average patients will need a repeat colonoscopy in 3–5 years, rather than the recommended 10 years if there are no polyps and no family history. Hyperplastic polyps, in general, are not a concern and do not turn into cancer. Adenomatous polyps can turn into cancer. Small polyps may be adenomas and will be removed during the colonoscopy. Histologic analysis is required to identify adenomatous polyps. A colonoscopy is the most sensitive and specific test for polyps and cancer, but there are factors that affect the effectiveness contributing to a variable miss rate for polyps and cancer.

56. Answer: 2

Rationale: Celiac sprue is a genetic disease of the small bowel that is caused by gluten intolerance. The diarrhea and cramping are related to the effects of malabsorption of gluten. Because of malabsorption, many patients have iron-deficiency anemia and can have elevated liver enzymes. Hepatitis B would produce elevated liver enzymes, but not the other listed symptoms. Salmonella infection could produce diarrhea and cramping, but not anemia. A bleeding ulcer could produce anemia, but not the other symptoms.

57. Answer: 1

Rationale: Nonalcoholic fatty liver disease (NAFLD) is associated with diabetes, hyperlipidemia, and obesity. The liver is storing excessive amounts of fat, which can, over time, cause inflammation of the liver. If the inflammation continues, the liver can become scarred, which can lead to cirrhosis. Autoimmune hepatitis is not common and affects women more than men; it would not be the primary differential. Celiac sprue is not associated with obesity or diabetes. Drug-induced liver disease is related to certain medications that can cause acute injury to the liver. Depending on the medications he is taking and the elevation of the enzymes, this diagnosis would be considered.

58. Answer: 3

Rationale: Abnormal villi found on the duodenal biopsy are the gold standard for diagnosis. A negative biopsy could mean the disease has not manifested, but the patient has the potential to develop celiac disease. The tissue transglutaminase antibody (tTG), IgA, and deamidated gliadin (DGP) are the most sensitive serologic tests for celiac disease. The antiendomysial antibody test (EMA IgA) is very specific for celiac disease, meaning if it is positive then it is likely the patient has celiac disease. However, it is not as sensitive for celiac disease, about 5%–10% will have a false negative test for celiac. With this patient, an EMAIgA could be tested and if positive that might explain the patient's results as a potential patient with celiac disease. It is thought that a positive tTG does not cause nonceliac gluten sensitivity. Removing gluten from the diet may improve the patient's symptoms. A strict gluten-free diet will normalize the biopsy findings and convert the antibodies to negative, but both tests would be affected and it could take 2–3 months or longer to have normal results. It is unlikely that a few weeks of a gluten-free diet would normalize the biopsy.

59. Answer: 2

Rationale: A common sequela of a viral infection is gastroparesis. The virus can affect the gastric pacer, causing it to malfunction and result in slow gastric emptying. Typical symptoms of nausea, decreased appetite, and early satiety occur because of the lingering of solid food in the stomach, which can be 4 hours or more. Typically, a stomach should empty in 1–2 hours for an average meal. Accumulation throughout the day can result in a full stomach that does not empty. These are not typical symptoms of an influenza infection. Vertigo causes nausea, but not the other symptoms. Although the patient may have taken ibuprofen for several days, it is less likely that an ulcer would have developed with a short course, but it should be in the differential.

60. Answer: 4

Rationale: The symptoms of cramping, diarrhea, and bloating are classic for irritable bowel syndrome (IBS) with diarrhea predominant. Abdominal pain is a symptom of IBS, but is not associated with rectal bleeding or fecal incontinence.

61. Answer: 1

Rationale: People with irritable bowel syndrome (IBS) can have many food triggers. The challenge is to identify the foods without having them avoid entire food groups. Simple sugars, specifically fermentable oligo-, di- and monosaccharides and polyols (FODMAPS) can cause symptoms of cramping, gas, bloating, and diarrhea. Rather than avoiding all fruits and vegetables, patients need to be aware of the most offending foods and carefully avoid those that cause a problem. Dairy products have lactose, which is not able to be broken down when someone is lacking some or all lactase, the enzyme needed for digestion of lactose. Although people have IBS and lactose intolerance, it should not be assumed the patient has both. Red meat and saturated fat can cause some problems, but are not prime offenders.

62. Answer: 3

Rationale: One of the ways patients can decrease the fat in the liver is to lose weight with exercise. It is important to treat hyperlipidemia because this is associated with fatty liver and statins should not be discontinued. Lowering cholesterol is not as effective as lowering saturated fats in the diet. Adding vitamin A as a supplement is controversial and excessive doses over 10,000 IU of vitamin A daily can cause or worsen liver damage.

63. Answer: 2

Rationale: *Norovirus* (*Norwalk*) can cause vomiting and diarrhea in adolescents and adults. The incubation period is short (18–72 hours) and the duration of symptoms is short, usually 24–48 hours. *Cytomegalovirus* rarely causes diarrhea and is commonly reactivated in patients after bone marrow transplant, late stages of HIV infection, and other immunocompromised situations. *Campylobacter* enteritis is the most common cause of bacterial diarrhea, especially in traveler's diarrhea and food poisoning. *Rotavirus* mainly affects infants 3–15 months of age in the winter months, causing excessive watery diarrhea.

64. Answer: 2

Rationale: A history of vaginal delivery of large babies and possible complications such as use of forceps can indicate she has weakened pelvic floor muscles and has lost the ability to maintain a closed external anal sphincter to control leakage. Typically, the development of incontinence can occur 20–30 years after the delivery. Diagnostic testing would include anorectal manometry and treatment with physical therapy and biofeedback may be helpful. While the past medical history should include the childbirth history, it is not necessarily obtained in detail and may not be relevant depending on the reason for the office visit. Stress can play a role in worsening many symptoms, it is less likely to be affecting her bowel control. A rectocele is a rectal prolapse into the vagina that can occur after delivery when the ligaments and muscles weaken. However, the main complaint with a rectocele is constipation, not stool leakage.

65. Answer: 3

Rationale: The location of the injury suggests a ruptured spleen. Hypovolemia can quickly occur as there can be a large amount of internal bleeding and is a medical emergency. The rupture occurs when there is a severe direct blow to the abdomen. Common causes of the trauma are motor vehicle accidents, contact sports, bicycle accidents, and domestic violence. Diseases such as lymphoma, infectious mononucleosis, and hemolytic anemia increase the risk of rupture. Although bowel and bladder injuries are possible with blunt trauma to the abdomen, the upper abdominal location, noted by the hematoma location, makes a spleen injury more likely. Older adolescents may complain of dizziness, fatigue, chest pain, and palpitations because of arrhythmias, but hematomas are not usually present.

Pharmacology

66. Answer: 1

Rationale: Eosinophilic esophagitis (EE) is an emerging disease that is increasingly recognized and prevalent. A typical presentation is dysphagia due to esophageal dysfunction, with symptoms of food sticking when swallowing. The diagnosis is made at endoscopy with biopsies of the esophagus showing eosinophilia in the squamous epithelium. EE is a chronic allergic/immune condition, identified in the past 20 years. Treatment includes corticosteroids, topical, but can include systemic as well if symptoms are persistent. An allergy evaluation is also recommended to determine if dietary factors are involved. Sucralfate has no role here. It is not well absorbed and mainly works to coat the mucosal lining and serve as a barrier to acids, enzymes, and bile salts. It can be helpful for symptom relief from peptic ulcer disease. H_2 RAs such as ranitidine and proton pump inhibitors (PPIs) such as omeprazole do not treat EE. Nonresponse to a PPI trial would lead to an endoscopy and diagnosis of EE.

67. Answer: 4

Rationale: Omeprazole is a proton pump inhibitor (PPI) that blocks all three pathways of acid production: histamine, gastrin, and acetylcholine, for up to 24 hours. Treatment with a PPI is recommended for patients who have frequent symptoms, at least several times a week. It is important to take the PPI on an empty stomach, and then eat 30–60 minutes after for maximum pH control. PPIs need food to work, and, if a second dose is required, it should be taken before the evening dose. Anticholinergics (hyoscyamine and others) will likely increase his symptoms by lowering the lower esophageal sphincter pressure. Anticholinergics are effective for the cramping of IBS. Ranitidine is a histamine 2 receptor antagonist (H_2 RA), which blocks one pathway for acid secretion, histamine, but there are two other pathways that continue to secrete hydrochloric acid. An H_2 RA can be effective for occasional symptoms, a few times a week or less, or as a short trial for new onset of symptoms.

68. Answer: 4

Rationale: Topical nitrate ointment applied twice daily for 6–8 weeks has been associated with healing of chronic anal fissure at least 50% of the time. It can also decrease rectal pain. The most commonly occurring side effect is headache in 20%–30% of the patients. Topical calcium channel blockers are also utilized but the data is insufficient to conclude healing superior to placebo. Sitz baths, psyllium, and bulking agents are first-line therapy for acute anal fissure and can be helpful for symptomatic relief. Topical lidocaine gel can provide some relief of pain but not effect healing. Analpram-HC is used to treat of symptoms of hemorrhoids, including pain, itching, and swelling. An anal fissure is a longitudinal tear in the midline of the anal canal, distal to the dentate line. An acute fissure looks like a simple tear in the anoderm while a chronic fissure is defined as lasting 8–12 weeks and has edema and fibrosis associated with it.

69. Answer: 3

Rationale: Goals of peptic ulcer disease (PUD) treatment include removal of offending agent, relief of pain, healing of ulcer, and cost effectiveness. In this case, the likely cause of her ulcer would be use of nonsteroidal anti-inflammatory drugs (NSAIDs). It is estimated that up to 25% of patients taking NSAIDs chronically will develop ulcer disease and 2%–4% will develop bleeding or perforation. Risk factors for NSAID-induced ulcers include: age greater than 65 years, high doses of NSAIDs, daily use, use of aspirin or anticoagulants or antiplatelet medications. Proton pump inhibitors (PPIs) heal 90% of duodenal ulcers after 4 weeks and 90% of gastric ulcers after 8 weeks, if *Helicobacter pylori (H. pylori)* is negative. PPIs, such as pantoprazole, are recommended for ulcers because these drugs provide faster pain relief and more rapid healing than H_2 RA because of their ability to decrease acid production. Clarithromycin, tetracycline, metronidazole, and bismuth (Pepto-Bismol) are some of the accepted treatments against active *H. pylori*–associated ulcers. Eradication of *H. pylori* requires a recommended regimen of acid blockers, antibiotics, and possibly bismuth in various combinations.

70. Answer: 4

Rationale: The best choice for this patient would be dexlansoprazole and celexicoxib. Treating a patient's arthritis pain with NSAIDs raises the risk of peptic ulcer disease. The body secretes prostaglandins to help protect the gastrointestinal (GI) mucosa lining that are blocked by cyclooxygenase-1 (COX-1) agents, such as ibuprofen and other NSAIDs that make this class of drugs risky. Utilizing an NSAID that is a cyclooxygenase-2 (COX-2) selective inhibitor (celecoxib, rofecoxib) is associated with significantly lower rates of ulcers, but this effect decreases if a patient is also taking aspirin, which this patient is likely taking for his heart disease. Proton pump inhibitors (PPI) have been shown to greatly reduce the development of gastric and duodenal ulcers. Combining a COX-2 inhibitor and PPI would offer the best protection while treating his pain. Additionally, there is some suggestion that taking NSAIDs, including COX-2 inhibitor agents, may increase the risk of cardiovascular thromboembolic events. The patient's health status may warrant a consult and close monitoring. An H_2 RA such as ranitidine may help prevent duodenal ulcers, but has not been shown to prevent gastric ulcers. Misoprostol is a synthetic prostaglandin E1 analog and when taken in full doses (200 mcg 4 times a day) has been shown to be very effective in preventing stomach ulcers when taken with NSAIDs, but is limited by gastrointestinal side effects (cramping and diarrhea) and compliance is poor given the dosing regimen. Lower doses of misoprostol (400–600 mcg/day) may be effective, but should not be used in pregnancy as it can induce labor. Sucralfate has not been shown to prevent gastric or duodenal ulceration.

71. Answer: 2

Rationale: If a person exposed to a patient known to be positive for hepatitis B has sufficient immunity to hepatitis B, no treatment is necessary. If this same person had not been vaccinated, in addition to initiation of the hepatitis B vaccine series, HBIG 0.06 mL/kg IM is also administered. If an exposed person has had an inadequate immune response to the hepatitis B vaccine series (negative antihepatitis surface antibody), a hepatitis B booster should be given.

72. Answer: 1

Rationale: Patients with gastric or duodenal ulcers due to *Helicobacter pylori (H. pylori)* can be successfully treated with triple-drug therapy: a proton pump inhibitor (bid for all except esomeprazole which is qd), clarithromycin and amoxicillin or metronidazole for 14 days (eradication rates 70%–85%). An alternative FDA-approved regimen is a quadruple regimen with a (qd or bid) or H_2 RA (bid), metronidazole, bismuth, and tetracycline for 10–14 days (eradication rates 75%–90%). Treatment should continue with a proton pump inhibitor for at least 2-4 weeks after to promote healing of the ulcer. After completion of *H. pylori* therapy, it is recommended that testing be done with the stool antigen for *H. pylori* at 8 weeks to assure eradication of the infection. The PPI would need to be stopped for 2 weeks before testing the stool, as there can be false negative results. Other treatment regimens have been suggested but eradication rates can vary. Cephalosporins are not included in any recommended regimens for *H. pylori.*

73. Answer: 2

Rationale: Mesalamine (5-aminosalicylic acid) therapy for patients with mild ulcerative colitis has been shown to improve symptoms and induce and maintain remission. It is an anti-inflammatory compound similar to aspirin, without the effects on platelets. There are several mesalamine products available, including rectal suspension and suppositories that can be very helpful for left-sided colitis. If no response is seen after 2–4 weeks, the addition of corticosteroids (prednisone) can be helpful, but they are not first-line therapy. Ciprofloxacin and metronidazole are typically used for gastrointestinal infections, including *Clostridium difficile,* which is common with ulcerative colitis.

74. Answer: 1

Rationale: To minimize the risk of a contact developing hepatitis A, which is spread by fecal-oral transmission, immunoglobulin 0.02 mL/kg should be given as soon as possible after exposure. It has not been shown to be effective if administered more than 2 weeks after exposure. Hepatitis B immune globulin (HBIG) is for hepatitis B.

75. Answer: 4

Rationale: For unvaccinated patients with exposure to hepatitis B, one dose of hepatitis B immune globulin (HBIG) is administered and the HBV series initiated. HBIG may be protective or may attenuate the severity of the illness if given within 7 days of exposure (adult dose of 0.06 mL/kg). If the patient thinks the individual may have been vaccinated, but does not know whether there was a response, the adult-gerontology primary care NP can test antihepatitis B surface antibody. Neither the HBe

antibody nor the viral load would be a first-line test. Because of the timing of appearance of the antibodies to hepatitis B, testing would need to be delayed.

76. Answer: 3

Rationale: The only contraindication to the hepatitis B vaccine is prior anaphylaxis or severe hypersensitivity to the vaccine or components of the vaccine.

77. Answer: 3

Rationale: Metronidazole 500 mg PO tid for 10 days is the first-line treatment for mild to moderate *Clostridium difficile* (CD) infection. Vancomycin would be second line, if there is no improvement in 5–7 days. He has no symptoms indicating severe disease which would include fever, abdominal tenderness, low albumin and creatinine, and leukocytosis >15,000 with a left shift of >20% neutrophils. For severe disease vancomycin would be the drug of choice. The regimen of vancomycin and IV metronidazole is reserved for severe complicated disease that can include hypotension, ileus, mental status changes, and need for admission to intensive care. The probiotics, *Lactobacilli acidophilus* and *L. casei,* have been suggested as helpful for infection and prevention control of CD infection, but the data on probiotics is insufficient at this time for a strong recommendation.

78. Answer: 3

Rationale: This is a common observation for a patient taking Pepto-Bismol. The patient may also experience a problem with discoloration of his tongue. The stool discoloration is not related to bleeding. Certain foods can affect the stool color, but bismuth is more likely the cause.

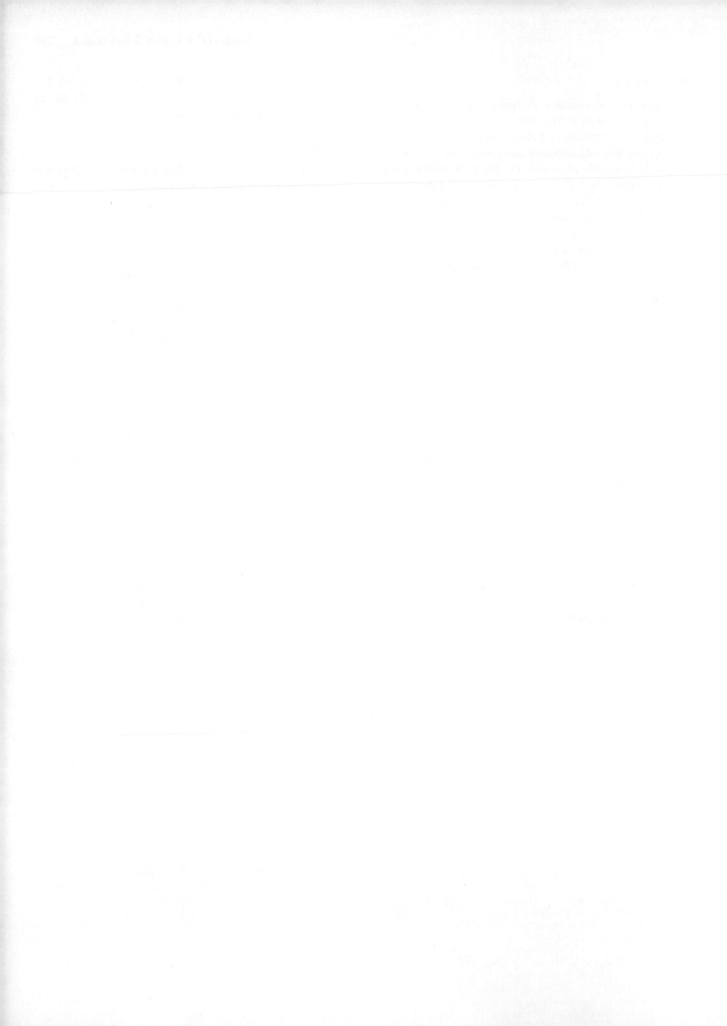

Hematology

13

Physical Examination & Diagnostic Tests

1. A male patient with iron deficiency would most likely present with which of the following lab values?
    1. Hct 30%, serum Fe 18, MCV 70, decreased transferrin, increased ferritin.
    2. Hct 22%, serum Fe 18, MCV 60, increased transferrin, increased ferritin.
    3. Hct 22%, serum Fe 18, MCV 70, increased transferrin, decreased ferritin.
    4. Hct 22%, serum Fe 18, MCV 90, decreased transferrin, increased ferritin.

2. On physical exam, a palpable, firm, nontender supraclavicular lymph node is noted on the left side of the body. The finding is consistent with a diagnosis of:
    1. Bacterial infection draining from the internal jugular chain.
    2. Thoracic or abdominal malignancy.
    3. Inflammation of the tonsils and adenoids.
    4. Non-Hodgkin lymphoma.

3. Which test is most important for diagnosing iron-deficiency anemia?
    1. Direct Coombs.
    2. Serum folate level.
    3. Serum ferritin.
    4. RBC count.

4. The term "shotty" is often used to describe lymph nodes that are:
    1. Tender, mobile, and >5 mm.
    2. Small and pellet-like.
    3. Discrete and cystic.
    4. Irregular, soft, and fixed to surrounding tissue.

5. A macrocytic, normochromic anemia is diagnosed in an older adult male patient. What should be the next test(s) ordered?
    1. Serum iron and TIBC levels.
    2. Bone marrow biopsy.
    3. Colonoscopy.
    4. Vitamin B_{12} and RBC/folate levels.

6. The adult-gerontology primary care NP would suspect disseminated intravascular coagulation (DIC) if the patient's laboratory results, including prothrombin time (PT), indicated:
    1. Increased PT, decreased platelet count, and decreased fibrinogen.
    2. Decreased PT, increased hematocrit, and increased fibrinogen.
    3. Increased platelet count, decreased hematocrit, and increased PT.
    4. Increased platelet count, increased hematocrit, and decreased PT.

7. When examining lymph nodes, the adult-gerontology primary care NP understands:
    1. Young adolescents are more likely to develop generalized lymphadenopathy than adults in response to a mild infection.
    2. Older adults frequently have enlarged, nontender supraclavicular and epitrochlear lymph nodes due to aging.
    3. Lymphadenopathy in an adult indicates acute or chronic infection and rarely malignancy.
    4. Enlarged neck lymph nodes in young adolescents with no other physical findings are highly suspicious of Burkitt lymphoma.

8. After confirming the diagnosis of iron-deficiency anemia in an older adult male patient based on CBC, peripheral smear, serum iron, TIBC, and serum ferritin, what would be the next essential test for the adult-gerontology primary care NP to order?
    1. Stool guaiac × 3.
    2. Prothrombin time/partial thromboplastin time (PT/PTT).
    3. Liver function tests.
    4. Endoscopy.

9. Evaluation of an older adult male patient reveals a macrocytic, normochromic anemia. Subsequent testing shows normal folate level and decreased vitamin B_{12} level. Further evaluation could include:
   1. Referral to a hematologist for a bone marrow biopsy.
   2. Assay for anti-IF antibodies.
   3. Upper gastrointestinal (GI) series.
   4. No tests are indicated at this time.

10. The most sensitive test for the diagnosis of sickle cell anemia is:
    1. CBC with a peripheral smear.
    2. Bone marrow biopsy and aspiration.
    3. Hemoglobin electrophoresis.
    4. Hemoglobin and hematocrit.

11. An older adult male patient presents to the office with complaints of fatigue, dizziness, decreased activity tolerance, and occasional bounding heart rate. Physical exam reveals pallor (including mucous membranes), tachycardia, and general appearance of lethargy. The adult-gerontology primary care NP orders CBC with differential, peripheral smear, serum iron, TIBC, and serum ferritin because there is a high index of suspicion for:
    1. Sideroblastic anemia.
    2. Pernicious anemia.
    3. Folic-acid-deficiency anemia.
    4. Iron-deficiency anemia.

12. Anemia of chronic disease would reveal which of the following laboratory findings?
    1. Decreased iron, decreased TIBC, and decreased serum ferritin.
    2. Decreased iron, decreased TIBC, and increased serum ferritin.
    3. Decreased iron, increased TIBC, and decreased serum ferritin.
    4. Decreased iron, increased TIBC, and increased serum ferritin.

13. A patient is planning a trip to a malaria-endemic area and will be receiving prophylactic medications. Which of the following medical conditions would warrant additional considerations by the adult-gerontology primary care NP?
    1. Gilbert syndrome.
    2. Von Willebrand disease.
    3. G6PD deficiency.
    4. Bernard-Soulier syndrome.

14. Which of the following statements is true concerning the leukemias?
    1. Liver function studies are decreased in the later stages of the disease process.
    2. Initial white blood cell (WBC) count is the most important predictor of prognosis.

3. Thrombocytopenia is rarely present.
4. The prognosis is better if a child is younger than 2 years.

15. In evaluating the laboratory findings for an older adult with iron-deficiency anemia, the adult-gerontology primary care NP expects:
    1. Low MCV and low reticulocyte count.
    2. High MCV and hemoglobin 12 g/dL.
    3. Normal MCV and hematocrit 34%.
    4. High MCV and normal reticulocyte count.

Disorders

16. An older adult client is diagnosed with leukemia and has constitutional symptoms of night sweats, unintentional weight loss, and fatigue with painless lymphadenopathy. What type of leukemia does this older adult client have?
    1. Acute lymphocytic leukemia.
    2. Chronic lymphocytic leukemia.
    3. Acute myelogenous leukemia.
    4. Chronic myelogenous leukemia.

17. Sickle cell anemia is caused by:
    1. Exposure to ionizing radiation.
    2. Genetically induced production of abnormal hemoglobin S.
    3. Deficiency of dietary folic acid.
    4. Long-term use of thiazide diuretics.

18. An adult patient presents to the adult-gerontology primary care NP with a history of erythrocytosis. One common complaint that could cause a serious complication for the patient is:
    1. A laceration.
    2. Vomiting and diarrhea.
    3. Coughing.
    4. Dizziness.

19. After the loss of his wife 5 months ago, a 67-year-old male patient began abusing alcohol. He has no prior medical problems and no history of alcoholism. Which of the following would be the most likely cause of new-onset anemia development in this patient?
    1. Liver cirrhosis.
    2. Thiamine deficiency.
    3. Folate deficiency.
    4. Cyanocobalamin deficiency.

20. A patient has a folic-acid-deficiency anemia. The adult-gerontology primary care NP teaches the patient to eat foods rich in folic acid, such as:
    1. Green leafy vegetables, nuts, and liver.
    2. Carrots, salmon, and avocados.
    3. Cottage cheese, yogurt, and skim milk.
    4. Lima beans, brussels sprouts, and potatoes.

21. Which three of the following statements are true about myelodysplastic syndromes?
    1. Affects predominantly older adults >65 years of age.
    2. Is primarily one disease that has a variable clinical presentation.
    3. Symptoms relate to bone marrow failure.
    4. Patients often become dependent on red blood cell transfusion.
    5. Immunosuppressive drug therapy is rarely indicated.

22. Which of the changes occurs in the RBC indices for pernicious anemia?
    1. Microcytic, normochromic.
    2. Microcytic, hypochromic.
    3. Normocytic, normochromic.
    4. Macrocytic, normochromic.

23. The adult-gerontology primary care NP knows which of the following is the most likely cause of acute hemolytic transfusion reactions?
    1. Contaminated blood products.
    2. ABO incompatibility.
    3. Immunoglobulin deficiency.
    4. Expired blood products.

24. Which statement is true concerning thalassemia?
    1. It is characterized by defective lymphocyte synthesis.
    2. Thalassemia minor does not require pharmacologic treatment.
    3. Thalassemia major is associated with high RBC counts and elevated serum iron.
    4. It is characterized with an acute onset of symptoms leading to leukocytosis.

25. An older adult who has acute myelogenous leukemia (AML) is undergoing cytotoxic chemotherapy treatment and has the following laboratory reports: elevated serum uric acid, serum potassium, and serum phosphate and a low serum calcium level. The WBC count is extremely elevated and on physical exam, there is noted lymphadenopathy and splenomegaly. What is most likely the cause?
    1. Disseminated intravascular coagulation (DIC).
    2. Leukostasis.
    3. Pancytopenia.
    4. Tumor lysis syndrome.

26. Iron-deficiency anemia is an example of:
    1. Macrocytic, normochromic anemia.
    2. Macrocytic, hypochromic anemia.
    3. Microcytic, hypochromic anemia.
    4. Normocytic, normochromic anemia.

27. An adult patient with pernicious anemia may present with which signs and symptoms?
    1. Peripheral neuropathy, ataxia, lethargy, and fatigue.
    2. Hepatomegaly, jaundice, and right upper quadrant pain.
    3. Hypertension, angina, and peripheral edema.
    4. Blurred vision, diplopia, and decreased vibratory sensation.

28. Anemia of chronic disease is a:
    1. Normochromic, normocytic anemia.
    2. Normochromic, microcytic anemia.
    3. Hypochromic, microcytic anemia.
    4. Hypochromic, macrocytic anemia.

29. A young adult presents to the clinic for a routine check-up. History is unremarkable, but on physical exam, the adult-gerontology primary care NP palpates an enlarged (2 cm), mobile, nontender, rubbery lymph node on the left posterior cervical chain. What is the adult-gerontology primary care NP's next step?
    1. Order a throat culture and monospot test.
    2. Refer to a surgeon for a lymph node biopsy.
    3. Order a STAT chest x-ray.
    4. No intervention is necessary at this time.

30. The adult-gerontology primary care NP understands that "B" symptoms associated with non-Hodgkin lymphoma (NHL) include:
    1. Bruising and bleeding.
    2. Peripheral edema, shortness of breath, and ascites.
    3. Fever, night sweats, and unexplained weight loss.
    4. Headache, fatigue, and weakness.

31. In teaching a patient with anemia to include foods rich in iron in the diet, the adult-gerontology primary care NP encourages the patient to eat:
    1. Cheese, milk, and yogurt.
    2. Red beans, whole-grain bread, and bran cereal.
    3. Tomatoes, cabbage, and citrus fruits.
    4. Beef, spinach, and peanut butter.

32. Anemia of chronic disease is associated with:
    1. Malnutrition and vitamin B_{12} deficiency.
    2. Infections, inflammation, and neoplasms.
    3. Traumatic injuries and folate deficiency.
    4. Excessive menstrual flow, trauma, and heredity.

33. The adult-gerontology primary care NP understands that most adult patients with Hodgkin lymphoma present with:
    1. Nausea, vomiting, and diarrhea.
    2. Night sweats, weight loss, and fever.
    3. Painless, movable mass in the neck, axilla, or groin.
    4. Hepatosplenomegaly with a painful mass in the mediastinum.

34. What is the most common leukemia found in the older adult, typically asymptomatic and characterized by median survival of about 10 years?
    1. Acute myelogenous.
    2. Chronic myelogenous.
    3. Acute lymphocytic.
    4. Chronic lymphocytic.

35. A female patient tells the adult-gerontology primary care NP they have a diagnosis of hemophilia A. What is the adult-gerontology primary care NP's understanding of the condition?
    1. Her mother was a carrier for the disease and her father had the disease.
    2. Both mother and father have the disease.
    3. Her mother was a carrier.
    4. Both grandparents were carriers of the disease.

36. Folic acid deficiency most often results from:
    1. Lead exposure.
    2. Poor dietary habits.
    3. Gastrointestinal bleeding.
    4. Genetic defect.

Pharmacology

37. A 65-year-old female is being discharged after a successful hip replacement. What is the minimum duration of therapy the adult-gerontology primary care NP would expect for postoperative DVT thromboprophylaxis with rivaroxaban (Xarelto)?
    1. 3–5 days.
    2. 5–7 days.
    3. 10–14 days.
    4. 14–21 days.

38. The adult-gerontology primary care NP determines that an adult male patient has an iron deficiency anemia and has ruled out gastrointestinal (GI) bleeding as the cause. The adult-gerontology primary care NP:
    1. Refers the patient to a hematologist.
    2. Orders iron dextran 50 mg IM weekly for 4 weeks and schedules the patient for weekly office visits for the injection.
    3. Prescribes ferrous sulfate 325 mg PO tid and schedules the patient to return in 1 month for a repeat CBC, serum iron, and TIBC.
    4. Schedules the patient to return in 6 months for additional stool guaiac testing.

39. A 56-year-old female patient requires emergent surgery. The patient has a history of atrial fibrillation and takes warfarin. Lab results reveal a PT/INR ratio of 2.7. The adult-gerontology primary care NP would expect to administer which of the following?

1. Tranexamic acid.
2. Vitamin K.
3. Fresh frozen plasma.
4. Vitamin K and fresh frozen plasma.

40. What information would the adult-gerontology primary care NP include in teaching a patient about the treatment of vitamin B_{12} deficiency following a total gastrectomy?
    1. The patient will be taking vitamin B_{12} tablets twice daily for 1 year.
    2. The patient will be taking oral folic acid supplements daily for life.
    3. The patient will receive monthly cyanocobalamin (vitamin B_{12}) injections for life (after being given daily weekly injections for the first month).
    4. The patient will require iron supplementation and monthly blood transfusions until the deficiency is corrected.

41. A 76-year-old female has been prescribed ciprofloxacin specifically due to bacterial susceptibility. She currently takes warfarin and has maintained therapeutic levels for the past 5 years. Her most recent INR was 2.3. The adult-gerontology primary care NP would expect to do which of the following?
    1. Bridge to heparin.
    2. Check INR within 1 week.
    3. Withhold warfarin.
    4. Increase warfarin dosage.

42. Treatment of anemia of chronic disease should include:
    1. Folic acid supplement 1 mg PO qd.
    2. Iron sulfate ($FeSO_4$) supplement 300 mg PO tid.
    3. Treatment of the underlying condition.
    4. Weekly epoetin alfa (Epogen) injections.

43. Which of the following would most likely need to be given to a patient with sickle cell anemia?
    1. Cyanocobalamin.
    2. Niacin.
    3. Thiamine.
    4. Folate.

44. The adult-gerontology primary care NP has prescribed elemental iron 6 mg/kg/day in three divided doses for a toddler diagnosed with iron-deficiency anemia. What instructions would the adult-gerontology primary care NP include for the parents?
    1. Give the iron with food to increase the absorption of the medication.
    2. Give the medication through a straw to decrease the staining of the teeth.
    3. Avoid foods containing ascorbic acid, which decreases absorption of the medication.
    4. If a dose is missed, double up on the next two doses.

45. The adult-gerontology primary care NP orders an oral iron supplement for an adult patient and is teaching the patient about foods to avoid that inhibit the absorption of iron. Which of the following four food items inhibit the absorption of iron?
    1. Eggs.
    2. Orange juice.
    3. Red meat.
    4. Soy protein.
    5. Milk.
    6. Coffee.

46. After initiating vitamin B_{12} therapy, the adult-gerontology primary care NP would expect which of the following at a 4-week follow-up visit to the clinic?
    1. Ferritin level of 40 ng/mL.
    2. Reduced RBCs, WBCs, and platelets.
    3. Increased macrocytosis and anisocytosis.
    4. Increased hemoglobin/hematocrit and reticulocyte count.

47. It is recommended to administer a 0.5 mL (25 mg) test dose of which medication?
    1. Nascobol (intranasal B_{12} gel).
    2. Folic acid.
    3. Iron dextran (INFeD).
    4. Ferrous sulfate (Feosol).

13 | Hematology Answers & Rationales

Physical Exam & Diagnostic Tests

1. Answer: 3

Rationale: Iron deficiency anemia is a hypochromic, microcytic anemia. Decreased iron stores (serum ferritin) are the hallmark of iron deficiency anemia along with increased transferrin. The liver compensates by increasing production of transferrin, which also increases total iron binding capacity (TIBC). Since iron stores are depleted, the percent of transferrin saturated with iron (% transferrin saturation) is decreased. Normal to increased iron stores (serum ferritin) with concurrent low-serum iron is the hallmark finding of anemia of chronic disease. Serum iron is decreased along with TIBC. Decreased iron, increased TIBC, and decreased serum ferritin contains the findings for iron-deficiency anemia.

2. Answer: 2

Rationale: A Virchow node in the left supraclavicular region is of concern because of the high correlation with abdominal or thoracic malignancy. Infections and inflammatory conditions produce tender, inflamed lymph nodes.

3. Answer: 3

Rationale: The serum ferritin correlates with total body iron stores because it is the major iron storage protein. Its value is reduced in iron-deficiency anemia. Direct Coombs measures in vivo red blood cell (RBC) coating by immunoglobulins and is positive in autoimmune hemolytic anemia, blood transfusion reactions, and drug-induced hemolysis. Serum folate measures the folic acid level in the blood.

4. Answer: 2

Rationale: "Shotty," or small and pellet-like, lymph nodes that are movable, cool, nontender, discrete, and less than 1 cm in diameter are usually considered normal and often represent enlargement of the lymph nodes following a viral infection. They feel like BBs or buckshot under the skin that move under the examiner's fingers when palpated. If shotty nodes are found in the epitrochlear or supraclavicular regions, they require additional evaluation. A fixed, or nonmovable, lymph node is cause for concern.

5. Answer: 4

Rationale: It is important to determine the type of macrocytic anemia so that the appropriate therapy can be ordered. Therefore, the vitamin B_{12} and RBC/folate levels would be ordered. These tests would determine whether the patient has a pernicious anemia (the most common type) or a folate deficiency (also common in older adult patients). Serum iron and total iron-binding capacity (TIBC) would be ordered if an iron-deficiency anemia was suspected (not in this case because this is a microcytic anemia). There is no indication for a colonoscopy. It would be premature to order a bone marrow biopsy without performing initial testing and potentially overlooking an easily treated condition (e.g., pernicious anemia, folate-deficiency anemia). Measurement of certain metabolites of vitamin B_{12}, methylmalonic acid and homocysteine, provide additional information to help identify the cause of the anemia.

6. Answer: 1

Rationale: Disseminated intravascular coagulation (DIC) is a complication of infection, malignancy, blood transfusions, liver disease, complications of pregnancy, and sometimes trauma. DIC is the inappropriate accelerated systemic activation of the coagulation cascade, resulting in simultaneous hemorrhage and thrombosis. Laboratory results would show increased PT and decreased platelet count and fibrinogen in response to the hemorrhage and clotting.

7. Answer: 1

Rationale: Young adolescents often have generalized lymphadenopathy in response to mild infections of the skin or respiratory tract. Palpable lymph nodes are generally not present in healthy individuals, but some may have small, discrete, nontender nodes that are not clinically significant. Enlarged lymph nodes may indicate infection, inflammation, and malignancy in both young adolescents and adults. Tender lymph nodes are noted with inflammatory processes. Hard, fixed, and painless lymph nodes may indicate a malignant process. A painless, firm supraclavicular or cervical lymph node is a common sign of Hodgkin disease in a young adolescent, not Burkitt lymphoma, in which the young adolescent has other associated symptoms depending on the system affected.

8. Answer: 1

Rationale: Stool guaiac testing would identify blood loss from the gastrointestinal tract—the most common cause of iron-deficiency anemia, along with menorrhagia in females. The other tests should be done if the stool guaiac results are positive. Finding the cause of the iron deficiency is paramount, and the stool guaiac test is an easy, noninvasive method of ruling out gastrointestinal bleeding as the cause.

9. Answer: 2

Rationale: The anti-intrinsic factor (anti-IF) or antiparietal cell antibody assay test is the currently accepted method to verify the diagnosis of pernicious anemia. The presence of anti-IF antibodies is highly specific for pernicious anemia. In the past, the Schilling test was used to determine the cause of the vitamin B_{12} deficiency. In pernicious anemia, it will be important to distinguish between inadequate intake (an intrinsic-factor deficiency) or a malabsorption problem. This will allow the practitioner to prescribe the most appropriate therapy for the patient. A bone marrow biopsy and an upper GI series are not indicated at this time.

10. Answer: 3

Rationale: Normal and abnormal hemoglobin can be detected by electrophoresis, which matches hemolyzed RBC material against standard bands for the various known hemoglobins, including hemoglobin S, the abnormal hemoglobin associated with sickle cell anemia. A CBC with peripheral smear and hemoglobin/hematocrit would not yield enough information to diagnose sickle cell anemia. Low hemoglobin, normal to increased MCV, increased MCHC, chronic reticulocytosis, mild-to-moderate anisocytosis, and poikilocytosis with numerous sickle cells and Howell-Jolly bodies would be noted on the CBC and differential. A bone marrow biopsy would not be necessary and would not indicate the presence of hemoglobin S.

11. Answer: 4

Rationale: This patient's clinical picture is a classic presentation for anemia. Further testing is needed to determine the type of anemia involved. The most common cause in older adult men is GI bleeding, which would cause an iron-deficiency anemia. The tests that were ordered would confirm or rule out this diagnosis. The peripheral smear is especially important in diagnosing the specific type of anemia, for example, hypochromic and microcytic. TIBC would be increased, serum ferritin and serum iron are decreased. If the smear ruled out the diagnosis of iron-deficiency anemia, it would lead the practitioner to other diagnoses (including the remaining choices) and the appropriate laboratory tests required for confirmation.

12. Answer: 2

Rationale: Normal to increased iron stores (serum ferritin) with concurrent low-serum iron is the hallmark finding of anemia of chronic disease. Serum iron is decreased along with total iron-binding capacity (TIBC). Decreased iron, increased TIBC, and decreased serum ferritin contains the findings for iron-deficiency anemia.

13. Answer: 3

Rationale: Malaria prophylaxis and treatment includes medications that are high risk of causing hemolytic anemia in patients with X-linked glucose-6-phosphate dehydrogenase (G6PD) deficiency. Patients who require primaquine for malaria prophylaxis must be screened for G6PD deficiency prior to administration. Excessive oxidative stress on RBC counts by medications such as primaquine, dapsone, and sulfa may induce hemolytic anemia.

14. Answer: 2

Rationale: The patient is at higher risk if initial WBC count >50,000 cells/mm³. Liver function studies and uric acid levels are increased. Approximately 75% of patients have marked thrombocytopenia with platelets <100,000 cells/mm³. Prognosis is poor for children <2 years and >10 years of age. The most likely diagnosis in children is acute lymphocytic leukemia (ALL). For adults, the most likely diagnosis is chronic lymphocytic leukemia (CLL), with the second most common type being acute myelogenous leukemia (AML).

15. Answer: 1

Rationale: The findings associated with iron-deficiency anemia include low mean corpuscular volume (MCV), decreased hemoglobin/hematocrit, and low reticulocyte count. Elevated MCV is associated with macrocytic anemias (e.g., pernicious anemia).

Disorders

16. Answer: 2

Rationale: Chronic leukocytic leukemia (CLL) is the most common leukemia in older adults caused by proliferation of immature lymphocytes. Patients with CLL can have variable clinical presentations including constitutional "B" symptoms, including night sweats, unintentional weight loss, and severe fatigue. Patients typically have painless lymphadenopathy and abnormal lab analysis with lymphocytosis, although neutropenia, anemia, and thrombocytopenia can be observed.

17. Answer: 2

Rationale: Sickle cell anemia is a genetic disorder characterized by the production of hemoglobin S, an anemia secondary to shortened erythrocyte survival, microvascular occlusion by sickle-shaped erythrocytes, and increased susceptibility to certain infections. Exposure to ionizing radiation has been associated with the development of certain malignancies, especially leukemia. A deficiency of dietary folic acid does not cause sickle cell anemia, although folic acid is used in the treatment of these patients to help increase hematopoiesis and aid in recovery from aplastic events. Long-term use of thiazide diuretics has been implicated in the development of hemolytic or aplastic anemias in rare cases.

18. Answer: 2

Rationale: Erythrocytosis (or polycythemia) can be worsened by dehydration from any cause, for example, vomiting and diarrhea. Coughing and dizziness will have no effect on the condition, and a laceration may actually improve the symptoms because of the blood loss.

19. Answer: 3

Rationale: Patients who abuse alcohol often develop macrocytosis (MCV >100 fL). Specifically, alcoholic patients often develop macrocytic anemia due to folate (vitamin B_9) and cyanocobalamin (vitamin B_{12}) deficiencies. Folate deficiency manifests within a few months due to relatively lower stores in the liver compared to cyanocobalamin. Additionally, older adults are at a higher risk for development of folate and cyanocobalamin deficiency related to food malabsorption.

20. Answer: 1

Rationale: Green leafy vegetables, oranges and orange juice, and nuts are excellent sources of folic acid. Also, cereals and breads are now fortified with folic acid. Be sure to stress that folate is heat labile and rapidly destroyed by prolonged cooking or food processing. The other foods are not significant sources of folic acid.

21. Answer: 1, 3, 4

Rationale: Myelodysplastic syndromes (MDSs) are a heterogeneous group of bone marrow disorders characterized by symptoms related to bone marrow failure and/or specific symptoms related to cytopenias (anemia, thrombocytopenia, neutropenia, etc.) that affects primarily older adults (age >65 years). MDS is not one disease but a diverse series of hematologic conditions that have variable clinical presentation. Immunosuppressive drug therapy is used for patients with MDS, with the primary goal of therapy being to improve quality of life. Patients often receive numerous red blood cell transfusions. When patients have received more than 20 red blood cell transfusions, patients become iron overloaded. With these patients, iron chelation becomes a consideration, because iron overload may contribute to both increased mortality and morbidity in early-stage MDS.

22. Answer: 4

Rationale: A macrocytic (MCV >100 fL), normochromic anemia resulting from atrophic gastric mucosa not secreting intrinsic factor is the definition of pernicious anemia. These indices could also include folic acid–deficiency anemia. Microcytic, normochromic, or hypochromic could include iron-deficiency anemia or anemia of chronic disease. Normocytic and normochromic could also include anemia of chronic disease.

23. Answer: 2

Rationale: Acute hemolytic transfusion reactions (AHTR) most often occur within the first 24 hours of blood product administration. The most common cause is due to clerical errors causing ABO incompatibility. Due to the serious risk of mortality associated with AHTR special attention to proper procedure, documentation, and communication should be observed.

24. Answer: 2

Rationale: Thalassemias are chronic, inherited anemias characterized by defective hemoglobin synthesis leading to a decreased RBC count, hypochromia (MCH <20 pg), microcytosis (MCV <70 fL), normal serum iron, and normal RBC distribution width (RDW) in thalassemia minor, which does not require pharmacologic treatment. This should be noted that although the RDW is usually normal, it can be elevated in about 50% of patients with thalassemia trait, which is in contrast to iron-deficiency anemia, where the RDW is almost always elevated (90%). Patients with thalassemia minor should not be given iron supplements to resolve anemia. Patients with thalassemia major are usually managed by a hematologist.

25. Answer: 4

Rationale. Tumor lysis syndrome occurs when a patient has a high WBC and is undergoing cytotoxic chemotherapy for the treatment of AML. It is characterized by the development of acute hyperuricemia, hyperkalemia, hyperphosphatemia, and hypocalcemia, with or without acute renal failure. It is the most common of all the oncologic emergencies. Other complications include leukostasis, DIC, and pancytopenia. Although AML is most often associated with DIC, it is characterized by a decreased platelet count, a prolonged prothrombin and partial thromboplastin time, and a decreased fibrinogen level with an elevation of fibrin degradation products. Leukostasis, blood sludging or stasis, occurs when the blood vessels become overcrowded with immature blast cells in patients with AML who have high WBC counts, which can lead to ischemia and infarcts in the pulmonary and cranial blood vessels. Pancytopenia is a drastic reduction in all types of blood cells (WBC, RBC, platelets) that can occur due to myelosuppression from cytotoxic chemotherapy.

26. Answer: 3

Rationale: Iron-deficiency anemia is a microcytic, hypochromic anemia. The RBCs are smaller (microcytic) because of the decrease in hemoglobin production caused by inadequate amounts of iron, which also makes the cell appear pale (hypochromic). The other selections describe other types of anemia, which would be determined by the peripheral smear.

27. Answer: 1

Rationale: Vitamin B$_{12}$ deficiency may result in neurologic signs and symptoms, including peripheral neuropathy, paresthesias, unsteady gait (ataxia), loss of proprioception, decreased vibratory sensation, lethargy, and fatigue. In the later stages of severe B$_{12}$ deficiency, spasticity, hyperactive reflexes, and presence of Romberg sign is noted because of the formation of a demyelinating lesion of the neurons of the spinal cord and cerebral cortex and presence of a beefy-red tongue. These findings are specific to pernicious anemia and must be assessed in all patients who present with anemia. The other signs and symptoms are not characteristic of pernicious anemia.

28. Answer: 1

Rationale: Anemia of chronic disease is a chronic normochromic, normocytic, and hypoproliferative anemia. There is normal production of hemoglobin, along with normal maturation of RBCs. The serum iron is low, ferritin level and TIBC elevated.

29. Answer: 2

Rationale: Lymphadenopathy as described, without evidence of infection, should always be referred to a surgeon for biopsy, the only definitive test to rule out a malignancy (a frequent cause of lymphadenopathy not caused by infectious processes). No signs or symptoms suggest the need for a throat culture, monospot test, or chest x-ray. Not intervening is inappropriate because the cause of lymphadenopathy needs to be determined.

30. Answer: 3

Rationale: This constellation of symptoms (fever, night sweats, and weight loss) is used in the staging of non-Hodgkin lymphoma (NHL), the presence of which is considered to be a poor prognostic indicator. The other symptoms may occur depending on the amount of disease involvement, but they are not considered "B" symptoms, also known as constitutional symptoms.

31. Answer: 4

Rationale: Beef, spinach, and peanut butter are iron-rich foods. The other options are examples of foods rich in calcium, fiber, and vitamin C, respectively.

32. Answer: 2

Rationale: Anemia or chronic disease is associated with infections (e.g., tuberculosis), chronic inflammatory conditions (e.g., systemic lupus erythematosus; rheumatoid arthritis), and malignancies. Excessive blood loss from menstrual flow or traumatic injuries would more likely cause an iron-deficiency anemia. Malnutrition can contribute to iron, vitamin B$_{12}$, and folate deficiencies.

33. Answer: 3

Rationale: Most patients with Hodgkin lymphoma present with a painless, movable mass in the neck, axilla, or groin. Constitutional symptoms may also occur, which include weight loss, persistent fever, and night sweats. Often the patient may experience pruritus and pain in the lymph node area after consuming alcohol (an unexplained finding). Hepatosplenomegaly presents with advanced disease.

34. Answer: 4

Rationale: Chronic lymphocytic leukemia (CLL) is found primarily in middle-aged and older adults (<10% of patients under age 50). Median age of diagnosis of CLL is 70 years, affecting more males than females. Acute myelogenous leukemia (AML) incidence increases with age with median age greater than 70 years. Chronic myelogenous leukemia (CML) occurs between 50 and 60 years. Acute lymphocytic leukemia (ALL) is most common in children and gradually increases in frequency in later life with the median age of 35–40 years.

35. Answer: 1

Rationale: Hemophilia A is characterized by a deficiency of factor VIII and is due to an X-linked chromosome recessive inheritance disorder. This means that males are almost exclusively affected with hemophilia and females are carriers. When a female has hemophilia, they are the offspring of a father with hemophilia and a mother who is a carrier. In the past, this rarely occurred because males with hemophilia rarely lived to adult reproductive age. Now with the availability of replacement factor VIII, male patients with hemophilia can live to reproductive age.

36. Answer: 2

Rationale: Folic acid deficiency most often results from dietary deficits and frequently affects the older adult, chronically ill, alcoholic patients, and food faddists (poor food selections). Pregnancy requires an increase in folic acid, as do disease states such as cancer, chronic inflammation, Crohn disease, rheumatoid arthritis, and malabsorption syndromes.

Pharmacology

37. Answer: 3

Rationale: The anticoagulant rivaroxaban (Xarelto) is a factor Xa inhibitor and is recommended for postoperative DVT thromboprophylaxis in hip and knee replacements. It should be started immediately after homeostasis has been achieved postoperatively for a minimum of 10–14 days. Therapy in some patients may be extended up to 35 days.

38. Answer: 3

Rationale: Treatment with iron orally for at least 6 months is necessary to correct both the anemia and the depleted body iron stores. Ferrous sulfate should be taken on an empty stomach 1 hour before meals. If the patient experiences GI symptoms, the dose can be reduced or the patient can take the iron with the meal; however, taking it with meals will reduce the delivery and absorption of the iron by 50%. Iron dextran (parenteral) may be used if the patient is unable to take PO medications or if the hemoglobin is less than 6 g/dL. The patient should have hemoglobin/hematocrit, iron, and total iron-binding capacity (TIBC) rechecked after 1 month on iron supplementation. If there is no improvement in all parameters, most notably a rise in the hemoglobin by 1 g/dL, the patient should be referred to a hematologist. Referral to a GI specialist or repeat of stool guaiac testing is unnecessary because there is no indication that this patient's condition is caused by bleeding.

39. Answer: 4

Rationale: Therapeutic levels of warfarin should be monitored with PT/INR. The goal of therapy should be between 2.0 and 3.0. Due to the half-life of warfarin (24–60 hours) patients undergoing elective procedures should stop taking warfarin a minimum of 5 days prior to surgery. Geriatric patients may often require additional 1–2 days to metabolize warfarin and normalize PT/INR levels. For more urgent correction monotherapy with vitamin K may be used but often requires 1–2 days. For immediate reversal of warfarin therapy both vitamin K along with fresh frozen plasma should be administered.

40. Answer: 3

Rationale: If the deficiency is not caused by inadequate intake, the patient will require lifetime supplementation of vitamin B_{12} (1000 μg of cyanocobalamin) by intramuscular injection to ensure absorption. In patients with irreversible malabsorption (total gastrectomy) and severe neurologic symptoms, parenteral therapy is indicated: 1000 μg/day for 7 days, and then 1000 μg weekly for 4 weeks, followed by 1000 μg monthly for life. The adult-gerontology primary care NP should keep in mind that high-dose, daily oral cyanocobalamin (1000–2000 μg) are as effective as monthly intramuscular injection and is the preferred route of initial therapy in most circumstances because it is cost-effective and convenient. Oral folic acid, iron, and blood transfusions would not treat the cause of the deficiency, and, therefore, the resulting anemia would not be corrected.

41. Answer: 2

Rationale: Warfarin is commonly affected by many medications including ciprofloxacin. PT/INR levels should be checked within 1 week of administration of ciprofloxacin due to the possibility for increased effects of warfarin.

42. Answer: 3

Rationale: Treatment of the underlying condition leads to resolution of the anemia of chronic disease. Folic acid and iron supplements are indicated for folate and iron-deficiency anemias, respectively. Epoetin alfa injections are indicated for conditions that affect erythropoiesis, including chronic renal failure, chemotherapy-induced anemia, and acquired immunodeficiency syndrome (AIDS). Patients with underlying iron-deficiency anemia and anemia of chronic disease may benefit from a trial of iron therapy.

43. Answer: 4

Rationale: Due to increased RBC turnover, folate supplementation is often required in patients with sickle cell anemia due to relatively low stores of the vitamin in the liver. Other supplementations may be indicated if dietary intake is insufficient but are given without iron. Deferoxamine or other iron chelators may be required in these patients due to a build-up of iron related to transfusions.

44. Answer: 2

Rationale: Iron medications can cause staining of the teeth, so it is a good practice to give the medication through a straw. It is best to give iron on an empty stomach (if tolerable) to increase absorption. Ascorbic acid increases absorption of iron. If a dose is missed, it is best to give the dose when it is remembered as long as it is not too close to the next dose. The next two doses would not be increased.

45. Answer: 1, 4, 5, 6

Rationale: The following foods inhibit the absorption of iron: soy protein, eggs, bran, dairy products, tea, and coffee. Foods that enhance the absorption of iron include those that are rich in ascorbic acid (vitamin C), citric acid, red meat, and leafy green vegetables.

46. Answer: 4

Rationale: In addition to a sense of well-being, improved appetite, and decreased neurologic symptoms (gait disturbances, peripheral neuropathy, paresthesias (numbness/tingling in fingers), and extreme weakness), the hemoglobin/hematocrit and reticulocyte count should increase with vitamin B_{12} therapy.

47. Answer: 3

Rationale: The use of IM or IV iron dextran (INFeD) is for patients who cannot tolerate oral supplementation or who have GI disease that limits oral absorption. Therapy should be initiated with an IV test dose of 0.5 mL (25 mg) to observe for anaphylaxis. It should be administered gradually over at least 30 seconds.

Urinary

14

Physical Examination & Diagnostic Tests

1. A basic urogenital evaluation in the older adult with complaints of new onset incontinence should include:
   1. History, physical exam, postvoid residual, and urinalysis (UA).
   2. Postvoid residual, blood urea nitrogen (BUN), serum creatinine, and UA.
   3. History, physical exam, serum glucose, BUN, serum creatinine, and UA.
   4. Urodynamic/endoscopic/imaging tests, UA, and serum creatinine.

2. Differential diagnoses for a patient presenting with flank pain and hematuria includes renal calculi, renal cell carcinoma, and hydronephrosis. Which one of the following diagnostic tools would be most useful in diagnosing this patient?
   1. Intravenous urography (IVU).
   2. Voiding cystourethrography.
   3. Intravenous pyelogram (IVP).
   4. Computed tomography (CT) urography.

3. A 39-year-old male bodybuilder is undergoing intense physical training. He tests his own urine using dipstick urinalysis in an attempt to measure his urinary ketones. He presents to the clinic inquiring about a single urinary analysis that indicated mild microscopic hematuria. Dipstick urinalysis today reveals no abnormalities other than ketones. What should the adult-gerontology primary care NP recommend?
   1. Reassurance.
   2. Evaluation for diabetes.
   3. Repeat urinalysis.
   4. Retrograde urethrogram.

4. Which of the following patients would be a good candidate for urodynamic studies (UDS)?
   1. Patient with history of stress incontinence and urge incontinence.
   2. Patient with recent surgery for bladder suspension.
   3. Patient with initial incontinence episode after total knee replacement.
   4. Older adult male with postvoid residual catheterization findings of 45 mL after 250-mL voiding.

5. The adult-gerontology primary care NP is evaluating blood chemistries on a patient who is experiencing an increase in blood pressure (BP). She has no previous history of hypertension or other chronic disease. Which serum laboratory value would be most concerning?
   1. Serum creatinine 4.2 mg/dL.
   2. Blood urea nitrogen (BUN) 30 mg/dL.
   3. Serum potassium 4.5 mEq/L.
   4. Serum osmolarity 290 mOsm/kg.

6. When taking a history on voiding patterns in adults, the adult-gerontology primary care NP should consider:
   1. Adults normally void q2–3h in a 24-hour period (8–12 times a day).
   2. Urge sensation to void occurs when the bladder fills to 200–300 mL.
   3. Normally, 15–20 minutes pass between first urge to void and reaching functional capacity.
   4. Adults typically reach functional (comfortable) capacity at 200–300 mL and normally experience some leakage if voiding is delayed.

7. The adult-gerontology primary care NP expects which findings on exam of an older adult patient with dehydration?
   1. Tongue furrows and skin tenting over the clavicle.
   2. Specific gravity of urine 1.004.
   3. Pulse rate 58 beats/min (strong, regular) and BP 100/62 mm Hg.
   4. Geographic tongue and reduced saliva pool.

8. A 68-year-old female returns for ongoing evaluation of *stress* incontinence that was thought to be associated with chronic urinary tract infections. She has been on low-dose trimethoprim-sulfamethoxazole (TMP-SMX, Bactrim) 40/200 mg for 6 months without resolution of her symptoms. This patient should be evaluated for:
   1. Pelvic organ prolapse.
   2. Dementia or a neuromuscular disorder.
   3. Environmental barriers in the home.
   4. Addition of a tricyclic antidepressant.

Disorders

9. A 65-year-old female explains to the adult-gerontology primary care NP that she has been having frequent and painful urination. A clean-catch urine specimen for routine urinalysis with culture and sensitivity is ordered. Laboratory results show 10^5 CFU/mL of *Escherichia coli* (*E. coli*) and 10^4 CFU/mL of *Staphylococcus epidermidis* (*S. epidermidis*). The adult-gerontology primary care NP's next step would be:
   1. Treat the *E. coli.*
   2. Order amoxicillin.
   3. Treat the *S. epidermidis.*
   4. Encourage citric fruit juices.

10. A young adult comes to the college student health clinic complaining of severe abdominal discomfort and bloody urine. An initial priority in the diagnostic workup would include:
    1. Intravenous pyelography to rule out a kidney stone.
    2. Straining all urine.
    3. Microscopic urine exam.
    4. 24-hour urine culture.

11. An older adult female client who is incontinent is in an extended care facility and is found to have a red and excoriated perianal area on exam. What would the adult-gerontology primary care NP advise the caregiver to avoid using on the skin in the perineal area?
    1. Petrolatum.
    2. Moisture-barrier films.
    3. Mild soap and water.
    4. Zinc oxide ointment.

12. Which plan would be most appropriate for an older patient with functional incontinence?
    1. Evaluate need for incontinence pads.
    2. Limit fluid intake in the evenings.
    3. Perform the Credé maneuver.
    4. Provide a bedside commode.

13. A 60-year-old man presents with recurrent urinary tract infections (UTIs) and low-grade fever. What is the most likely cause?
    1. Balanitis.
    2. Epididymitis.
    3. Chronic bacterial prostatitis.
    4. Benign prostatic hypertrophy.

14. A 78-year-old female returns to the office after a 6-day stay in the hospital for new-onset heart failure. Her chief complaint is urinary incontinence. Which one of the following is a possible cause for her new-onset urinary incontinence?
    1. Poor pelvic support causing hypermobility of the base of the female bladder.
    2. Lower urinary tract problems, such as carcinoma.
    3. Cystocele or uterine prolapse.
    4. Ingestion of certain medications, such as sedatives, diuretics, anticholinergics, and α-adrenergic agents.

15. Which statement characterizes functional incontinence?
    1. Leakage of urine during activities that increase abdominal pressure, such as coughing, sneezing, and laughing.
    2. Mainly caused by factors outside the urinary tract, especially immobility, that prohibit proper toileting habits.
    3. Characterized by the inability to delay urination, with an abrupt and strong desire to void.
    4. Occurrence of incontinence with over distention of bladder.

16. What are the two most common pathogens in community-acquired UTIs?
    1. *Klebsiella pneumoniae.*
    2. *Proteus mirabilis.*
    3. *Staphylococcus saprophyticus.*
    4. *Escherichia coli.*
    5. *Staphylococcus aureus.*
    6. *Streptococcus pyogenes.*

17. A healthy 66-year-old female presents with cystitis. The adult-gerontology primary care NP would expect which of the following findings?
    1. No symptoms noted.
    2. Acute onset of chills, fever, flank pain, headache, malaise, and costovertebral angle tenderness.
    3. Complaints of dysuria, urgency, frequency, nocturia, and suprapubic heaviness.
    4. Signs and symptoms of fever, irritability, decreased appetite, vomiting, diarrhea, constipation, dehydration, and jaundice.

18. Fifteen days after completion of a course of antibiotics for a UTI, a 66-year-old female returns to the clinic with reoccurring symptoms. Recurrent UTIs in women are caused by relapse or reinfection. The adult-gerontology primary care NP understands the following about relapse.
    1. It is less common than reinfection and occurs within 2 weeks of completing drug therapy for the infection.
    2. It is responsible for most recurrent UTIs in women.
    3. May result from residual urine after voiding due to prolapsed uterus or bladder or lack of estrogen.
    4. Can be treated with the same medication regimen used for the original infection.

19. The adult-gerontology primary care NP understands the following about pyelonephritis:
    1. Young adults with severe illness may present with altered mental state and absence of fever.
    2. Patients complain of localized flank/back pain combined with systemic symptoms, such as fever, chills, and nausea.
    3. Requires hospitalization for most cases including parenteral antibiotic therapy.
    4. Requires no follow-up.

20. What is the term given to the type of urinary incontinence associated with conditions such as Parkinson disease or Alzheimer disease?
    1. Stress incontinence.
    2. Urge incontinence.
    3. Functional incontinence.
    4. Overflow incontinence.

21. A 37-year-old male patient presents to the outpatient clinic complaining of anuria for 1 day. He recently had complaints of nausea, diarrhea, abdominal pain, and a low-grade fever for 3 days, which he states started improving yesterday. Physical exam reveals no abnormalities. Lab analysis reveals hemoglobin 10.1 g/dL, hematocrit 26%, and platelets 90,000 mm^3. Urinalysis is unable to be obtained initially. Which of the following should the adult-gerontology primary care NP suspect?
    1. Urinary retention.
    2. Viral syndrome.
    3. Nephrotic syndrome.
    4. Hemolytic uremic syndrome.

22. A 67-year-old white man presents to the clinic with a uric acid renal calculi. Knowing that the alkaline-ash, low-purine diet is difficult for patients to adhere to, which other option should the adult-gerontology primary care NP consider?
    1. Monitor the patient for another episode.
    2. Discuss the alkaline-ash, low-purine diet in detail with the patient.

3. Start the patient on a xanthine oxidase inhibitor and monitor serum uric acid level.
4. Refer the patient to a urologist.

23. A 60-year-old male patient presents with complaints of blood in his urine; he denies dysuria or abdominal pain. The adult-gerontology primary care NP obtains UA to confirm hematuria. There is no evidence of infection. What is the priority diagnosis in the list of differentials?
    1. Cancer of the prostate.
    2. Prerenal failure.
    3. Renal calculi.
    4. Renal cell carcinoma.

24. The adult-gerontology primary care NP is taking the history of a patient who has been diagnosed with renal calculi. What information in the history would include a precipitating factor in the development of renal calculi?
    1. Increased incidence of UTIs over the past 3 years.
    2. Drinking 6–8 ounces of milk daily.
    3. History of fractured femur and prolonged bed rest.
    4. High intake of citrus fruit and high-fiber carbohydrates.

25. An older adult patient is diagnosed with renal failure. Lipid panel is noted to be within normal limits as does the patient's glycosylated hemoglobin. Which one of the following is most likely the cause of his renal failure?
    1. History of MI with severe hypotensive episode.
    2. Advanced prostatic hypertrophy with hematuria.
    3. Renal vascular changes secondary to long history of diabetes.
    4. Exposure to carbon tetrachloride at the job site.

26. An adult-gerontology primary care NP recognizes which factor as contributing to the development of prerenal azotemia?
    1. History of a hypovolemic shock.
    2. Extended treatment of an infection with gentamicin (Garamycin).
    3. Acute pyelonephritis with subsequent glomerulonephritis.
    4. Renal vascular changes secondary to atherosclerotic disease.

27. The adult-gerontology primary care NP teaching a female patient about bladder health would include which three of the following guidelines:
    1. Drink at least six to eight glasses of water per day.
    2. Avoid doing Kegel exercises.
    3. Avoid constipation.
    4. Consider weight loss, if incontinence occurs.
    5. Have at least one cup of coffee or tea daily.

28. Which one of the following objective findings on a 52-year-old male is consistent with a diagnosis of benign prostatic hyperplasia (BPH)?
    1. Elevated PSA.
    2. Gross hematuria.
    3. A nodular firm prostate palpated on digital rectal exam (DRE).
    4. A smooth enlarged prostate palpated on DRE.

29. Which two situations should the adult-gerontology primary care NP refer to a urologist?
    1. Patient with a smooth enlarged prostate palpated on digital rectal exam (DRE).
    2. Patient with a nodular firm prostate palpated on DRE.
    3. If initial treatment for BPH is not effective.
    4. When the patient with BPH develops a UTI.

30. Which three of the following objective findings are characteristics of nephrotic syndrome?
    1. Hematuria.
    2. Peripheral edema.
    3. Proteinuria.
    4. Hypoalbuminemia.
    5. Hypolipidemia.
    6. Decreased coagulation.

31. Early signs of renal damage in patients with diabetes mellitus and hypertension include which two of the following?
    1. Increased BUN.
    2. Increase in serum creatinine.
    3. Presence of proteinuria.
    4. Decrease in GFR.
    5. Hematuria.
    6. Elevated A1C.

32. A 47-year-old female patient complains of frequent urination. Physical exam reveals no abnormalities. She has a history of bipolar disorder controlled with lithium and states she "takes her medications somewhat regularly." Which of the following should the adult-gerontology primary care NP suspect?
    1. Central diabetes insipidus.
    2. Nephrogenic diabetes insipidus.
    3. Diabetes mellitus.
    4. Primary polydipsia.

33. A 75-year-old white female patient presents to the clinic with her husband, her primary caregiver. She has a history of multiinfarct dementia (MID), likely from a long history of untreated hypertension. Her husband reports that for the past 2 days she has been agitated and increasingly confused, and he has not been able to redirect her. He denies the addition of new medications or over-the-counter herbal supple-

ments. What would the adult-gerontology primary care NP suspect?
    1. New infarct.
    2. Worsening of dementia.
    3. Urinary tract infection.
    4. Underlying stress to caregiver.

Pharmacology

34. A 69-year-old male patient with renal failure receives dialysis once per week. Results from his most recent lab results include phosphorus 6.6 mg/dL, potassium 5.0 mEq/L, and sodium 133 mEq/L. Which of the following medications should be administered to control the imbalance?
    1. Insulin.
    2. Sevalamer (Renagel).
    3. Magnesium citrate.
    4. Sodium bicarbonate.

35. A patient is diagnosed with benign prostatic hypertrophy. Which medication should be recognized by the adult-gerontology primary care NP as likely to aggravate this condition?
    1. Glyburide (DiaBeta).
    2. Oral buspirone (Buspar).
    3. Inhaled ipratropium (Atrovent).
    4. Ophthalmic timolol (Timoptic).

36. A 67-year-old female patient presents with weakness. Available lab results include: leukocytes 5200/mm³, hemoglobin of 7.6 g/dL, and hematocrit of 22.7%. She has a history of nondialysis dependent chronic kidney disease (CKD). Which of the following medications would the adult-gerontology primary care NP expect to be administered?
    1. Epoetin alfa (Procrit).
    2. Filgrastim (Neupogen).
    3. Sargramostim (Prokine).
    4. Sevelamer (Renvela).

37. A 69-year-old female patient reports worsening stress incontinence. Which one of the following agents would be useful in treating her symptoms?
    1. Propantheline (Pro-Banthine) 15 mg before meals; 30 mg at bedtime.
    2. Oxybutynin 2.5 mg three to four times a day.
    3. Doxepin (Sinequan) 10–25 mg once a day initially to maximum total daily dose of 25–100 mg.
    4. Conjugated estrogen (Premarin) 0.3–1.25 mg/day orally or vaginally and medroxyprogesterone (progestin) 2.5–10 mg/day continuously or intermittently.

38. A 56-year-old female patient presents to the outpatient health clinic with complaints of urgency and vaginal pruritis. A urinalysis reveals 100,000 CFU/mL gram-negative rods. The patient history includes no prior urinary tract infections, but that she has multiple allergies including sulfa and penicillin medications. Which of the following three medications would be best indicated for this patient?
    1. Nitrofurantoin (Marcrodantin) 100 mg PO once.
    2. Nitrofurantoin (Macrodantin) 100 mg PO bid for 5 days.
    3. Trimethoprim/sulfamethoxazole (TMP/SMZ) 160/800 mg PO daily for 3 days.
    4. Trimethoprim/sulfamethoxazole (TMP/SMZ) 160/800 mg PO daily for 7 days.
    5. Ciprofloxacin (Cipro) 500 mg PO bid for 7 days.
    6. Fosfomycin (Monurol) 3000 mg PO once.

39. To decrease the production of uric acid stones, the adult-gerontology primary care NP orders which medication?
    1. Allopurinol (Zyloprim).
    2. Indomethacin (Indocin).
    3. Bethanechol (Urecholine).
    4. Colchicine (Colcrys).

40. A 70-year-old woman is treated with oxybutynin for her urinary frequency and urgency. The NP would explain to the patient she will probably experience:
    1. Increased sensitivity to sunlight.
    2. Dizziness on standing.
    3. Dry mouth and increased thirst.
    4. Increased bruising.

41. An older adult male in an assisted living facility begins to experience urinary incontinence. The adult-gerontology primary care NP is reviewing his medication list and finds that the following three medications may be responsible for this new onset:
    1. Temazepam (Restoril) 30 mg PO at bedtime.
    2. Nitrofurantoin (Macrodantin) 150 mg PO at bed-time.
    3. Diazepam (Valium) 5 mg PO prior to MRI.
    4. Polyethylene glycol 3350 (MiraLax) 1 capful in water or juice daily as needed.
    5. Amitriptyline (Elavil) 75 mg PO at bedtime for postherpetic neuralgia.
    6. Tramadol (Ultram) 50 mg PO every 8 hours as needed for pain.

42. The adult-gerontology primary care NP has selected low dose trimethoprim-sulfamethoxazole (TMP-SMZ) for treatment of chronic UTI in an adult female patient. Which two parameters should be evaluated before administration of TMP-SMZ?
    1. Creatinine clearance (>50 mL/min).
    2. Levels of serum alanine aminotransferase (ALT).
    3. Current medications that include anticoagulants.
    4. History of allergic reactions to sulfa-based medications.
    5. Serum BUN.

43. A patient with recurrent calcium oxalate renal calculi can be treated with which of the following medications to aid in the prevention of stone formation?
    1. Triamterene (Dyrenium).
    2. Furosemide (Lasix).
    3. Hydrochlorothiazide (HCTZ).
    4. Acetazolamide (Diamox).

44. A 66-year-old man with a history of renal calculi presents with complaints of severe flank pain radiating to his groin area. He is also experiencing nausea and vomiting, and his temperature is 99°F (37.2°C). What is the best initial therapy that the adult-gerontology primary care NP can provide?
    1. Ketorolac 30 mg IM.
    2. Ibuprofen (Advil) 600 mg PO q6h.
    3. Increase fluid intake and strain all urine.
    4. Trimethobenzamide (Tigan) 250 mg PO.

45. The adult-gerontology primary care NP is prescribing nitrofurantoin (Macrodantin) for a young woman who is experiencing problems with UTIs. What specific directions should be given to the patient regarding administration of nitrofurantoin?
    1. Take with food and expect brownish discoloration of urine.
    2. Do not take with milk products; take on empty stomach for better absorption.
    3. Take four times a day until symptoms have subsided for at least 24 hours.
    4. Do not take acetaminophen (Tylenol) or ibuprofen (Advil) with nitrofurantoin.

46. An adult woman presents with complaints of burning on urination, frequency, and urgency. Phenazopyridine (Pyridium) is prescribed. What specific directions should the adult-gerontology primary care NP provide for the patient regarding phenazopyridine?
    1. May discolor contact lenses; if sclerae begin to turn yellow, return to the office.
    2. Always take on an empty stomach to increase absorption.
    3. Do not take any medication containing aspirin or salicylate.
    4. May interfere with effectiveness of mini-pill for birth control.

47. The adult-gerontology primary care NP is reviewing lab results from several patients during inpatient service. Upon review of a urinalysis of a 67-year-old male it is discovered that muddy brown granular casts are present. The adult-gerontology primary care NP would be most concerned about which of the following medications that can lead to this?
    1. Furosemide (Lasix).
    2. Amphotericin (Ambisome).
    3. Gentamicin (Garamycin).
    4. Ibuprofen (Motrin).

48. A 64 year-old-male is being evaluated for severe protein-uria. Which of the following three medications would the NP suspect as the most likely causative agent(s) for nephrotic syndrome?
    1. NSAIDs.
    2. Losartan (Cozaar).
    3. Captopril (Capoten).
    4. Penicillamine (Cuprimine).
    5. Vancomycin (Vancocin).

49. When prescribing oxybutynin for the patient with stress incontinence symptoms, which disorder in the patient's medical history must the adult-gerontology primary care NP consider before prescribing?
    1. Diabetes.
    2. Cough.
    3. Narrow-angle glaucoma.
    4. Gallstones.

50. A 65-year-old female patient visits the clinic for urinary incontinence. She complains that she has been frequently losing small volumes of urine with no urge for micturi-tion. She also confirms nocturnal wetting. She has a his-tory of uncontrolled diabetes and peripheral neuropathy. Which of the following medications would the NP select for this patient's symptoms?
    1. Bethanechol (Urecholine).
    2. Atropine.
    3. Hyoscyamine (Levsin).

4. Mirtazapine (Remeron).
5. Dicyclomine (Bentyl).

51. A patient with no history of allergies presents with an uncomplicated urinary tract infection. When considering fluoroquinolones for the treatment, the adult-gerontology primary care NP correctly understands that:
    1. A fluoroquinolone, such as ciprofloxacin, is the drug of choice for urinary tract infections.
    2. Fluoroquinolones are preferable to both nitrofuran-toin and trimethoprim/sulfamethoxazole due to high levels of antibiotic resistance.
    3. Fluoroquinolones are considered safe in pregnancy.
    4. Fluoroquinolones should be used cautiously due to potential serious side effects.

52. Angiotensin-converting enzyme (ACE) inhibitors are rec-ommended for slowing the progression of chronic renal disease, but are contraindicated in the following disorder:
    1. Cardiovascular disease.
    2. Hypertension.
    3. Diabetes.
    4. Renal artery stenosis.

53. A frail older adult female presents for annual physical exam. Her comprehensive metabolic panel (CMP) re-veals a GFR of 38; previous year her GFR was 64. Which one of the following medications should be eliminated from her profile?
    1. Ibuprofen (Motrin).
    2. Levothyroxine (Synthroid).
    3. Metoprolol tartrate (Lopressor).
    4. Clopidogrel (Plavix).

54. A 72-year-old male patient is scheduled for an angiogram. His list of medications is as follows. Which should the adult-gerontology primary care NP be concerned about?
    1. Glyburide (DiaBeta).
    2. Metformin (Glucophage).
    3. Captopril (Capoten).
    4. Temazepam (Restoril).

14 | Urinary Answers & Rationales

Physical Exam & Diagnostic Tests

1. Answer: 1

   Rationale: A basic evaluation of urinary incontinence should include a history and physical; there are systemic reasons for incontinence, which include neurological, gastrointestinal, as well as genitourinary/reproductive organ impairments. Measurement of postvoid residual either by pelvic ultrasound (bladder scan) or catheterization is done to determine retention and potential overflow incontinence. Urinalysis (UA) may indicate urinary tract infection as the cause of incontinence. The other tests may be performed based on the findings from the initial evaluation including 3-incontinence questionnaire (3IQ) and voiding diaries.

2. Answer: 4

   Rationale: Computed tomography (CT) urography has become the most useful diagnostic tool in different urinary tract abnormalities, such as complex congenital anomalies, trauma, infection, and tumors. The use of CT urography in different anomalies including vascular, parenchymal, and urothelial evaluation has a great impact in management of patients. CT urography has many disadvantages over intravenous urography (IVU), including its high cost and the higher radiation dose, but it is more effective than IVU at visualizing the structures of the kidney.

3. Answer: 1

   Rationale: Transient microscopic hematuria on dipstick analysis is a common finding and does not warrant further investigation unless significant risk factors are present. False positive results on urinary dipstick analysis are commonly caused by exercise, contaminated samples, or menstruation. Significant or nontransient hematuria would warrant lab microscopic urinalysis for evaluation of myoglobinuria and other disorders.

4. Answer: 1

   Rationale: The optimal patients for urodynamic studies (UDS) include those who have not had prior incontinence surgery or who have clear symptoms of stress or urge incontinence. Urodynamic testing is a group of tests that examine how well the bladder, sphincters, and urethra are storing and releasing urine. Most urodynamic tests focus on the bladder's ability to hold urine and empty steadily and completely. Urodynamic tests can also show whether the bladder is having involuntary contractions that cause urine leakage. Postvoid residual volume may be seen in an older adult male patient.

5. Answer: 1

   Rationale: The primary concern in the patient is the elevated serum creatinine level of 4.2 mg/dL. All the other blood chemistry values are within normal limits. The patient should be referred to a nephrologist immediately because of the elevated creatinine level. The adult-gerontology primary care NP, in addition to completing a history and physical, should order a parathyroid hormone level, liver function tests, lipid and renal panels, CBC, and magnesium/calcium levels. Having these laboratory tests completed will assist the nephrologist in determining the cause of the patient's renal failure. A review of the patient's medications should be initiated to determine whether she is taking any medications that are nephrotoxic including angiotensin-converting enzyme (ACE) inhibitors. Nephrotoxic medications should be discontinued. The patient's family history may be reviewed to rule out familial kidney disorders (e.g., Alport syndrome, polycystic kidney disease).

6. Answer: 2

   Rationale: Adults normally void four to six times in a 24-hour period (q4–6h). Most adults usually do not awaken to void at night unless they have a medical problem (e.g., benign prostatic hypertrophy, urge incontinence, or diuretic therapy). The feeling of the bladder filling occurs at about 90–150 mL, with the first urge sensation at 200–300 mL. Normally, 1–2 hours pass between the first urge to void and reaching functional capacity. Adults typically reach functional (comfortable) capacity at 300–600 mL and should *never* experience leakage if voiding is delayed.

7. Answer: 1

   Rationale: Signs of dehydration in the older adult are skin tenting over the clavicle, concentrated urine (specific gravity >1.025), oliguria, sunken eyes, lack of axillary moisture, orthostatic blood pressure (BP) changes, tachycardia, dry mucous membranes of mouth and nose, and absent or small saliva pool. In the obese older adult patient who has lost weight, tenting of the forehead is not always a reliable clinical sign because of excessive loss of subcutaneous fat. As the older patient becomes dehydrated, aqueous humor of the eye also decreases. Gentle palpation of the eyeball will reveal a boggy versus a firm eyeball, a useful assessment tool in these patients. It is important to examine the mouth because it reveals reliable assessment data in the older adult suspected of dehydration. A geographic tongue (patchy papillary loss that causes a maplike appearance) should not be confused with tongue furrows and tongue coating.

8. Answer: 1

Rationale: Stress incontinence in postmenopausal women is associated with weakness in the pelvic floor that can lead to pelvic organ prolapse; multiparity is a key factor. Dementia is associated with overflow incontinence. Environmental barriers put one at risk for functional incontinence and the addition of tricyclic antidepressants or any hypnotic or sedative can cause retention leading to overflow incontinence.

Disorders

9. Answer: 1

Rationale: *Escherichia coli (E. coli)* is the most common organism causing urinary tract infections (UTIs) in women, and counts of 10^5 CFU/mL are diagnostic. Counts of 10^2–10^3 CFU/mL should be considered positive and indicate treatment when it is *E. coli. E. coli* will likely respond to trimethoprim-sulfamethoxazole (Septra DS) or any suitable, sensitive antiinfective agent, and the patient should also be treated for the UTI. *Staphylococcus epidermidis (S. epidermidis)* is normal skin flora and is likely a contaminant because of an inappropriate clean-catch specimen collection technique.

10. Answer: 3

Rationale: The adult-gerontology primary care NP suspects UTI and needs to confirm the diagnosis with microscopic urine exam to identify white blood cells (WBCs) and bacteria. If no WBCs or bacteria are seen, a noncontrast CT or ultrasound should be ordered to rule out a kidney stone, which is also part of the differential diagnosis.

11. Answer: 2

Rationale: Although effective in protecting healthy skin from urine, moisture-barrier films often contain alcohol and can burn and irritate denuded skin and therefore should be used sparingly. If the perineal area is already red and excoriated, using a moisture-barrier film is contraindicated. Each time the patient is changed, the caregiver should cleanse the perineal area with mild soap and water, and then apply a thin layer of petrolatum or zinc oxide to treat the irritant dermatitis. The addition of vitamin C 250 mg and zinc 220 mg daily will aid the healing process. Once the perineal area is healed, vitamin C and zinc should be discontinued.

12. Answer: 4

Rationale: Functional incontinence is the inability to toilet appropriately because of impaired mobility. Ensuring that the patient has the appropriate equipment in the home (bedside commode, walker, wheelchair, accessible bathroom, and clothing that is easily removed) will assist the patient in maintaining independence. The patient may also benefit from scheduled toileting every 2 hours to reduce "accidents." Often these patients become socially isolated and depressed because of their concern about an accident in public. The adult-gerontology primary care NP should explore all options available. Evaluating the need for incontinence pads is effective with stress incontinence. Limiting fluid intake in the evenings to reduce nocturnal incontinence is appropriate for urge incontinence. Performing the Credé maneuver is appropriate for overflow incontinence.

13. Answer: 3

Rationale: The patient likely has chronic bacterial prostatitis, which is difficult to treat because the bacteria reside in prostatic calculi and corpora amylacea. Chronic bacterial prostatitis requires 3–4 months of therapy with trimethoprim-sulfamethoxazole (Septra DS) or a quinolone (e.g., ciprofloxacin) to prevent urinary symptoms, although care should be taken when prescribing quinolones in patients because of risks of Achilles tendon rupture and other potential side effects.

14. Answer: 4

Rationale: This patient has reversible transient urinary incontinence most likely due to excessive urine and/or new pharmacological agents, as a result of her recent hospitalization. Reversible transient urinary incontinence can be caused by **D**elirium, **I**nfection, **A**trophic vaginitis or urethritis, **P**harmaceuticals (sedative-hypnotics, diuretics, anticholinergics, α-adrenergic agents, and calcium channel blockers), **P**sychiatric disorders (psychosis, depression), **E**xcessive excretion (urine, hyperglycemia), **R**estricted mobility, and **S**tool impaction (**DIAPPERS** is the acronym). Poor pelvic support is a possible cause of stress incontinence. Urge incontinence, or the inability to delay urination with a sudden and powerful urge to void, is a possible result of lower urinary tract problems. A prolapsed uterus or bladder can cause overflow incontinence with over distention of the bladder.

15. Answer: 2

Rationale: Functional incontinence is the inability to toilet appropriately because of impaired mobility. Stress incontinence is leakage from the bladder during activities that increase intra-abdominal pressure and, therefore, pressure on the bladder, forcing urine leakage. Urge incontinence is an inability to delay urination, with a strong, abrupt urge to void, caused by bladder hyperactivity or hypersensitive bladder. The patient often has little warning before urine passes out of the bladder. Incontinence with overdistention of the bladder is called overflow incontinence, caused by an underactive or noncontracting detrusor muscle or by bladder outlet or urethral obstruction. It is characterized by frequent urination in small amounts.

16. Answer: 3, 4

Rationale: *E. coli* is the pathogen in 80% of community-acquired UTIs. Gram-positive *Staphylococcus saprophyticus (S. saprophyticus)* is the second most common pathogen in 15% of community-acquired UTIs. *Klebsiella pneumoniae (K. pneumoniae)* and *Proteus mirabilis (P. mirabilis)* are also possible pathogens. In hospital settings, *E. coli* is less prevalent. *Staphylococcus aureus* infections typically are not associated with UTIs, but are found more often with skin (impetigo; mastitis), lung (pneumonia), bone (osteomyelitis), and blood vessel (thrombophlebitis) infections. Enterococci and group B streptococci rarely cause cystitis.

17. Answer: 3

Rationale: Cystitis in adults usually presents with dysuria, urgency, frequency, nocturia, and suprapubic heaviness. Acute onset of chills, fever, flank pain, headache, malaise, and costovertebral angle tenderness are common in pyelonephritis in adults.

18. Answer: 1

Rationale: Relapse is an uncommon cause of recurrent UTIs in women and occurs within 2 weeks of completion of antibiotic therapy. It may need to be treated for 2–12 weeks. Reinfection is the cause of most UTIs in women and may be caused by residual urine resulting from a prolapsed uterus or bladder or by lack of estrogen in perimenopausal women. If the patient has up to two UTIs a year, single-dose or 3-day antibiotic therapy may be used.

19. Answer: 2

Rationale: Pyelonephritis is characterized by localized flank/back pain, costovertebral angle tenderness, combined with systemic symptoms, such as fever (100.4°F [38°C]), chills, and nausea. In older adults, mental status changes and absence of fever is noted. Suggested follow-up is by telephone contact within 12–24 hours of initiation of antibiotic therapy and at 2 weeks and 3 months for posttreatment urine cultures. Outpatient therapy is usually how the patient is followed for mild to moderate illness (not pregnant, no nausea/vomiting; fever and pain not severe), uncomplicated, and tolerating oral hydration and medications. Most patients can be treated as outpatients. With extremes of age (older adult) and severe illness inpatient treatment is indicated.

20. Answer: 2

Rationale: Urge incontinence, an established incontinence versus transient incontinence, is associated with conditions such as Parkinson disease or Alzheimer disease and involves the central nervous system causing detrusor motor and/or sensory instability. Urge incontinence is the involuntary leakage accompanied by or immediately preceded by urgency.

21. Answer: 4

Rationale: Hemolytic uremic syndrome (HUS) is most often caused by Shiga toxin-producing *Escherichia coli* (STEC) or *Shigella* and less commonly by *Streptococcus pneumoniae.* Urinary symptoms and thrombocytopenia in HUS typically do not manifest until several days after the presentation of nausea, vomiting, and diarrhea (which is often bloody). Immediate supportive therapy is indicated including transfusions and dialysis based on the severity of symptoms.

22. Answer: 3

Rationale: Although discussing the alkaline-ash, low-purine diet with the patient is appropriate, most patients, when they learn how difficult the diet is to follow, will be noncompliant with the diet even though they realize they risk developing another uric acid renal calculi. Increasing fluid intake (2–3 L/day) and alkalinization of urine (with potassium citrate or potassium bicarbonate) is also important in the treatment plan. Starting the patient on a xanthine oxidase inhibitor (allopurinol, febuxostat) and monitoring to ensure that the serum uric acid level remains at normal levels will control the incidence of uric acid stones while allowing the patient freedom without such strict dietary restrictions. Monitoring the patient for another episode is inappropriate because the serum uric acid is likely elevated and a repeat incident is likely imminent. Referral to a urologist is inappropriate at this time because there is no acute episode and the patient does not have recurrent stone formation.

23. Answer: 4

Rationale: Painless hematuria, flank pain, and a palpable abdominal renal mass are the classic triad of symptoms in the patient with renal cell carcinoma. Men over the age of 50 with a history of smoking that have painless hematuria almost always have a diagnosis of renal cell carcinoma. There is no evidence of renal failure (oliguria; edema). Renal calculi would be characterized by both hematuria and flank pain, but no abdominal mass. Prostate cancer often presents with the other symptoms of benign prostatic hypertrophy, along with anorexia and bone pain (occurs with metastasis).

24. Answer: 3

Rationale: A sedentary lifestyle or episodes of immobilization can predispose a patient to the development of renal calculi. UTIs usually do not precipitate problems with renal calculi; however, the presence of renal calculi will predispose the patient to UTIs. Milk intake of 6–8 oz daily is not excessive and will not predispose a patient to renal calculi, and increased intake of citrus and high-fiber carbohydrates is good for the patient's dietary needs. However, excess intake of vitamin C can cause hyperoxaluria and predispose a patient to renal stones.

25. Answer: 2

Rationale: Postrenal azotemia results from development of an obstructive problem distal to the kidney, as seen in advanced prostatic hypertrophy with hematuria, bladder tumor, or pelvic mass. A severe hypotensive episode, often seen after acute myocardial infarction (MI), is considered prerenal. The vascular changes resulting from diabetes and the exposure to nephrotoxic chemicals are considered intrarenal disease.

26. Answer: 1

Rationale: The precipitating factor in prerenal failure is most often an incident that precipitated renal ischemia, such as hypovolemic shock. Treatment with nephrotoxic medications such as gentamicin (Garamycin), pyelonephritis, and renal vascular changes are causes of intrarenal failure or intrinsic renal disease.

27. Answer: 1, 3, 4

Rationale: Routinely performing Kegel (pelvic floor) exercises should be taught because they assist in maintaining strong pelvic floor musculature. Weak pelvic floor musculature may contribute to urinary incontinence, especially with activity. Recommend weight loss if patient is overweight and incontinence occurs. The adult-gerontology primary care NP should include teaching about avoiding dietary substances that can irritate the bladder, such as caffeine, alcohol, and spicy foods.

28. Answer: 4

Rationale: A smooth symmetrically enlarged prostate palpated on digital rectal exam (DRE) is noted on physical exam of a patient with benign prostatic hypertrophy (BPH). An elevation in prostate specific antigen (PSA) can be found in prostate cancer as well as BPH, but is not diagnostic for either. Gross hematuria may be found in men over the age of 60 with BPH because of the chronicity of the disorder that leads to chronic cystitis. A nodular firm prostate is indicative of prostate cancer.

29. Answers: 2, 3

Rationale: Subsequent testing by a urologist is done if cancer is a concern, which is suspected when the prostate is nodular and firm, or if the patient does not improve with medication management. The subsequent testing may include uroflometry to help diagnose obstruction, a cystometrogram that measures bladder compliance for patients with suspected neurologic disease, and a cystoscopy to determine whether surgical intervention is required for obstruction or cancer. Often, one of the symptoms that accompany initial diagnosis of BPH is a urinary tract infection (UTI). Unless the patient develops chronic UTIs, the adult-gerontology primary care NP can treat UTI with routine antibiotics.

30. Answers: 2, 3, 4

Rationale: Nephrotic syndrome is damage to the kidneys that is caused by disorders that lead to increased protein in the urine (>3.5 g/day) and to a subsequent decrease in serum albumin, which leads to peripheral edema (third spacing). Other objective findings include an increase in lipids because of an increase in synthesis of very low-density lipoproteins (VLDL) as well as cholesterol and triglycerides. This leads to lipiduria, which is the sloughing of tubular cells containing fat. Increased coagulation occurs, along with reduced kidney function.

31. Answers: 3, 4

Rationale: The earliest indication of renal damage from diabetes is the presence of microalbuminuria, because of this all patients with diabetes should have this tested annually, beginning at the time of diagnosis of type 2 diabetes and 5 years after diagnosis of type 1 diabetes. A decrease in GFR is also noted. Diabetic nephropathy is characterized by proteinuria, hypertension, edema, and renal insufficiency. BUN and serum creatinine may not elevate until 50% of renal function is lost. Hematuria is not usually found. Elevated A1C is related to diabetic control and not specifically indicative of renal damage, although consistently high levels do correlate with the long-term complication of nephropathy.

32. Answer: 2

Rationale: Lithium is a mood stabilizer with an unknown mechanism of action. Toxicity of lithium is measured when serum levels rise above 1.5 mEq/L (1.5 mmol/L). Lithium prevents the ability to concentrate the urine with elevated levels causing, central nervous system changes, polyuria, and most severely nephrogenic diabetes insipidus (DI). More frequent urination may be controlled by administering lithium in a once-daily regime, while treatment of nephrogenic DI requires immediate intervention, cessation of the medication, and close monitoring of sodium levels.

33. Answer: 3

Rationale: Acute onset of increased confusion, inability to redirect, and increased agitation indicate an infection, likely a UTI, in the older adult patient with dementia. The adult-gerontology primary care NP should obtain a UA and empirically treat for UTI until the UA results are received. Because the patient has no neurologic symptoms (e.g., weakness; flaccidity), a new infarct is unlikely. Acute confusion is not a sign of worsening dementia because dementia is a gradual process. The caregiver bringing the patient with this acute problem would not indicate underlying caregiver stress, which usually presents when persons complain of stress to their own primary care provider.

Pharmacology

34. Answer: 2

Rationale: Hyperphosphatemia is often seen in patients with chronic kidney disease (CKD) as GFR declines below 25–40 mL/min. In addition to dietary restriction of phosphates, phosphate binders such as sevelamer (Renagel) and calcium carbonate are routinely administered. Controlling hyperphosphatemia in CKD has been associated with decreased mortality. As patients with CKD have a further decline of GFR with associated hyperphosphatemia, increasing frequency or duration of dialysis is also indicated.

35. Answer: 3

Rationale: Benign prostatic hypertrophy is a common cause of urinary retention in older men. Inhaled ipratropium is an atropine-like bronchodilator used to treat chronic bronchitis, and its anticholinergic agent may aggravate urinary retention. Neither glyburide (oral antihyperglycemic) nor buspirone (oral antianxiety agent) has an effect on the urinary system. Timolol is a topical agent used to treat glaucoma and does not have a systemic effect.

36. Answer: 1

Rationale: Chronic kidney disease often results of a loss of erythropoietin as GFR decreases. This increases the risk of anemia. After evaluating and ensuring iron levels are appropriate, initiation of therapy with an erythropoiesis-stimulating agent is appropriate. Initiation of therapy is typically considered at hemoglobin levels <9 g/dL for nondialysis dependent patients (<10 g/dL if dialysis dependent), especially if the patient is near transfusion levels. Treatment is at 4-week intervals and should be reduced or stopped if hemoglobin is >11 g/dL due to adverse side effects.

37. Answer: 4

Rationale: Combination hormone replacement therapy using conjugated estrogen (Premarin) 0.3–1.25 mg/day orally or vaginally and medroxyprogesterone (progestin) 2.5–10 mg/day continuously or intermittently can be useful for management of stress incontinence. Propantheline and oxybutynin may be useful in urge incontinence; research is limited on their use for stress incontinence. Doxepin (Sinequan) is a tricyclic antidepressant and is used infrequently.

38. Answer: 2, 5, 6

Rationale: First line treatment options for uncomplicated cystitis or urinary tract infections without recent or recurrent infections include trimethoprim-sulfamethoxazole (TMP-SMX), nitrofurantoin, and fosfomycin. There are other outpatient treatment options including fluoroquinolones, like ciprofloxacin, as well as beta-lactam antibiotics. These should only be selected if known contraindications exist such as allergy, renal failure, known antibiotic resistance, or suspicion of pyelonephritis. Nitrofurantoin is administered for a minimum of 5 days but is avoided in renal failure (GFR <30). TMP-SMX is contraindicated in this patient due to sulfa allergy but is normally indicated 160/800mg (double strength) PO bid for 3 days. TMP-SMX should be avoided if a patient has recurrent UTIs or has taken TMP-SMX within the past 3 months. Ciprofloxacin is acceptable but in 2016 the FDA advised against first line systemic use in uncomplicated UTIs for patients with other treatment options. Fosfomycin is acceptable as a one-time treatment but is contraindicated in patients with suspicion of pyelonephritis.

39. Answer: 1

Rationale: To decrease the formation of uric acid stones, a urinary alkylating agent, such as allopurinol, is frequently used. As standard practice, the adult-gerontology primary care NP should check the patient's serum uric acid level monthly for 3 months to ensure the levels are decreasing to normal ranges, and then annually once serum uric acid levels are normalized. Indomethacin is used for its antiinflammatory properties in the treatment of gout. Urecholine is a cholinergic agent that stimulates the bladder to contract, which improves urine flow. Colchicine is an antigout medication also used for its antiinflammatory properties.

40. Answer: 3

Rationale: Oxybutynin produces anticholinergic effects, and dry mouth is a common side effect. Because this patient is an older adult, the adult-gerontology primary care NP should review the patient's list of medications to verify that no other medications will exacerbate dry mouth. If another medication will increase this side effect (e.g., diuretic), the practitioner should advise the patient of methods to relieve the dry mouth, such as hard candy or chewing gum. The patient may also be taking other medications with anticholinergic side effects, which could be increased with the addition of oxybutynin to the point the patient could be at risk for falls. Careful review of the patient's medication list is essential before adding a new drug. The other reactions are not consistent with oxybutynin administration.

41. Answer: 1, 3, 5

Rationale: Sedatives and hypnotics (temazepam and diazepam) lead to sedation and muscle relaxation in all groups, but particularly in the older adult population; central nervous system (CNS) changes from aging may lead to increased muscle relaxation, with the addition of a sedative-hypnotic leading to urinary incontinence. Antidepressants (amitriptyline) have anticholinergic effects and lead to sedation. CNS changes and the addition of antidepressants with anticholinergic side effects will increase muscle relaxation in the older adult patient and contribute to urinary incontinence. Antibiotics and laxatives have not been implicated in the development of urinary incontinence in older patients. Opioids (tramadol) increase the tone in the urinary bladder sphincter, leading to urinary retention. Nitrofurantoin (Macrodantin) is on the Beers List and should not be prescribed for an older adult.

42. Answer: 1, 4

Rationale: Trimethoprim-sulfamethoxazole (TMP-SMZ) is contraindicated if renal function is impaired, antibacterial concentration in the urine is inadequate, or patient is allergic to sulfa medications. To treat chronic UTI, the adult-gerontology primary care NP would consider low trimethoprim-sulfamethoxazole (TMP-SMZ) as treatment. Using this low dose in the adult patient should not cause serum or tissue accumulation of the drug. Liver function studies may be indicated if the patient experiences adverse reactions to the medication. Anticoagulants have not been reported to cause significant drug interactions. The BUN test is not a sensitive indicator of renal creatinine clearance.

43. Answer: 3

Rationale: Hydrochlorothiazide (HCTZ) decreases the risk of forming calcium oxalate stones because of decreased renal calcium excretion, or hypocalciuria. Hypercalcemia is a possible side effect of this medication. Furosemide, acetazolamide, and triamterene may increase the risk of formation of calcium oxalate stones by causing hypercalciuria. It is important to note that HCTZ may subsequently increase the risk of gout and/or uric acid stone formation due to hyperuricemia.

44. Answer: 1

Rationale: The severe pain of renal calculi should be addressed before other treatments or diagnostics. Narcotics and now nonsteroidal antiinflammatory drugs (NSAIDs) are commonly used for pain relief. In most randomized, blinded studies of NSAIDs versus narcotics, NSAIDs have shown equal or greater efficacy for pain relief, shorter duration to pain relief, with equal or fewer side effects. Ketorolac works at the peripheral site of pain production rather than on the CNS and based on clinical findings, has been proven to be as effective as opioid analgesics, with fewer adverse effects. Ketorolac is only indicated for short-term therapy and is contraindicated in patients with renal failure. Due to an increased risk of bleeding, it is not given concurrently with other NSAIDs and should be used with caution in patients > age 65.

45. Answer: 1

Rationale: The most important side effects of nitrofurantoin are gastrointestinal upset, which can be decreased if the medication is taken with food or milk, and brown discoloration of the urine. The patient should continue taking nitrofurantoin for at least 3 days after sterile urine is obtained. If applicable to the patient, the drug may interfere with the efficacy of oral contraceptives.

46. Answer: 1

Rationale: The adult-gerontology primary care NP should advise the patient that if she experiences yellow discoloration of the sclerae while taking phenazopyridine, she is to return to the office immediately. This may indicate poor renal excretion and requires a renal workup (renal panel, parathyroid and thyroid-stimulating hormone, serum magnesium/calcium, and a 24-hour urine for creatinine clearance) and possible referral to a nephrologist. Phenazopyridine should be administered with food, and no drug interactions occur with aspirin or oral contraceptives.

47. Answer: 3

Rationale: Muddy brown granular casts are indicative of acute tubular necrosis (ATN). ATN is the most common cause of acute kidney injury and is the result of intrinsic (renal) damage of the tubules most often due to ischemia. Leading causes include sepsis, hypotension, rhabdomyolysis, contrast agents, as well as aminoglycosides. Renal damage due to aminoglycosides like gentamicin is often after administration for 5–7 days and is relatively uncommon compared to other causes of ATN. Furosemide, amphotericin, and ibuprofen are often implicated in acute interstitial nephritis and urinalysis would more likely appear with WBCs and/or WBC casts in addition other symptoms.

48. Answer: 1, 3, 4

Rationale: Membranous nephropathy is the most common cause of nephrotic syndrome in adults and is caused by many factors including medications. Common medications implicated in causing nephrotic syndrome include heavy metals, heroin, NSAIDs, captopril, as well as penicillamine. Patients developing proteinuria while taking these medications should withhold the medication and be monitored for other signs of nephrotic syndrome.

49. Answer: 3

Rationale: Oxybutynin is contraindicated in patients with narrow-angle glaucoma (angle-closure glaucoma). Patients with open-angle glaucoma may take this medication. Anticholinergics may increase the pressure within the eye, which puts the patient at risk for progression of the glaucoma, which is blindness.

50. Answer: 1

Rationale: This patient most likely has overflow urinary incontinence. Overflow incontinence is due to an inability to contract the detrusor muscle of the bladder or a bladder outlet obstruction. The patient also likely has decreased sensation or genitourinary autonomic neuropathy bladder due to uncontrolled diabetes. Other causes of overflow incontinence include anticholinergic medications, neuropathic diseases, and physical obstruction due to pelvic organ prolapse, strictures, severe constipation or BPH in men. A post void residual urine should be obtained and will likely exceed 100 mL. Treatment options include removing the offending agent and/or self-catheterization, which is typically the best treatment. Medical options include cholinergic agents like bethanechol and alpha-blockers such as terazosin and doxazosin. Dicyclomine is an antispasmodic used to treat irritable bowel syndrome. Mirtazapine is an antidepressant. Hyoscyamine (Levsin) is an antispasmodic used to treat bowel or bladder cramping.

51. Answer: 4

Rationale: Although fluoroquinolones are a common and generally effective treatment for urinary tract infections, these drugs received a black box warning in 2016 due to potential side effects, such as tendon ruptures, peripheral neuropathy, and central nervous system effects. Therefore, fluoroquinolones should not be used for minor infections as a first-line agent. Fluoroquinolones should not be used in pregnancy.

52. Answer: 4

Rationale: Angiotensin-converting enzyme (ACE) inhibitors increase pressure within the kidney in renal artery stenosis, causing an increase in serum creatinine and potassium. ACE inhibitors have protective properties for patients with cardiovascular disease, hypertension, and diabetes.

53. Answer: 1

Rational: Ibuprofen (Motrin) is a nonsteroidal antiinflammatory agent with risk of renal toxicity and should be avoided in patients with preexisting or renal impairment. Levothyroxine is metabolized predominantly in the liver. Metoprolol is a beta blocker and has little effect on the kidneys, unlike the ACE inhibitors. Clopidogrel works on the liver and also has little effect on the kidneys.

54. Answer: 2

Rational: Metformin is contraindicated in patients with heart failure, liver failure, and impaired renal function. It is contraindicated for 2 days prior to and 2 days after receiving intravenous (IV) radiographic contrast. Metformin combined with IV contrast dye puts the patient at risk for fatal lactic acidosis. Baseline glomerular filtration rate (GFR) should be documented. Captopril is an ACE inhibitor that is renal protective until GFR is noted to be worsening. Glyburide and temazepam minimally affect the renal function, and there is no need to hold these medications prior to the study.

15

Male Reproductive

Physical Examination & Diagnostic Tests

1. Which of the following circumstances is ideal for ordering a prostate specific antigen (PSA) laboratory test?
   1. A 41-year-old white male with no family history of prostate cancer who "just wants to know if he might have it."
   2. A 60-year-old man with new onset lower urinary tract symptoms, such as increased urgency and frequency of urination and painful urination.
   3. A 55-year-old male presenting with new symptoms of erectile dysfunction.
   4. A 72-year-old male who recently completed a course of antibiotics for prostatitis.

2. Which organ is not palpable on physical exam of a male patient?
   1. Vas deferens.
   2. Testes.
   3. Epididymis.
   4. Cowper glands.

3. During a sports physical, an adolescent asks the adult-gerontology primary care NP if he should be doing testicular self-exams. The nurse correctly tells him:
   1. Testicular self-exams are needed if you have a strong family history of testicular cancer.
   2. Testicular self-exams should be done in the shower once a month.
   3. The United States Preventive Services Task Force no long recommends testicular self-exam.
   4. Testicular self-exam has been replaced by regular ultrasound screenings of asymptomatic men.

4. The proper technique for examining for a scrotal hernia is to:
   1. Listen to the scrotum for bowel sounds.
   2. Transilluminate the scrotum and expect the presence of a transilluminating mass.
   3. Invaginate the scrotum with the index finger and follow the spermatic cord, assessing for the presence of bowel pushing through the inguinal ring.
   4. Check visually for the presence of a bulge; if no bulge is noted, there is no scrotal hernia present.

5. Review of a laboratory report indicating elevated serum gonadotropin would raise suspicion of which disorder?
   1. Seminal vesiculitis.
   2. Vas deferens disease.
   3. Testicular disease.
   4. BPH.

6. Which of the following structures can be palpated during an external exam of a male patient?
   1. Epididymis.
   2. Cowper ducts.
   3. Seminal vesicles.
   4. Ejaculatory ducts.

7. What would be most helpful in diagnosing gynecomastia?
   1. History and physical.
   2. Liver function test.
   3. Thyroid function test.
   4. Mammogram.

8. The correct position in which to place a healthy adult male patient to examine the rectum and prostate is:
   1. Left lateral Sims position with right knee flexed and left leg extended.
   2. Supine position with hips and legs flexed and feet positioned on the examining table.
   3. Modified knee-chest position with patient prone and knees flexed under hips.
   4. Leaning over the exam table with chest and shoulders resting on the table.

9. How is prostate cancer appropriately diagnosed?
   1. An elevated PSA.
   2. Upon palpating a nodule during a digital rectal exam.
   3. Biopsy via transrectal ultrasonography.
   4. An elevated prostatic acid phosphatase.

10. Which statement is correct about the PSA test?
    1. PSA can be elevated in patients with BPH.
    2. PSA is not elevated in patients with prostatitis.
    3. Prostatic massage will not elevate PSA levels.
    4. PSA does not increase in recurrence of prostate cancer.

11. The United States Preventive Services Task Force recommends against routine screening for prostate cancer screening because:
    1. There is a high mortality rate from prostate cancer regardless of screening.
    2. There is harm associated with a high number of false positives.
    3. Digital rectal exam is shown to be superior to serological testing.
    4. Ultrasonography is now the screening of choice.

12. When examining the scrotum of a dark complexion male, a normal finding is:
    1. Symmetric scrotal sac with two movable testes.
    2. Smooth, rubbery, saclike surface that is sensitive to gentle compression.
    3. Asymmetric sac with left side lower than right side.
    4. Reddish color that is darker than body skin with sebaceous cysts.

Disorders

13. A 45-year-old male presents with a several-week history of feeling pain in the scrotum that worsens with coughing, lifting, and straining. He states that his scrotum feels "full" at the end of the day. The adult-gerontology primary care NP would be suspicious of:
    1. A spermatocele.
    2. An inguinal hernia.
    3. Epididymitis.
    4. Testicular torsion.

14. A 49-year-old male smoker presents to the clinic with complaints of painless gross hematuria. What is the most serious problem that needs to be considered by the adult-gerontology primary care NP?
    1. Bladder cancer.
    2. Benign prostatic hypertrophy.
    3. Erectile dysfunction.
    4. Urinary tract infection.

15. A 65-year-old male presents with well-controlled hypertension and diabetes mellitus. He is a nonsmoker. He has been married for 35 years, is monogamous, and reports that his relationship with wife is good. He complains of new onset erectile dysfunction. First-line therapy for erectile dysfunction includes:
    1. Relationship counseling.
    2. Oral phosphodiesterase-5 inhibitors.

3. Intraurethral injections of alprostadil (Caverject).
4. Use of a vacuum device.

16. What finding is indicative of testicular torsion?
    1. Scrotal swelling with tenderness that occurs only after age 40.
    2. Sudden onset of pain with a firm, tender mass in the scrotum.
    3. A scrotum that transilluminates.
    4. Cremasteric reflex.

17. A 57-year-old male suffers blunt trauma to the penis. He complains of pain and an inability to urinate. Which of the following should be the adult-gerontology primary care NP's priority?
    1. Insertion of an indwelling catheter.
    2. Insertion of an intermittent catheter.
    3. Insertion of a suprapubic catheter.
    4. Order a retrograde urethrogram.

18. On a routine physical exam, a patient expresses concern over the observation that one side of his scrotum is larger than the other side. He states that it has been getting larger for the past few months and that the scrotum is smaller in the morning and enlarges through the day. He has felt a heaviness in the scrotum, denies any acute pain, but does confirm some discomfort in his lower back. He reports no history of trauma to the scrotal area. On exam, the adult-gerontology primary care NP confirms the enlargement. Further exam reveals that the scrotum will transilluminate and that manual manipulation of the scrotum does not cause pain. What is the initial diagnosis for the patient?
    1. Hydrocele.
    2. Orchitis.
    3. Epididymitis.
    4. Traumatic injury.

19. A 47-year-old male presents with pain of his right knee and discomfort when grasping objects with his hands for 14 days. He reports a low-grade fever of 100.4°F (38°C) for the last 5 days as well as dysuria 5 days ago. He is sexually active with multiple partners and does not use barrier protection. For which of the following organisms should the adult gerontology NP begin immediate treatment?
    1. *Treponema pallidum*.
    2. *Neisseria gonorrhoeae*.
    3. *Staphylococcus aureus*.
    4. *Chlamydia trachomatis*.

20. Which statement is correct concerning circumcision?
    1. Circumcision is helpful in preventing phimosis.
    2. Circumcision is a cause of paraphimosis.
    3. Balanoposthitis is the direct result of circumcision in older men.
    4. Circumcision increases the incidence of cancer of the penis.

21. A 31-year-old male presents with his fifth diagnosis of gonorrhea in the past 3 years and affirms he completed all treatment regimens as prescribed. Which of the following is an appropriate next step by the adult-gerontology primary care NP to evaluate the cause of recurrent infections?
    1. Safe sex education.
    2. Screening for complement deficiency.
    3. Intravenous treatment of the resistant gonococcal infection.
    4. Behavioral therapy for sex addiction.

22. Acute epididymitis is characterized by:
    1. Absence of dysuria.
    2. Nonenlarged scrotum.
    3. Tenderness over epididymis.
    4. Lack of abdominal pain.

23. In a 70-year-old man, which of the following bacteria is likely responsible for epididymitis?
    1. *Escherichia coli.*
    2. *Treponema pallidum.*
    3. *Neisseria gonorrhoeae.*
    4. *Chlamydia trachomatis.*

24. Which of the following is true about hypogonadism?
    1. Usually presents with decreased libido.
    2. May cause an increase in muscle mass.
    3. It causes an increase in body hair.
    4. Does not contribute to infertility.

25. Which of the following is a common cause of impotence?
    1. The use of antihypertensives.
    2. Dietary supplements.
    3. Masturbation.
    4. It is a natural part of aging.

26. Which action is true about the prostate?
    1. Secretes fluid that is acidic.
    2. Secretes fluid that is alkaline.
    3. Secretes androgens.
    4. Produces sperm.

27. An older adult man presents to the clinic with complaints of difficulty voiding and hematuria. The digital rectal exam reveals a firm prostate about 5 cm in diameter, asymmetric, with firm nodules. The PSA level is 14. The next action is to:
    1. Medicate with finasteride (Proscar) 5 mg PO daily and reevaluate in 3 months.
    2. Advise patient to avoid caffeine, alcohol, and over-the-counter decongestants.
    3. Obtain a urinalysis to determine presence of infection and amount of hematuria.
    4. Refer to urologist for biopsy and diagnostic evaluation for prostatic cancer.

28. A 20-year-old male patient presents with scrotal pain. A suspected diagnosis that requires immediate referral is:
    1. Testicular torsion.
    2. Hydrocele.
    3. Epididymitis.
    4. Inguinal hernia.

29. The adult-gerontology primary care NP has been following an older adult patient who has been treated for BPH with behavioral modifications (limiting fluids before bedtime, avoiding caffeine and alcohol, etc.) and taking an alpha-1 blocker. Select two indications for referral to a urologist.
    1. Urinary tract infection.
    2. Urinary retention.
    3. Prostatic bleeding.
    4. Increased urinary flow rate.
    5. PSA level below 4 ng/mL.

30. An adult male patient is being evaluated for dysuria, fever, and perineal pain. The physical exam by the adult-gerontology primary care NP reveals a distended bladder. Which of the following should be avoided?
    1. Urine culture.
    2. Prostate massage.
    3. Cultures for gonorrhea and chlamydia.
    4. CBC.

31. An older adult male presents with a history of burning on urination and difficulty urinating that has been increasing over the past few days. He often has to void a short time later to fully empty his bladder. A digital rectal exam reveals an enlarged prostate. What is the most likely diagnosis considered by the adult-gerontology primary care NP?
    1. Bladder cancer.
    2. Testicular torsion.
    3. Benign prostatic hypertrophy.
    4. Renal failure.

32. The patient with localized prostate cancer will exhibit which symptoms?
    1. Hesitancy, frequency, and dysuria.
    2. Fatigue, severe constipation, and dysuria.
    3. Hematuria, nocturia, and weight loss.
    4. Myalgia, confusion, and lethargy.

33. A young patient presents with a complaint of a feeling of fullness in the scrotum. Physical exam reveals a round, soft, nontender, nonadherent, bluish testicular mass resembling a "bag of worms." No variation in size occurs with respiration or Valsalva maneuver. The mass transilluminates and is located anterior to the testes. The most likely diagnosis is:
    1. Varicocele.
    2. Hernia.
    3. Tumor.
    4. Spermatocele.

34. An uncircumcised patient presents with a complaint of not being able to retract the foreskin over the glans penis. What is the most likely diagnosis?
    1. Lateral phimosis.
    2. Phimosis.
    3. Peyronie disease.
    4. Paraphimosis.

35. A middle-aged patient complains of a tight band causing a dorsal curvature of the penis and shortening of the penis both with and without an erection. What is the most likely diagnosis?
    1. Phimosis.
    2. Lateral phimosis.
    3. Lateral paraphimosis.
    4. Peyronie disease.

36. A middle-aged, uncircumcised patient presents with tender or pruritic, red pinpoint pustules and papules on the prepuce and glans. The most likely diagnosis is:
    1. Peyronie disease.
    2. Balanitis.
    3. Phimosis.
    4. Paraphimosis.

37. A male patient is diagnosed with balanitis. The most likely cause is:
    1. Candidiasis.
    2. Herpes genitalis.
    3. Lichen planus.
    4. Psoriasis.

38. A male patient presents with a complaint of sexual dysfunction. The adult-gerontology primary care NP understands that sexual dysfunction is impairment of:
    1. Erection only.
    2. Emission only.
    3. Ejaculation only.
    4. Erection, emission, or ejaculation.

39. A man presents with a complaint of dysuria, an edematous scrotum, tenderness over the epididymis, and abdominal pain. What is the most likely diagnosis for the patient?
    1. Testicular torsion.
    2. Vas deferens inflammation.
    3. Epididymitis.
    4. Balanitis.

40. The adult-gerontology primary care NP knows that erectile dysfunction is:
    1. Primarily psychological in origin.
    2. Unusual in older men.

3. The persistent inability to achieve and maintain an erection adequate for sexual intercourse.
4. The physiologic dysfunction when smooth muscle contracts, causing a lack of adequate amount of blood in the penis to render a rigid, larger penis.

41. Priapism is classified as which type of sexual dysfunction?
    1. Erection.
    2. Emission.
    3. Ejaculation.
    4. Priapic.

42. Which of the following is correct in response to a patient's question concerning a possible cause of testicular cancer?
    1. Syphilis.
    2. Gonorrhea.
    3. Cryptorchidism.
    4. Balanitis.

43. A male patient complains of impotence. Which of the following may be a contributing factor?
    1. Antihypertensive drugs.
    2. Sexual intercourse.
    3. Rheumatoid arthritis.
    4. Frequent masturbation.

44. A 16-year-old boy presents with gynecomastia. The adult-gerontology primary care NP knows that it is likely:
    1. A result of hypogonadism.
    2. Caused by medication.
    3. Due to the hormonal imbalances of adolescence.
    4. An aggressive form of breast cancer.

45. Which is true of prostate cancer?
    1. Rarely diagnosed in men >50 years of age.
    2. Soft, indiscrete, symmetric nodules of the prostate.
    3. Obstructive symptoms rarely present.
    4. Firm prostate, often with hard nodules.

46. Which symptoms would be most concerning about a possible diagnosis of prostate cancer in a male over 50 years of age?
    1. Hesitancy, dribbling, and urgency.
    2. Decreased force of urine stream.
    3. Pain and feeling of a full bladder.
    4. Urinary symptoms coupled with pain in the hips or back.

47. Which statement is correct concerning testicular cancer?
    1. It is a common problem in men over age 50.
    2. It is directly related to testicular trauma.
    3. It always presents suddenly with pain.
    4. It is primarily found in young men.

48. Which of the following is true about acute bacterial prostatitis?
    1. Characterized by recurrent urinary tract infections.
    2. Involves an ascending infection of the urinary tract.
    3. Always occurs in men under age 30.
    4. Usually treated with 1 month of antibiotics.

49. Which of the following is true of orchitis?
    1. Is rarely viral.
    2. The lesion transilluminates.
    3. Is relatively painless.
    4. Can be associated with a worsening epididymitis.

50. A patient has nongonococcal urethritis (NGU). The adult-gerontology primary care NP understands that:
    1. No related problems occur if NGU is untreated.
    2. Patients with NGU are often asymptomatic.
    3. NGU is easily differentiated from gonococcal urethritis on physical exam.
    4. There is a very purulent discharge with a foul odor.

51. What organism is the most common cause of nongonococcal urethritis (NGU) in men?
    1. *Chlamydia trachomatis.*
    2. *Neisseria gonorrhoeae.*
    3. *Escherichia coli.*
    4. *Streptococcus faecalis.*

52. Which test is a useful tumor marker for testicular cancer?
    1. Alpha-fetoprotein (AFP).
    2. Prostate-specific antigen (PSA).
    3. Prostatic acid phosphatase (PAP).
    4. Alkaline phosphatase (ALP).

53. The most common viral causative agent of orchitis is:
    1. Arbovirus.
    2. Echovirus.
    3. Mumps.
    4. Rubeola.

54. What are common symptoms of benign prostatic hypertrophy (BPH)?
    1. Dribbling, hesitancy, loss of stream volume and force, and recurrent urinary tract infections.
    2. Dysuria, urgency, frequency, nocturia, and suprapubic heaviness or discomfort.
    3. Obstructive symptoms, such as a weak urine stream, abdominal straining to void, hesitancy, incomplete bladder emptying, and terminal dribbling.
    4. Acute onset of fever, chills, flank pain, headache, malaise, costovertebral angle tenderness, and possibly hematuria.

55. A 25-year-old patient with a history of sickle cell disease complains of a sudden problem with erections that are not sexually oriented. He is currently experiencing a painful erection and he is unable to void. The adult-gerontology primary care NP determines the treatment of choice is:
    1. Morphine sulfate and bed rest.
    2. Immediate referral to a urologist.
    3. Increased hydration for sickle cell crisis.
    4. Determination of PSA level.

56. The adult-gerontology primary care NP is speaking with a group of male teenagers who are most concerned about symptoms associated with gonorrhea. Which of the following would the adult-gerontology primary care NP include in the discussion?
    1. Reddish lesions may appear on the palms of the hands and soles of the feet.
    2. Men may observe a rash over the body of the penis.
    3. Urinary dribbling may result from irritation of the urinary tract.
    4. Painful urination results from inflammation of the urethra.

57. A 17-year-old boy comes into the clinic with complaints of sudden, severe scrotal pain radiating inguinally. He has no difficulty voiding and has some nausea but no vomiting. Examination reveals scrotal edema and erythema. The scrotum on the affected side is slightly higher than the unaffected side, and the cremasteric reflex is negative. What would the adult-gerontology primary care NP determine as the best treatment for the patient?
    1. Bed rest with ice pack and scrotal elevation.
    2. Warm scrotal pack and return to clinic the next day.
    3. Immediate referral to a urologist.
    4. Schedule for an ultrasound in the morning.

58. A 65-year-old uncircumcised man presents to the clinic with complaints of a painless "bump" on his penis, difficulty retracting the foreskin, and serosanguineous drainage from beneath the foreskin. The adult-gerontology primary care NP must first consider a possible diagnosis of:
    1. Balanitis.
    2. Penile cancer.
    3. Herpes.
    4. Penile trauma.

59. What is considered a major contributing factor in erectile dysfunction?
    1. Diet high in vitamin C.
    2. Diabetes mellitus.
    3. Allergies.
    4. Low-sodium diet.

60. A 30-year-old male presents with a macular-papular rash on his body, including the soles of his feet and his palms. He is also complaining of fatigue, fever, malaise, and swollen lymph nodes. On further questioning, it is revealed that the illness began several weeks ago with several papules on his penis. The adult-gerontology primary care NP suspects:
    1. Herpes simplex.
    2. Granuloma inguinale.
    3. Gonorrhea.
    4. Syphilis.

61. Which of the following sexually transmitted infections often begins with a prodrome of headaches, fever, malaise, and myalgia?
    1. Genital herpes.
    2. Granuloma inguinale.
    3. Gonorrhea.
    4. Syphilis.

62. Which of the following clinical presentations are commonly associated with genital herpes?
    1. Vesicular lesions on an erythematous base.
    2. Chancres on the penis.
    3. Purulent urethral discharge.
    4. Small, flattened papules and larger verrucous lesions.

63. Which of the following is true of testicular cancer?
    1. It affects hundreds of thousands of adolescent boys each year.
    2. It has a high mortality rate.
    3. Early detection via testicular self-exam improves morbidity and mortality.
    4. Cryptorchidism is a risk factor for testicular cancer.

64. A 15-year-old male presents with complaints of severe scrotal pain for the past 2 hours. The scrotum is swollen and extremely tender; palpation of the epididymis is not possible. What does the adult-gerontology primary care NP recognize as the immediate treatment?
    1. Narcotic analgesics and bed rest.
    2. Warm packs and scrotal support.
    3. Antibiotics, ice packs, and analgesics.
    4. Referral to a surgeon for evaluation.

Pharmacology

65. Which of the following is correct regarding short-acting phosphodiesterase-5 inhibitors, such as sildenafil (Viagra) or vardenafil (Levitra)?
    1. They work best in combination with a large, fatty meal.
    2. They should be taken 30 minutes to an hour before intercourse.
    3. They are the only class of medications that is effective for treating erectile dysfunction.
    4. They work in all men.

66. Common side effects of phosphodiesterase-5 inhibitors include:
    1. Erections lasting longer than 4 hours.
    2. Headaches, flushing, and dyspepsia.
    3. Nausea and vomiting.
    4. Rash, itching, and loss of appetite.

67. An important contraindication to phosphodiesterase-5 inhibitors is:
    1. Selective serotonin reuptake inhibitors.
    2. Beta blockers.
    3. Nitrates.
    4. Thiazide diuretics.

68. A patient has been taking doxazosin (Cardura) 2 mg PO daily for 3 weeks for treatment of BPH. He returns to the clinic and is complaining of feeling dizzy when he stands up. Which action would the adult-gerontology primary care NP take?
    1. Determine blood pressure with patient lying down, standing, and sitting.
    2. Order urinalysis to determine hematuria and presence of bacteria.
    3. Review with patient his symptoms over the past 3 weeks.
    4. Perform digital rectal exam to determine if prostate is smaller than previously noted.

69. A 74-year-old male patient has benign prostatic hypertrophy (BPH) and stage 1 hypertension. Which of the following medications would be the most appropriate selection to possibly treat both disorders?
    1. Tamsulosin (Flomax).
    2. Finasteride (Proscar).
    3. Doxazosin (Cardura).
    4. Tadalafil (Cialis).

70. In planning treatment for a patient with balanitis, the adult-gerontology primary care NP orders:
    1. Rest, ice, and elevation.
    2. Massage therapy.
    3. Antifungal agents.
    4. Emergency circumcision.

71. A 28-year-old man presents with complaints of fever, low back pain, perineal pain, and intense pain on voiding. Rectal exam reveals a tender, swollen, firm, warm prostate. Based on the patient's symptoms, the treatment of choice is:
    1. Ceftriaxone (Rocephin) 250 mg IM × 1, followed by doxycycline 100 mg PO bid × 10 days.
    2. Tetracycline (Achromycin) 250 mg PO qid × 10 days.
    3. Amoxicillin (Amoxil) 500 mg PO tid × 14 days.
    4. Erythromycin (Ilosone) 250 mg PO q6h × 24 days.

72. Which of the following side effects is common in a 56-year-old patient taking tamsulosin (Flomax)?
    1. Constipation.
    2. Decreased ejaculate.
    3. Anorgasmia.
    4. Hypertension.

73. A 70-year-old man complains of scrotal pain with dysuria and frequency that has been increasing over the past 2 weeks. Physical exam reveals extreme scrotal tenderness and swelling, urethral discharge, and testes normal in size and position. UA reveals pyuria. What is the treatment of choice for the patient?
    1. Nitrofurantoin (Macrodantin) 100 mg PO qid × 14 days.
    2. Levofloxacin (Levaquin) 750 mg PO qd × 10 days.
    3. Doxazosin (Cardura) 1 mg PO qd × 10 days.
    4. Oxybutynin (Ditropan) 5 mg PO tid × 10 days.

74. Finasteride (Proscar) is prescribed for a 50-year-old man who is experiencing a problem with urination secondary to an enlarged prostate. The adult-gerontology primary care NP would teach the patient that while he is taking this medication, it is important to:
    1. Increase his fluid intake.
    2. Restrain from sexual activity.
    3. Take special precautions around women of childbearing age.
    4. Increase intake of folic acid.

75. A 75-year-old patient is diagnosed with chronic bacterial prostatitis and the adult-gerontology primary care NP selects ciprofloxacin (Cipro) as the treatment. How should the ciprofloxacin be prescribed for this patient?
    1. 500 mg PO bid × 10 days.
    2. 500 mg PO tid × 3 days, then 500 mg PO bid × 10 days.
    3. 500 mg PO bid × 21 days.
    4. 500 mg PO bid × 30–45 days.

76. Which of the following would be considered an initial treatment for Peyronie disease?
    1. Surgery.
    2. Pentoxifylline (Trental).
    3. Circumcision.
    4. Oxybutynin (Ditropan).

15 | Male Reproductive Answers & Rationales

Physical Exam & Diagnostic Tests

1. Answer: 2

Rationale: A prostate specific antigen is most appropriate to order for a man who presents with lower urinary tract symptoms, which could be indicative of either benign prostatic hyperplasia or prostate cancer. Due to low sensitivity and specificity, the prostatic specific antigen should not be used as a screening test in most men. A man with lower urinary tract symptoms and an elevated prostate specific antigen should be referred to urology for further evaluation.

2. Answer: 4

Rationale: Cowper glands (bulbourethral glands) are located near the prostate and beside the urethra near the base of the penis. These internal glands are nonpalpable. The testes, vas deferens, and epididymis are all palpable on exam.

3. Answer: 3

Rationale: Neither testicular self-exam nor clinical exam is recommended by the United States Preventive Services Task Force due to low incidence of disease and the potential harm from anxiety and testing procedures. Similarly, the American Academy of Family Physicians, American Academy of Pediatrics, and the American Cancer Society do not recommend testicular self-exams. Testicular cancer is a low-incidence disease with a high cure rate even in advanced disease.

4. Answer: 3

Rationale: Invaginating the scrotum with the index finger and following the spermatic cord, assessing for the presence of bowel pushing through the inguinal ring is the correct way to assess for a hernia penetrating into the scrotum. Inguinal hernias do not transilluminate, as they are solid. An inguinal hernia is not always observable on inspection.

5. Answer: 3

Rationale: Gonadotropin is often elevated in testicular disease, whereas prostate surface antigen (PSA) is elevated in diseases of the prostate, such as benign prostatic hypertrophy (BPH), prostate inflammation, and prostate cancer.

6. Answer: 1

Rationale: The epididymis is palpable, whereas the ducts and glands are not. The comma-shaped epididymis is palpated on the posterolateral surface of each testis. The seminal vesicles (pair of glands) lie behind the urinary bladder in front of the rectum. These vesicles join the ampulla of the vas deferens to form the ejaculatory duct.

7. Answer: 1

Rationale: A complete history and physical usually provide the cause of gynecomastia without further testing, since it can be caused by medication, starving and refeeding, or lack of androgen production (atrophying testes), which changes the estrogen/androgen ratio. Serologic tests are considered only when the history and physical exam suggests other disorders. It is common in adolescents.

8. Answer: 4

Rationale: For patient comfort and ease of exam, the healthy ambulatory adult is asked to lean over the exam table with his chest and upper body resting on the table. Although left lateral Sim position is correct, it is the position used for examining a patient who is confined to bed or requests an alternative to standing.

9. Answer: 3

Rationale: The standard for diagnosing prostate cancer is a biopsy obtained by a urologist via transrectal ultrasonography. An elevated PSA is usually present during prostate cancer, but can also be present in noncancerous disorders, such as benign prostatic hyperplasia. A nodule palpated on exam is suggestive of prostate cancer, but is not diagnostic. Prostatic acid phosphatase is an enzyme present in prostate cancer that is an older test for prostate cancer and is also present in other diseases and when taking some medications.

10. Answer: 1

Rationale: PSA can be elevated in patients with benign prostatic hypertrophy (BPH) and those with prostatitis, as well as after prostate gland massage. PSA does increase with the increasing burden of the tumor, as in recurrent prostate cancer.

11. Answer: 2

Rationale: Prostate cancer has a low mortality regardless of screening, as only 2.8% of men will die of the disease. Over 80% of PSAs are false positives and not attributed to prostate cancer. Biopsies to rule out prostate cancer can cause anxiety, pain, bleeding, and urinary dysfunction. Digital rectal exam (DRE) and ultrasonography have not been proven to be effective methods of detecting prostate cancer.

12. Answer: 3

Rationale: The scrotal sac is asymmetric. In darker complexion men, the scrotal skin is often darker than the body. On all men, the scrotal surface may be coarse with small lumps on the skin, which are sebaceous or epidermoid cysts that may have an oily discharge.

Disorders

13. Answer: 2

Rationale: An inguinal hernia presents with the stated symptoms, along with a bulge in either the groin or scrotum that becomes more obvious when standing. Epididymitis symptoms result from inflammation and lead to scrotal pain and swelling. Testicular torsion is characterized by an acute onset of pain, which is often during a period of inactivity with nausea and vomiting. A spermatocele is a fluid-filled mass, often painless, and arises from the epididymis and is usually benign.

14. Answer: 1

Rationale: Gross hematuria in a patient over 40 years old should be considered as possible bladder cancer until proven otherwise. Smoking increases the patient's risk of bladder cancer.

15. Answer: 2

Rationale: Oral phosphodiesterase-5 inhibitors are a safe, effective, and reasonable first-line therapy for erectile dysfunction (ED). The class includes commonly known drugs such as sildenafil (Viagra), vardenafil (Levitra), adalafil (Cialis), and avanafil (Stendra). Patients should be educated on side effects and proper use prior to first administration. Relationship issues can compound or cause erectile dysfunction and should be investigated as a part of the initial evaluation. Second-line therapies for the treatment of ED include intraurethral suppositories, intracavernous injections, and vacuum pump devices. If the patient has only difficulty in maintaining an erection, a constriction band or a vacuum device are the least invasive and least expensive of the current treatment options for this condition.

16. Answer: 2

Rationale: The sudden pain in testicular torsion is not relieved when the involved testicle is elevated to relieve pressure. Transillumination is associated with cystic masses, such as a hydrocele. The cremasteric reflex is usually absent. Testicular torsion is most common among neonates and adolescents, with the highest incidence during puberty.

17. Answer: 4

Rationale: After stabilization of any life-threatening injuries, patients with suspected urethral trauma should be evaluated with a retrograde urethrogram. Once urethral patency has been established, a urinary catheter can be placed.

18. Answer: 1

Rationale: The lack of pain, increase in size of scrotal contents, and transillumination are characteristic of a hydrocele. Orchitis and epididymitis are usually characterized by pain; orchitis is most often associated with parotitis or mumps. There is no history of injury, and the scrotum is usually nontender to palpation.

19. Answer: 2

Rationale: A high suspicion of disseminated gonococcal infection (DGI) resulting from an untreated infection by the bacteria *Neisseria gonorrhoeae* should be treated. DGI presents rarely in patients and includes a triad of tenosynovitis, arthritis, and dermatitis. Variable symptoms of DGI include dysuria, penile discharge, and low-grade fever. Treatment includes ceftriaxone and azithromycin or doxycycline as well as evaluation for other sexually transmitted infections.

20. Answer: 1

Rationale: Circumcision can be helpful in preventing chronic or severe phimosis and paraphimosis because both are a retraction dysfunction of the prepuce. In phimosis, the foreskin is too tight to be retracted backward over the glans penis. In paraphimosis, once the foreskin has been retracted behind the glans penis, it is too constricted to return to a position of covering the glans penis. Balanoposthitis is inflammation of the foreskin in an uncircumcised male.

21. Answer: 3

Rationale: Patients with recurrent *Neisseria* infections should be evaluated for a deficiency of the complement system. Late components of the complement pathway (C5–C9) place patients at high risk of contracting infections by *Neisseria* organisms, especially meningitis. Other reasons for recurrent infections include failure to treat the patient's partner and continued high-risk sexual activity. Safe sex education is indicated in all patients.

22. Answer: 3

Rationale: Acute epididymitis is characterized by an acute scrotal pain, dysuria, and enlarged unilateral scrotum with abdominal pain. Scrotal pain is relieved when the involved testicle is elevated.

23. Answer: 1

Rationale: In men over age 35, the most likely cause of epididymitis is *Escherichia coli (E. coli)*. These men usually have benign prostatic hypertrophy or urinary tract disorders that make them more susceptible to *E. coli*. Sexually active men under age 35 are more likely to have epididymitis because of a sexually transmitted infection, such as *Neisseria gonorrhoeae* or *Chlamydia trachomatis*. *Treponema pallidum* is the causative agent of syphilis.

24. Answer: 1

Rationale: A man with primary hypogonadism will often present with low energy and decreased libido. These same men will often have gynecomastia because of the low or absent production of gonadotropin. Men with hypogonadism often have decreased body hair, which may result in decreased need for shaving. Males with Klinefelter syndrome (chromosomal abnormality with karyotype of 47,XXY–47,XXXXY) is the most common genetic cause of male hypogonadism, with failure of both spermatic function and virilization.

25. Answer: 1

Rationale: Impotence can be commonly caused by antihypertensives, particularly beta blockers and diuretics. Other causes of impotence are diabetes, trauma, and vascular and psychological disorders.

26. Answer: 2

Rationale: The prostate secretes an alkaline fluid that helps sperm survive in the acidic environment of the female reproductive tract. Androgens are produced by Leydig cells of the testes. Sperm are produced in the seminiferous tubules of the testes.

27. Answer: 4

Rationale: The digital rectal exam (DRE) findings and elevated levels of PSA are the primary indicators of prostatic cancer and should be thoroughly evaluated by a urologist. The other options are directed toward treatment of BPH and should be considered only after prostatic cancer has been ruled out.

28. Answer: 1

Rationale: Testicular torsion can be successfully treated with immediate diagnosis and surgical intervention. Delayed diagnosis may lead to loss of the testicle. Hydrocele, epididymitis, and inguinal hernias also require referral, but do not require immediate attention.

29. Answer: 2, 3

Rationale: The adult-gerontology primary care NP should make a referral to a urologist when symptoms of urinary retention or prostatic bleeding occur. Other indications for referral include the appearance of intractable symptoms related to obstruction, recurrent or persistent urinary tract infection, increase in postvoid residual, very low urinary flow rate, and any significant changes caused by prostatic obstruction or bladder calculi.

30. Answer: 2

Rationale: In suspected acute prostatitis, only a rectal exam should be performed, if at all. Vigorous massage must be avoided because of the risk of inducing bacteremia. Although diagnostically helpful, palpation of the prostate in acute disease can be quite painful. Urine culture, urethral cultures for gonorrhea and chlamydia, and an elevated white blood cell count may be helpful in making the diagnosis.

31. Answer: 3

Rationale: BPH is often seen in men over age 50. Bladder cancer should be ruled out as a diagnosis in any patient presenting with microscopic or gross hematuria.

32. Answer: 1

Rationale: All the symptoms listed can be found in the patient with prostate cancer, but only the symptoms of hesitancy, frequency, and dysuria are localized. The patient often is asymptomatic.

33. Answer: 1

Rationale: A varicocele presents as described, whereas a hernia may transilluminate, and bowel sounds sometimes can be auscultated in the scrotum. Hernias vary in size with Valsalva maneuver. Tumors are solid and, therefore, do not transilluminate.

34. Answer: 2

Rationale: Phimosis is a retraction disorder of the penile foreskin or prepuce. It can occur at any age and is usually the result of poor hygiene and chronic infection (the foreskin cannot be retracted back over the glans penis). Paraphimosis is the inability to retract the foreskin from behind the glans penis.

35. Answer: 4

Rationale: Peyronie disease is a fibrotic condition that causes a lateral curvature of the penis during erection. Most patients simply require reassurance. Some patients with more severe symptoms may require surgical intervention.

36. Answer: 2

Rationale: Inflammation of the glans penis and prepuce (balanitis) can be associated with poor hygiene and is often found in men with poorly controlled diabetes.

37. Answer: 1

Rationale: Candidiasis is the usual cause of balanitis and is often found in men with poorly controlled diabetes.

38. Answer: 4

Rationale: In sexual dysfunction, erection, emission, or ejaculation may not be functioning because of multifactorial causes, such as medications, vascular disorders, neuropathy, and trauma. Peyronie disease and priapism are examples of erection dysfunction.

39. Answer: 3

Rationale: Epididymitis presents as described. Testicular torsion does not usually present with dysuria, although if there is any doubt, an ultrasound should be immediately performed.

40. Answer: 3

Rationale: This is the correct definition of erectile dysfunction (ED). The incidence of erectile dysfunction increases significantly in men as they age, particularly at age 60 and over. It involves a dysfunction in the hemodynamic mechanism of smooth muscle relaxation that increases blood flow in the penis and ultimately causes venous trapping (compression of subtunical venules) and rigidity. Patients who present with vascular ED are at a higher risk for cardiovascular events.

41. Answer: 1

Rationale: Priapism is a condition of prolonged penile erection related to venous obstruction and unrelated to sexual arousal. Although rare, men with sickle cell disease are at greatest risk. Men with erections lasting longer than 4 hours are at increased risk for impotence and should be evaluated immediately by a urologist.

42. Answer: 3

Rationale: Patients with undescended testicles are more prone to developing testicular cancer. The other conditions listed are not causes of testicular cancer.

43. Answer: 1

Rationale: Antihypertensive drugs, such as propranolol (Inderal LA), can cause impotence. Other common causes include cardiovascular disease, diabetes, smoking, prostate surgeries, antidepressants, and depression.

44. Answer: 3

Rationale: Gynecomastia in adolescent boys is most likely a result of hormonal imbalances experienced during puberty. In older men, it is frequently caused by medications, such as spironolactone and H2 blockers. In adolescents, the condition requires reassurance that it rarely persists beyond the age of 17.

45. Answer: 4

Rationale: Prostate cancer is usually found in men over age 65 and causes rapid onset of urinary obstructive symptoms. Palpation reveals a firm, enlarged, hard prostate. Advanced stages may include complaints of bone pain.

46. Answer: 4

Rationale: Urinary symptoms coupled with pain in the hips or back are concerning for metastatic prostate cancer. It is difficult to differentiate between BPH and prostate cancer based on symptoms alone. Prostate cancer usually has no symptoms in early stages.

47. Answer: 4

Rationale: Although rare, testicular cancer is primarily found in men under age 40 and presents as a scrotal mass with or without pain. It is commonly mistaken for epididymitis. It is second to leukemia as the most common cause of cancer in adolescent boys and is the most common cancer in men age 20–40. Trauma is not a causal factor. Men with a history of cryptorchidism are at significantly increased risk.

48. Answer: 2

Rationale: Acute bacterial prostatitis is caused by an infection in the urinary tract moving up the urethra into the prostate. The most common organisms are *Escherichia coli, Pseudomonas,* and *Enterococcus.* The condition tends to occur in men ages 30 to 50, but can be associated with BPH in older men. Chronic bacterial prostatitis is characterized by recurrent urinary tract infections. The usual antibiotic course is 2 weeks in acute prostatitis and is 1 to 3 months for chronic prostatitis.

49. Answer: 4

Rationale: Orchitis can be either bacterial or viral in nature. The viral form is often caused by mumps and the bacterial form of the disease is often as a result of *Escherichia coli,* spread from a worsening epididymitis. The disorder can range from being uncomfortable to painful, and often presents with constitutional symptoms.

50. Answer: 2

Rationale: Nongonococcal urethritis (NGU) is often asymptomatic and is difficult to diagnose. NGU typically has a clear discharge and usually is caused by chlamydia. Gonococcal urethritis produces a yellow, purulent discharge. If there is a discharge, NGU is difficult to differentiate from gonorrhea without a culture. Epididymitis and reactive arthritis are also associated with untreated chlamydial infection of the urogenital tract.

51. Answer: 1

Rationale: *Chlamydia trachomatis* is the most common organism in male patients with NGU.

52. Answer: 1

Rationale: Alpha-fetoprotein (AFP), lactate dehydrogenase (LDH), and human chorionic gonadotropin (hCG) are all useful tumor markers for testicular cancer.

53. Answer: 3

Rationale: The mumps virus is responsible for causing orchitis. Arbovirus and echovirus are implicated in meningitis and encephalitis. Rubeola is associated with complications of otitis media, pneumonia, croup, and encephalitis.

54. Answer: 3

Rationale: Obstructive symptoms are common in BPH. Dribbling, hesitancy, loss of normal urine stream, and recurrent urinary tract infections are present in chronic bacterial prostatitis. Dysuria, urgency, frequency, nocturia, and suprapubic heaviness are common symptoms of cystitis. Fever, chills, flank pain, headache, malaise, and costovertebral angle tenderness of acute onset with or without hematuria are indications of pyelonephritis.

55. Answer: 2

Rationale: This is considered a urologic emergency because of the inability to void and because the circulation to the penis may be compromised. The patient should be referred immediately to a urologist.

56. Answer: 4

Rationale: Dysuria is one of the most common complaints of young men with gonorrhea. No lesions, rash, or urinary dribbling accompanies the yellow discharge.

57. Answer: 3

Rationale: The symptoms described are consistent with testicular torsion. This is an emergent surgical problem, and the patient should be referred immediately.

58. Answer: 2

Rationale: The patient's age, presentation, and uncircumcised state put him at risk for the relatively rare condition of penile cancer. Balanitis does not present with a serosanguineous drainage. Human papillomavirus (HPV) is frequently associated with this type of cancer.

59. Answer: 2

Rationale: Diabetes is a common contributor to erectile dysfunction because of the impaired circulation.

60. Answer: 4

Rationale: This patient has classic symptoms of secondary syphilis. Granuloma inguinale also presents with ulcerative lesions on the penis and lymphadenopathy, but lacks the maculopapular rash and the systemic symptoms associated with syphilis. In this stage, syphilis is particularly infectious.

61. Answer: 1

Rationale: Many patients with genital herpes experience a prodrome of constitutional symptoms with their primary infection. In syphilis, systemic symptoms appear weeks to months after the genital lesions. Gonorrhea and granuloma inguinale are not typically associated with constitutional symptoms.

62. Answer: 1

Rationale: Vesicular lesions on an erythematous base are typical of genital herpes. Later in the course of the outbreak, the blisters break and leave a painful sore. Chancres on the penis are associated with syphilis. Purulent urethral discharge is found in those with gonorrhea or chlamydia infection. Small, flattened papules are associated with genital warts.

63. Answer: 4

Rationale: Testicular cancer affects around 8500 men per year in the United States. Treatment is effective and there are fewer than 400 who will die of the disease. The United States Preventive Services Task Force recommends against screening for testicular cancer because it is unreliable, is of low incidence, and false-positives cause anxiety. A major risk factor for testicular cancer is cryptorchidism (undescended testicles).

64. Answer: 4

Rationale: This involves the differential diagnosis between epididymitis and testicular torsion. Ultrasound is the preferred diagnostic test. Irreversible damage will be done to the testicles if torsion is not released in 3–4 hours. Time should not be wasted with other treatments if torsion is strongly suspected.

Pharmacology

65. Answer: 2

Rationale: Phosphodiesterase-5 inhibitors should be taken 30 to 60 minutes prior to intercourse. Large, fatty meals interfere with absorption and should be avoided. Although this class of medications works best for treating erectile dysfunction, there are other medications that can be prescribed by a urologist should they not prove to be effective.

66. Answer: 2

Rationale: Common side effects of phosphodiesterase-5 inhibitors include headaches and flushing due to vasodilation. Erectile dysfunction lasting longer than 4 hours is rare but should be promptly evaluated in an emergency room or by a urologist.

67. Answer: 3

Rationale: Patients who are on phosphodiesterase-5 inhibitors cannot concurrently take nitrates due to dangerous effects of synergistic vasodilation. Patients who are on selective serotonin reuptake inhibitors, nitrates, and thiazide diuretics often find that phosphodiesterase-5 inhibitors are effective for treating erectile dysfunction.

68. Answer: 1

Rationale: Doxazosin is also used as an antihypertensive agent; the patient may be experiencing orthostatic hypotension. The other options are directed toward evaluating his BPH, which has already been diagnosed.

69. Answer: 3

Rationale: Doxazosin is indicated as treatment in both BPH and hypertension due to its favorable side effect. Both tamsulosin and doxazosin are alpha 1 blockers. Tamsulosin has a low potential to cause hypotension and syncope. Finasteride, a 5-alpha-reductase inhibitor, is indicated for treatment of BPH. Tadalafil is a phosphodiesterase-5 (PDE-5) inhibitor indicated for BPH and erectile dysfunction.

70. Answer: 3

Rationale: Topical antifungals, such as clotrimazole, are appropriate for mild-to-moderate disease. Oral agents, such as metronidazole or fluconazole, can also be used to treat this disorder.

71. Answer: 1

Rationale: The patient is presenting with classic symptoms of acute bacterial prostatitis. The treatment of choice is IM ceftriaxone plus oral tetracycline.

72. Answer: 2

Rationale: Tamsulosin (Flomax) is an alpha-1 blocker indicated for use in benign prostatic hypertrophy. Common side effects include syncope due to orthostatic hypotension, dizziness, decreased ejaculate, and loss of libido. Patients should be reassured that the decreased volume of ejaculate is not worrisome.

73. Answer: 2

Rationale: The patient is presenting with classic symptoms of epididymitis. The treatment of choice is a fluoroquinolone, such as levofloxacin or ciprofloxacin. Nitrofurantoin is a urinary antiseptic, doxazosin is given for BPH, and oxybutynin is indicated for incontinence or enuresis.

74. Answer: 3

Rationale: Finasteride has some risk to women of childbearing age. It is important that women of childbearing age not be exposed to the sperm of a patient taking finasteride. These women and pregnant women should avoid handling crushed tablets. Exposure can cause fetal abnormalities.

75. Answer: 4

Rationale: The recommended treatment is for at least 30–45 days to prevent recurrence. Patients may require continued suppression therapy for an extended period.

76. Answer: 2

Rationale: Pentoxifylline (Trental) 400 mg PO bid is a reasonable choice in a patient with moderate curvature of the penis. Vitamin E is also commonly used. Oxybutynin (Ditropan) is used to treat symptoms of overactive bladder. Surgical treatment is indicated for patients in the chronic phase when the fibrosis has stabilized and if the deformity significantly limits or interferes with sexual intercourse; otherwise, medical management is more helpful during the initial or acute phase.

16

Female Reproductive

Physical Examination & Diagnostic Tests

1. Which two patients should have a Papanicolaou (Pap) smear test performed by the adult-gerontology primary care NP?
   1. An 18-year-old female patient who is not sexually active.
   2. A 45-year-old female patient who denies sexual activity but has two children.
   3. A 21-year-old female patient who denies sexual activity.
   4. A 16-year-old female patient who is not sexually active.

2. An adult-gerontology primary care NP has just reviewed bone mineral density (DEXA) report for a 65-year-old postmenopausal woman and noted normal findings. Which interval timeframe should be utilized for repeated DEXA screening so as to have more predictive value with regard to fracture risk?
   1. Greater than 2 years.
   2. DEXA should be performed on an annual basis.
   3. In 2 years from the date of the initial screening test.
   4. There is no need for repeated testing.

3. When obtaining a cervical specimen for a conventional Pap smear, the adult-gerontology primary care NP:
   1. Lubricates the speculum with a non–water-soluble lubricant to assist in the insertion of the instrument.
   2. Uses a cotton-tipped applicator when obtaining the cervical cells from a prenatal patient.
   3. Uses warm water to lubricate the speculum to assist in the insertion of the instrument.
   4. Completes the bimanual portion of the exam first in order to determine the relative position of the cervix to assist in the comfortable insertion of the speculum.

4. To promote patient comfort before performing a pelvic exam, the adult-gerontology primary care NP:
   1. Asks the patient to bear down slightly as the speculum is inserted.
   2. Has the patient empty her bladder.

   3. Explains each step of the procedure in a calm manner.
   4. Carefully reassures the patient that the exam will only take a few minutes.

5. What finding is considered a normal surface characteristic of the cervix?
   1. Small, yellow, raised round area on cervix.
   2. Red patches with occasional white spots.
   3. Friable, bleeding tissue at opening of cervical os.
   4. Irregular granular surface with red patches.

6. The primary role of a breast ultrasound is to:
   1. Screen for breast cancer.
   2. Definitively diagnose breast cancer.
   3. Determine if a breast lesion is cystic or solid.
   4. Locate small lesions before surgery.

7. The screening bone mineral density (DEXA) report ordered for a 60-year-old postmenopausal woman shows a result of −1.5 SD (standard deviation) at the hip. She gives a past history of myocardial infarction (MI) 1 year ago and wrist fracture at age 32. What option would *not* be considered for this patient?
   1. Counsel on smoking cessation and alcohol consumption.
   2. Initiate therapy with continuous conjugated estrogen 0.625 mg and medroxyprogesterone acetate (MPA) 2.5 mg.
   3. Initiate therapy with raloxifene (Evista).
   4. Encourage weight-bearing exercises and increased calcium intake.

8. When is the optimal time to perform a hysterosalpingogram (HSG)?
   1. During menses.
   2. Immediately after ovulation.
   3. After menses, but before ovulation.
   4. 3–4 days before menses.

9. Which statement about mammography is *false*?
   1. Mammography detects all breast cancers.
   2. Mammography should be accompanied by a breast exam.
   3. Negative mammography should not delay biopsy of a clinically suspicious mass.
   4. Mammography is a cost-effective method to screen for breast cancer.

10. The use of potassium hydroxide (KOH) when doing a wet mount assists in the diagnosis of:
    1. Bacterial vaginosis and candida vaginitis.
    2. Trichomoniasis and chlamydia cervicitis.
    3. Syphilis and gonorrhea.
    4. Herpes simplex and condyloma.

11. Which three factors, if noted in a patient's medical history, would alert the adult-gerontology primary care NP to an increased risk for development of osteoporotic fractures?
    1. Patient is a smoker.
    2. No parental history of hip fractures.
    3. Body mass index (BMI) has been stable for several years at 23.9.
    4. History of rheumatoid arthritis.
    5. Progressive loss of height noted by measurement within last 2 years.

12. The adult-gerontology primary care NP is reviewing the laboratory results of an 18-year-old patient seen recently for a Pap smear: Classification: high-grade squamous intraepithelial lesion; endocervical cells seen; adequate smear. The adult-gerontology primary care NP phones the patient and tells her which of the following?
    1. "Your Pap smear was normal. Follow up in 1 year, or sooner if problems arise."
    2. "Your Pap smear shows invasive cancer. I would like you to see a gynecologic oncologist for treatment."
    3. "Your Pap smear shows abnormal tissue that needs to be evaluated. Please schedule an appointment for a colposcopy."
    4. "Your Pap smear shows a minor abnormality. Sometimes this can signify a disease process just beginning. Please schedule another Pap smear in 4 months for follow-up."

13. A 27-year-old patient reports the desire to become pregnant. She and her husband have had regular, unprotected intercourse for more than 1 year. The adult-gerontology primary care NP completes a thorough history and gynecologic exam, which appear normal. What diagnostic test might be ordered early in the workup?
    1. Hysterosalpingogram.
    2. Tests for antisperm antibodies.
    3. Semen analysis.
    4. Endometrial biopsy.

14. For which of the following women does the National Osteoporosis Foundation (NOF) recommend a screening bone DEXA scan? Select two responses.
    1. A 48-year-old white woman who smokes and has excessive alcohol intake.
    2. A 50-year-old woman having irregular menstrual cycles.
    3. A 51-year-old woman on long-term corticosteroid therapy.
    4. A 54-year-old woman receiving hormone replacement therapy (HRT).
    5. A 45-year-old woman who plays tennis regularly and recently fractured her ulna while playing.

15. When describing the findings from a normal breast exam, what would the adult-gerontology primary care NP document on the patient record?
    1. Left nipple everted, several coarse black hairs arising from areola, enlarged axillary lymph nodes palpated bilaterally, tender nodes in supraclavicular area.
    2. No dimpling or retraction; 1-cm hard, fixed, stellate mass noted next to nipple with scant nipple discharge; no pain or tenderness on palpation.
    3. Right breast slightly larger and denser than left with no nipple discharge, right areola dark pink in color and inverted, left areola dark brown in color and everted, breasts tender to palpation with no axillary nodes noted.
    4. Pendulous breasts with no dimpling, retraction, nipple discharge, or areas of discoloration; numerous small nevi near areola with Montgomery tubercles noted, no supraclavicular or axillary lymph nodes palpated.

16. In an infertility workup, what is the best way to evaluate ovulation?
    1. Hysterosalpingogram.
    2. Postcoital test.
    3. Endometrial biopsy.
    4. Basal body temperature (BBT) chart.

17. The adult-gerontology primary care NP is reviewing the laboratory results of a 61-year-old patient seen recently for a Pap smear: atrophic changes, scant endocervical cells, and adequate smear. She has been treated for breast cancer with mastectomy and tamoxifen (Nolvadex). She has never received hormone replacement therapy (HRT). What is appropriate for the adult-gerontology primary care NP to tell the patient when she phones her with her results?
    1. "Your Pap smear is slightly abnormal. I would recommend the use of some estrogen vaginal cream nightly for 3 weeks, then return to the office to have the Pap smear repeated."
    2. "Your Pap smear is normal, but shows a mild thinning of the tissue. This is to be expected in someone who is postmenopausal and not on hormones, and it does not pose a threat to your health. Please return to the office in 1 year for your annual exam, or sooner if needed."

3. "Your Pap smear shows that you don't have enough endocervical cells. Please make an appointment for endocervical curettage."

4. "Your Pap smear is abnormal. This could signify a disease state of the cervix. Please schedule a colposcopy at your earliest convenience."

18. Which test is the "gold standard" for the diagnosis of chlamydial infection?
    1. Use of KOH wet mount "whiff" test.
    2. Presence of inflammatory cells in Pap smear.
    3. Direct fluorescent antibody (DFA) test.
    4. Culture with special media and collection technique.

19. The adult-gerontology primary care NP is discussing mammography with a group of women and providing the recommendation from the American Cancer Society. What important information should the adult-gerontology primary care NP include in the discussion?
    1. A mammogram should be done annually for all women of childbearing age.
    2. All women age 40 years and older should have a mammogram annually.
    3. A mammogram should be done annually after pregnancy if the woman does not breastfeed.
    4. A mammogram should be done only if the woman has breast pain or nipple retraction.

20. Which is the *most* accurate statement regarding a reactive serologic test for syphilis?
    1. All reactive serologic tests require confirmation with a treponemal test.
    2. Reactive serologic tests are highly suspicious for active syphilis.
    3. A false-positive serologic test, although rare, can be unnecessarily traumatizing to a patient.
    4. A reactive serologic test most likely implies the need for re-treatment.

21. In the workup for a patient with secondary amenorrhea, the prolactin serum assay results show a level of 24 ng/mL. Appropriate management includes:
    1. Administering medroxyprogesterone acetate (MPA; Provera) 10 mg PO bid × 5 days.
    2. Referral to a specialist.
    3. Recording the results as WNL (within normal limits).
    4. Assessment for nipple discharge.

22. In the evaluation of a young adult with amenorrhea and normal secondary sex characteristics, the purpose of the progesterone challenge is to determine the presence of:
    1. Endogenous estrogen.
    2. Thyroxine.
    3. Prolactin.
    4. Adequate body fat.

23. A patient comes to the office complaining of fatigue, breast tenderness, abdominal bloating, fluid retention, and irritability about a week before onset of her menses. This has been occurring for the past 4 months. What is the most important information for the adult-gerontology primary care NP to obtain to assist in determining the diagnosis of premenstrual syndrome (PMS)?
    1. Point in menstrual cycle when symptoms occur.
    2. Severity of symptoms.
    3. Number and frequency of symptoms over past 4 months.
    4. Presence or absence of anxiety or depression.

24. A 65-year-old woman reports to the clinic stating she has been experiencing intermittent vaginal bleeding over the last 2 months. Her last menstrual period was more than 10 years ago. Her last Pap smear at the clinic 9 months ago was within normal limits (WNL). She is not taking any hormonal products. She is sexually active with occasional complaints of dyspareunia. What is the *most* appropriate response of the adult-gerontology primary care NP at this time?
    1. Order complete blood count and thyroid-stimulating hormone and repeat Pap smear.
    2. Schedule laparoscopy.
    3. Schedule endometrial biopsy.
    4. Schedule pelvic/transvaginal ultrasonography.

Normal Gynecology

25. An adult-gerontology primary care NP is reviewing information about follicle-stimulating hormone (FSH) in female patients. Place or drag/drop the phase in order of sequence from highest to lowest levels of FHS under normal physiological conditions.
    1. Follicular phase.
    2. Luteal phase.
    3. Ovulation phase.
    4. Postmenopausal women.

26. The endometrial cycle is often described in three phases. Select the correct phases:
    1. Follicular, menstrual, and luteal.
    2. Proliferative, luteal, and menstrual.
    3. Follicular, secretory, and menstrual.
    4. Proliferative, secretory, and menstrual.

27. The adult-gerontology primary care NP understands that premenstrual syndrome (PMS) occurs with greatest frequency and severity in the:
    1. Late luteal phase.
    2. Follicular phase.
    3. Proliferative phase.
    4. Ovulatory phase.

28. Which three hormones are released from the anterior pituitary gland?
    1. Follicle-stimulating hormone (FSH).
    2. Luteinizing hormone (LH).
    3. Oxytocin.
    4. Prolactin.
    5. Antidiuretic hormone (ADH).

29. What is the primary function of follicle stimulating hormone (FSH)?
    1. Stimulation of maturation of ovarian follicles.
    2. Milk secretion.
    3. Triggering ovulation.
    4. Inhibiting release of luteinizing hormone (LH) from the pituitary gland.

30. How is the term *menopause* best defined?
    1. Cessation of ability for natural reproduction.
    2. Completion of 12 months of amenorrhea after last menstrual period.
    3. Follicle stimulating hormone (FSH) level of 30 and estradiol level of 30.
    4. Last menstrual period.

31. In the ovarian cycle, what phase begins with ovulation and ends with the onset of menses?
    1. Follicular phase.
    2. Ovulation.
    3. Proliferative phase.
    4. Luteal phase.

32. Which is not a risk factor for heart disease in the postmenopausal female?
    1. Regular exercise.
    2. Cigarette smoking.
    3. Hormone replacement therapy.
    4. Diabetes mellitus.

33. An adult patient's last menstrual period (LMP) was 2 months ago. She has had an intrauterine device (IUD) in place for the last 4 months. She is complaining of nausea, fatigue, breast tenderness, and abdominal bloating. Physical exam reveals the following:
    • Abdomen: no abnormalities noted.
    • Pelvic: cervix—positive Chadwick sign, IUD strings protruding from cervical os.
    • Uterus: enlarged and nontender.
    • Adnexae: nontender, without mass and no cervical motion tenderness.
    What is the most likely diagnosis?
    1. Uterine fibroid.
    2. Ovarian cancer.
    3. Dislodged IUD.
    4. Pregnancy.

34. Which of the following clinical symptoms would occur in response to vaginal changes during menopause?

1. Increase in acidity causing pelvic discomfort.
2. Increased vaginal discharge because of increased lubrication.
3. Hypertrophy of vaginal tissue leading to pelvic discomfort.
4. Increased likelihood to develop urinary tract infections due to change in vaginal flora.

35. What function do the Bartholin glands have in reproduction?
    1. Prevent vaginitis by maintaining adequate pH.
    2. Prepare the mucous plug that occurs during early pregnancy.
    3. Produce an alkaline secretion that enhances sperm viability.
    4. Produce small amounts of hormones necessary for ovulation.

36. Which is not a risk factor for osteoporosis?
    1. Cigarette smoker.
    2. White race.
    3. Alcohol consumption.
    4. Obesity.

37. A young woman complains to the adult-gerontology primary care NP that she is experiencing headaches, irritability, decreased appetite, and fatigue about 1 week before menses. Appropriate management includes which of the following?
    1. Treat premenstrual syndrome (PMS) with increased protein and salt in the diet.
    2. Incorporate daily aerobic exercise and dietary changes into her lifestyle.
    3. Order complete blood count (CBC), comprehensive metabolic panel, and urinalysis.
    4. Supplement her diet with an additional 1–2 g of vitamin C.

38. A middle-aged female presents with abnormal uterine bleeding. A hormonal profile reveals increased follicle stimulating hormone (FSH) and luteinizing hormone (LH) levels. What is the most likely cause for these findings?
    1. Hypothalamic disorder.
    2. Onset of climacteric.
    3. Premature ovarian failure.
    4. Anterior pituitary disorder.

39. A 29-year-old patient presents to the adult-gerontology primary care planning clinic for her annual exam. She had a tubal ligation postpartum 6 months ago. She has been feeling tired, is nauseated, and is slowly gaining weight. She had one menses postpartum, 4 months ago. The adult-gerontology primary care NP notes the following on physical exam:
    • Abdomen: bowel sounds × 4, soft, no hepatosplenomegaly, palpable mass in lower abdomen measures 14 cm, no tenderness.

- Pelvic: Bartholin/urethral/Skene glands (BUS) normal; cervix: os closed, smooth pink mucosa.
- Bimanual: uterus enlarged, nontender, smooth contours, no cervical motion tenderness.
- Adnexae: not palpable.

What is the likely diagnosis?
1. Pregnancy.
2. Uterine fibroid.
3. Premature menopause.
4. Colon cancer.

40. Which physical finding would be present in a patient with a clinical diagnosis of uterine fibroids?
    1. Diarrhea.
    2. Shoulder pain.
    3. Increased blood flow during menses.
    4. Amenorrhea.

41. Menopause occurs at a mean age of 51 years. Which of the following factors has been linked to influencing the age at which menopause occurs?
    1. Use of oral contraceptives.
    2. Socioeconomic status.
    3. Age at menarche.
    4. Smoking.

Gynecologic Disorders

42. A female patient presents to the clinic with complaints of pelvic pressure and discomfort. When questioned about her menstrual cycle, the patient relates a history of heavy bleeding recently. Age of menarche was 16. Pelvic examination of the uterus reveals a bicornuate uterus. The adult-gerontology primary care NP suspects that the patient may have:
    1. Premenstrual syndrome.
    2. Secondary dysmenorrhea.
    3. Pelvic inflammatory disease.
    4. Dyspareunia.

43. An adult-gerontology primary care NP is discussing therapeutic management with a patient who is being actively treated for polycystic ovarian syndrome (PCOS). Which finding would indicate that the disease has progressed?
    1. Positive pregnancy test.
    2. Hemoglobin A1c level is 5.4%.
    3. Blood pressure reading 150/92 mmHg.
    4. Menstrual period lasts between 5 and 7 days.

44. During a yearly physical exam, an adult-gerontology primary care NP asks a woman if she has any problems or questions about sexual function or activity. Initially, the patient hesitates, but with further questioning and discussion, she states that she is unsure if she has ever experienced an orgasm. The adult-gerontology primary care NP suspects:
    1. Vaginismus.
    2. Primary orgasmic dysfunction.
    3. Secondary orgasmic dysfunction.
    4. Dyspareunia.

45. The adult-gerontology primary care NP is talking with a young women who has been diagnosed with herpes simplex type 2. In discussing her care, it would be important for the adult-gerontology primary care NP to include what information?
    1. The initial lesions are usually worse than lesions that occur with outbreaks at a later time.
    2. Her sexual partner will not contract it if she does not have sex when the lesions are present.
    3. This condition can be treated and cured if she takes all of the antibiotics for 2 weeks.
    4. If she becomes pregnant in the future, she will need to have a cesarean delivery.

46. The definition of bacterial vaginosis is:
    1. A syndrome resulting from homeostatic disruption in the vagina.
    2. Vaginitis caused by a flagellated protozoan.
    3. A bacterial sexually transmitted infection that can be symptomatic or asymptomatic.
    4. A virus characterized by recurrent outbreaks and remissions.

47. A 22-year-old married patient complains of severe dysmenorrhea. Her gynecologic exam is normal. Which management protocol is preferred?
    1. Assess for contraceptive interest and, if interested, suggest use of oral contraceptives (OCs).
    2. Suggest use of a prostaglandin synthetase inhibitor.
    3. Suggest use of over-the-counter ibuprofen.
    4. Assess exercise patterns and use of relaxation techniques.

48. Which is not a criterion for the diagnosis of bacterial vaginosis?
    1. Positive amine test (whiff test).
    2. Presence of clue cells.
    3. Vaginal pH >4.5.
    4. Presence of pseudohyphae.

49. A patient with a history of dilation and curettage (D&C) after a first-trimester spontaneous abortion and subsequent amenorrhea would lead the adult-gerontology primary care NP to a working diagnosis of which of the following?
    1. Polycystic ovarian syndrome.
    2. Asherman syndrome.
    3. Hypogonadism.
    4. Premature ovarian failure.

50. The LH/FSH ratio in polycystic ovarian syndrome (Stein-Leventhal syndrome) is:
    1. 1.5:1.
    2. 3:1.
    3. 6:1.
    4. 1:3.

51. What are common findings in a patient with polycystic ovarian syndrome?
    1. Weight loss, dental caries, and amenorrhea.
    2. Hyperprolactinemia and galactorrhea.
    3. Dysmenorrhea, nodules palpated on bimanual exam, and infertility.
    4. Chronic irregular menses, hirsutism, and increased abdominal girth.

52. What is the most common cause of dysfunctional uterine bleeding?
    1. Thyroid disorder.
    2. Blood dyscrasia.
    3. Anovulation.
    4. Uterine tumor.

53. A 30-year-old patient presents with scant pubic hair, minimal breast development, absent cervix, and uterus with a 46,XY karyotype. Which diagnosis would the adult-gerontology primary care NP suspect?
    1. Turner syndrome.
    2. Müllerian agenesis.
    3. Testicular feminization.
    4. Gonadal dysgenesis.

54. The most common cause of a breast mass in patients ages 15–25 is:
    1. Fibroadenoma.
    2. Intraductal papilloma.
    3. Infiltrating lobular carcinoma.
    4. Fibrocystic breast syndrome.

55. An effective treatment for primary dysmenorrhea is:
    1. Nonsteroidal antiinflammatory drugs (NSAIDs).
    2. Tranquilizers.
    3. Progestins.
    4. Steroids.

56. What is a cause of secondary amenorrhea?
    1. Testicular feminization.
    2. Hypogonadotropic hypogonadism.
    3. Congenital absence of uterus.
    4. Extreme exercise.

57. A young woman comes into the clinic for a well-woman checkup. She states that, about 3 weeks ago, she had a sore on her labia that went away. It was not particularly painful, did not itch, and apparently caused no residual prob-

lems. The adult-gerontology primary care NP would treat this patient by:
    1. Ordering the treponemal-specific test (FTA-ABS).
    2. Swabbing the area of the lesion for a viral culture.
    3. Advising her to notify her sexual contacts to determine if they have had any symptoms.
    4. Ordering nystatin (Mycostatin) cream to be applied to the area three or four times a day.

58. Which is not a risk factor for the development of cervical cancer?
    1. Human papillomavirus (HPV).
    2. Virginal status.
    3. Multiple sexual partners.
    4. Previous high-grade squamous intraepithelial lesion (HSIL).

59. A young woman is complaining of tenderness and burning of her vulva. On exam, the vulva is edematous and excoriated. The adult-gerontology primary care NP performs a wet mount preparation of the vaginal secretions. It reveals pseudohyphae and spores. The diagnosis for this patient is:
    1. Vulvovaginal candidiasis.
    2. Chlamydial infection.
    3. Bacterial vaginosis.
    4. Gonorrhea.

60. The leading cause of mortality in women with genital cancer, excluding breast, is:
    1. Ovarian cancer.
    2. Endometrial cancer.
    3. Cervical cancer.
    4. Vulvar/vaginal cancer.

61. A young woman presents with complaints of an irritation in the vaginal area. This is the first time it has occurred. On vaginal exam, the cervix is inflamed and friable. Flagellated protozoa are seen on the wet mount. The most likely diagnosis is:
    1. Trichomoniasis.
    2. Cervicitis.
    3. Chlamydial infection.
    4. Bacterial vaginosis.

62. A 26-year-old female patient presents to the emergency department complaining of gradual onset of abdominal pain. The pain started in the periumbilical region and is now in the right lower quadrant, accompanied by nausea, anorexia, constipation, and low-grade fever. Physical exam confirms the diagnosis of acute appendicitis. What diagnostic studies are least useful in confirming this diagnosis?
    1. Complete blood count (CBC) with differential.
    2. Flat plate of abdomen, kidneys-ureter-bladder (KUB).
    3. Pelvic ultrasound.
    4. Pregnancy test.

63. Which is not a risk factor for endometrial cancer?
    1. Obesity.
    2. Oral contraceptive use.
    3. Unopposed estrogen use.
    4. Advancing age, >50 years.

64. Which statement is true regarding the diaphragm?
    1. May be inserted up to 24 hours before intercourse.
    2. May be inserted any time up to 6 hours before intercourse.
    3. Should be removed within 1 hour after intercourse.
    4. Should not be left in place longer than 24 hours.

65. A contraceptive method associated with an increase in urinary tract infections (UTIs) is the:
    1. Intrauterine device.
    2. Diaphragm.
    3. Norplant.
    4. Oral contraception.

66. Which is not a risk factor for ovarian cancer?
    1. Family history of ovarian cancer.
    2. Advancing age, >50 years.
    3. Oral contraceptive use.
    4. Positive *BRCA-2* gene.

67. What is the most common female genital malignancy, excluding the breast?
    1. Ovary.
    2. Endometrium.
    3. Cervix.
    4. Vulva/vagina.

68. A 20-year-old college student presents to urgent care with new onset of painful sores in the vulva. These erupted yesterday and are associated with exquisite pain, fever, and flulike symptoms of headache, general body aches, and mild dysuria. She has a new sexual partner. The exam reveals vesicular lesions covering the labia, extreme tenderness of external genitalia to palpation, normal Bartholin glands (BUS), normal vaginal inspection with mild leukorrhea, normal cervical mucosa, and slightly tender, minimally enlarged inguinal lymph nodes bilaterally. What is the likely diagnosis?
    1. Gonorrhea.
    2. Chlamydial infection.
    3. Herpes simplex virus.
    4. Lymphogranuloma venereum.

69. A 21-year-old patient is seen for her annual gynecologic exam. She is sexually active, rarely uses condoms for sexually transmitted disease (STD) prevention, and has multiple sexual partners. She smokes one pack of cigarettes per day, admits to a sedentary lifestyle, and eats two meals per day, most often at fast-food restaurants. Her exam is negative for any abnormalities. Her family history and personal medical history are negative for major disease. She has no menstrual abnormalities; her last menstrual period was 1 week ago. The adult-gerontology primary care NP has done her Pap smear. Which would not be appropriate for this patient?
    1. Cultures for gonorrhea and *Chlamydia*.
    2. Laboratory testing of glucose, cardiac risk profile, and thyroid stimulating hormone (TSH).
    3. Human immunodeficiency (HIV) titer and rapid plasma reagin (RPR).
    4. Counseling on safe sex practice and contraceptive information.

70. Which are considered to be three risk factors in the development of breast cancer?
    1. Early menopause.
    2. High-fat diet.
    3. Advancing age.
    4. Early menarche.
    5. Nonproliferative fibroadenomas.

71. A 32-year-old female patient, G2 T1 P1 A0 L2, is seen in the clinic by the adult-gerontology primary care NP for her annual exam and is requesting information on preconception counseling. She has been taking oral contraceptives (OCs) for 3 years without complications. During the past year she has started an exercise program at a health club 5 days a week and is eating three nutritionally sound meals daily. She has lost 33 lbs and is now at her ideal body weight. She quit her job as a postal worker and now stays home with her children. As part of her preconception care, what should the adult-gerontology primary care NP recommend?
    1. Start prenatal vitamins with folic acid.
    2. Discontinue exercise.
    3. Update measles-mumps-rubella (MMR) vaccine.
    4. Start genetic counseling due to advanced maternal age.

72. The initial workup for abnormal uterine bleeding should include:
    1. Referral for diagnostic dilatation and curettage (D&C).
    2. Referral for endometrial biopsy to rule out cancer.
    3. Complete blood count (CBC), pregnancy test, and endocrine studies.
    4. Coagulation studies and sexually transmitted disease (STD) cultures.

73. Which is not a risk factor for breast cancer?
    1. History of maternal breast cancer, premenopausal onset.
    2. First pregnancy after age 35.
    3. Late menopause, after age 54.
    4. Fibrocystic breast disease.

74. A 21-year-old female patient presents for her first well-woman exam. She has never been sexually active. Her family history and past medical history are negative for any gynecologic diseases. Her menses occur every 28 days, lasting 5 days, with a relatively moderate flow and no significant abdominal cramps. Her physical exam/visit today should include which tests?
    1. Pap smear.
    2. Cultures for gonorrhea and *Chlamydia*.
    3. Stool hemoccult.
    4. Baseline mammogram.

75. What is the leading cause of death for women in the United States?
    1. Breast cancer.
    2. Colon cancer.
    3. Heart disease.
    4. Stroke.

76. Reactive cellular changes noted on a Pap smear are most often associated with:
    1. Inflammation.
    2. Use of estrogen vaginal cream.
    3. Drying artifact.
    4. Use of oral contraceptives (OCs).

77. Risk factors for cervical cancer include:
    1. Pregnancy after age 35.
    2. Viral exposure.
    3. Low parity.
    4. Prolonged contraceptive use.

78. What is the most common cancer in women in the United States?
    1. Breast cancer.
    2. Colon cancer.
    3. Malignant melanoma.
    4. Lung cancer.

79. A 48-year-old patient presents to the clinic complaining of hot flashes, no menses for 14 months, insomnia, crying spells, irritability, decreased libido, and fatigue. At the end of her history and physical, she begins to cry and tells the adult-gerontology primary care NP that she "thinks she's going crazy." She then begs the adult-gerontology primary care NP to tell her what is wrong. Which action is inappropriate for the adult-gerontology primary care NP to do at this point?
    1. Obtain laboratory tests, including follicle stimulating hormone (FSH) and luteinizing hormone (LH).
    2. Discuss hormone replacement therapy (HRT), including risks and benefits and short- and long-term treatment strategies.
    3. Provide antidepressant therapy and a referral for counseling sessions for depression.
    4. Provide written information regarding menopause and options for treatment of symptoms.

80. Care for a patient with chancroid should include:
    1. Screening for HIV as well as syphilis.
    2. Mandatory notification and treatment of all sexual partners.
    3. Screening for lymphogranuloma venereum.
    4. Culture for gonorrhea.

81. During her annual exam, a 35-year-old patient complains of recent breast changes. She states that her breasts are painful and frequently feel "lumpy." Because of this, she has stopped doing monthly breast self-exam (BSE), believing BSE is a "waste of time." What would be the most appropriate advice for the adult-gerontology primary care NP to give to this patient?
    1. Stress the importance of the woman knowing the normal look and feel of her breasts and to report any changes.
    2. Suggest she at least do BSE every 2 months.
    3. Suggest she start having mammograms to establish some baseline data about her breasts.
    4. Determine when her breasts are nontender and least "lumpy," and change her BSE schedule.

82. During a breast exam on a young woman, palpation reveals a painless, 2-cm lobular mass in the right breast that is firm and freely mobile. Appropriate management includes:
    1. Continued observation and rechecking in 3 months.
    2. Referral for a mammogram.
    3. Referral for probable surgical excision.
    4. Detailed family history to determine breast cancer risk.

83. A woman with bilateral breast implants asks if it is really necessary to do monthly breast self-exam (BSE) because she "does not know what to feel for." The most appropriate response would be:
    1. Suggest she involve her sexual partner in assessing her breasts on a regular basis.
    2. Review the steps in BSE until she feels comfortable with the process.
    3. Acknowledge the difficulty of doing BSE after implant surgery.
    4. Explain the usefulness of regular mammograms for implant patients.

84. An adult patient comes to the clinic complaining of abnormal vaginal discharge (dark watery brown) along with postcoital bleeding. The adult-gerontology primary care NP suspects the possibility of cancer of the cervix. During the vaginal exam, suspicious physical results would be:
    1. Soft, sill-shaped cervix.
    2. Very firm cervix with an ulcer.
    3. Vague lower abdominal discomfort.
    4. Tender, enlarged lymph nodes.

85. A postmenopausal patient is worried about pain in the upper outer quadrant of her left breast. The adult-gerontology primary care NP should:
    1. Do a breast exam and order a mammogram.
    2. Explain that the pain is related to hormone fluctuations, and order laboratory studies.
    3. Reassure the patient that pain is not a presenting symptom of breast cancer, and check for proper fit of the brassiere.
    4. Teach the patient breast self-exam (BSE).

86. A 22-year-old female patient comes to the adult-gerontology primary care NP's office with a complaint of 1 day of fever of 102°F (38.9°C), a diffuse macular rash, vomiting, headache, and decreased urine output. The history obtained by the adult-gerontology primary care NP must include:
    1. Whether the patient's immunizations are up to date.
    2. If the patient is currently menstruating.
    3. If the patient has a history of tuberculosis.
    4. What type of contraception the patient uses.

87. A young female patient presents to the adult-gerontology primary care NP's office with a complaint of abdominal pain. Which differential diagnosis should be ruled out given that the patient is of child-bearing age and could lead to increased morbidity and mortality if not treated promptly?
    1. Irritable bowel syndrome.
    2. Cholelithiasis.
    3. Pyelonephritis.
    4. Ectopic pregnancy.

88. A young adult patient presents with a history of vaginal itching and heavy white discharge. The patient gives a history of no sexual activity. On exam, the adult-gerontology primary care NP finds a red, edematous vulva and white patches on the vaginal walls. The discharge has no odor. The adult-gerontology primary care NP expects which factors in the patient's history?
    1. Vegetarian diet.
    2. Recent diarrhea.
    3. Early menopause.
    4. Recent antibiotic use.

89. A young patient comes to the office complaining of vaginal bleeding. The patient states that she has used five tampons in the past 3 hours. She admits to sexual activity and takes oral contraceptives (OCs). On further questioning, the patient states that she started her last pack of OCs "about 2 weeks late." The adult-gerontology primary care NP should:
    1. Perform a STAT urine pregnancy test.
    2. Perform a STAT complete blood count (CBC).
    3. Discuss proper use of OCs.
    4. Send the patient for a pelvic sonogram.

90. The adult-gerontology primary care NP knows that the majority of breast cancers occur in which area of the breast?
    1. Upper inner quadrant.
    2. Upper outer quadrant.
    3. Beneath the nipple and areola.
    4. Lower outer quadrant.

91. The patient presents with abnormal uterine bleeding and has been found to have endometrial cancer. She returned to the adult-gerontology primary care NP because she does not understand how this is possible when the Pap smear 6 months ago was negative. What is the adult-gerontology primary care NP's best response?
    1. "Uterine cancer develops quickly."
    2. "Pap smears are difficult to read, and mistakes can happen."
    3. "Pap smears are not useful in detecting uterine cancers in most cases."
    4. "The previous Pap smear did not have an adequate sample."

92. A postmenopausal woman is seen in the office with complaints of frequent urination, stress incontinence, vaginal dryness, and dyspareunia. Her last menstrual cycle was 6 years ago, and she elected not to take hormone replacement therapy (HRT). She has increased her intake of soy products. What is the most common cause of her symptoms?
    1. Urinary tract infection.
    2. Cystocele.
    3. Bacterial vaginitis.
    4. Atrophic vaginitis.

93. While assessing a 16-year-old girl, the adult-gerontology primary care NP was asked about douching. What information would be used in the adult-gerontology primary care NP's teaching plan?
    1. Douching during menstruation is safe.
    2. Daily douching is important because the patient has copious vaginal discharge.
    3. Hypoallergenic douches include flavored or perfumed types.
    4. Douching removes natural mucus and upsets normal vaginal flora.

94. A high school athlete presents to the clinic with concerns regarding her menstrual periods. She states she has not had a period in the past 2 months. She has been in training and running about 3 miles a day for the past 3 months. She has lost approximately 15 lbs. Her height is about 63 inches, and she currently weighs 100 lbs. What is the best response by the adult-gerontology primary care NP?
    1. Determine the patient's percentage of body fat and body mass.
    2. Obtain follicle stimulating hormone (FSH) serum levels.
    3. Determine serum levels of human chorionic gonadotropin (hCG).
    4. Order thyroid function tests.

95. During a gynecologic examination at the adult-gerontology primary care planning clinic, an underweight 17-year-old presents with bruising around her upper torso and genitalia. She is minimally interactive and avoids eye contact as much as possible. Priority intervention should focus on:
    1. Lab work to rule out bleeding disorder.
    2. Nutritional assessment to determine possible anemia.
    3. Determination of possible physical abuse.
    4. Finding out if she has a support system.

Pharmacology

96. A female patient has received treatment for *Trichomonas vaginalis* and completed the course of therapy but the patient remains symptomatic. Which two findings might prompt the adult-gerontology primary care NP that the patient has not been compliant with treatment?
    1. Patient states that she had a few alcohol drinks during the course of therapy.
    2. Uses cotton underwear as an undergarment.
    3. Did not douche during the course of therapy.
    4. Took 2 g dose of metronidazole (Flagyl) as a single dose as opposed to 500 mg twice a day dosage for 7 days.
    5. Patient reports that she has not abstained from sexual intercourse.

97. A 42-year-old female patient presents to the office with complaints of dysuria, urinary frequency, and urgency. These symptoms began early this morning. She leaves a clean-catch midstream urine specimen, which shows white blood cells (WBCs) too numerous to count (TNTC)/high-power field (HPF), 4–5 red blood cells (RBCs)/HPF, and positive nitrites. A urine culture will be ready in 3 days. Which three of the following medications might be prescribed for an uncomplicated lower urinary tract infection (UTI)?
    1. Phenazopyridine (Pyridium) 200 mg 1 tab PO tid × 2 days.
    2. Trimethoprim-sulfamethoxazole (TMP-SMX; Septra DS) 1 tab PO bid × 5 days.
    3. Ceftriaxone (Rocephin) 1 g IM.
    4. Nitrofurantoin (Macrobid) 1 tab PO bid × 5 days.
    5. Neomycin 1 g PO q6h × 5 days.

98. The results of the Women's Health Initiative (WHI) provided evidence-based data that have led to new guidelines in assessing the risk/benefit ratio for initiation of hormone replacement therapy (HRT) in postmenopausal women. Which statement is not correct?
    1. HRT is indicated for the treatment of menopausal symptoms, such as vasomotor and urogenital symptoms.

2. HRT should be continued for primary prevention of coronary heart disease.
3. HRT can be continued for the prevention of postmenopausal fractures due to osteoporosis.
4. HRT should be limited to the shortest duration consistent with treatment goals and benefits in consideration with risks in the individual woman.

99. A 46-year-old female patient is being seen in the clinic by the adult-gerontology primary care NP. She was last seen 2 weeks ago for an upper respiratory tract infection and was treated with amoxicillin (Amoxil) 250 mg PO tid × 10 days. She completed her medication last week, but now is aware of vaginal itching and has cottage cheese–like vaginal discharge. She states that she has never experienced such intense itching. She is in a mutually monogamous relationship. Her last menstrual period was 2 weeks ago. Her partner had a vasectomy 2 years ago. Wet mount with KOH shows negative whiff test, rare clue cells, positive lactobacilli, positive hyphae and spores, few WBCs, and no trichomonads. She is leaving tomorrow for a week-long cruise. She is not taking any medications and has no known drug allergies. The adult-gerontology primary care NP knows that the best treatment for this problem is:
    1. Metronidazole (Flagyl) 500 mg PO bid × 7 days.
    2. Clindamycin (Cleocin) vaginal cream one applicator full vaginally hs × 7 days.
    3. Fluconazole (Diflucan) 150 mg 1 tab PO one time.
    4. Hydrocortisone (Cortaid) 1% cream sparingly bid × 7 days.

100. A 25-year-old patient presents with complaints of a malodorous vaginal discharge, which is described as white and watery. She douches with vinegar and water every 2 weeks. She uses a diaphragm for contraception. She and her boyfriend have been sexually active for 2 years, using condoms for sexually transmitted disease prevention with every act of coitus. She denies any dyspareunia. Her last menstrual period was 1 week ago, and there are no noted changes in her normal menstrual pattern. Her wet mount with KOH results show a positive whiff test, too numerous to count clue cells/high-power field, no lactobacilli, no hyphae or spores, no trichomonads, and few WBCs. What is the diagnosis and treatment for this patient?
    1. *Chlamydia*; doxycycline (Vibratabs) 100 mg PO bid × 10 days.
    2. *Candida albicans*; terconazole (Terazol 7) vaginal cream 1 applicator hs × 7 days.
    3. Herpes simplex type 2; acyclovir (Zovirax) 200 mg PO q4h × 5 days.
    4. Bacterial vaginosis; metronidazole (Metrogel) vaginal gel 1 applicator hs × 5 days.

101. A 55-year-old patient, G2 T2 P0 A0 L2, is being seen in the clinic for her annual exam. She went through a natural menopause 5 years ago and has never been interested in hormone replacement therapy (HRT). She smokes one pack per day and does no formal exercise. Her family history is positive for osteoporosis in her mother, positive for myocardial infarction (MI) in her father, and negative for cancer. She has a normal physical exam today and had a negative mammogram yesterday. She is now interested in HRT, but wants to know her alternatives. Which choice has *not* been clinically proven for prevention of osteoporosis?
    1. Estradiol (Estrace) 0.5 mg 1 tab PO qd and micronized progesterone (Prometrium) 100 mg 1 tablet PO qd.
    2. Weight-bearing exercise three times weekly.
    3. Discontinue cigarette smoking.
    4. Wild Mexican yam cream applied to skin tid.

102. A young woman is seen in the sexually transmitted disease (STD) clinic. She noticed some itchy bumps in the vulvar area and is concerned that they could be cancer. On careful inspection, the adult-gerontology primary care NP notes five cauliflower-like, warty, pinkish lesions in the lower introitus. Two smaller lesions nestled anterior to hymeneal ring of vagina and cervix fail to reveal any abnormalities. Wet mount with KOH is negative. Culture for gonorrhea and *Chlamydia* was obtained, Pap smear done, and HIV titer and RPR drawn. Which is not an appropriate treatment for this patient?
    1. Podophyllin (Podoben) application; wash off in 6 hours with soap and water.
    2. Trichloroacetic acid application; do not wash off.
    3. Cryotherapy with liquid nitrogen to lesions.
    4. Benzathine penicillin 2.4 million units IM weekly × 3 weeks.

103. A young adult complaining of vaginal itching, thick yellow mucous discharge, and urinary discomfort is seen in the urgent care unit by the adult-gerontology primary care NP. She is sexually active and uses condoms with only one of her two partners. On physical exam, the abdomen is negative; pelvic exam reveals the Bartholin glands (BUS) within normal limits, cervix with mucopurulent discharge from the os, and mucosa friable to palpation; bimanual exam is negative. Cultures were taken, but are not yet available. Wet mount with KOH reveals a negative whiff test, few clue cells, too numerous to count WBCs/high-power field, no yeast, and no trichomonads. What is the likely diagnosis and appropriate treatment?
    1. *Chlamydia;* azithromycin (Zithromax) 1 g PO single dose.
    2. *Chlamydia;* ceftriaxone (Rocephin) 125 mg IM.
    3. Herpes simplex virus; acyclovir (Zovirax) 200 mg 1 cap PO q4h × 5 days.
    4. Trichomoniasis; metronidazole (Flagyl) 2 g PO single dose.

104. A 52-year-old woman presents for her annual gynecologic exam from her primary care provider. She received a hysterectomy with ovarian conservation at age 40 for uterine fibroids and dysfunctional uterine bleeding. She has been taking oral estrogen (conjugated equine estrogen 0.625 mg) hormone replacement therapy (HRT) for 1 year. Although HRT has definitely reduced the discomfort of hot flashes, vaginal dryness, and mood swings from insomnia, she still experiences flashes and some night sweats. Her diagnostic lipid panel shows total cholesterol 180; LDL 112; HDL 52; and triglycerides 325. What, if any, change might be considered in her medication regimen?
    1. No change should be considered at this time.
    2. Decrease estrogen dosage to 0.3 mg daily.
    3. Recommend stopping estrogen therapy.
    4. Suggest changing route of administration to transdermal.

105. An adult female patient is seen in the family planning clinic for a consultation on contraception. She is using oral contraceptives (OCs) but forgets to take them because her work schedule changes every week; she is looking for an effective method that will be easy to remember. She has been married for 14 years, is G2 T2 P0 A0 L2, and is a nonsmoker. She has a negative past history for major diseases and a negative gynecologic history for abnormalities. She has never been treated for a sexually transmitted disease (STD) and is in a mutually monogamous relationship. She is needle phobic and faints when she has to have blood drawn. What contraceptive method would be a good choice for the patient?
    1. Depo-Provera injection every 3 months.
    2. Implantation system for 5 years.
    3. Intrauterine device (IUD).
    4. Diaphragm.

106. A young woman is seen at the family planning clinic by the adult-gerontology primary care NP. The patient wants birth control pills but has heard that oral contraceptives (OCs) are "dangerous to one's health." When asked for clarification, she lists weight gain, ovarian cancer, heavy or irregular periods, and infertility. After saying, "I can see that you are concerned about your health," what would be appropriate for the adult-gerontology primary care NP to tell the patient?
    1. "There are a lot of fallacies about birth control pills. They actually are thought to reduce the risk of ovarian cancers and to help regulate the bleeding, and they are not associated with causing infertility. There can be a minor increase in body weight of 3 to 5 pounds."
    2. "Perhaps you would be better off trying the implantation system or Depo-Provera."
    3. "What you have heard is true. They can be dangerous to your health, and many women experience these problems."
    4. "There are a lot of fallacies about birth control pills. Ovarian cancer and infertility are risks when taking the pills, but they do not cause weight gain or bleeding changes during periods. Pap smears done every year will detect such problems as ovarian cancer."

107. An adult female patient is taking oral contraceptives (OCs). She calls into the clinic with complaints of bleeding through the first 2 weeks of every package of pills. She has been taking this pill for 4 months at the same time every day. Her present OC is a low-dose monophasic pill. She is not taking any other medications and denies any adverse effects from the OCs. She would prefer to keep taking the OCs if possible. The adult-gerontology primary care NP's advice should include:
    1. Discontinue the pills and do not restart them. Use an alternative contraceptive method.
    2. Change to a higher dosage, and higher progestational agent.
    3. Try taking the pills early in the morning on an empty stomach to improve their metabolism.
    4. There is no cause for concern; breakthrough bleeding is a normal side effect of OCs.

108. An adult female patient is seen by the adult-gerontology primary care NP at the family planning clinic. The patient notes heavy, irregular menses and an increase in facial acne and facial/abdominal hair growth over the past few years. She is G1 T1 P0 A0 L1 and is not planning future pregnancies. After a normal pelvic exam, she decides she wants oral contraceptives (OCs). What is a good choice for this patient?
    1. Loestrin 1/20.
    2. Triphasil.
    3. Demulen 1/35.
    4. OCs are inappropriate for this patient.

109. A 41-year-old patient is seen for her 6-week postpartum exam by the adult-gerontology primary care NP. She is breastfeeding without difficulty and plans to continue for a year. She wants to begin using a contraceptive and plans no further pregnancies. Which of the following is an inappropriate choice for this patient?
    1. Depo-Provera 150 mg IM every 3 months.
    2. Intrauterine device (IUD).
    3. Progestin-only oral contraceptive (OC).
    4. Combination OC.

110. A 38-year-old patient is seen for her 6-week postpartum exam by the adult-gerontology primary care NP. The patient was breastfeeding for a short time but discontinued 4 weeks ago. Her menses have resumed. She is contemplating another pregnancy in about a year, but if she became pregnant before then, she "wouldn't mind." She is seeking contraception. She smokes one pack per day. Her exam is normal, with the uterus well involuted. Which of the following is contraindicated in this patient?
    1. Progestasert intrauterine device (IUD).
    2. Oral contraceptives.
    3. Depo-Provera injection.
    4. Condoms and spermicide.

111. A 22-year-old female patient presents to the urgent care department and is seen by the adult-gerontology primary care NP. She is complaining of abdominal pain, low-grade fever, and mucopurulent vaginal discharge. Her symptoms began 3 days ago and are worsening. She has a new sexual partner and has not yet used condoms with him. Her menses just ended; she is taking oral contraceptives. She denies nausea, vomiting, or anorexia. Her exam reveals findings consistent with pelvic inflammatory disease (PID). Cultures are taken for gonorrhea and *Chlamydia*. Which of the following represents an inappropriate treatment plan for the adult-gerontology primary care NP to follow?
    1. Ceftriaxone (Rocephin) 250 mg IM.
    2. Doxycycline (Vibratabs) 100 mg PO bid × 10 days.
    3. Complete blood count (CBC), erythrocyte sedimentation rate (ESR).
    4. Hospitalization.

112. What is the primary role of progestins in prescribing postmenopausal hormone replacement therapy (HRT)?
    1. Reduce side effects of estrogen-related breast tenderness.
    2. Provide endometrial protection against hyperplasia.
    3. Stabilize mood swings and reduce hot flashes.
    4. Reduce occurrence of breakthrough bleeding.

113. An older female patient is seen by the adult-gerontology primary care NP for her annual exam. She has been on hormone replacement therapy (HRT) for 6 months, having started herself on the pills left over by her deceased mother. She brings the pills, which she wants to keep taking, and requests a prescription for Estrace 1 mg daily.

She has an intact uterus, is in excellent health, and denies any complaints. She does not have any contraindications to the use of HRT. Her exam is normal. Which represents an incorrect and potentially dangerous plan for the adult-gerontology primary care NP to follow?
1. Endometrial biopsy.
2. Prescription for Estrace 1 mg daily plus medroxyprogesterone acetate (Provera) 2.5 mg daily.
3. Prescription for Estrace 1 mg daily.
4. Instruct patient on the risks and benefits of HRT.

114. An older adult patient is seen for follow-up to discuss her hormone replacement therapy (HRT) that she began 3 months ago. She needs a refill on her HRT but is not sure "if it is working right." She continues to feel hot flashes, moodiness, and decreased libido, and has many sleep disturbances. She is taking Premarin 0.625 mg daily and Provera 2.5 mg daily. She denies any vaginal bleeding. Which is *not* an acceptable choice for the patient?
    1. Premarin 0.9 mg 1 tab PO qd and Provera 5 mg 1 tab PO qd days 1–12.
    2. Premarin 0.9 mg 1 tab PO qd and Provera 5 mg 1 tab PO qd days 16–25.
    3. Premarin 0.3 mg 1 tab PO qd and Provera 2.5 mg 1 tab PO qd.
    4. Premarin 1.25 mg 1 tab PO qd and Provera 10 mg 1 tab PO qd days 1–12.

115. Which is *not* a contraindication to the use of hormone replacement therapy (HRT) in the postmenopausal woman?
    1. Recent deep vein thrombosis.
    2. Chronic active hepatitis.
    3. Controlled hypertension.
    4. Undiagnosed abnormal genital bleeding.

116. A young adult patient presents to the clinic with complaints of a malodorous, yellowish vaginal discharge and vulvovaginal itching. She has never had a gynecologic exam and is extremely apprehensive. She is sexually active and has had a new sexual partner for 2 months. She states that they use condoms "most of the time" and are not interested in alternate forms of contraception at this time. Her last menstrual period was 1 week ago. Her wet mount with KOH shows few clue cells, moderate lactobacilli, few WBCs, no yeast, and too numerous to count mobile trichomonads. Appropriate treatment for this patient would include:
    1. Metronidazole (Flagyl) 2 g PO single dose.
    2. Metronidazole (Metrogel) vaginal cream 1 applicator hs × 5 days.
    3. Fluconazole (Diflucan) 150 mg PO single dose.
    4. Terconazole (Terazol) vaginal cream 1 applicator hs × 7 days.

117. Which dose of conjugated equine estrogen (Premarin) is the minimal effective dose to prevent osteoporosis?

1. 0.3 mg.
2. 0.625 mg.
3. 0.9 mg.
4. Premarin is inappropriate.

118. A single woman presents for contraceptive counseling, expressing preference for a diaphragm. Which factor in her history would make a diaphragm a poor choice?
    1. Three urinary tract infections (UTIs) in the past year.
    2. Strong desire to avoid pregnancy.
    3. Last two Pap smears showing atypical cells.
    4. Nulliparous cervix.

119. Combination oral contraceptives (OCs) prevent pregnancy primarily by:
    1. Decreasing fallopian tube motility.
    2. Thinning of cervical mucus.
    3. Suppressing ovulation.
    4. Causing inflammation of the endometrium.

120. A young adult patient is hesitant to be fitted for an intrauterine device (IUD) because of strong anti-abortion views and asks for the NP's opinion. Which explanation least accurately describes an IUD's probable action?
    1. Slows transport of ovum through the fallopian tube, causing it to age and die in transit.
    2. Prevents effective implantation of a fertilized ovum.
    3. Action is no different than that of a spermicide.
    4. Slows transport of sperm.

121. What is a unique advantage of a Progesterone T intrauterine device (IUD)?
    1. Lowest failure rate of IUDs.
    2. May be left in place for up to 10 years.
    3. Decreases menstrual blood loss and dysmenorrhea.
    4. Must be replaced annually.

122. An older female patient is seen by the adult-gerontology primary care NP for her annual exam and needs a refill on her hormone replacement therapy (HRT). She is feeling well and has not voiced concerns. The patient had a total abdominal hysterectomy and bilateral salpingo-oophorectomy 2 years ago for benign fibroids. Her exam is normal. She takes conjugated estrogen (Premarin) 0.625 mg days 1–25 and medroxyprogesterone acetate (Provera) 10 mg from days 16–25. What changes would be appropriate for the adult-gerontology primary care NP to make in the HRT regimen?
    1. No changes needed; the patient is doing well on the present regimen.
    2. Premarin 0.625 mg daily and discontinue the Provera.
    3. Premarin 0.625 mg daily and Provera 2.5 mg daily.
    4. Premarin 0.625 mg days 1–25 and Provera 5 mg days 16–25.

123. Which statement about progestin-only pills is true?
     1. Women who are breastfeeding should not use pro-
        gestin-only pills.
     2. Ovulation suppression is as effective with progestin-
        only pills as with combination oral contraceptives
        (OCs).
     3. There is an increased incidence of functional ovarian
        cysts.
     4. The risk of ectopic pregnancy is lower for women using
        progestin-only pills.

124. Before prescribing hormone replacement therapy (HRT),
     which clinical approach should have the highest priority?
     1. The decision about use should rest primarily with
        the patient after providing appropriate education and
        counseling.
     2. For most women, the benefits of HRT far outweigh
        any possible side effects, so HRT should be actively
        encouraged.
     3. Involving the sexual partner in the counseling ses-
        sion is likely to lead to a higher compliance rate for
        HRT.
     4. Education regarding HRT should include a thor-
        ough review of risk factors and possible side effects
        to avoid liability issues.

125. The most common side effect associated with depome-
     droxyprogesterone (DMPA; Depo-Provera) is:
     1. Nausea.
     2. Acne.
     3. Menstrual cycle changes.
     4. Increased menstrual cramps.

126. What information should the adult-gerontology prima-
     ry care NP include when teaching a patient about taking
     alendronate (Fosamax)?
     1. Take it midmorning.
     2. Take with food.
     3. Take with a full glass of orange juice.
     4. Remain upright after taking medication.

127. The addition of a progesterone to an estrogen regimen
     in a postmenopausal woman with a uterus reduces the
     risk of:
     1. Endometrial cancer.
     2. Cervical cancer.
     3. Gallbladder disease.
     4. Breast cancer.

128. The single-dose treatment of choice for trichomoniasis
     is:
     1. Azithromycin (Zithromax) 1 g PO.
     2. Ofloxacin (Floxin) 500 mg PO.
     3. Metronidazole (Flagyl) 2 g PO.
     4. Clindamycin (Cleocin) 300 mg PO.

129. A 25-year-old woman comes into the office with com-
     plaints of profuse malodorous discharge. The adult-
     gerontology primary care NP makes a diagnosis of
     bacterial vaginosis, and then would:
     1. Advise the patient to notify her sexual contacts re-
        garding the diagnosis.
     2. Treat the problem with metronidazole (Flagyl) 2 g
        for one dose.
     3. Initiate treatment with doxycycline (Vibramycin)
        100 mg PO bid × 7 days.
     4. Determine the presence of pregnancy before initiating
        a course of treatment.

130. A young woman who is taking a low-dose oral con-
     traceptive (OC) calls the clinic in a panic, stating that
     she forgot her pill 2 days ago. She is taking phenytoin
     (Dilantin) for seizure activity and has been seizure free
     for over a year. She asks, "What should I do about my
     pills?" What would be the adult-gerontology primary
     care NP's most appropriate response?
     1. "Take the forgotten dose today along with the regular
        dose."
     2. "See your physician for advice about the Dilantin."
     3. "Continue the pills, but use another contraceptive
        through the rest of this cycle."
     4. "Come to the clinic for a 'morning-after' pill."

131. A vaginal culture has confirmed the presence of a
     chancroid in a homeless woman who presented with a
     painful genital ulcer. The treatment regimen of choice
     should be:
     1. Ceftriaxone (Rocephin) 250 mg IM single dose.
     2. Erythromycin (E-Mycin) 500 mg PO qid × 7 days.
     3. Metronidazole (Flagyl) 2 mg PO single dose.
     4. Clindamycin (Cleocin) 2% vaginal cream 1 applica-
        tor × 5 days.

132. You are counseling a 49-year-old woman who had
     her last menstrual period 10 months ago. She is ex-
     periencing some hot flashes and night sweats and
     is not sleeping well. These symptoms are affecting
     her ability to work effectively because she finds her-
     self tired and "cranky." She does not want hormone
     replacement therapy. Which of the following evi-
     dence-based alternative measures is most accurately
     described?
     1. Venlafaxine (Effexor SR) has been effective in
        reducing hot flashes in randomized controlled
        trials.
     2. Raloxifene (Evista) has demonstrated a significant
        reduction in hot flashes compared with placebo in
        clinical trials.
     3. Black cohosh (*Cimicifuga racemosa*) has been report-
        ed as efficacious in treating menopausal symptoms in
        many large, controlled trials.

4. Isoflavones, specifically soy, have been shown in studies to be significantly more effective than placebo in reducing hot flashes.

133. A 65-year-old postmenopausal female has been treated with alendronate (Fosamax) for 6 years. Current screening indicates no increase in risk factors. Based on clinical guidelines, which treatment option would the adult-gerontology primary care NP suggest to the patient?
    1. Discontinue medication at this time.
    2. Switch medication from oral to intravenous route in order to maintain adequate coverage.
    3. Add vitamin D 500 IU daily to treatment regimen.
    4. Increase calcium supplementation to 1500 mg per day.

134. A young woman presents to the office for evaluation of abdominal pain. The patient admits to recent sexual activity and states that she does not have her partner use condoms. On exam, the adult-gerontology primary care NP finds vaginal discharge and cervical motion tenderness. Besides sending cultures to the laboratory, the adult-gerontology primary care NP's treatment plan for the patient would also include which two medications?
    1. Penicillin G 2.4 million units IM.
    2. Metronidazole (Flagyl) 500 mg PO bid × 7 days.
    3. Ceftriaxone (Rocephin) 125 mg IM.
    4. Azithromycin (Zithromax) 1 g PO.
    5. Acyclovir (Zovirax) 400 mg PO bid × 7 days.

135. Which information about hormone replacement therapy (HRT) should the adult-gerontology primary care NP understand when discussing HRT with patients?
    1. Estrogen replacement delays the onset of menopause.
    2. Estrogen and progesterone cause vasomotor symptoms.
    3. Estrogen decreases the risk of osteoporosis.
    4. Estrogen replacement with progesterone increases risk of ovarian cancer.

16   Female Reproductive Answers & Rationales

Physical Exam & Diagnostic Tests

1. Answer: 2, 3

Rationale: Based on current cervical screening guidelines, Papanicolaou (Pap) smear tests should be performed on female patients aged 21 and older regardless of sexual activity.

2. Answer: 1

Rationale: Recommendations made by the U.S. Preventative Services Task Force (USPSTF) with regard to screening intervals to establish better risk fracture prediction suggest intervals longer than the minimum of 2 years.

3. Answer: 3

Rationale: Lubricants, other than water, should not be used if a cervical specimen is being obtained for conventional Papanicolaou (Pap) smear analysis; some can alter the appearance of the cells and affect cytologic accuracy. For a liquid-based Pap test, in addition to the use of water, the posterior blade of the speculum may also be lubricated with a small amount of water-based lubricant before insertion. The endocervical cell retrieval is diminished with use of a cotton-tipped applicator and is not recommended in any female patient regardless of pregnancy status. The bimanual exam is performed after the internal vaginal exam.

4. Answer: 2

Rationale: To aid in the exam, an empty bladder provides comfort for the patient and assists the adult-gerontology primary care NP in making a more accurate assessment during the bimanual portion of the exam. Asking the patient to bear down slightly while the speculum is inserted and explaining each step of the procedure helps reduce the patient's anxiety, which ultimately may help achieve comfort.

5. Answer: 1

Rationale: A nabothian cyst (Naboth follicle) is a small, white or yellow, raised, round area on the cervix and is considered to be a normal variant. The surface of the cervix should be smooth and may have a symmetric, reddened circle around the os (squamocolumnar epithelium, or ectropion). The other options are all unexpected, abnormal findings.

6. Answer: 3

Rationale: A breast ultrasound is used to determine whether a lesion is solid or cystic. Ultrasound misses 50% of lesions <2 cm. The test is not sensitive enough to be used for routine screening and cannot replace mammography. The definitive diagnosis of breast cancer is the breast biopsy.

7. Answer: 2

Rationale: The World Health Organization defines osteoporosis as a bone mineral density T-score below −2.5 SD and osteopenia as a T-score between −1 and −2.5. The woman has early signs of osteopenia. She is not a candidate for HRT (estrogen + MPA) because of her past cardiovascular history. Raloxifene has been shown to prevent the progression of osteoporosis and, as a selective estrogen-receptor modulator (SERM), may be a good alternative to HRT. The other two lifestyle modifications are important counseling issues to reduce the risk of developing osteoporosis.

8. Answer: 3

Rationale: The hysterosalpingogram (HSG) is used to document the presence of a normal uterine cavity and the patency of the fallopian tubes. A contrast dye is injected into the uterus and radiographs are taken to assess anatomy. The best time to do this test is 2–5 days after menses, but before ovulation.

9. Answer: 1

Rationale: Approximately 10% of breast cancers are not seen mammographically.

10. Answer: 1

Rationale: KOH lyses epithelial and white blood cells, making it easier to visualize *Candida albicans* (yeast). *Candida* cells are resistant and remain intact. KOH also assists with diagnosing bacterial vaginosis by alkalinizing vaginal discharge, causing a distinct fishy odor. This is a positive amine or whiff test.

11. Answer: 1, 4, 5

Rationale: Smoking, history of rheumatoid arthritis, and progressive loss of height in an individual indicate an increased risk for the development of osteoporotic fracture. No parental history of hip fractures and a body mass index (BMI) stable within normal range do not support evidence of increased risk of osteoporotic fracture.

12. Answer: 3

Rationale: The Pap smear is a screening test for cervical cancer and precancerous states. The diagnostic test needed to confirm the diagnosis of a high-grade lesion is the colposcopy with guided biopsies. The results of this test are clearly abnormal and must be addressed. Waiting a year could be deleterious to the patient's health. This is not a Pap smear report that one would choose to redo in 4 months; the patient needs a diagnostic test, not another screening test. Because this is not a diagnosis of cervical cancer on this Pap smear, referral to a gynecologic oncologist is premature at this time.

13. Answer: 3

Rationale: All the tests listed may be included in the workup for infertility. Because male factors account for 35%–40% of infertility, a semen analysis should be done early in the workup. HSG and endometrial biopsy require scheduling at specific times of the menstrual cycle. Tests for antisperm antibodies would be done if the postcoital test revealed abnormalities.

14. Answer: 1, 3

Rationale: The National Osteoporosis Foundation (NOF) has conducted cost analyses on the value of screening bone DEXAs for evaluation of bone mineral density (BMD). The NOF reports that BMD testing is cost effective for postmenopausal women ages 50–60 who have other risk factors for development of osteoporosis, including lifestyle factors of minimal exercise, smoking, excessive alcohol intake, and low calcium intake. Other risk factors include genetic history of disease, slender physical frame, premature menopause, hyperthyroidism, multiple myeloma, rheumatoid arthritis, chronic renal disease, corticosteroid use, and long-term anticonvulsant therapy. The woman with the history of long-term corticosteroid therapy would meet the NOF criteria.

15. Answer: 4

Rationale: Long-standing nevi and Montgomery tubercles are normal findings; pendulous breast is only a description of size, which is important to note. Enlarged lymph nodes and tender supraclavicular nodes are potential cause for concern. A fixed stellate mass with nipple discharge is not normal, and although asymmetry might be normal, the different colors of the areolae and unilateral nipple inversion could represent a problem.

16. Answer: 4

Rationale: The basal body temperature (BBT) chart is an easy and inexpensive tool to evaluate for ovulation. Patients should be instructed on the first visit how to use a BBT thermometer and record the findings on a BBT chart. The remaining answers are usually included in an infertility workup, but do not evaluate the presence of ovulation.

17. Answer: 2

Rationale: Atrophic changes on the cervix of a postmenopausal woman are to be expected, as is the paucity of endocervical cells. Because of her past medical history of breast cancer, she is not a candidate for the use of estrogen vaginal cream, and the Pap smear interpretation is not abnormal. Endocervical curettage is used as a biopsy technique for sampling tissue from the endocervical canal; however, it is not appropriate to recommend this invasive procedure for someone with scant endocervical cells, but rather for one with abnormal endocervical cells. Because this Pap smear report is not really classified as abnormal, there is no need to recommend a diagnostic procedure for the patient.

18. Answer: 4

Rationale: Culture is a definitive method of diagnosis. It is a collected cervical specimen, and the results take about 2–6 days to obtain. Blood titers and a urine screen can also be used to diagnose a chlamydial infection. The direct fluorescent antibody (DFA) is fast and has good sensitivity and specificity.

19. Answer: 2

Rationale: Mammography is recommended annually by the American Cancer Society for all women 45 to 54 years of age based on average risk. Currently, the US Preventive Services Task Force has a draft recommendation of screening mammography every other year beginning at age 50. There is no place for annual mammographic testing for all women of childbearing age. Breastfeeding does not preclude the use of mammography, and screening is not done only for breast symptoms.

20. Answer: 1

Rationale: Serologic tests are used as screening tests, but positive results require follow-up with a treponemal test to detect specific antibodies.

21. Answer: 2

Rationale: Serum prolactin assay levels >20 ng/mL indicate the need for medical referral, usually to an endocrinologist. The most common cause of hyperprolactinemia and galactorrhea is a pituitary tumor or lesion of the hypothalamus. Other causes include hypothyroidism, medications (narcotics, tranquilizers, and antihypertensives), and oral contraceptives.

22. Answer: 1

Rationale: A positive withdrawal bleed after a progesterone challenge indicates adequate levels of endogenous estrogen. A serum prolactin level should be obtained as part of the amenorrhea workup in addition to a serum pregnancy test. A diagnosis of anovulation can be made on the basis of the successful withdrawal bleed and normal prolactin levels. Low body fat and abnormal thyroxine levels can also lead to amenorrhea, but do not affect the progesterone challenge test.

23. Answer: 1

Rationale: The occurrence of the symptoms during the luteal phase of the cycle (following ovulation) will assist the adult-gerontology primary care NP in making the diagnosis of premenstrual syndrome (PMS). Having the patient keep a calendar to track her symptoms for three cycles is helpful in making the diagnosis and measuring successful treatment. Severity of symptoms, although important, is not the most important information.

24. Answer: 3

Rationale: If bleeding resumes after 1 year of amenorrhea in a postmenopausal woman or persists longer than 6 months after HRT initiation, further evaluation is necessary. The most common cause of this abnormal finding is endometrial atrophy, but more serious pathology must be definitively ruled out. An endometrial biopsy should be scheduled to further evaluate the cause of bleeding.

Normal Gynecology

25. Answer: Correct sequence from highest to lowest levels: 4, 3, 1, 2

Rationale: The highest level of follicle-stimulating hormone (FSH) is found during the postmenopausal period in women. Ovulation phase follows, then follicular phase, and finally luteal phase.

26. Answer: 4

Rationale: The uterine lining first proliferates, and then prepares for implantation. During the secretory phase, glandular epithelium develops, further enhancing the lining. If no fertilized egg arrives for implantation, the lining sloughs off; this is the menstrual phase.

27. Answer: 1

Rationale: Premenstrual syndrome (PMS) occurs approximately 5–11 days before onset of menses (late luteal phase) and subsides within 1–2 days of menses onset. This phase is progesterone dominant. The follicular phase is estrogen dominant.

28. Answer: 1, 2, 4

Rationale: Oxytocin and antidiuretic hormone (ADH) are released from the posterior pituitary. FSH, LH, and prolactin are all released from the anterior pituitary gland. The other hormones released from the anterior pituitary are thyroid-stimulating hormone, adrenocorticotropic hormone, and growth hormone.

29. Answer: 1

Rationale: Follicle stimulating hormone (FSH) stimulates the maturation of ovarian follicles, resulting in a dominant follicle. Milk secretion depends on prolactin. The production and release of LH is regulated by estrogen. Lutenizing hormone (LH) is responsible for ovulation.

30. Answer: 2

Rationale: Menopause is one point in time and is defined after 12 months of amenorrhea, following the final menstrual period. In postmenopause, follicle stimulating hormone (FSH) levels rise 10-fold to 15-fold with marked reductions in estradiol, but other menstrual irregularities can create a variation in these levels. Therefore these levels are not considered the best definition for menopause.

31. Answer: 4

Rationale: The ovarian cycle is divided into three phases. The follicular phase begins on the first day of menses and continues until day 14, when ovulation usually occurs. Immediately after ovulation, the empty follicle begins to enlarge and develops into a corpus luteum, which releases increasing amounts of progesterone. If implantation does not occur, the corpus luteum regresses, causing the onset of menses. This phase, from ovulation to menses, is the luteal phase.

32. Answer: 1

Rationale: Regular exercise and a healthy diet reduce the risk for heart disease in postmenopausal women. As many as 30% of all coronary events are associated with tobacco use. HRT increases the risk of cardiovascular disease. Diabetes increases the mortality from cardiovascular disease two to four times compared with nondiabetic patients.

33. Answer: 4

Rationale: Pregnancy is the most likely diagnosis in this patient, given the list of symptoms and physical findings. She could have a uterine fibroid, but it is not contributing to the symptoms listed. Ovarian cancer could present with nausea, fatigue, and abdominal bloating, but would not cause the enlarged uterus or the positive Chadwick sign. A dislodged IUD will usually change the position of the IUD, decreasing visibility of the strings or causing the IUD itself to be expelled into the vagina or endocervical canal.

34. Answer: 4

Rationale: During menopause, vaginal flora changes leading to an increased likelihood for pathogenic growth and urinary symptoms. Vaginal tissue becomes more alkaline, drier (decreased lubrication), and thinner.

35. Answer: 3

Rationale: Maintaining an alkaline pH is important to promote viability of sperm that are deposited into the vaginal vault.

36. Answer: 4

Rationale: Obesity is not a risk factor for osteoporosis. Cigarette use, white race, and alcohol consumption, among others, are considered risk factors for osteoporosis.

37. Answer: 2

Rationale: Conservative management for PMS includes daily exercise, stress reduction, dietary changes, and reassurance that her symptoms are valid should help the patient gain more control. A low-salt diet is encouraged; when necessary, a diuretic may be used for fluid retention. The use of vitamins B_6, A, and E may be helpful as well. Laboratory studies are not indicated here but might be helpful if the symptoms were sustained throughout the menstrual cycle.

38. Answer: 2

Rationale: As the function of the ovaries declines and the amount of circulating estrogen begins to fall, the middle-aged woman may begin to experience the symptoms typically associated with menopause. The body's feedback system will attempt to stimulate the ovaries and increase estrogen level. FSH and LH levels rise in response to these efforts.

39. Answer: 1

Rationale: Pregnancy is the most likely diagnosis, requiring a pregnancy test and pelvic ultrasound to confirm it. Even though the patient has had a tubal ligation, failure rates of 1 in 300 have been reported. This patient could have uterine fibroids, but these do not generally present with this symptom complex and are not associated with amenorrhea, although they do cause uterine enlargement. Premature menopause could cause all these symptoms, including amenorrhea, but not the enlarged uterus. Colon cancer can present with these symptoms and could be responsible for an abdominal mass, but not for uterine enlargement or amenorrhea.

40. Answer: 3

Rationale: Uterine fibroids are associated with heavy menstrual blood flow which can be prolonged. Constipation, pelvic, leg, and back pain are also associated with uterine fibroids.

41. Answer: 4

Rationale: The age of menopause has fluctuated little over the past several centuries, even though life expectancy has increased. Of the options, only smoking has been found to cause an earlier menopause (average 1.5 years). Research shows a direct correlation among number of cigarettes smoked, number of years of smoking, and age at menopause. Nulliparity and epilepsy have also been associated with an earlier age at menopause.

Gynecologic Disorders

42. Answer: 2

Rationale: Secondary dysmenorrhea is associated with clinical symptoms that are due to anatomical abnormalities in the pelvis. Premenstrual syndrome presents with both physical and psychological clinical symptoms which typically occur prior to menses. Pelvic inflammatory disease is an infectious process that affects uterine and pelvic structures that can impact fertility. Dyspareunia is pain experienced during intercourse.

43. Answer: 3

Rationale: Complications associated with polycystic ovarian syndrome (PCOS) include hypertension, increased glucose levels, and infertility. Hemoglobin A1c level between 4% and 5.6% is within normal range as is a menstrual period lasting between 5 and 7 days.

44. Answer: 2

Rationale: Dyspareunia is painful intercourse, and vaginismus is painful vaginal spasms on penetration. Primary orgasmic disorder is when an individual has never achieved orgasm, usually a lifelong problem. Secondary orgasmic dysfunction refers to an acquired problem of loss of orgasmic function after an individual has experienced orgasm.

45. Answer: 1

Rationale: The initial outbreak is usually the worst. It can be transmitted even when there is no lesion present, and it cannot be cured. Vaginal delivery is allowed if there are no genital lesions at the time of labor.

46. Answer: 1

Rationale: Bacterial vaginosis results when the normal environment in the vagina is disrupted. The normal vaginal lactobacilli are decreased or absent, and there is an overgrowth of many different types of anaerobic bacteria. Trichomoniasis is caused by a flagellated protozoan, and gonorrhea is caused by a bacterium and may be asymptomatic. The virus that causes recurrent outbreaks of genital lesions is herpes simplex type 2 (HSV-2).

47. Answer: 1

Rationale: Oral contraceptives (OCs) will reduce prosta-glandin production, which is thought to be the primary cause of dysmenorrhea.

48. Answer: 4

Rationale: The criteria for the diagnosis of bacterial vagi-nosis are characteristic milky homogeneous discharge, pH >4.5, amine odor (positive whiff test) with addition of potassium hydroxide (KOH), and presence of epithelial cells studded with coccobacilli that obscure the borders (clue cells). Pseudohyphae are present in candidiasis.

49. Answer: 2

Rationale: In Asherman syndrome, a normally function-ing uterus has been damaged and scarred secondary to instrumentation, usually a dilation and curettage (D&C). Ovulation may be occurring normally, but no endome-trium is built up and, therefore no endometrium is shed (menstruation does not occur). Pregnancy, as well as the other diseases listed, should be ruled out in this patient.

50. Answer: 2

Rationale: The LH/FSH ratio in polycystic ovarian syn-drome is 3:1. The normal LH/FSH ratio is 1.5:1.

51. Answer: 4

Rationale: The criteria for the diagnosis of polycys-tic ovarian syndrome include menstrual irregular-ity, increased body weight, hirsutism, androgen excess evidenced by laboratory studies and physical find-ings, chronic anovulation, and multiple bilateral ovar-ian cysts. Weight loss, dental caries, and amenorrhea would be more common in anorexia nervosa/bulimia. Hyperprolactinemia and galactorrhea are found with a prolactin-secreting pituitary tumor. Dysmenorrhea, nodules palpated on bimanual exam, and infertility are associated with endometriosis.

52. Answer: 3

Rationale: Anovulation causes 90% of dysfunctional uterine bleeding. The lack of progesterone allows for asynchronous, excessive proliferation of the endometri-um to take place. This tissue is fragile, and the normal hemostatic mechanism is altered. Thyroid disease, blood dyscrasias, and uterine tumors can mimic dysfunctional uterine bleeding and must be excluded.

53. Answer: 3

Rationale: A female-appearing person with a 46,XY kar-yotype has androgen insensitivity syndrome, or testicular

feminization. This maternal X-linked recessive disorder accounts for approximately 10% of all cases of amenor-rhea, and these persons appear normal until puberty. These patients present with amenorrhea, scant or absent pubic hair, and abnormal or no breast development. Per-sons with müllerian abnormalities have a normal XX karyotype with abnormalities of fallopian tubes, uterus, and upper vagina occurring in fetal development. In Turner syndrome, congenital absence of ovaries results from loss of one X chromosome.

54. Answer: 1

Rationale: The most common breast mass in young wom-en <30 years old is the fibroadenoma. This benign breast mass is the third most common breast mass after fibro-cystic changes and carcinoma. Fibrocystic breast changes are seen most commonly in women 30–50 years old. Intra-ductal papilloma is a wartlike growth located in the mam-mary duct and occurs in women 40–50 years old. Malig-nant breast neoplasms occur most frequently in women over 40 and are rarely seen in women 15–25 years old.

55. Answer: 1

Rationale: Nonsteroidal antiinflammatory drugs (NSAIDs) inhibit prostaglandin synthesis and are effective agents in primary dysmenorrhea. The other agents listed have not demonstrated effectiveness in primary dysmenorrhea. Other measures to decrease discomfort are exercise, re-laxation techniques, heat application, and low-dose OCs.

56. Answer: 4

Rationale: Secondary amenorrhea is defined as no menses for three-cycle lengths or 6 months in a woman with pre-viously established menses. Exercise can cause an increase in estrogen and endorphin levels, which influences the re-lease of gonadotropin-releasing hormone (GnRH). Without appropriate GnRH release, follicle stimulating hormone and luteinizing hormone are not released adequately, resulting in anovulation, which may lead to amenorrhea. The other conditions listed are causes of primary amenorrhea.

57. Answer: 1

Rationale: This has the characteristics of a syphilitic le-sion and needs to be evaluated. Only after determining the presence or type of sexually transmitted infection can it be treated effectively. The herpes viral culture should be done while the lesion is present and the fluid from the vesicles can be obtained.

58. Answer: 2

Rationale: A person who has never engaged in coital ac-tivity is not considered at risk for cervical cancer because exposure to human papillomavirus (HPV) is unlikely. In addition to other factors not listed, the presence of HPV, multiple sexual partners, and previous high-grade squamous intraepithelial lesion (HSIL) are considered to be risk factors in the development of cervical cancer.

59. Answer: 1

Rationale: The pseudohyphae and spores on the wet mount with KOH are diagnostic for candida infection. *Chlamydia trachomatis* is diagnosed by direct immunofluorescent assay or by chlamydial culture. Gonorrhea is diagnosed by cervical culture, and bacterial vaginosis has microscopic findings of clue cells and positive amine odor.

60. Answer: 1

Rationale: Cancer of the ovary is the leading cause of death from female genital cancer, excluding the breast, in the United States.

61. Answer: 1

Rationale: Flagellated protozoan confirms the diagnosis of trichomoniasis. Chlamydial infection is best diagnosed by direct immunofluorescent assay or culture. Bacterial vaginosis is diagnosed by wet mount revealing clue cells and positive amine test. Inflammatory cervicitis is generally asymptomatic and will not cause vaginal irritation.

62. Answer: 3

Rationale: The pelvic ultrasound is not a useful test for appendicitis because it does not allow for adequate exam of the appendix. The CBC with differential is useful because of the expected rise in white blood cells seen in this inflammatory state. The flat plate of the abdomen and kidney-ureters-bladder (KUB) are helpful to determine the extent of the problem and to rule out other diagnoses. Because pregnancy can cause these symptoms if complicated by an ectopic state, the practitioner should consider it as part of the differential diagnosis.

63. Answer: 2

Rationale: Oral contraceptives (OCs) have been shown to reduce the risk of endometrial cancer. Obesity, unopposed estrogen use, and advanced age, in addition to others not listed here, are considered to be risk factors for developing endometrial cancer.

64. Answer: 4

Rationale: The diaphragm may be inserted up to 2 hours before intercourse and should be removed no sooner than 6 hours after intercourse has ended. It should not be left in place longer than 24 hours.

65. Answer: 2

Rationale: Urethral discomfort and recurrent urinary tract infections (UTIs) are associated with diaphragm use and are the most common reasons for discontinuing use and changing birth control methods.

66. Answer: 3

Rationale: Oral contraceptive (OC) use has been shown to reduce the risk of ovarian cancer. Family history of ovarian cancer, advancing age, and positive *BRCA-2* gene are considered risk factors for developing ovarian cancer.

67. Answer: 2

Rationale: Endometrial cancer is the most common female genital cancer with ovarian cancer causing the most deaths annually. Endometrial cancer is more common than ovarian cancer and is easier to cure with just surgery alone. Because ovarian cancer is usually diagnosed in a later stage, the condition is more difficult to cure.

68. Answer: 3

Rationale: Herpes simplex virus type 2 (HSV-2) typically presents dramatically in the newly infected primary outbreak. Gonorrhea generally is associated with a mucopurulent vaginal discharge and is not accompanied by vesicular lesions. Chlamydial infection may be associated with dysuria and, unless accompanied by pelvic inflammatory disease (PID), is not generally accompanied by fever or body aches and is not associated with vesicular lesions. Lymphogranuloma venereum is a rare disease classically accompanied by pustular enlargement of the lymph nodes, particularly the inguinal nodes. It is associated not with vesicles, but buboes.

69. Answer: 2

Rationale: Screening blood studies for glucose, cardiac risk profile, and TSH in this age group without any stated risk factors is not cost effective and is of little value. The patient can be better served with a discussion regarding diet and exercise. Because this patient is at risk for STDs, counseling and testing for these is a reasonable approach. Contraceptive information educates the patient and allows her to make wiser choices in her family planning.

70. Answer: 2, 3, 4

Rationale: High-fat diet, advancing age, and early menarche have been identified as risk factors in the development of breast cancer. Early menopause and nonproliferative fibroadenomas have not been associated with the development of breast cancer.

71. Answer: 1

Rationale: The use of prenatal vitamins with folic acid before conception has been found to reduce the risk of neural tube defects in the fetus. It is important for the patient to continue her exercise program, although some discussion about the type of exercise and any limitations are important once pregnancy is achieved. Because the patient has had two previous pregnancies, it is likely that her rubella immune status has been determined; if she is found to not be immune to rubella, an MMR vaccination should be recommended. This patient is not of advanced maternal age and, therefore, does not require genetic counseling for this reason.

72. Answer: 3

Rationale: Baseline laboratory work should be obtained to determine the presence of anemia, possible pregnancy, and endocrine dysfunction.

73. Answer: 4

Rationale: Fibrocystic breast disease is not a risk factor for breast cancer. In addition to others, those listed in the other options are considered to be risk factors for breast cancer.

74. Answer: 1

Rationale: The recommended age for a female to begin screening Pap smears is at the onset of sexual activity or at 21 years of age. Because this patient is 21 years old and has not yet had her first Pap smear, this would be the most appropriate test to perform. It is not necessary to perform STD screening on patients who have not been sexually active. Stool guaiac (hemoccult) testing and mammography are not recommended as screening procedures in the young adult.

75. Answer: 3

Rationale: Heart disease remains the leading cause of death for women in the United States.

76. Answer: 1

Rationale: Reactive cellular changes are most often associated with inflammation, including typical repair. Other causes include atrophy with inflammation (atrophic vaginitis), IUD use, radiation, and diethylstilbestrol exposure in utero. Oral contraceptives (OCs) do not cause reactive changes, and estrogen vaginal cream may be used to improve atrophy.

77. Answer: 2

Rationale: Cervical cancer has been directly linked with high-risk types of human papillomavirus (HPV). Pregnancy after age 35, low parity, and prolonged contraceptive use are not risk factors for cervical cancer.

78. Answer: 1

Rationale: Breast cancer is the most common cancer in women in the United States. Lung cancer mortality is higher than that for breast cancer.

79. Answer: 3

Rationale: These symptoms are classic for menopausal syndrome, although some depressive symptoms are listed. Antidepressant therapy and counseling for depression at this stage of treatment is not appropriate. Testing, teaching, and treatment in this case should be aimed at the menopause. The depressive symptoms will undoubtedly improve with greater understanding and treatment of the menopausal symptoms.

80. Answer: 1

Rationale: Chancroid is well established as a cofactor for HIV transmission. Chancroid is a sexually transmitted infection of the genitals that is caused by the bacteria, *Haemophilus ducreyi*. It is characterized by an open sore or ulcer and can be transmitted from skin-to-skin contact with an infected person. It should be noted that is rarely seen in the United States, but occurs more in third-world countries.

81. Answer: 1

Rationale: According to the American Cancer Society, women should be advised of the benefits and limitations of monthly breast self-exam (BSE) and should be aware of how their breasts normally look and feel and to report any new breast changes.

82. Answer: 2

Rationale: Symptoms are most likely indicative of benign fibroadenoma. Mammography is indicated. Surgical excision is unlikely for a young woman.

83. Answer: 2

Rationale: This patient needs to become more knowledgeable about the normal feel of implants as well as her own breast tissue. Mammography is not a substitute for breast self-exam (BSE).

84. Answer: 2

Rationale: A very firm cervix along with a cervical lesion/ulcer is suspicious for cancer of the cervix, which can be confirmed with a Pap smear.

85. Answer: 1

Rationale: This complaint is an indication for clinical breast exam and mammography. Although uncommon, breast pain can be a presenting symptom for breast cancer. Teaching breast self-exam (BSE) is important, but not the most important action at this point. Hormonal fluctuations can explain breast pain, as can excessive caffeine intake, but should be a diagnosis of exclusion after ruling out malignancy.

86. Answer: 2

Rationale: Toxic shock syndrome occurs primarily in menstruating women ages 12–24 who use tampons. The diagnosis is made with the presence of fever over 102°F (38.9°C), macular rash, hypotension, and involvement of three or more organ systems.

87. Answer: 4

Rationale: Ectopic pregnancies, if not diagnosed and treated promptly can lead to increased morbidity and mortality accounting for up to 4% of all pregnancy related deaths. This is especially evident if the death occurred during the first trimester.

88. Answer: 4

Rationale: Almost half of all vaginal infections are caused by candidiasis. The majority of women who develop the infection have recently taken antibiotics. It is not a sexually transmitted infection.

89. Answer: 1

Rationale: It is important to evaluate the patient for threatened abortion as soon as possible. It is most likely too soon for the CBC to reflect blood loss. A pelvic sonogram takes longer than a urine pregnancy test, and the patient must be immediately referred for a D&C if her pregnancy test is positive.

90. Answer: 2

Rationale: The most common site for breast cancer occurrence is the upper outer quadrant (Tail of Spence), followed by the area beneath the nipple.

91. Answer: 3

Rationale: Pap smears are crucial for the detection of cervical cancer, but do not diagnose uterine cancer. In the early stages, uterine cancer can be asymptomatic and would not be detectable even on bimanual exam.

92. Answer: 4

Rationale: Vulvovaginal changes, such as atrophic vaginitis, often become apparent and bothersome several years after the last menstrual period (LMP) in women not receiving estrogen therapy. Insufficient data are available to demonstrate that isoflavones have a positive effect on vaginal symptoms. Vaginal lubricants are therapeutic in relieving symptoms of vaginal dryness. If nonprescription remedies do not provide relief and no contraindications exist, estrogen (often topical) is the treatment of choice.

93. Answer: 4

Rationale: Douching is never necessary. It changes the normal pH and upsets the normal vaginal flora. Douching during menstruation could cause "retrograde menstruation," a potential precursor to endometriosis. Copious vaginal discharge can be a symptom of infection and warrants workup.

94. Answer: 3

Rationale: Pregnancy is the most common cause of amenorrhea in young women. It is important to rule out pregnancy by obtaining a serum human chorionic gonadotropin (hCG) level in patient with a problem of amenorrhea, even if she is very athletic. Interviewing the patient regarding her sexual practices is unreliable. The presence or absence of pregnancy should be determined before other diagnostic studies.

95. Answer: 3

Rationale: The presence of bruising, particularly on genitalia, should raise suspicion of abuse. Combined with her nonverbal behavior, the bruising should prompt the adult-gerontology primary care NP to explore the possibility of abuse.

Pharmacology

96. Answer: 1, 5

Rationale: Recommended treatment for *T. vaginalis* is metronidazole (Flagyl), which can be delivered as a single dose (2 g) or as 500 g dose, twice a day for 7 days. During the course of therapy, both alcohol and sexual activity avoidance are recommended. As the patient relates drinking and sexual activity, this is indicative of noncompliance with treatment therapy. Use of cotton underwear and avoiding douching are part of the treatment plan.

97. Answer: 1, 2, 4

Rationale: TMP-SMX and nitrofurantoin are both effective against UTI. Phenazopyridine helps make the patient more comfortable until the antibiotic reaches effective levels for treatment. Ceftriaxone is an effective drug for complicated UTI, but is unnecessary in an uncomplicated lower UTI. Neomycin is an aminoglycoside and would not be used for an uncomplicated UTI, but rather for severe systemic infections and preoperatively to sterilize the bowel for intestinal surgery.

98. Answer: 2

Rationale: The Women's Health Initiative (WHI) study was stopped early because after 5.2 years, in the opinion of the Safety/Data Monitoring Board, the health risks for the women on the study (mean age 63) taking estrogen plus progestin exceeded the benefits. Women taking estrogen/progestin were at higher risk for developing MIs, strokes, and thromboemboli as well as developing breast cancer than women taking placebo. However, women taking HRT were less likely to have a fracture caused by osteoporosis and less likely to develop colorectal cancer. The study did not address the shorter term use of HRT for treatment of menopausal symptoms, the primary indication for initiating the therapy. This landmark study stresses the need for providers to discuss the risks/benefits of initiating or continuing HRT with postmenopausal women.

99. Answer: 3

Rationale: Fluconazole is now approved for a single-dose oral treatment of uncomplicated vulvovaginal candidiasis. It is the most convenient approach for this patient, who is unlikely to be compliant with vaginal creams, given the upcoming travel. She does not have contraindications to its use. Metronidazole and clindamycin are for bacterial vaginosis, not *Candida* infections. Hydrocortisone is a topical steroid used for inflammatory dermatologic conditions, and although it may help the itching, it would not treat the candidiasis.

100. Answer: 4

Rationale: Metronidazole vaginal gel is the treatment of choice for bacterial vaginosis in the nonpregnant female. The presence of clue cells, and the associated malodorous discharge and absence of lactobacilli, are markers for the diagnosis of bacterial vaginosis.

101. Answer: 4

Rationale: Although some authors may recommend herbal treatments for menopausal symptoms, no controlled studies have been done on disease prevention. Traditional allopathic Western medicine supports the use of HRT for the prevention of osteoporosis. Weight-bearing exercise and increased calcium intake have been shown to help maintain bone health. Cigarette smoking increases the risk for bone loss. This patient can reduce her risk by quitting smoking.

102. Answer: 4

Rationale: Benzathine penicillin 2.4 million units IM is the treatment of choice for syphilis, but this patient has condyloma acuminatum, not condyloma latum. Topical use of podophyllin, trichloroacetic acid, and cryotherapy are all accepted treatment modalities for condyloma acuminatum.

103. Answer: 1

Rationale: *Chlamydia* often presents this way (dysuria, mucopurulent discharge, and cervical friability). The treatment of choice in ambulatory care settings is single-dose azithromycin 1 g PO. Another treatment dose regime would be 250 mg IM of ceftriaxone for a chlamydial infection, not 125 mg, plus doxycycline 100 mg PO for 14 days with or without metronidazole 500 mg PO bid for 14 days. Herpes simplex virus will present with painful vesicles in the vulvovaginal region and is treated with acyclovir 200 mg 1 cap PO q4h × 5 days for recurrences. Trichomoniasis can present this way, but trichomonads on the wet mount are absent. Therapy for trichomoniasis is single-dose metronidazole 2 g PO.

104. Answer: 4

Rationale: A hepatic effect due to the first-pass metabolism in the liver occurs with oral estrogen products. A 25% increase in triglycerides has been associated with this route of administration. Because transdermal estrogen is not dependent on gastrointestinal absorption or affected by the first-pass metabolic effect, this option should be considered. A discussion regarding risks/benefits of continuing HRT is appropriate from the primary provider. Because the patient is only 52 years old and is still experiencing menopausal symptoms, reducing the most common dosage or stopping the medication, unless significant risks are apparent, is probably not the most therapeutic option.

105. Answer: 3

Rationale: The IUD would be a good choice for this patient because it is extremely effective (>99%). Maintenance is minimal, and no injections are involved for insertion or removal. The Depo-Provera injections, although extremely effective as well (>99%), require an injection every 3 months, which could lead to decreased patient compliance. The system of implants is also very effective (>99%) but also requires injections for insertion and removal, which this patient is trying to avoid. The diaphragm is a noninvasive contraceptive that is effective (88%), but requires her to be more active in its use. None of these methods is contraindicated for this patient, but an attempt should be made to help her choose one with which she is likely to be comfortable.

106. Answer: 1

Rationale: The adult-gerontology primary care NP should try to determine what the patient has heard and dispel the fallacies if possible. Recent research supports the protective benefit of OCs against ovarian cancer as well as endometrial cancer. Amount of menstrual bleeding usually is decreased and the cycle regulated. Minimal weight fluctuations are reported. Infertility is not associated with OC use. To suggest either implantation system or Depo-Provera injections to someone who voices concerns about irregular menses or weight gain is sure to lead to an unhappy patient because these are common side effects of both methods. Pap smears do not screen for ovarian cancer.

107. Answer: 2

Rationale: Changing to a pill with a stronger progestational agent or changing to a different progestational agent often will resolve the problem of bleeding irregularities with OCs. Many choices are available regarding the dose or strength of an OC, and her problem likely can be resolved with a different pill. Taking the pills at a different time of day or on an empty stomach will do nothing to resolve the stated problem, which is not breakthrough bleeding, but rather prolonged bleeding, probably secondary to poor endometrial support. If a change is not made in the pills, the patient will continue to bleed and may eventually develop anemia.

108. Answer: 3

Rationale: An OC such as Demulen 1/35, is a good choice for women with more androgenic characteristics because of its strong estrogenic effect with moderate progestational effect. Loestrin 1/20 is a poor choice; the weaker dose of estrogen and progestin may not adequately support her endometrium and will not have a positive effect on this patient's androgenic characteristics. Triphasil is a triphasic pill and does have a positive progestational effect that should support the endometrium, but the progestin in this OC tends to be slightly more androgenic, which is undesirable in this patient.

109. Answer: 4

Rationale: Combination OCs are not recommended for breastfeeding mothers because of the potential effect on decreasing milk quantity and quality. Progestin-only OCs are approved for nursing mothers because no deleterious effect on milk quantity or quality have been shown. Depo-Provera and the IUD are also accepted contraceptive methods for lactating females.

110. Answer: 2

Rationale: OCs are contraindicated in a cigarette smoker age 35 years or older. No contraindication exists to the use of Depo-Provera injection in the cigarette smoker. The Progestasert IUD would probably be a good IUD choice for this patient because it is only approved for 1 year's use and is safe in a cigarette smoker. The only contraindication to condoms and spermicide is allergy to either substance.

111. Answer: 4

Rationale: It is not necessary to hospitalize the patient with acute pelvic inflammatory disease (PID) who is not vomiting or pregnant. If she does not respond well to outpatient treatment, hospitalization may be recommended. The medications listed are the accepted treatment of choice for outpatient management of PID and should be started before lab results are available, based on the patient's clinical presentation. The CBC and ESR are helpful to track the WBC count and inflammatory response of the body.

112. Answer: 2

Rationale: Unopposed estrogen in a woman with an intact uterus increases her risk of endometrial hyperplasia and progression to endometrial cancer. Women who have taken unopposed estrogen for more than 3 years have a fivefold increased risk of endometrial cancer compared with women not on this regimen. The addition of progesterone to the regimen provides uterine protection. However, the progestin component of HRT is responsible for the breakthrough bleeding, a chief complaint at the initiation of therapy that may lead to discontinuance of the drug. Some women also are intolerant of progestins, which have been linked to irritability.

113. Answer: 3

Rationale: The use of unopposed estrogen in the patient with an intact uterus could put her at risk for endometrial hyperplasia or cancer. The addition of a progestin protects the endometrium adequately. The patient is an excellent candidate for endometrial biopsy to document the status of the endometrium. This patient also needs to be educated on the risks and benefits of HRT.

114. Answer: 3

Rationale: Lowering the dose of the estrogen would not help this patient's symptoms. The other dosage regimens listed are all acceptable choices for this patient, proving that there are many effective ways to utilize HRT, allowing for individualization of the regimen to the patient.

115. Answer: 3

Rationale: Well-controlled hypertension is not a contraindication to the use of HRT.

116. Answer: 1

Rationale: Metronidazole 2 g PO in a single dose is the treatment of choice for trichomoniasis. Metronidazole vaginal cream does not effectively treat vaginal trichomoniasis. Fluconazole and terconazole are treatments for vaginal candidiasis.

117. Answer: 1

Rationale: A dose of 0.3 mg of conjugated equine estrogen (Premarin) is the minimal effective dose to prevent osteoporosis. Hormone replacement therapy (HRT) helps maintain bones, but this effect only lasts as long as HRT is taken. Because of the risks for cardiovascular disease from using HRT, it is no longer recommended for osteoporosis prevention. Other methods of osteoporosis prevention include regular exercise, smoking cessation, and sufficient calcium (1200–1500 mg of elemental calcium) and vitamin D (400–800 IU) daily.

118. Answer: 1

Rationale: The diaphragm predisposes many women to UTIs. Some women are sensitive to the contraceptive cream or jelly. The diaphragm has been associated with toxic shock syndrome, so its use should be avoided during menses, and it should not be left in place longer than 24 hours.

119. Answer: 3

Rationale: The primary mechanism of action of oral contraceptives (OCs) is suppression of ovulation. Ovulation is suppressed in 95%–98% of patients. Should ovulation occur, the other mechanisms of action likely to prevent conception are thickening of cervical mucus, causing the endometrium to become atrophic and making the uterine environment unfavorable for implantation.

120. Answer: 3

Rationale: Although still unproven conclusively, mechanisms of action for IUDs include prevention of blastocyst implantation by inducing low-grade endometritis, the copper's effects on enzymes, progesterone's actions on the endometrium, and inhibition of sperm/ovum migration.

121. Answer: 3

Rationale: A progesterone-releasing IUD acts to decrease blood loss and cramping. Progesterone-releasing IUDs thicken the cervical mucus, thicken the endometrium, and inhibit ovulation. Copper-containing IUDs can increase bleeding and dysmenorrhea. There are two hormonal IUDs available; one works for 3 years and the other for 5 years. The copper IUD can stay in place for up to 10 years.

122. Answer: 2

Rationale: The patient no longer requires Provera to protect the endometrium from the potential effects of estrogen; therefore the progestin can be discontinued and the patient given continuous estrogen therapy without concern. The other dosage regimens listed are appropriate for a HRT patient with an intact uterus.

123. Answer: 3

Rationale: The progestin-only pill does not consistently suppress ovulation. This suppression only occurs in 40%–60% of cycles, which makes the progestin-only pill less effective than combination oral contraceptives (OCs). Mechanisms of action that contribute to the progestin-only pill's effectiveness include creating an atrophic endometrium and possibly altering tubal physiology by decreasing ovum transport. Progestin-only pills contain no estrogen and are a good choice for the breastfeeding woman. There is an increased incidence of functional ovarian cysts.

124. Answer: 1

Rationale: Informed consent is essential. The pros and cons of HRT should be explained, but the choice is up to the patient.

125. Answer: 3

Rationale: Depo-Provera is frequently associated with menstrual cycle changes. In fact, irregular bleeding is the most frequently cited reason for discontinuation. These menstrual changes range from heavy, irregular bleeding to spotting and even amenorrhea. Nausea and acne are usually effects of estrogen and are not seen with Depo-Provera.

126. Answer: 4

Rationale: Patients taking alendronate are instructed to take the medication on awakening, 30 minutes before eating, and with a full glass of water. Patients should be instructed to remain upright to prevent esophageal irritation. Taking medication with food (reduces bioavailability by 40%), coffee, orange juice (decreases bioavailability by 60%), or after eating significantly reduces absorption.

127. Answer: 1

Rationale: Women with a uterus taking unopposed exogenous estrogen have an increased risk of endometrial cancer. The addition of progesterone decreases this risk. The addition of progesterone may prompt bleeding, which many women view unfavorably. Progesterone does not affect cervical cancer, breast cancer, or gallbladder disease.

128. Answer: 3

Rationale: Metronidazole in a single 2-g dose is the treatment of choice for trichomoniasis. An alternative is giving the 2 g in divided doses the same day to reduce nausea and improve compliance.

129. Answer: 4

Rationale: Metronidazole is the treatment of choice for bacterial vaginosis. However, pregnancy should be ruled out before beginning treatment because metronidazole should not be used if the woman may be pregnant. The sexual partners do not require treatment, and doxycycline is not the drug of choice.

130. Answer: 3

Rationale: This patient requires added protection through this cycle because of the low-dose oral contraceptive (OC). Phenytoin may also decrease the effectiveness of OCs, especially low-dose forms.

131. Answer: 1

Rationale: Because of the patient's homeless status, the adult-gerontology primary care NP needs to use a single-dose treatment. Erythromycin, although a correct medication, is a poor dosing choice for this patient.

132. Answer: 1

Rationale: The most accurate answer is venlafaxine. This combination serotonin and norepinephrine reuptake inhibitor has been found to reduce hot flashes at doses of 25–150 mg/day in several clinical trials. Although many individuals consider the "natural" over-the-counter products to be safer than prescription drugs, these products can have pharmacologic effects and side effects. Use of these drugs by patients should be questioned at the time of the exam. Critics argue that the trials studying black cohosh (*Cimicifuga racemosa*) have been too small, uncontrolled, and not randomized to provide evidence-based information on the herb's efficacy and safety. Soy has been found to be moderately effective in reducing hot flashes, but comparable results have been seen in the placebo groups as well. A side effect of raloxifene, used to prevent postmenopausal osteoporosis, is hot flashes.

133. Answer: 1

Rationale: Patients who have low fracture risk after being treated with alendronate (Fosamax) for at least 5 years qualify for a drug holiday as the effects of the medication are still present. There is no need to switch the route of medication. Vitamin D supplementation should be within 800 to 1000 IU per day. Calcium supplementation greater than 1200 mg per day maybe associated with increased risk of complications ranging from kidney stones to cardiac events.

134. Answer: 3, 4

Rationale: The most common cause of PID in sexually active women is gonococcal infections. These infections are often accompanied by *Chlamydia,* and usually both are treated.

135. Answer: 3

Rationale: HRT may be considered for short-term use (3–4 years) to alleviate menopausal symptoms and the risk of osteoporosis in high-risk patients. The ovarian cancer risk may increase for women using estrogen alone for 10 years or longer. Current data are insufficient to know if combination HRT has the same risk. HRT reduces colorectal cancer risk.

Mental Health

Psychosocial Examination & Diagnostic Tests

1. The mental status exam enables the adult-gerontology primary care NP to identify:
   1. Intelligence quotient (IQ) and reasoning.
   2. Abstract thinking and memory functioning.
   3. Reasoning and coordination.
   4. Memory functioning and IQ.

2. **QSEN** The adult-gerontology primary care NP understands the following concerning direct questioning about intimate partner violence in the home:
   1. Direct questioning should be avoided for fear of offending the patient.
   2. It should be a routine component of history taking with female patients.
   3. Direct questioning should be used only when there are obvious findings noted on physical exam.
   4. It should be used only once a year when the patient is seen for a routine physical exam.

3. A patient with a history of psychiatric problems arrives at the clinic shouting that he is a messenger of God and knows the meaning of the prophecies in Revelations. This behavior is assessed as:
   1. A delusion.
   2. A hallucination.
   3. Magical thinking.
   4. An illusion.

4. A tool used to screen adolescents for alcoholism is the:
   1. CRAFFT.
   2. CAGE questionnaire.
   3. PACES tool.
   4. HITS screening tool.

5. An assessment of a patient experiencing auditory hallucinations would most likely reveal:
   1. Patient mumbling to self, tilted head, eyes darting back and forth.
   2. Performance of obsessive-compulsive rituals of turning off and on a radio, talking to self.
   3. Hyperactivity, expansive mood, easy distractibility.
   4. Cool, aloof, unapproachable, avoiding enclosed areas.

6. CAGE is a screening instrument for which disease process?
   1. Glaucoma.
   2. Depression.
   3. Alcoholism.
   4. Diabetes.

7. When receiving records from another agency, the adult-gerontology primary care NP notes on the summary sheet that the patient has a dual diagnosis. This means the patient has:
   1. Both manic and depressive symptoms of bipolar affective disorder.
   2. Two closely related psychiatric disorders (e.g., panic disorder and bulimia nervosa).
   3. Coexistence of both a psychiatric disorder (e.g., depression) and a substance abuse disorder (e.g., alcohol dependence).
   4. Coexistence of a personality disorder (e.g., borderline personality) and a psychiatric disorder (e.g., panic disorder).

8. When you the adult-gerontology primary care NP asks the patient to tell you the meaning of a proverb or metaphor, you are assessing which of the following?
   1. Impaired judgment.
   2. Memory.
   3. Abstract reasoning.
   4. Level of consciousness.

9. While completing the history on an older adult, the adult-gerontology primary care NP understands that when a patient "makes up stories or answers" to questions, it is known as:
   1. Perseveration.
   2. Confabulation.
   3. Echolalia.
   4. Alcoholic encephalopathy.

10. **QSEN** In taking a history from a patient with depression, which is the most important question for the adult-gerontology primary care NP to ask?
    1. Have you ever experienced hallucinations, delusions, or illusions?
    2. Have you ever been hospitalized in a psychiatric facility?
    3. Do you regularly take antidepressants or other medications?
    4. Have you thought about or attempted suicide?

11. The adult-gerontology primary care NP asks the patient to follow a series of short commands to assess:
    1. Judgment.
    2. Abstract reasoning.
    3. Attention span.
    4. Cooperation.

12. A common laboratory finding associated with bulimia nervosa is:
    1. Hyperkalemia.
    2. Hypochloremia.
    3. Elevated liver enzymes.
    4. Platelet abnormalities.

13. The adult-gerontology primary care NP is testing recent memory on an older adult client. Select the response that can be used to test for recent memory.
    1. Ask the patient to recall three items after a delay of 3–5 minutes.
    2. Ask the patient to solve a simple math problem.
    3. Ask the patient to name the past four presidents.
    4. Ask the patient his or her mother's maiden name.

14. An 85-year-old woman comes in with her daughter with the primary complaint of worsening confusion over 6 months. The adult-gerontology primary care NP has already ordered a urine analysis and it was negative. The basal metabolic panel was unremarkable. Complete blood count showed a mild anemia. What other tests might the adult-gerontology primary care NP consider ordering for this patient?
    1. A1C, folic acid, TSH.
    2. TSH, lipid panel, vitamin B_{12}, vitamin D.
    3. Folic acid, vitamin B_{12}, TSH.
    4. Lipid panel, A1C, vitamin D.

15. The adult-gerontology primary care NP knows drug tolerance is suggested when a patient gives a history of:
    1. Reduced effects with the same dose of the drug.
    2. Less of the medication produces the desired effects.
    3. No withdrawal symptoms when the drug is stopped.
    4. Increasing side effects with an increase in the dose of the drug.

16. When doing a mental status exam, which questions would be helpful to assess the patient for the ability to think abstractly?
    1. Can you repeat the following numbers: 1, 3, 5, 7, 9?
    2. What is today's date?
    3. How are a carpet and a hardwood floor alike?
    4. Can you tell me the names of three past US presidents?

Psychiatric Disorders

17. An older adult patient is experiencing a recent onset of confusion. The adult-gerontology primary care NP is trying to determine whether the confusion is related to depression or dementia. In evaluating the patient, what specific assessment finding would be helpful in making this distinction?
    1. Determining whether confusion worsens in the evening.
    2. Assessing early morning agitation, hyperactivity, and insomnia.
    3. Noting signs of anger, hostility, and loss of control.
    4. Assessing reality distortions and preoccupation with family matters.

18. **QSEN** A patient calls the clinic and asks to speak to the adult-gerontology primary care NP. When the adult-gerontology primary care NP answers the telephone, the patient states that he is going to commit suicide. The priority goal is to:
    1. Refer the patient to an appropriate treatment facility.
    2. Encourage ventilation of angry and depressed feelings.
    3. Assess the lethality of the suicide plan.
    4. Establish rapport with the patient.

19. During an intake interview with a 26-year-old man diagnosed with generalized anxiety disorder, the adult-gerontology primary care NP might observe what type of behavior?
    1. An inflated sense of self.
    2. Constant relation to future events.
    3. Inability to concentrate and irritability when questioned.
    4. Nervousness and fear of the adult-gerontology primary care NP during the interview.

20. An older adult woman answers the adult-gerontology primary care NP's questions by mumbling in low tones with answers that seem inappropriate. What would be initial findings associated with a diagnosis of dementia?
    1. Sees people floating across the ceiling of her room.
    2. Has problems with cognition and confusion.
    3. Hears voices at night telling her to change her clothes.
    4. Shows fear when the nurse makes any movements toward her.

21. An older patient comes to the office with the complaint of confusion. The daughter is concerned that her mother is developing Alzheimer disease. Which of these assessments would indicate the patient is experiencing delirium versus dementia?
    1. The confusion has been slowly developing.
    2. The confusion started after the patient started taking over-the-counter cimetidine (Tagamet).
    3. The patient's attention span has been affected.
    4. The patient's memory has been impaired.

22. When the adult-gerontology primary care NP talks with a patient about his chemical dependency, the patient states, "I wish I would have never used cocaine. It has ruined my life!" What would be the most appropriate response by the adult-gerontology primary care NP?
    1. "You should think before you do something."
    2. "Things will work out, don't worry."
    3. "It sounds like you've thought a lot about your cocaine use."
    4. "You shouldn't be so hard on yourself. You can change."

23. The adult-gerontology primary care NP would expect which symptoms in a patient with a diagnosis of schizophrenia?
    1. High energy with varying sleep patterns and nonstop conversation.
    2. Extreme and frequent mood swings with hyperactivity and difficulty concentrating.
    3. Paranoia, delusions, hallucinations, and diminished self-care.
    4. Antisocial behavior, manipulative, charismatic, and ability to lie convincingly.

24. Dementia can be distinguished from delirium because:
    1. Dementia lasts days to weeks compared to delirium, which lasts months to years.
    2. Dementia is often associated with medications or systemic illness.
    3. Dementia exhibits a disturbance in attention that is not present in delirium.
    4. Dementia is a chronic medical condition and delirium is an acute illness.

25. An older adult patient is brought to the adult-gerontology primary care NP by his family for evaluation of increasing confusion over the past few days. The patient has a history of dementia; however, the family states that there is a definite change. What course of action would the adult-gerontology primary care NP consider?
    1. Help the family look for a nursing home.
    2. Order an MRI scan.
    3. Order a noncontrast head CT.
    4. Order a urinalysis (UA).

26. **QSEN** A middle-aged, upper-middle class, married woman presents to your clinic for the third time in 2 months with a complaint of headache, gastrointestinal upset with abdominal pain, and difficulty sleeping. Past exams have been essentially negative. You suspect the patient suffers from depression, but she has been reluctant to complete even the briefest of screenings for this. Today, the patient requests "something for sleep" again stating that she "doesn't have time to take a bunch of tests." Which tentative diagnosis seems most likely?
    1. Hypochondriasis.
    2. Domestic violence.
    3. Addiction.
    4. Irritable bowel syndrome.

27. An older adult patient was taken to the clinic in a confused state that began suddenly 24 hours ago. She fails to be oriented to person, time, or place. She was incontinent of urine because of her confusion. She looks apathetic and is drowsy. The adult-gerontology primary care NP would suspect:
    1. Delirium.
    2. Dementia.
    3. Depression.
    4. A psychotic disorder.

28. **QSEN** Which of the following groups of patients fall under mandatory reporting laws for abuse and neglect in a majority of states in the United States?
    1. Children, adult women, dependent older adults.
    2. Children, disabled individuals, adult women.
    3. Disabled individuals, adult women, dependent older adults.
    4. Children, disabled individuals, dependent older adults.

29. Which patient statement would be the most reassuring when considering early diagnosis of dementia?
    1. "I have forgotten where I put my keys about three times in the past year."
    2. "I have been in three little car accidents in the past few years."
    3. "My family tells me I am forgetful and don't cook like I should."
    4. "I remember my prom dress, but I can't remember what I had for lunch."

30. Physical findings of cocaine abuse include:
    1. Bradycardia, miosis, hypertension.
    2. Hypertension, tachycardia, tremor.
    3. Hypotension, bradycardia, abdominal cramps.
    4. Decreased level of consciousness, tachycardia, excessive salivation.

31. What three behaviors meet the criteria for alcohol use disorder in the Diagnostic and Statistical Manual of Mental Disorders, Fifth Edition (DSM-V):
    1. Repeated arrests for drunk driving.
    2. Multiple absences from work due to substance use.
    3. Chronic anxiety attacks.
    4. Recurrent arguments with spouse about his/her drinking behavior.
    5. Obsessively washing hands.

32. **QSEN** An older adult patient's wife is concerned about her husband's increasing confusion and agitation. Not only has he exhibited symptoms of increased confusion, but he also is unable to care for his physical needs. He has been incontinent of urine and feces and sometimes is totally unaware of other people. What would be an assessment priority for the patient?
    1. Evaluate changes in social habits.
    2. Assess for hallucinations and impaired reality testing.
    3. Evaluate his orientation to person, place, and time.
    4. Determine if he is experiencing a problem with impaired judgment.

33. **QSEN** A 42-year-old male comes in to the office with his friend. The friend states that he found the patient confused with some shaking and seeing things that are not there. The patient typically drinks two six packs of beer every day. The patient decided to stop drinking 2 days ago. Vital signs show elevated blood pressure, fever, and tachycardia. The adult-gerontology primary care NP transfers the patient to the hospital as he:
    1. Is overdosing on heroin.
    2. Has thyroid storm.
    3. Is septic from pneumonia.
    4. Has delirium tremens.

34. What four items are risk factors for a major depressive disorder in an adult?
    1. Female gender.
    2. Male gender.
    3. Lack of social support.
    4. Married women.
    5. Married men.
    6. Family history of depression.

35. A patient is transferred to the alcohol treatment unit from the emergency room. What is important to include in the therapeutic milieu during detoxification?
    1. Keep the environment adequately lit to diminish hallucinations.
    2. Keep a radio or television on in the room to assist in maintaining orientation.
    3. Speak quietly when in the room to avoid overstimulation.
    4. Keep the suction equipment available in case of seizures.

36. While taking a history, the adult-gerontology primary care NP is aware that the following drug is most commonly first used by an adolescent:
    1. Nicotine.
    2. Alcohol.
    3. Marijuana.
    4. Crystal methamphetamine.

37. In evaluating a 16-year-old female patient, which symptom would indicate anorexia nervosa?
    1. Refuses to discuss questions pertaining to food.
    2. Reflects a positive body image.
    3. States she is eating very well but has episodes of vomiting.
    4. The family states she refuses to stop her severe dieting.

38. A 16-year-old adolescent boy is 54 inches in height. The adult-gerontology primary care NP identifies the following as a positive, effective coping behavior:
    1. Acts as the class clown.
    2. Has a rehearsed reply to teasing comments.
    3. Spends most of his free time watching television.
    4. Has predominantly friends that are short statured.

39. The adult-gerontology primary care NP is examining an older adolescent who has been a long-term intravenous cocaine user. What other findings would alert the adult-gerontology primary care NP to a frequent complication?
    1. Epistaxis and chronic rhinorrhea.
    2. Cardiac arrhythmias and hypertension.
    3. Chest congestion and wheezing.
    4. Hepatitis and cellulitis.

40. The adult-gerontology primary care NP is comparing the typical signs of depression in the adolescent with the adult patient. The depressed adolescent would present with:
    1. Lonely feelings.
    2. Sad, flat affect.
    3. Anger and acting-out behavior.
    4. Feelings of powerlessness and anxiety.

41. While interviewing a teenager to determine her level of health, the adult-gerontology primary care NP recognizes symptoms of anorexia nervosa. Which characteristics of anorexia nervosa would be noted in the admission assessment interview?
    1. Below-to-average intelligence.
    2. Increased libido.
    3. Vigorous daily exercise.
    4. Tachycardia.

42. A teenage female patient is brought to the adult-gerontology primary care NP for evaluation by her grandmother with whom she lives. The teenager has been vomiting and her grandmother believes that she is becoming confused. The

grandmother relates that the patient has been upset lately over a breakup with her boyfriend. What will the adult-gerontology primary care NP investigate as a possible cause for the teenager's symptoms?
1. Appendicitis.
2. Ectopic pregnancy.
3. Drug overdose.
4. Sexually transmitted disease.

43. A teenager comes to the office of the adult-gerontology primary care NP and states that she was raped several hours ago by her boyfriend. The immediate action taken by the adult-gerontology primary care NP is:
    1. Perform a pelvic examination to determine injuries to the patient.
    2. Accompany her to the emergency department for an exam.
    3. Send her immediately for counseling to help her deal with this situation.
    4. Call the patient's parents so they can be with her.

44. While interviewing an adolescent female presenting with her mother for birth control counseling and examination, you detect signs of family tension. During the physical exam, while the mother is out of the room, the daughter admits to frequent marijuana use and occasional drinking. What assessment information would most confirm the presence of active or potential violence in the home?
    1. Signs of general neglect.
    2. Injuries at different stages of healing.
    3. Patient's response to a direct question.
    4. Admitted fear of mother's boyfriend.

45. The adult-gerontology primary care NP's physical exam on an adolescent is as follows: disheveled appearance, 5-lb weight loss since the last visit 2 months ago, pulse strong and regular at 128, + 4 deep tendon reflexes, nasal mucosa erythematous and ulcerated. His mother relates that he has been getting in trouble at school, avoids the adult-gerontology primary care, has no appetite, and is not sleeping much at night. The adult-gerontology primary care NP suspects drug use of:
    1. Heroin.
    2. Marijuana.
    3. LSD.
    4. Crack cocaine.

Pharmacology

46. **QSEN** A patient has been receiving fluphenazine (Prolixin) for the past 3 weeks. The adult-gerontology primary care NP's assessment notes the following: temperature elevated 105.8°F (41°C), marked muscle rigidity, agitation, and confusion. The adult-gerontology primary care

NP understands these findings are often associated with the diagnosis of:
1. Acute dystonia.
2. Tardive dyskinesia.
3. Neuroleptic malignant syndrome.
4. Extrapyramidal disorder.

47. The preferred antidepressant for an older adult patient is:
    1. Amitriptyline (Elavil).
    2. Citalopram (Celexa).
    3. Trazodone (Desyrel).
    4. Haloperidol (Haldol).

48. A patient has been referred to the adult-gerontology primary care NP. The patient's medical history reveals long-term use of benzodiazepines, which the patient considers harmless. The adult-gerontology primary care NP understands that benzodiazepines can:
    1. Cause drug dependency.
    2. Produce nephrotoxicity.
    3. Lead to functional damage of the cardiopulmonary system.
    4. Cause profound dissociative personality problems.

49. Which medication group is considered first-line treatment for anxiety disorders in older adult patients?
    1. Benzodiazepine.
    2. Selective serotonin reuptake inhibitor (SSRI).
    3. Tricyclic antidepressants.
    4. Atypical antipsychotics.

50. An older female has a diagnosis of dementia and is taking haloperidol (Haldol) 2 mg every evening. The adult-gerontology primary care NP observes her engaging in a restless, repetitive movement with her legs. She states that, not only does she have ongoing movement, but she also feels jittery. The adult-gerontology primary care NP would interpret this activity to be:
    1. Ataxia.
    2. Akathisia.
    3. Agitation.
    4. Dyskinesia.

51. The adult-gerontology primary care NP is prescribing an antidepressant medication for an older adult. What is an important consideration about starting doses?
    1. Reduce starting doses by 50%.
    2. Reduce starting doses by 10%.
    3. Increase starting doses by 25%.
    4. Order the normal therapeutic dose.

52. What is the best initial treatment plan for a sleep disorder in the older adult patient?
    1. Medicate with amitriptyline (Elavil).
    2. Medicate with trazodone (Desyrel).
    3. Discuss the importance of naps daily.
    4. Decrease noise and light in the environment.

53. The adult-gerontology primary care NP is aware that patients taking atypical antipsychotics have a higher risk of which three conditions?
    1. Weight loss.
    2. Hypercholesterolemia.
    3. Diabetes.
    4. Metabolic syndrome.
    5. Pulmonary infection.

54. An older adult patient presents with a new symptom of acute confusion over the last 24 hours. Which assessment would be a priority for the adult-gerontology primary care NP to evaluate during the exam?
    1. Medication review.
    2. Electrocardiogram.
    3. Mini-mental status exam.
    4. Thyroid profile.

55. The adult-gerontology primary care NP is aware that the following class of drugs is most likely to precipitate a hypertensive crisis in the older adult:
    1. Narcotic analgesics.
    2. Monoamine oxidase (MAO) inhibitors.
    3. Barbiturates.
    4. Phenothiazines.

56. The adult-gerontology primary care NP knows that the following class of drugs would have the greatest effect on memory in the older adult patient:
    1. Phenothiazines.
    2. Tricyclic antidepressants.
    3. Benzodiazepines.
    4. MAO inhibitors.

57. The adult-gerontology primary care NP understands that adolescents who use LSD:
    1. Experience withdrawal symptoms within 24 hours.
    2. Will quickly become addicted.
    3. Experience flashbacks and depression.
    4. Experience disorientation and delusional feelings.

58. Of the following antidepressants, which one has the most sedating side effects, making it a good sleeping agent?
    1. Fluoxetine (Prozac).
    2. Doxepin (Sinequan).
    3. Trazodone (Desyrel).
    4. Paroxetine (Paxil).

59. In the management of acute alcohol withdrawal delirium, which three drugs would the adult-gerontology primary care NP consider using?
    1. Bupropion (Wellbutrin).
    2. Chlordiazepoxide (Librium).
    3. Lorazepam (Ativan).

    4. Citalopram (Celexa).
    5. Thiamine.
    6. Chlorpromazine (Thorazine).

60. Which three laboratory results would be important to assess before placing a patient on lithium?
    1. TSH, T4, T3.
    2. Fasting lipids.
    3. BUN, creatinine.
    4. Electrolytes.
    5. ESR.
    6. ALT, AST, LDH.

61. **QSEN** A patient comes to the rural clinic having taken an undetermined amount of heroin. Before transferring the patient to a psychiatric treatment facility, the adult-gerontology primary care NP anticipates the drug of choice for an opioid overdose is:
    1. Clonidine (Catapres).
    2. Methadone (Dolophine).
    3. Naloxone (Narcan).
    4. Naltrexone HCl (Revia).

62. Benzodiazepines are useful in the treatment in which three of the following disorders:
    1. Alcohol withdrawal.
    2. Schizophrenia.
    3. Anxiety.
    4. Obsessive-compulsive disorder.
    5. Seizures.
    6. Bipolar affective disorder.

63. **QSEN** When starting a psychotropic medication in the older adult, a good rule of thumb is:
    1. Start low, go slow.
    2. Higher doses are almost always needed.
    3. Side effects of psychotropic medications will usually not impact other medications.
    4. The same adult dosages can be used initially without any problems.

64. A patient is a 20-year, two-pack-a-day smoker with a history of chronic bronchitis. In addition to counseling, what is the prescription to give the patient who wishes to stop smoking?
    1. Nicotine polacrilex (Nicorette) gum 2-mg piece, chew for 30 minutes, q1–2h × 6 weeks, then q2–4h × 3 weeks, then q4–8h × 3 weeks, and then discontinue.
    2. Nicotine patch (Nicoderm) 21 mg/24 hr qd × 6 weeks, then 14 mg/24 hr qd × 2 weeks, then 7 mg/24 hr qd × 2 weeks, and then discontinue.
    3. Bupropion HCl (Zyban) 150 mg qd × 3 days, then 150 mg bid for 7–12 weeks, and then to stop smoking when medication is started.
    4. Nicotine patch (Nicoderm) 14 mg/24 hr qd × 6 weeks, then 7 mg/24 hr qd × 6 weeks, and then discontinue.

65. A young woman tells the adult-gerontology primary care NP that she no longer wants to be on sertraline (Zoloft). She had a traumatic event a few years ago but has been doing much better and has a strong support structure from family and friends. The adult-gerontology primary care NP advises her to:
    1. Stop taking the medication.
    2. Taper the dose slowly.
    3. Keep taking the medication.
    4. Switch to citalopram (Celexa).

66. A patient with bipolar disorder is on divalproex sodium (Depakote) for mania. What test(s) would the adult-gerontology primary care NP monitor?
    1. Liver function test and CBC.
    2. Pulmonary function test.
    3. Electrocardiogram.
    4. Urinalysis with culture and sensitivity.

67. An 82-year-old male, who is on a stable dose of furosemide (Lasix) for heart failure, comes in with complaints of feeling down for the last year after losing his wife. After assessing the patient, the adult-gerontology primary care NP diagnoses the patient with depression and starts the patient on citalopram (Celexa). The adult-gerontology primary care NP knows the patient is at risk for:
    1. Hypernatremia.
    2. Hyponatremia.
    3. Hyperkalemia.
    4. Hypokalemia.

68. A 75-year-old female comes to see the adult-gerontology primary care NP to follow-up on an upper respiratory infection that she has had for 1 week. She has been taking diphenhydramine (Benadryl). The adult-gerontology primary care NP knows this is a poor medication for older adult patients because diphenhydramine (Benadryl) can cause:
    1. Confusion.
    2. Prolonged QT.
    3. Bradycardia.
    4. Hypertension.

69. **QSEN** What is the maximum dose of citalopram (Celexa) for a patient over 60 years old?
    1. 40 mg once daily by mouth.
    2. 20 mg twice daily by mouth.
    3. 20 mg once daily by mouth.
    4. 10 mg once daily by mouth.

70. The adult-gerontology primary care NP understands the following about the use of benzodiazepines in the older adult:
    1. Withdrawal symptoms may occur within 24 hours of abruptly stopping the medication.
    2. Adverse effects are minimal and rarely lead to falls or other injury.
    3. Long-acting medications (e.g., chlordiazepoxide [Librium]) are preferred over the shorter-acting medications (e.g., lorazepam [Ativan]).
    4. Larger doses are needed to maintain therapeutic levels for the anxious or agitated patient.

17 Mental Health Answers & Rationales

Psychosocial Exam & Diagnostic Tests

1. Answer: 2

   Rationale: The mental status exam provides a basic assessment of the patient's intellectual functioning (reasoning, abstract thinking, and memory). The intelligence quotient (IQ) is determined by neuropsychological evaluation. Coordination is part of a neurologic exam and can be tested by rapid alternating movements and heel-to-shin or finger-to-nose tests.

2. Answer: 2

   Rationale: Given the high prevalence of intimate partner violence with women more likely to report intimate partner violence than men and the lack of harm and potential benefits of screening, routine screening is recommended for all patient visits. For those patients who screened positive, the adult-gerontology primary care NP should offer resources, reassure confidentiality, and provide close follow-up.

3. Answer: 1

   Rationale: Delusions are false, fixed beliefs that can be of a persecutory or grandiose nature. In this instance, the patient is experiencing a delusion of grandeur. Often older adults with a diagnosis of dementia will have delusions, which worsen with acute illnesses. A person may have delusions as a symptom of a disorder, such as schizophrenia. They may also occur as part of a delusional disorder, such as grandiose, jealousy, persecutory, somatic, or mixed. A hallucination is a false sensory experience. An illusion is a misinterpretation of reality. Magical thinking is when the patient feels that his or her thoughts or wishes can control other people.

4. Answer: 1

   Rationale: The CRAFFT Screening Test (Car, Relax, Alone, Forget, Friends, Trouble) is a behavioral health screening tool that consists of a series of six questions developed to screen adolescents for high-risk alcohol and other drug use disorders simultaneously. The CAGE questionnaire is a screening tool that asks four questions and is a widely used for screening adults about problem drinking and potential alcohol problems. Physical Activity Enjoyment Scale (PACES) is a reliable tool for assessing enjoyment of physical activity and has been used with all age groups. HITS is a screening tool and scale that stands for Hurt, Insult, Threaten, and Scream that consists of four questions to assess risk for intimate partner violence.

5. Answer: 1

   Rationale: The patient experiencing auditory hallucinations will often look out into space and act as if he or she is listening to someone talking. This is associated with behaviors such as tilting the head, mumbling, and eye movement.

6. Answer: 3

   Rationale: CAGE (Cut down, Annoyed, Guilty, Eye opener) is a screening instrument used to alert providers to possibility of alcoholism.

7. Answer: 3

   Rationale: Dual diagnosis involves both a psychiatric diagnosis and a substance abuse diagnosis.

8. Answer: 3

   Rationale: Abstract thinking is the ability to think about concepts, objects, principles, and ideas that are not physically present. Using a metaphor or an analogy is an example of assessing abstract thinking, for example, "America is a melting pot." Judgment refers to the person's capacity to make good decisions and act on them. Memory is the ability to recall something.

9. Answer: 2

   Rationale: Patients who experience confabulation are fabricating events or situations to fill in gaps in their memory, usually in a plausible way. Confabulation is a common symptom of alcohol amnesic disorder, or Korsakoff syndrome. Echolalia is the parroting or automatic, meaningless repeating of another's words. Perseveration is the involuntary persistent repetition of an idea or response (e.g., patient keeps repeating the same phrase over and over).

10. Answer: 4

    Rationale: Although it is important to know whether the patient has ever experienced hallucinations, delusions, or illusions and had ever been hospitalized in a psychiatric facility, the single most important factor to ascertain is whether or not the patient has contemplated suicide. In addition, determination of a specific plan and the means to do it are also involved in the questioning about suicidal ideation. Asking a patient whether or not he or she is suicidal does not increase the risk of the patient committing suicide. It is also important for the adult-gerontology primary care NP to determine whether the patient regularly takes antidepressants or other medications. Patients may have stopped taking their antidepressant, causing an acute exacerbation of their depression, or starting another medication that may be causing an increase in their depression.

11. Answer: 3

Rationale: A patient's attention span is the length of time the patient can keep their thoughts and interest fixed on something. Although patient cooperation is a necessity for following a series of short commands, it is not measuring attention span. Abstract thinking is the ability to think about concepts, objects, principles, and ideas that are not physically present. Judgment refers to the person's capacity to make good decisions and act on them.

12. Answer: 2

Rationale: The other abnormalities are not usually associated with bulimia. Hypochloremia is associated with the purging (self-induced vomiting). Other fluid and electrolyte imbalances that may be seen include hyponatremia, hypokalemia, and metabolic alkalosis and acidosis.

13. Answer: 1

Rationale: Recent memory is tested by asking the patient to recall something after a brief delay. Testing for remote memory is usually related to historical events (past presidents or maiden name). Thinking and cognition can be assessed by asking the patient to solve a simple math problem.

14. Answer: 3

Rationale: It is appropriate to check for other conditions that cause confusion, such as hypothyroidism and folic acid and vitamin B_{12} deficiency. The other tests listed are important for patient health but will not help determine the cause of confusion.

15. Answer: 1

Rationale: Drug tolerance exists when the same dose of the drug produces reduced effects, and is usually seen with the development of physical dependence on any medication. Addiction occurs when there is a deep-seated psychological need for the drug/medication.

16. Answer: 3

Rationale: Abstract thinking requires the patient to compare and tell how two things are alike or different, involving the thought process that is oriented toward the development of an idea without application to a particular object; it is independent of space and time. Today's date assists to determine orientation, the names of past presidents assists to demonstrate long-term memory, and repetition of numbers assists to demonstrate short-term memory.

Psychiatric Disorders

17. Answer: 1

Rationale: Confusion can occur in both dementia and depression. However, with dementia, symptoms worsen at night and are commonly referred to as sundowning. Additionally, the adult-gerontology primary care NP must also ensure that the increased confusion is not a result of an acute illness. Often the only sign or symptom the demented older adult may present with is confusion. Usually the culprit is a urinary tract infection. The adult-gerontology primary care NP should order a urine analysis to ensure that the confusion is not the result of an acute illness and is reversible.

18. Answer: 4

Rationale: The adult-gerontology primary care NP must first establish trust and rapport with the caller before an assessment can be made. If rapport is not established, the patient will hang up the phone. The adult-gerontology primary care NP understands that, by keeping the patient talking, he or she is prevented from acting out the suicidal threat.

19. Answer: 3

Rationale: Impaired concentration and irritability are major characteristics of generalized anxiety disorder. Other symptoms of generalized anxiety disorder include excessive anxiety and worry; inability to control the worry and restlessness; easily fatigued; difficulty concentrating; muscle tension; and sleep disturbance. Patients often pace the exam room because of their irritability; they are more focused on the here and now and have low self-esteem.

20. Answer: 2

Rationale: Confusion and cognitive function problems (e.g., short-term memory loss) are initial signs of dementia. Other signs of early-stage Alzheimer dementia include time and spatial disorientation, poor judgment, personality changes, depression or withdrawal, and perceptual disturbances. The severity of the symptoms depends on what stage of cognitive degeneration the patient is manifesting. The other options are characteristic of hallucinatory experiences and may occur later. This patient may also be exhibiting signs and symptoms of an acute illness. The culprit is commonly a urinary tract infection and the adult-gerontology primary care NP should order a urinalysis to ensure that that cause of the confusion is not related to a reversible cause.

21. Answer: 2

Rationale: Cimetidine (Tagamet) is not tolerated well in the older adult patient and should be avoided, as reversible central nervous system effects can occur, such as disorientation, mental confusion, agitation, psychosis, depression anxiety, and hallucinations. It is important to obtain a thorough history of all over-the-counter medications, as well as those prescribed. Any time a new medication is added to an older adult patient's medication regimen, an abrupt onset of confusion must be reviewed closely, because it may be attributed to the new medication or a drug-drug interaction with an existing medication. Another possibility is the onset of an acute illness, which often manifests as acute confusion in the older adult patient. Most often the culprit is a UTI; therefore in addition to a careful medication review, obtaining a urinalysis could also rule out a UTI. When a patient has true dementia, the onset of confusion develops slowly, over a longer period of time and not acutely, which would indicate that there is another underlying problem causing the acute confusion. Attention span and memory may be affected in each diagnosis.

22. Answer: 3

Rationale: The adult-gerontology primary care NP's statement acknowledges the patient's feelings and is open ended, which promotes open discussion and helps the patient clarify feelings and thoughts. Telling the patient to think before doing something is condescending and punitive. Telling the patient to not worry and things will work out offers false reassurance. When the adult-gerontology primary care NP tells the patient to not be so hard on himself or herself, it tends to discount the patient's feelings.

23. Answer: 3

Rationale: The characteristics of schizophrenia are paranoia, delusions, tangential thought, suspiciousness, disorganized behavior, and hallucinations.

24. Answer: 4

Rationale: Dementia lasts for months to years and the patient never recovers. Delirium is an acute process that is often associated with medications or a systemic illness, and is reversible once the acute problem is addressed and resolved.

25. Answer: 4

Rationale: One of the most common reasons for an acute change in mental status in the demented older adult patient is an acute infection. This is usually a urinary tract infection (UTI). Usually, the demented older adult patient is incontinent, and, because of the changes of aging, does not recognize the normal signs or symptoms of a UTI (burning, urgency, frequency, and suprapubic tenderness). Older adults also do not typically run elevated temperatures. The adult-gerontology primary care NP should order a UA to ensure that an acute infectious process is not the cause of the acute confusion. The adult-gerontology primary care NP should also conduct a medication review to ensure that no new medications have been added or that no new over-the-counter or herbal medications have been added because this is the second major reason for acute confusion in the older adult patient.

26. Answer: 2

Rationale: The indicators to domestic violence in this case are the multiple vague physical complaints without supporting objective data, the suspected depression, and the reluctance to wait around in the clinic for extended periods of time. This patient is on the verge of disclosing if a provider would only ask her about domestic violence.

27. Answer: 1

Rationale: Based on the state of acute confusion and the incontinence, she is experiencing delirium. This is most likely secondary to sepsis, with the source of infection being a urinary tract infection. The fact that she has mental status changes (disoriented to person, place, or time, in addition to the acute confusion, delirium, and incontinence) gives you the clues to sepsis. Dementia is more insidious versus acute. Depression and psychosis are not consistent with the assessments. The major symptoms in depression would include loss of interest, sleep disorder, decreased appetite, loss of concentration, inactivity, guilt, lack of energy, and potential suicidal thoughts. Psychotic disorders include thoughts and behavior indicating the patient is not in touch with reality.

28. Answer: 4

Rationale: The laws in most states require the reporting of suspected or actual abuse and neglect of any person considered to be dependent or with a reduced ability to make life choices. Children, disabled individuals, and dependent older adults fall into these categories. Very few states require reporting for adult women unless a weapon is involved; this is a different situation, requiring a report.

29. Answer: 1

Rationale: Patients admitting to forgetfulness are not as much of a concern for the diagnosis of cognitive impairment as those who have been in motor vehicle accidents or deny any level of memory loss. Dementia is associated with loss of short-term/recent memory more than long-term/remote memory loss.

30. Answer: 2

Rationale: Bradycardia and excessive salivation are not found with cocaine abuse. There are no drug antagonists that can be used for cocaine overdose, although benzodiazepines are used to treat effects of cocaine toxicity such as seizures, tachycardia, and hypertension. Naloxone is given to reduce the concurrent toxic effects of other narcotic drugs that may be in the patient's body system but is not effective against cocaine toxicity.

31. Answer: 1, 2, 4

Rationale: Chronic anxiety attacks and obsessive-compulsive disorder behaviors are not part of the Diagnostic and Statistical Manual of Mental Disorders, Fifth Edition (DSM-V) criteria for alcohol use disorder.

32. Answer: 4

Rationale: Although all of the items listed are appropriate to assess in the patient, it is most important to determine judgment. If he cannot make safe judgments, he is at high risk for unsafe behaviors, such as driving, walking along the sidewalk, running the bath water, etc.

33. Answer: 4

Rationale: Delirium tremens is severe alcohol withdrawal that typically develops 24–72 hours after the last drink. The patient may be confused and disoriented and have hallucinations, tremors, elevated blood pressure, tachycardia, a rise in body temperature, and tonic-clonic seizures. A patient with heroin overdose may also be confused, but he or she would have hypotension, slowed respirations, and a decreased pulse. A patient septic from pneumonia may present with cough, chills, low oxygen saturation, fever, hypotension, and tachycardia. Thyroid storm is severe hyperthyroidism that presents with elevated temperature, weakness, sweating, confusion, tachycardia, and gastrointestinal symptoms.

34. Answer: 1, 3, 4, 6

Rationale: The risk factors for depression include the following: female gender, history of depression, unmarried men, married women, within 6 months of having a baby, pain, lack of social support, medical illness, substance abuse, and a negative or traumatic event.

35. Answer: 1

Rationale: The patient needs to be able to easily interpret his surroundings. Shadows or areas of poor lighting will increase the hallucinations. When in the room, it is important to speak in clear tones and make sure to include the patient in the conversations to decrease the paranoia and feelings that people are talking about him or her. Radio and television may provide too many stimuli and may not be of any assistance in maintaining orientation. Suction equipment is for physical safety, not therapeutic milieu.

36. Answer: 1

Rationale: Nicotine is known as the "gateway drug" and is commonly the first drug used by adolescents.

37. Answer: 4

Rationale: Adolescents with anorexia nervosa will severely reduce their nutritional intake by dieting constantly on high fiber and low calories. They usually have an inappropriate body image and may admit to occasional episodes of vomiting.

38. Answer: 2

Rationale: Role playing and planning a rehearsed reply to teasing comments about short stature are helpful tools to deal with this issue. Although humor can be effective, constantly clowning around for attention is not positive coping behavior. Withdrawal (e.g., watching television or reading) is not effective coping and may indicate depression. Spending time and associating only with younger adolescents who are his height is not a positive coping behavior and may hinder normal maturation.

39. Answer: 4

Rationale: More than 50% of intravenous cocaine users develop hepatitis, phlebitis, endocarditis, and acquired immunodeficiency syndrome. Epistaxis, rhinorrhea, and nasal congestion are seen most often in intranasal users of cocaine. Chest congestion, wheezing, and eventual emphysema occur with chronic free-base (crack) smokers. Although cardiac arrhythmias, hypertension, and respiratory arrest can occur, they are not the common complications.

40. Answer: 3

Rationale: Adolescents often act out to protect themselves from feelings of vulnerability and dependency. It is important to evaluate signs of anger and frustration in the adolescent because the significance of the behavior may indicate symptoms of depression. Adults who are depressed typically display findings noted in the other three options.

41. Answer: 3

Rationale: People with anorexia nervosa will exercise up to 4 hours a day. They are above average intelligence in most cases, suffer from bradycardia, and have decreased libido.

42. Answer: 3

Rationale: The grandmother's concern is warranted. In teenage girls, the most common form of suicide attempt is by drug overdose. The combination of vomiting and confusion suggests a drug overdose, and the adult-gerontology primary care NP should run a toxicology screen.

43. Answer: 2

Rationale: This patient should be examined by emergency department personnel, many of whom are specially trained to collect the evidence needed to testify in court about rape. The exam should not be done in the office unless the adult-gerontology primary care NP has been trained in evidence collection and has a rape evidence collection kit. The exam must be done quickly, before evidence is destroyed. The patient decides who should be called for support. Although she is encouraged to call her parents, she is also offered the support of rape crisis and other resources.

44. Answer: 4

Rationale: Although all answers may contribute to an adult-gerontology primary care NP's suspicion of family violence, the admission of genuine fear of a household member is considered an excellent indicator of actual or potential violence and the level of danger in a home. The adult-gerontology primary care NP should involve social services to assist the adolescent female in this situation.

45. Answer: 4

Rationale: Often, the first indication of drug use in adolescents is a sudden change in behavior or school performance. Symptoms of heroin use are constricted pupils, respiratory depression, needle tracks, and poor nutrition. Symptoms of marijuana use are slow reflexes, tachycardia, conjunctival injection, nasal congestion, and increased appetite. Symptoms of LSD use are dilated pupils, reddened eyes, hypertension, increased appetite, and hallucinations. The use of central nervous system stimulants, like crack cocaine, leads to hypertension, weight loss, anorexia, insomnia, hyperreflexia, and a perforated or ulcerated nasal septum.

Pharmacology

46. Answer: 3

Rationale: The patient is experiencing a rare problem called neuroleptic malignant syndrome. The patient would require immediate referral and hospitalization. This can also occur with the medication prochlorperazine. Acute dystonia, parkinsonism, and akathisia are associated with extrapyramidal disorder or acute movement disorder. Tardive dyskinesia occurs late in therapy and is often irreversible. Slow, wormlike movements of the tongue are the earliest symptom, followed by grimacing, lip smacking, and involuntary limb movements.

47. Answer: 2

Rationale: The favorable side effect profile of citalopram (Celexa), which is an SSRI, makes it a useful antidepressant

in the older adult because it has a short half-life. Amitriptyline (Elavil) has the most anticholinergic and sedating side effects of the antidepressants. There may be pronounced effects on the cardiovascular system (hypotension). Geropsychiatrists agree it is best to avoid amitriptyline (Elavil) in the older adult; however, low dose (10 mg, PO every evening) is low cost and can be effective at controlling neuropathic pain. Trazodone (Desyrel) is very sedating for the older adult patient but can be used for insomnia and for behavioral issues with dementia patients. Haloperidol (Haldol) is an antipsychotic medication and is not to be used at all in long-term care facilities.

48. Answer: 1

Rationale: Physical dependence can occur, even with low doses of benzodiazepines. This is a particular problem in the older adult, who is sensitive to low dose ranges. If possible, it is better to slowly taper the patient from benzodiazepines; often they can be tapered to a much lower dose.

49. Answer: 2

Rationale: Antidepressants, such as selective serotonin reuptake inhibitors (SSRIs) and serotonin-norepinephrine reuptake inhibitors (SNRIs), are considered first-line treatment for anxiety disorders. Benzodiazepines are not helpful in the older adult patient due to problems associated with this class of medications, including increased risk of falls, confusion, and memory problems. Tricyclic antidepressants (TCAs) and older monoamine oxidase inhibitors have indications for management of some of the anxiety disorders but are not considered first line because of tolerability and carry a high risk of cardiac dysrhythmias. Atypical antipsychotics are not first-line therapy and include significant side effects (metabolic syndrome, extrapyramidal effects, sedation), which can be problematic for the older adult.

50. Answer: 2

Rationale: Akathisia is a feeling of restlessness and can be challenging to distinguish from anxiety. The adult-gerontology primary care NP should slowly taper the patient from the haloperidol (Haldol) 2 mg; it is possible that she may not need the medication or that one of the newer atypical antipsychotics would be more effective with a lesser side effect profile. Patients may complain of a feeling of muscular quivering. Ataxia is a disorder wherein muscular incoordination occurs with voluntary muscular movements. Agitation is a general assessment that may be part of the psychotic behavior. Dyskinesia is a defect in voluntary movement.

51. Answer: 1

Rationale: It is important to reduce starting doses of antidepressants by 50% in older adults, people with impaired renal function, or those especially sensitive to side effects.

52. Answer: 4

Rationale: Correction of environmental factors and treatment of underlying iatrogenic and medical problems should be addressed initially. Amitriptyline (Elavil) can cause excessive somnolence. Trazodone (Desyrel) may be of particular use when sleep disturbance is prominent; however, it does not address the best initial plan. The goal is to begin with good sleep hygiene before pharmacologic therapy. Eliminating naps during the day may be useful in facilitating sleep.

53. Answer: 2, 3, 4

Rationale: The atypical antipsychotics, such as clozapine (Clozaril), olanzapine (Zyprexa), quetiapine (Seroquel), have been linked to weight gain, dyslipidemia, diabetes, metabolic syndrome, and accelerated cardiovascular disease. Weight loss and pulmonary infections are not associated with atypical antipsychotic medication use.

54. Answer: 1

Rationale: Drug-drug interactions are a common cause of acute confusion in the older adult patient. This medication review assessment can minimize the need to do further costly interventions if the patient only needs medication adjustment. The other options should be included in the plan after the medication review history is completed and has been ruled out as a potential problem. The adult-gerontology primary care NP must always consider that an acute illness, such as a urinary tract infection, may be the cause of acute confusion. A urinalysis should also be obtained because the patient can quickly progress to sepsis.

55. Answer: 2

Rationale: In combination with tyramine-rich foods that have undergone an aging process such as cheese, wine, beer, salami, and yogurt, catecholamines are released from the nerve endings, causing a hypertensive crisis. The other drugs listed cause hypotension.

56. Answer: 3

Rationale: The benzodiazepines cause sedation and decreased attention, which, in turn, affect the memory. Although phenothiazines and antidepressants may also cause sedation, they do not affect memory.

57. Answer: 3

Rationale: Flashbacks, depression, and psychotic behavior can occur with lysergic acid diethylamide (LSD) use.

There are no withdrawal symptoms or physical dependence associated with use; however, tolerance develops quickly. Commonly, the adolescent remains oriented but experiences hallucinations and altered bodily sensations.

58. Answer: 3

Rationale: Trazodone (Desyrel) has sedation as a side effect, which has made it less popular as an antidepressant; however, it is commonly prescribed for insomnia.

59. Answer: 2, 3, 5

Rationale: Lorazepam (Ativan) is a short-acting benzodiazepine and may be used in acute alcohol withdrawal delirium. Chlordiazepoxide (Librium) is also a benzodiazepine and can be used for acute alcohol withdrawal. Thiamine (B_1) deficiency is often seen with alcoholism and should be given as a supplement. Citalopram (Celexa) and bupropion (Wellbutrin) are antidepressants and are not used in acute alcohol withdrawal. Chlorpromazine (Thorazine), which is an antipsychotic, would not be used in the management plan.

60. Answer: 1, 3, 4

Rationale: Lithium has adverse side effects on renal, cardiac, and thyroid function. Baseline electrolytes are also important to obtain. It is not important to evaluate liver function, fasting lipids, and ESR before initiating treatment with lithium.

61. Answer: 3

Rationale: Naloxone (Narcan) is a narcotic antagonist and is used for the reversal of narcotic depression, including respiratory depression. Clonidine (Catapres) is a central-acting α_2-agonist and is indicated for treatment of hypertension. Methadone is used in the treatment of opioid addiction. The Food and Drug Administration (FDA) has placed methadone in a special drug category that allows medically supervised administration of the drug to addicts with chronic, intractable addiction to heroin. In addition, methadone can be used for pain management. The therapeutic classification of naltrexone (Revia) is as a narcotic detoxification adjunct.

62. Answer: 1, 3, 5

Rationale: Seizures, alcohol withdrawal, and anxiety are commonly treated with benzodiazepines. They are not the first drug of choice for obsessive-compulsive disorder; selective serotonin reuptake inhibitors are usually used. Schizophrenia and bipolar affective disorder are treated with antipsychotics.

63. Answer: 1

Rationale: The rule of thumb for starting medications in the older adult patient is to start low and go slow; therefore doses should be reduced by 30%–50% to start therapy and gradually increased as necessary. Adverse effects are likely to occur because of slowed drug metabolism, which occurs with aging. These include hypotension, arrhythmias, and sedative and anticholinergic effects.

64. Answer: 2

Rationale: A highly nicotine-dependent patient benefits from intense counseling and prescription of alternative nicotine delivery during the smoking cessation process. The nicotine patch is usually the preferred form of replacement because the gum is noncontinuous and withdrawal symptoms may occur during nonchewing times. The nicotine patch delivers a fixed dose of nicotine on a continual basis, is applied once daily, and eliminates the gastrointestinal upset that often occurs with the gum. If this patient insisted on using the gum, the dose should be 4 mg, not 2 mg. A nicotine patch with 14 mg is too low a dose to start on this patient and is not the correct dosing schedule. Underdosing can cause patients to start smoking again. Zyban (bupropion HCl) would be used in conjunction with the nicotine patch, and patients are to quit smoking 1–2 weeks after starting the Zyban, not immediately.

65. Answer: 2

Rationale: When stopping a selective serotonin reuptake inhibitor (SSRI), such as sertraline (Zoloft), it is important to taper the dose over at least 2 weeks. Stopping the medication abruptly can lead to flulike symptoms. There is no need to continue the medication or switch to a different antidepressant because the patient was assessed for safety and it is reasonable to stop the medication. The adult-gerontology primary care NP should make a follow-up appointment to assess how the patient is doing off the medication.

66. Answer: 1

Rationale: Divalproex sodium (Depakote) is an antiepileptic used to treat seizures, mania in bipolar disorder, and prevent migraine headaches and is used for agitation in dementia patients. Divalproex sodium (Depakote) can cause hepatotoxicity, especially in the first 6 months of starting the medication. It can also cause thrombocytopenia and pancreatitis in some incidences.

67. Answer: 2

Rationale: Selective serotonin reuptake inhibitors (SSRIs), such as citalopram (Celexa), can lead to hyponatremia from syndrome of inappropriate antidiuretic hormone (SIADH). The patient is at particular risk because he is an older adult and is on furosemide (Lasix). The patient may be at risk for hypokalemia secondary to furosemide (Lasix), but it is not aggravated with the addition of citalopram (Celexa).

68. Answer: 1

Rationale: Diphenhydramine (Benadryl) is an antihistamine with anticholinergic properties. Anticholinergic drugs may cause confusion, urinary retention, orthostatic hypotension, tachycardia, dry mouth, constipation, sedation, and blurred vision. Anticholinergic drugs are particularly dangerous in the older adult because they can lead to falls and confusion.

69. Answer: 3

Rationale: The maximum dose of citalopram (Celexa) for a patient older than age 60 is 20 mg. Celexa has a risk of prolonged QT interval, which can lead to torsades de pointes. Torsades de pointes is a ventricular dysrhythmia that can lead to sudden death.

70. Answer: 1

Rationale: Benzodiazepines should be tapered in all patients but especially in the older adult. Withdrawal symptoms may include sweating, vomiting, muscle cramps, tremors, and/or seizures. Rebound or withdrawal symptoms occur within 24 hours in patients taking the shorter-acting medications and may not occur for several days in patients taking long-acting medications. The adverse effects of oversedation—dizziness, confusion, and orthostatic hypotension—contribute to falls and other injuries in the older adult. Short-acting medications are preferred. Typically, larger doses are not needed but rather small initial doses with gradual increases.

18

Research & Theory

Research

1. The adult-gerontology primary care NP has determined that the current policy and procedures for diagnosing and stabilizing new diabetic patients need to be updated to reflect current evidence-based practice (EBP) standards. Using the Stetler's Model of Research Utilization to Facilitate EBP, what is the first step in using research evidence to promote EBP?
   1. Phase II: Validation.
   2. Phase I: Preparation.
   3. Phase V: Evaluation.
   4. Phase IV: Translation/Application.

2. An adult-gerontology primary care NP has read a nursing research article in which there were no statistically significant findings. In interpreting these findings, what would be the adult-gerontology primary care NP's most appropriate response?
   1. "Because there were no statistically significant findings, there are no relationships between the study groups."
   2. "Because there were no statistically significant findings, there is no reason to conduct similar studies."
   3. "Because there were no statistically significant findings, further study is warranted to compare results."
   4. "Because there were no statistically significant findings, the sample size was too large."

3. The best explanation of the peer review process in research is:
   1. To ensure that the manuscript is well written.
   2. To determine whether the manuscript provides additional information on the content subject area.
   3. To provide edits for grammar and formatting in the submitted manuscript.
   4. To begin to learn how to analyze research and data findings.

4. What is the primary purpose of utilizing evidence-based practice in clinical research and practice management?
   1. Increasing the amount of credible resources that can be used in clinical decision making.
   2. To further advance the peer review process.
   3. To provide quality care to patients by closing the gap between theory, experience, and best practice guidelines.
   4. To arrive at a consensus of opinion.

5. In a recent study, the researcher reports that "the statistical analysis used was Pearson's product-moment correlation." Based on this information, when is it appropriate to use Pearson's product-moment correlation as the statistical analysis for analyzing data in research? Select two responses.
   1. Pearson's product-moment correlation can be used for comparing interval or ratio levels of measurement among two or more variables.
   2. Pearson's product-moment correlation actually determines if a causal relationship exists between one or more variables.
   3. Pearson's product-moment correlation can be used only when there is a single variable.
   4. Pearson's product-moment correlation is used to identify the relationship between two or more variables.

6. When might a qualitative research design be employed over a quantitative or mixed methods research design?
   1. Qualitative research is the preferred methodology for exploring and understanding a particular phenomenon of interest.
   2. Qualitative research does not require rights of research subjects to be protected.
   3. Qualitative research will provide precise measures for statistical analysis.
   4. Qualitative research ensures tight control during data collection and data analysis.

7. A patient's serum sodium on postsurgical day 1 was 132 mEq/L, on postsurgical day 2 was 136 mEq/L, and on postsurgical day 3 was 137 mEq/L. What is the mean for the patient's serum sodium value?
   1. 132 mEq/L.
   2. 136 mEq/L.
   3. 135 mEq/L.
   4. 145 mEq/L.

8. An adult-gerontology primary care NP is reviewing a research article which refers to a study of elderly patients who receive different treatment protocols regarding fall risk assessments. Based on this information, what type of research design is being represented?
   1. Historical.
   2. Experimental.
   3. Correlational.
   4. Descriptive.

9. Variance is a key statistical concept. How would current research methods change if there were no variance?
   1. Nurse researchers would need to increase the sample size in all research studies to 100 research subjects or greater.
   2. Because current research methods do not depend on the presence of variance, researchers would not need to change current methods.
   3. Nurse researchers would need to decrease the sample size of all research studies to 15 research subjects.
   4. Because current research methods are based on the presence of variance, researchers would not be able to use current methods.

10. An adult-gerontology primary care NP is reviewing an assessment tool to determine whether the tool should be used in the clinical practice setting. Which statistical measure would indicate that the tool can be used?
    1. Two-tailed t-test.
    2. Descriptive statistics.
    3. Cronbach's alpha.
    4. Factor analysis.

11. An adult-gerontology primary care NP understands that an incidence rate is (select two responses):
    1. Often a percentage and describes the characteristics of a population.
    2. A sensitive indicator of the changing health of a community.
    3. The number of new cases of a disease in those exposed to a disease.
    4. The number of cases of a specific disease or condition in a population at a specified point in time relative to the population at the same point in time.
    5. The occurrence of new cases of a disease or condition in a population over a period of time relative to the size of the population at risk for the disease of condition in the same time period.

12. A community screening for hypertension revealed 15 patients previously diagnosed with hypertension and 22 new cases for a total of 37 cases. What is this called?
    1. Case-fatality rate.
    2. Incidence rate.
    3. Incidence proportion.
    4. Prevalence rate.

13. A state public health region reported 21 cases of influenza in adults 65 years of age and older to date this year, with two adults who died. The total population for this geographic region is 11,533 of whom 4420 are adults 65 years of age and older. What is the prevalence rate of influenza in the region thus far in the current year?
    1. 1.8/1000.
    2. 2/1000.
    3. 21/1000.
    4. 4.7/1000.

14. What are the five major sequential steps in evidence-based practice (EBP)?
    1. Establish a patient relationship, perform a health assessment, make a diagnosis, devise a plan of care, perform prescribed treatments, and evaluate efficacy of the treatments.
    2. Identify the problem and generate a clinical question, conduct a literature review of scholarly research articles, critically appraise published research, implement useful findings in practice and clinical decision making, and disseminate findings.
    3. Review the popular literature; review the institution's policy and procedures; summarize the findings from the literature review, policies, and procedures; and evaluate applicability of the study findings to practice setting.
    4. Review the patient's lab reports, complete a thorough health assessment, diagnose, collaborate with the healthcare provider in developing a treatment plan, implement the treatment, and evaluate the efficacy of the treatment.

15. An adult-gerontology primary care NP is planning to conduct a study to examine the efficacy of a high-protein, high-fiber diet in weight reduction of obese patients. The adult-gerontology primary care NP develops the following research question to guide the study: *What is the effect on the weight of obese patients who follow a high-protein, high-fiber diet compared with the weight of obese patients who do not follow a high-protein, high-fiber diet over a 12-week period?*
    What is the independent variable and dependent variable in the research question?
    1. The independent variable is the 12-week timeframe and the dependent variable is the high-protein, high-fiber diet.
    2. The independent variable is the high-protein, high-fiber diet and the dependent variable is the patients' weight.

3. The independent variable is the patients' weight and the dependent variable is the high-protein, high-fiber diet.

4. The independent variable is the high-protein, high-fiber diet and the dependent variable is the 12-week timeframe.

16. The adult-gerontology primary care NP is evaluating research reports on the efficacy of cognitive-behavioral therapy (CBT) on anxiety in patients with Alzheimer disease. When reviewing the literature, which type of research study does the adult-gerontology primary care NP recognize as the highest level of evidence?

    1. A qualitative research study using a grounded theory approach.
    2. A quantitative research study using a correlational research design.
    3. A quantitative research study using a randomized-controlled trial design.
    4. A qualitative research study using a phenomenologic approach.

17. When the adult-gerontology primary care NP determines whether being exposed to secondhand smoke leads to lung cancer in a group of residential home patients with another group of residential patients that have not been exposed to secondhand smoke, the adult-gerontology primary care NP is determining the:

    1. Prevalence rate.
    2. Incidence rate.
    3. Confidence interval.
    4. Relative risk.

18. The state public health department reported a total of 423 cases of tuberculosis between 2014 and 2016. During that same time, 17 deaths were attributed to tuberculosis. Based on this information, what is the death-to-case ratio?

    1. 4.05.
    2. 2.08.
    3. 2.48.
    4. 4.01.

19. The adult-gerontology primary care NP is conducting a meta-analysis on the effectiveness of patient teaching on how to use a metered-dose-inhaler (MDI) in the treatment of asthma patients. Which three statements are accurate concerning a meta-analysis?

    1. Assesses clinical effectiveness of health care interventions.
    2. Provides a precise estimate of the treatment effect.
    3. Focuses on a few targeted studies with homogeneity.
    4. Adds potential bias to the review of specific research studies.
    5. Provides a qualitative review of pertinent research literature.
    6. Provides highest level of evidence due to statistical analysis and integration of many studies.

20. The adult-gerontology primary care NP is working with a team of colleagues on a research study that will involve patients. The research team understands that what must be included in the written consent to participate?

    1. Role of the primary research investigator.
    2. Anticipated date for publication of the completed research report.
    3. Assurance of patient privacy and confidentiality.
    4. Number of previously published research studies about this topic.

21. An adult-gerontology primary care NP is trying to determine if a group of elderly patients are at increased risk for falls and wants to design a research study to examine the concerns of both patient and family member relative to the impact that falls in the elderly population have on physical and emotional life style changes. What type of research design should be employed?

    1. Quantitative research design looking at number of falls and hospital admissions as a result of complications.
    2. Mixed methods design looking at physical variables related to falls, hospital admissions, and focus group discussions to allow for exchange of information related to feelings.
    3. Qualitative research using focus groups to obtain information for analysis.
    4. Quasi-experimental design to examine relationships among participants.

22. The adult-gerontology primary care NP understands that when determining whether to incorporate a new procedure into a clinical practice based on the findings of a recent quantitative research study, which of the following should be considered (select two responses)?

    1. Statistical significance of the findings.
    2. Statistical relevance of the findings.
    3. Statistical software program used.
    4. Statistical background of the researcher.
    5. Methodological limitations of the study.

23. The adult-gerontology primary care NP understands that both descriptive and inferential statistics are used in research. However, their purposes are different in that (select two responses):

    1. Inferential statistics are used for assigning participant code numbers.
    2. Descriptive statistics are used for assigning participant code numbers.
    3. Descriptive statistics are used to provide information about the study sample.
    4. Inferential statistics are used for hypothesis testing.
    5. Descriptive statistics are used for hypothesis testing.

24. The adult-gerontology primary care NP is preparing to participate in a research study and is considering the key differences between qualitative and quantitative research designs. The NP discovers, upon review, that the key differences between these two research designs include:
    1. Qualitative research is a process in which the researcher attempts to stay far removed from the process to control for potential bias.
    2. Quantitative research design aims to search for themes collected during the research process.
    3. Qualitative research methods utilize research questions and/or hypotheses to test for relationships or cause and effect.
    4. Quantitative researchers employ controls during the research process to minimize impact to the results of the study.

25. The scientific method for conducting research uses the null hypothesis, which is statistically based. What is the correct format for stating the null hypothesis?
    1. There is no relationship between the independent and dependent variables.
    2. There is a significant relationship between the independent and dependent variables.
    3. There is a moderate relationship between the independent and dependent variables.
    4. There is an opposite relationship between the independent and dependent variables.

26. When evaluating claims made on advertisements, such as "Drug X has been used for 5 years with over 1 million doses administered in the United States, Canada, and Great Britain. Drug X stops heartburn, aids in digestion, and prevents esophageal reflux, and is the 'treatment of choice' to relieve GERD," the adult-gerontology primary care NP realizes that the claim is:
    1. Invalid; there is no control or comparison group, and no statistics are stated.
    2. Valid; there are sufficient numbers of users who have had success.
    3. Invalid; the level of significance is not mentioned to be at the 0.05 level or higher.
    4. Valid; as the Hawthorne effect clearly demonstrates the relationship between the drug and the outcome.

27. The adult-gerontology primary care NP is critiquing several research articles to evaluate causality of an intervention to improve patient health. The NP will consider what three questions to evaluate causality?
    1. Did the independent variable(s) have an impact on the dependent variable(s)?
    2. Did the influence of the intervention occur before the outcome?
    3. Did the researcher provide their credentials in the study report?
    4. Did the researcher control for extraneous variable(s) that may have impacted the effect?

28. What is the difference between univariate and multivariate studies?
    1. Number of subjects in the sample.
    2. Number of statistical hypotheses.
    3. Number of sites for collecting data.
    4. Number of variables being studied.

29. The adult-gerontology primary care NP is compiling monthly statistics for the practice. One piece of data that is collected is the ethnicity of patients. What level of measurement data can be used to analyze the variable of ethnicity?
    1. Nominal level.
    2. Ordinal level.
    3. Interval level.
    4. Ratio level.

30. Quantitative research articles provide a section containing descriptive findings because descriptive data analysis:
    1. Provides the basis for making inferences about the findings.
    2. May yield statistically significant findings that were unexpected.
    3. Provides a clearer understanding of study participants and variables.
    4. Is conducted for predicting patient outcomes in nursing settings.

31. An adult-gerontology primary care NP is compiling statistics at the end of the month for an older adult patient population with coronary artery disease. The adult-gerontology primary care NP and physician in the general practice want to know the average total cholesterol level of their patients. Which would be the most appropriate statistical measure of the average cholesterol level for the patient population?
    1. The mean.
    2. The median.
    3. The mode.
    4. The range.

32. An adult-gerontology primary care NP is evaluating research articles for a research utilization project. The majority of the articles report that randomization was used. The practitioner understands that the purpose of randomization in many quantitative research studies is to:
    1. Be sure that subjects can choose whether they receive the intervention or not.
    2. Select research subjects who fit certain demographic criteria.
    3. Attempt to control for threats to internal validity by allowing research subjects to choose either the control or treatment group.
    4. Attempt to control for threats to internal validity by randomly assigning research subjects to either a control or treatment group.

33. The ability to predict outcomes of care is desirable both in research and in practice. If an adult-gerontology primary care NP wanted to determine the impact of the independent variables of exercise and diet on the dependent variable of blood pressure, which statistical analysis method would be most appropriate to analyze the clinical data?
    1. Descriptive statistics.
    2. Paired t-test.
    3. Multiple regression.
    4. Chi-squared (χ^2) test.

34. Quantitative research articles are being evaluated by an adult-gerontology primary care NP for an evidence-based practice project. What four steps are essential in providing a critical appraisal of a quantitative research article?
    1. Read the discussion section.
    2. Identify the strengths and limitations of the study.
    3. Examine the professional and educational background of the research author(s).
    4. Examine the presentation and organization of the research article.
    5. Evaluate the study's contribution to nursing knowledge.

Theory

35. Which statement provides a best practice approach towards the development of nursing theory?
    1. Nursing theory should be integrated with other disciplines so as to arrive at a consensus of opinion.
    2. Nursing theory must be based solely on relevant clinical practice.
    3. Continued research must be encouraged to support the body of nursing research as a professional discipline.
    4. Realignment of nursing theory to focus solely on middle range theory.

36. Which concept is noted in the metaparadigm of nursing?
    1. Environment.
    2. Homeostasis.
    3. Evidence-based practice.
    4. Stress.

37. Martha Rogers' theory of principles of homeodynamics focuses on several principles that explain how individuals interact with the environment. Which of the following three principles are included in Rogers' theory of principles of homeodynamics?
    1. Carative factors.
    2. Resonancy.
    3. Primary prevention.
    4. Integrality.
    5. Helicy.

38. An adult-gerontology primary care NP is conducting a home safety assessment of an elderly couple, because the couple's adult children are concerned their parents are no longer able to live independently. The couple are of advanced age (ninth decade of life). The wife is legally blind with macular degeneration. The spouse has heart failure and mitral valve stenosis; his cardiac condition is worsening and he now requires continuous oxygen therapy. During the home visit, the couple express that they no longer find enjoyment in life, because they cannot do the activities they previously were able to do before becoming ill. Based on the patient case scenario, what type of nursing theory could be applied here?
    1. Neuman's Systems Model.
    2. Watson's Theory of Caring.
    3. King's Theory of Goal Attainment.
    4. Johnson's Behavioral System Model.

39. Using the Transtheoretical Model (TTM) as a framework for a behavioral change process, the adult-gerontology primary care NP knows that the patient who has expressed a desire to quit smoking, has begun to examine their tobacco use, and is weighing the pros and cons of quitting is in which stage of change?
    1. Precontemplation.
    2. Contemplation.
    3. Determination or preparation.
    4. Action.

40. King's Theory of Goal Attainment specifically focuses on:
    1. Effective communication between patient, family, and healthcare provider.
    2. Reducing stressors that may contribute to illness and disease.
    3. Interaction, transactions, and mutually shared outcomes between the nurse and patient.
    4. The nurse assisting the patient with improving and meeting self-care needs.

41. The theoretic basis for nursing practice is:
    1. A recent development in nursing practice.
    2. Developed from the medical model.
    3. Traced back to Florence Nightingale.
    4. Unrelated to the practice of nursing.

42. The verification of the more abstract nursing theories (e.g., of Martha Rogers) is often hampered by:
    1. Lack of adequate instrumentation for the theoretical concepts.
    2. Prior studies that did not support the theory.
    3. Lack of adequate settings for conducting experiments.
    4. Prior studies that were conducted in other countries.

43. The adult-gerontology primary care NP is aware that basing nursing practice on nursing theory contributes to the professionalization of nursing practice by (select two responses):
    1. Exploring relationships between person, health, environment, and nursing.
    2. Limiting the choice of treatments for patients, families, and communities.
    3. Determining what type of patients will be seen by the adult-gerontology primary care NP.
    4. Providing a consistent perspective for providing nursing care to patients.

44. Which nursing theory focuses on the transaction interaction between nurse and patient?
    1. Watson's Theory of Caring.
    2. Neuman's Systems Model.
    3. Martha Roger's Science of Unitary Beings.
    4. King's Theory of Goal Attainment.

45. An adult-gerontology primary care NP has decided to incorporate a theoretic nursing model into the ambulatory care practice, which emphasizes patients doing as much as possible independently to maintain their own health. Which nursing model is most applicable to this setting?
    1. Orem's Self-Care Deficit Theory of Nursing.
    2. Roy's Adaptation Model.
    3. Roger's Science of Unitary Human Beings.
    4. King's Theory of Goal Attainment.

46. Which of the following nursing theorists is considered to have general systems theory as the philosophic orientation to her model?
    1. Callista Roy.
    2. Martha Rogers.
    3. Rosemarie Parse.
    4. Betty Neuman.

47. Which nursing conceptual model addresses interventions in terms of primary, secondary, and tertiary prevention?
    1. Roy's Adaptation Model.
    2. Neuman's Systems Model.
    3. Levine's Conservation Model.
    4. Johnson's Behavioral System Model.

48. Which nursing model focuses on a concept that explores the individual's desire to improve health and well-being?
    1. Watson's Theory of Caring.
    2. Neuman's Systems Model.
    3. Pender's Health Promotion Model.
    4. Roy's Adaptation Model.

49. The adult-gerontology primary care NP is planning to conduct an educational program to facilitate smoking cessation in a group of adult smokers. The adult-gerontology primary care NP will employ interventions that facilitate the participant's recognition of the health risk associated with continued smoking to facilitate the participant's desire to utilize the proposed interventions to improve overall health. Based on the goals and desired outcomes of the educational program, the adult-gerontology primary care NP knows that the most appropriate theoretic model to guide the development of the program would be:
    1. Roy's Adaptation Model.
    2. The Health Belief Model.
    3. The Conservation Model.
    4. The Intersystem Model.

50. Many biologic theories have been developed to explain aging. Which theory supports the idea of "biological clock"?
    1. Programmed Aging Theory.
    2. Autoimmune Theory.
    3. Wear-and-Tear Theory.
    4. Oxidative Stress Theory.

51. The adult-gerontology primary care NP is reviewing nursing theories that utilize the nursing metaparadigm. The adult-gerontology primary care NP knows that the nursing metaparadigm is composed of which four concepts?
    1. Person.
    2. Research.
    3. Environment.
    4. Nursing.
    5. Health.
    6. Education.

52. Utilizing the framework of Benner's Theory of Novice to Expert, which statement describes an adult-gerontology primary care NP who is just starting his or her professional practice but has over 10 years' experience as a registered nurse?
    1. Advanced beginner.
    2. Expert.
    3. Novice.
    4. Proficient.

53. The adult-gerontology primary care NP is discussing methods to facilitate independence with a patient who has recently had a stroke, who is experiencing residual hemiplegia. The adult-gerontology primary care NP is using which concept of Orem's Self-Care Deficit Theory during this interaction?
    1. Universal self-care requisites.
    2. Developmental self-care requisites.
    3. Health deviation self-care deficits.
    4. Nursing system.

54. The adult-gerontology primary care NP is working in a culturally diverse medical clinic and would like to develop an educational program to facilitate improvement in health in the patient population. Based on the patient population and the purpose of the program, which of the following nursing theorists would be most appropriate to consider when developing the educational program?
    1. Calista Roy.
    2. Dorothea Orem.
    3. Margaret Newman.
    4. Madeleine Leininger.

55. The adult-gerontology primary care NP is working with a group of colleagues to develop a research study that will use Roy's Adaptation Model as the theoretic framework to guide the development of the study. Which three theoretic concepts will the team be sure to include in the study?
    1. Adaptation.
    2. Cognator subsystem.
    3. Exploitation phase.
    4. Contextual stimuli.

56. An adult-gerontology primary care NP has been practicing for 2 years in the current role. Professional role evaluations have indicated that the practitioner is assuming an interactive role in the interdisciplinary team, demonstrating leadership skills and management skills with minimal direction. Based on the framework of Benner's Theory of Novice to Expert, the practitioner is functioning at which practice level?
    1. Competent.
    2. Expert.
    3. Proficient.
    4. Advanced beginner.

57. The adult-geriatric NP understands that psychosocial theories of aging began with an emphasis on role theory and activity theory, often called the "first generation of theories" on aging. As theory evolved, other theoretic ideas (second generation of theories) were expanded. Select four theories that are considered part of the second generation of theories.
    1. Critical theory.
    2. Modernization theory.
    3. Age-stratification theory.
    4. Disengagement theory.
    5. Continuity theory.
    6. Feminism theory.

18 | Research & Theory Answers & Rationales

Research

1. Answer: 2

   Rationale: As a first step in using research to promote EBP, the adult-gerontology primary care NP would identify the purpose, intent, and goals to make a practice change based on evidence. Under Stetler's model, the first phase (preparation), involves identifying the purpose, focus, and outcomes for a proposed practice change. Phase II involves a critical appraisal of the literature on the proposed topic and would occur after the purpose and goals of the practice change have been identified. Phase IV involves implementing the research evidence into practice and Phase V involves evaluation of the practice change; neither phase would be used before reviewing and implementing the evidence into practice.

2. Answer: 3

   Rationale: The lack of significant findings is an important piece of information in the study findings. Particularly when findings are not statistically significant, additional studies need to be conducted about this topic to determine if the data is inconclusive. Threats to validity may cause a relationship to exist between study groups with no statistically significant findings. Ideally, changes in practice are based on the findings of more than one study, and a small sample size makes it more difficult to find statistically significant findings, not a large sample size.

3. Answer: 2

   Rationale: The peer review process exists across all disciplines in that the expectation is that the peer review process will help to determine if the provided research adds to the body of knowledge, is logically presented, well designed, and scientifically based. Although a manuscript should be well written, an excellent writing style alone in contrast to a research design with flaws is not acceptable. Individuals who participate in the peer review process do not have to provide editorial edits for grammar and formatting. Additionally, requirements in terms of clinical, research, and/or academic experience are required to be able to participate in the peer review process, thus it is not a beginning learning activity to understand how to analyze research and data findings.

4. Answer: 3

   Rationale: The primary purpose of utilizing evidence-based practice (EBP) in clinical research and practice management is focused on the ability to provide quality care to patients by closing the gap between theory, experience, and best practice guidelines. Although credible resources are important, this relates more to the systematic process and ranking of research. The peer review process is also used in conjunction with EBP, but again this relates to the evaluation process rather than the primary purpose. Lastly, arriving at a consensus of opinion relates to the overall evaluation of the presented research. It is not an expectation of purpose.

5. Answer: 1, 4

   Rationale: Pearson's product-moment correlation is the preferred statistical analysis to use for variables that consist of ratio or interval levels of measurement; whereas, Spearman's correlation would be an appropriate statistical test to use when the research variables are ranked. Pearson's product-moment correlation also identifies the relationships between variables, not causal relationships between variables. Two or more variables are used for Pearson's product-moment correlation.

6. Answer: 1

   Rationale: The purpose of qualitative research designs is to learn more about a particular phenomenon of interest by exploring the beliefs, values, and experiences of individuals. Qualitative designs do not yield precise measures, are usually not analyzed statistically, and carry the same concerns about the rights of subjects as all other research designs. Quantitative research designs ensure tight control over data collection and analysis.

7. Answer: 3

   Rationale: The mean is an average of the blood chemistry values. To find the mean, the lab values are added, and then divided by the number of numbers.

   $$\text{Example: } 132 + 136 + 137 = 405\,; 405 \div 3 = 135$$

8. Answer: 2

   Rationale: Based on the provided information, the research design is based on quantitative methods using an experimental approach as there are different treatment protocols being provided. Historical design is an example of qualitative research looking at prior information in terms of predicting possible future outcomes. Correlational design is an example of quantitative research looking at relationships between specific factors within a sample group. Descriptive design is an example of quantitative research providing information about specific factors in a data set providing summary information.

9. Answer: 4

Rationale: All current research and statistical analysis methods rely on the presence of variance or variation. Variance is a statistical measure used to identify how spread out scores are from the mean. If variance is no longer present, current methods could no longer be used. If there is no variance, a sample of one would be adequate.

10. Answer: 3

Rationale: Cronbach's alpha is a statistical tool that helps to determine reliability by examining internal consistency. A two-tailed t-test is a statistical measurement based on observation of two independent groups. Descriptive statistics provides information related to data sets. Factor analysis is used to assess relative effects of variables as to which is most important.

11. Answer: 2, 5

Rationale: The incidence rate is the occurrence of new cases of a disease or condition in a population over a period of time relative to the size of the population at risk for the disease of condition in the same time period. Incidence rates are helpful for monitoring short-term changes in a disease (influenza, chickenpox, measles, etc.) and are a sensitive indicator of the changing health of a community because the rate captures the fluctuations of a disease. A prevalence rate is the number of cases of a specific disease or condition in a population at a specified point in time relative to the population at the same point in time. An attack rate is the number of new cases of a disease in those exposed to the disease.

12. Answer: 4

Rationale: Prevalence is a measure of disease that allows the adult-gerontology primary care NP to determine a person's likelihood of having a disease. A prevalence rate is the total number of cases of a disease existing in a population divided by the total population at a point in time. The incidence rate is a measure of the frequency with which a disease occurs in a population over a period of time. Case-fatality rate refers to the proportion of persons with a disease who die from it. Incidence proportion refers to the proportion of the population that develops an illness or disease during an outbreak.

13. Answer: 4

Rationale: A prevalence rate is the total number of cases of a disease existing in a population divided by the total population. The formula to calculate is:

$$\frac{number\ of\ existing\ cases}{total\ population} \times 1000$$

The number of existing cases is 21 and the total geriatric population is 4420.

14. Answer: 2

Rationale: Identify the problem and generate a clinical question, conduct a literature review of scholarly research articles, critically appraise published research, implement useful findings in practice and clinical decision making, and disseminate findings contain the published steps of evidence-based practice. All other options are nursing actions taken on behalf of the patient (in no particular order).

15. Answer: 2

Rationale: The independent variable is the measure that can be manipulated in a study; the high-protein, high-fiber diet. The dependent variable is the response from the independent variable and is measurable, for example, the obese patients' weight. The population of interest is the obese patient and the length of the study is 12 weeks.

16. Answer: 3

Rationale: A randomized-controlled trial is one of the highest levels of evidence in determining if a cause and effect relationship exists between an experimental intervention (treatment) and dependent variable (outcome). By randomizing participants into either a control or treatment group, rigor is increased. A quantitative correlational research design examines the relationship between one or more variables; correlational research does not predict causality. Qualitative research designs are lower on the hierarchal level of evidence pyramid as they do not attempt to predict causality or determine the effectiveness of an intervention.

17. Answer: 4

Rationale: The relative risk or risk ratio (RR) is a measure of the risk of a certain event (getting lung cancer) happening in one group exposed to a factor (secondhand smoke) compared to the risk of the same event happening in another group not exposed to a factor. A prevalence rate is the total number of cases of a disease existing in a population divided by the total population. The incidence rate is a measure of the frequency with which a disease occurs in a population over a period of time. The confidence interval describes the amount of uncertainty associated with a sample estimate of a population parameter, usually at a 95% level, and assists in representing how good an estimate is.

18. Answer: 4

Rationale: The death-to-case ratio is the number of deaths caused by a certain disease during a specific period of time divided by the number of new cases of that disease identified during the same time period and is calculated as follows:

$$\frac{\text{Number of deaths caused by a disease during specific time period}}{\text{Number of new cases of the same disease identified during the same time period}} \times 100$$

19. Answer: 1, 2, 6

Rationale: A meta-analysis is a summary of a number of independent studies focused on one question or topic, and uses a specific statistical methodology to synthesize the findings in order to draw conclusions about the area of focus that ultimately seeks new knowledge, as well as confirming knowledge, from existing research data. It is used to assess clinical effectiveness of health care interventions and is helpful in providing a precise estimate of a treatment or intervention outcome. Meta-analysis provides level I evidence, which is considered the highest level of evidence, as it statistically analyzes and integrates the results of many independent studies. An effective, robust meta-analysis aims for complete coverage of all relevant studies, examines for the presence of heterogeneity in the studies, and explores the studies' main findings using sensitivity analysis. Meta-analysis, when carried out as a rigorous systematic review, can overcome inherent bias by offering an unbiased synthesis of the empirical data. Meta-analyses offer a systematic and quantitative (not qualitative) approach to synthesizing research evidence to analyze clinical interventions.

20. Answer: 3

Rationale: By federal law, the rights of human research subjects must be protected. Patients must be assured of their privacy and confidentiality through informed consent. The researchers may include the other information; however, it is not required by federal law.

21. Answer: 2

Rationale: The situation described relates to looking at both physical and emotional components of the subject groups and as such a mixed methods design should be employed that looks at both physical and emotional variables across the population. Descriptive statistics (quantitative) would be needed to look at number of falls and hospital admissions as a result of complications but this is just one aspect of the research design. Similarly, only using focus groups (qualitative) would not address the other relevant factors expressed by the adult-gerontology

primary care NP. A quasi-experimental design would not be applicable in this situation for it would not address the information as provided and there is no attempt to control for variables.

22. Answer: 1, 5

Rationale: In published research reports, of the options listed, statistical significance of the findings and methodological limitations of the study are consistently reported by researchers. The statistical significance of a study's findings provides consumers of research with information about the likelihood that the results may have occurred by chance. It is also equally important to have knowledge of a study's limitations, such as sample size, to determine whether the findings could be applicable in a different population or setting. The clinical relevance is considered, not the statistical relevance. The specific statistical software program used does not make a difference because all are based on the same statistical formulas. Researchers frequently work with statistical consultants, so a researcher's background is not a limitation to a published study.

23. Answer: 3, 4

Rationale: Neither type of statistics is used to assign participant code numbers. Descriptive statistics utilize statistical methods to describe the study sample and variables. Inferential statistics are utilized for hypothesis testing to analyze data from a sample to determine whether the study findings could be generalized to an entire population.

24. Answer: 4

Rationale: Quantitative researchers remain as removed from the research process as possible and employ controls to mitigate influencing test results or introducing potential bias. Quantitative research tests for relationships and cause an effect through a statistical analysis and reporting to test hypotheses or research questions. Qualitative researchers are integrated into the research process and through analysis of dialogue and observations search for themes.

25. Answer: 1

Rationale: The correct format for the null hypothesis is "There is no relationship between the independent and dependent variables." If a relationship does exist, the null hypothesis would be rejected. The alternate or research hypothesis may take the other forms.

26. Answer: 1

Rationale: Even though the claims detail extensive use of "Drug X," there must be statistical evidence reported.

Additionally, randomization, as demonstrated through the use of control or comparison groups, should be implemented that will render a level of significance. The Hawthorne effect is a limitation and threat to a study's validity, as the study participants' behaviors and responses are changed because of being in the study, not necessarily from the intervention or treatment performed.

27. Answer: 1, 2, 4

Rationale: When evaluating for causality, the consumer of research should consider the following: did the intervention precede the effect, did the intervention impact the outcome, and what, if any, impact did extraneous variable(s) have on the effect. Although the experience and credentials of the researcher are important when evaluating the strength of the study, they have little influence on the interventions(s) and outcomes of the study.

28. Answer: 4

Rationale: Variate refers to the number of variables in the study. A univariate study has one variable and a multivariate study has two or more variables. Variate does not relate to the number of participants, hypotheses, or a description of the study setting.

29. Answer: 1

Rationale: The variable of ethnicity is categorical data or nominal-level data. Ordinal level measurements are also categorized, but the categories can be ranked. Interval-level measurements of data are categorized, ranked, and have equal interval scales where the distance between intervals is always the same. Ratio-level measurement has all of the criteria as interval-level data but also has an absolute zero point.

30. Answer: 3

Rationale: Descriptive data analysis organizes the data, and it facilitates understanding of the participants who participated in the study and variables of the study. Descriptive statistics cannot be used for significance testing or for making inferences; inferential statistics are used. Predictions or causality are made from studies that use inferential statistics.

31. Answer: 1

Rationale: In light of the fact that the practitioner is looking for the average, the mean would provide for the average of all values. The median is the middle score, the mode is the most frequent score, and the range provides the difference between the highest and lowest scores in a set.

32. Answer: 4

Rationale: Randomization is a research technique used to increase the amount of control and reduce potential

threats of internal validity in any research design. The other three options do not decrease potential threats to internal validity.

33. Answer: 3

Rationale: Of the options, only multiple regression examines the relationship between two or more independent variables on a dependent variable. Descriptive statistics provides information about the study variables and sample. A paired t-test is used to determine differences between two groups (e.g., control and experimental group) on an outcome. Chi-squared (χ^2) test compares whether the frequency in each category is different from what would be expected by chance.

34. Answer: 2, 3, 4, 5

Rationale: In conducting a critical appraisal of quantitative research, it is important to determine the strengths and limitations of the study, evaluate the credentials of the researcher author(s), evaluate the organization and completeness of the research report, and evaluate the contribution of the study to nursing knowledge. In a critical appraisal, the reader should read and evaluate the entire study, not just one section, such as the discussion.

Theory

35. Answer: 3

Rationale: The best practice approach towards the development of nursing theory is to build upon research that directly relates to the professional discipline of nursing. Although it is important to work with other disciplines, integration of nursing theory should not be subject to restriction and limitation. Nursing theory should be based on both hypothesis-generating as well as experience-generating issues. No one theoretic model should be used for any professional discipline for it will limit/restrict original thought.

36. Answer: 1

Rationale: The metaparadigm of nursing focuses on the concepts of person, health, nursing, and environment. Homeostasis, evidence-based practice, and stress are not defined as part of the four concepts.

37. Answer: 2, 4, 5

Rationale: Resonancy, integrality, and helicy are principles of homeodynamics that Rogers' developed and defined to explain how individuals interact with their environment. Carative factors refer to Jean Watson's 10 carative factors under the Theory of Human Caring, and primary prevention relates to Neuman's Systems Model.

38. Answer: 4

Rationale: Johnson's Behavioral System Model is applicable to this case scenario because it involves an elderly couple conflicted with their current state of health and independence. There are eight subsystems associated with Johnson's Behavioral System Model. The individual's internal and external environment can be attributed to a disruption of one or more subsystems. To achieve balance of the subsystem, goal-setting and implementing interventions at the specific affected subsystem are undertaken. Neuman's Systems Model focuses on health promotion and prevention. Watson's Theory of Caring and King's Theory of Goal Attainment are not as applicable to the patient's case scenario.

39. Answer: 2

Rationale: The Transtheoretical Model developed by Prochaska and DiClemente is used to conceptualize the process of intentional behavior change, such as quitting smoking, losing weight, or exercising regularly. There are five steps: precontemplation (not ready), contemplation (getting ready), determination or preparation (ready), action (change is made), maintenance (sustains change). The patient who expresses a desire to quit smoking, has begun to examine tobacco use, and is weighing the pros and cons of quitting is in the contemplation stage.

40. Answer: 3

Rationale: King's Theory of Goal Attainments focuses on human interaction between the nurse and patient. During this interaction, information sharing and mutual patient goal-setting occurs between the nurse and patient. Although King's Theory focuses on communication, additional factors make up King's Theory. Minimizing stressors in the patient's environment refers to Neuman's Systems Model. Orem's Self-Care Theory focuses on assisting the patient with meeting self-care needs.

41. Answer: 3

Rationale: The theoretic basis for nursing practice began with Florence Nightingale and has been used in practice and research for more than a century. Nursing theories are specifically developed for nursing.

42. Answer: 1

Rationale: The lack of adequate tools and instruments for theoretic concepts is a major roadblock in many areas of research, and particularly so with the more abstract theories. Prior studies always provide information about the theory, even when conducted in other countries. The setting of the study plays no role in testing the theory.

43. Answer: 1, 4

Rationale: Theory-based practice contributes the consistent perspective that permits the comparison of care across settings. This practice does not necessarily limit treatments or determine patient types. Theory-based practice specifically eliminates reliance on the medical model and provides nursing with a method to explain and explore the relationships between phenomena specific to nursing; specifically, the following four concepts (person, health, environment, and nursing).

44. Answer: 4

Rationale: King's Theory of Goal Attainment focuses on the transactional interactions between the nurse and the patient. The other theories do not examine transactional relationships between the nurse and patient as the primary measurement parameter. Watson's Theory of Caring focuses on health promotion and restoration applied to the delivery of nursing care. Neuman's Systems Model examines the individual in the context of environmental systems. Martha Roger's Science of Unitary Beings focuses on nursing phenomenon characteristics.

45. Answer: 1

Rationale: Orem's theory focuses on the patient participating in their own health care. Roy's model focuses on adaptation. Roger's theory focuses on the synchronicity between the patient and the environment. King's theory is focused on the patient and nurse working together to achieve health-related goals.

46. Answer: 4

Rationale: Neuman's Systems Model is based on general systems theory. Roy's Adaptation Model is based on stress and adaptation as the framework. The theories of Martha Rogers and Rosemarie Parse are based on a humanistic developmental framework.

47. Answer: 2

Rationale: Betty Neuman identified the need to implement nursing interventions through the use of one or more of three modalities: primary, secondary, and tertiary prevention. Roy, Levine, and Johnson do not employ these concepts in their nursing models.

48. Answer: 3

Rationale: Pender's Health Promotion Model explores the concept of health promotion in which the individual seeks to improve health. Watson, Neuman, and Roy do not focus on the concept of health promotion.

49. Answer: 2

Rationale: The Health Belief Model recognizes that an individual's desire to employ health promoting interventions is directly related to their perceived risk of developing a negative outcome if the intervention is not employed. The Intersystem Model, the Conservation Model, and Roy's Adaptation Model do not employ the risk and benefit concepts to facilitate participation in improving health or participating in health promotion activities.

50. Answer: 1

Rationale: The Programmed Aging Theory postulates that each cell had a preprogrammed life span, that is, the biological clock; the number of cell reproductions were limited. The wear-and-tear theory proposes that cellular errors were the result of "wearing out" over time because of continued use, in which the damage was caused by pollutants and metabolic by-products, that is, free radicals. Oxidative stress theory postulates that stress appears to be random and unpredictable, varying from one cell to another, from one person to another. Oxidative stress theories and their associated mitochondrial theories of aging are among the most studied and most widely accepted. The autoimmune theory postulates that aging is a result of an accumulation of damage due to changes in the activities and function of the immune system (immunosenescence), which leads to the decreased ability of lymphocytes to withstand oxidative stress and appears to be a key factor in the aging process.

51. Answer: 1, 3, 4, 5

Rationale: The nursing metaparadigm is composed of four concepts: person, environment, health, and nursing. Research and education are not concepts within the nursing metaparadigm.

52. Answer: 3

Rationale: Even though the individual has clinical work experience as a registered nurse, the fact that the individual is beginning/assuming an advanced practice role would indicate, according to Benner's Theory of Novice to Expert, that they would be classified as a novice. An advanced beginner would have some experience within the advanced practice role. An expert level would represent the highest level of knowledge, skill integration, and application in practice. A proficient level would indicate flexibility and fluid use of nursing judgment.

53. Answer: 3

Rationale: Health deviation self-care deficits relate to facilitating self-care when a health care deficit exists. Universal self-care requisites relate to general human needs.

Developmental self-care deficits refer to necessary developmental processes that occur throughout life. Nursing systems, according to Orem's Self-Care Deficit Theory, refers to the relationship between the nurse and the patient.

54. Answer: 4

Rationale: Madeleine Leininger's Theory of Transcultural Nursing explores cultural diversity and aims to recognize similarities and differences with various cultures and the role of nursing in working with these cultures in the healthcare setting. Calista Roy's Adaptation Model, Dorothea Orem's Self-Care Deficit Theory, and Margaret Newman's Health as Expanding Consciousness Theory all explore the interrelationship of nursing and the patient, but only Leininger's Theory of Transcultural Nursing explores the aspect of cultural diversity in addition to these concepts.

55. Answer: 1, 2, 4

Rationale: Adaptation, cognator subsystem, and contextual stimuli are all theoretic concepts of Roy's Adaptation Model and should be addressed in a study in which the model serves as the theoretic framework. The exploitation phase is a theoretic concept associated with Peplau's Art and Science of Nursing theory and would not be addressed in a study guided by Roy's Adaptation Model.

56. Answer: 1

Rationale: The noted findings of assuming an interactive role within the interdisciplinary team, demonstrating leadership and management skills with minimal direction, point to the level of competency. An expert would represent the highest level of knowledge, skill integration, and application in practice. A proficient level would indicate flexibility and use of nursing judgment. An advanced beginner would have some experience within the advanced practice role but would still rely on other guidelines.

57. Answer: 2, 3, 4, 5

Rationale: There are six theories that are considered second generation theories and include disengagement, continuity, age-stratification, social exchange, modernization, and gerotranscendence theories. Critical theory, feminism, and postmodernism theories are a third generation of theoretic development related to aging that have a phenomenologic approach using qualitative methods and understanding of the individual about the aging person.

19

Professional Issues

Legal and Ethical

1. Which three statements are accurate regarding adult-gerontology primary care NP competencies established by the American Association of Colleges of Nursing (AACN) 2010 standards?
   1. Preparation for patient care should occur across the adult-older lifespan.
   2. Practitioner provides direct care to patients.
   3. Disease management is limited to commonly occurring clinical diagnoses.
   4. Practice management focuses primarily on health promotion measures.
   5. Young adults are included in the practice population.

2. Which authority regulates the scope of practice of adult-gerontology primary care NPs?
   1. Federal law.
   2. Academic institutions.
   3. Individual state law.
   4. Individual practice settings.

3. An adult-gerontology primary care NP is obtaining informed consent for a 78-year-old female patient with a clinical diagnosis of dementia for a minor incision and drainage procedure. Which option would provide best practice for obtaining informed consent?
   1. Have the patient sign the form.
   2. Inquire as to whether there is an individual who is a power of attorney (POA) for the patient.
   3. Have the patient sign the form in the presence of a witness who can substantiate informed consent and that information has been provided.
   4. Reschedule the procedure until next week when the patient's daughter can be contacted.

4. What priority action should the adult-gerontology primary care NP take when assessment findings on an older adult patient indicate potential physical abuse during a scheduled office visit?
   1. Admit patient to the hospital for observation.
   2. Review patient's chart to see if there were any other documented findings that would indicate abuse.
   3. Report case to appropriate agency based on state law.
   4. Arrange for home health to assess and monitor patient.

5. An occurrence-form professional liability insurance policy is preferred because:
   1. The amount of insurance money available to pay a claim increases with each renewal of the policy.
   2. The policy proceeds are available to pay claims regardless of when the claim is reported to the carrier.
   3. The carrier will be notified of a potential claim during the policy period.
   4. The coverage is broader than that provided by a claims-made policy form.

6. Early reporting of a potential professional liability claim is advantageous because:
   1. Insurance carriers have a 10-day reporting window, after which the coverage is canceled.
   2. Documents and witnesses needed to defend the claim are more likely to be available at the time of the event.
   3. Insurance premiums will be reduced with a good-faith showing of cooperation with the carrier.
   4. Risk management personnel require such reporting in order to comply with Joint Commission on the Accreditation of Healthcare Organizations (JCAHO) mandates.

7. An adult-gerontology primary care NP's nursing license may be in jeopardy if:
   1. The adult-gerontology primary care NP appropriately delegates medication administration to a trusted registered nurse (RN) employee, who administers a fatal dose.
   2. The adult-gerontology primary care NP delegates patient assessment tasks to a licensed practical nurse (LPN), who has been "floated" to the outpatient clinic for the day.
   3. The adult-gerontology primary care NP provides nursing care services consistent with established standards of practice in the jurisdiction.
   4. The medical assistant in the supervising physician's office exceeds the scope of her authority, but the adult-gerontology primary care NP takes prompt action to correct the problem.

8. A 46-year-old mentally challenged man has been diagnosed with colon cancer. Consent for his corrective surgery should be obtained from:
   1. The patient himself.
   2. The patient's 84-year-old mother, who is his closest relative.
   3. The patient's court-appointed guardian.
   4. The administrator of the group home where the patient lives.

9. A family member calls the office to speak to the adult-gerontology primary care NP who is taking care of her father who is 65 years old and has since left the office. The family member asks for specific information related to the patient's medical history and clinical diagnosis. What action should be taken at this time by the adult-gerontology primary care NP?
   1. Answer all of the questions that the family member has with regard to the patient.
   2. Acknowledge the family member's concerns but do not answer any questions as there is nothing listed on the chart to indicate that the patient has given consent to release information.
   3. Call the patient at home and ask if the patient gives consent to answer the family member's questions.
   4. Contact the patient and have him come back to the office to fill out a medical release of information form.

10. An adult-gerontology primary care NP has a 75-year-old female patient with metastatic cancer. Her affairs are in order; she has arranged all her finances and her own funeral rites. She has systematically secured enough barbiturates to successfully end her life. The patient asks the practitioner to mix the drugs for her in some pudding to make them palatable for ingestion. What would be the adult-gerontology primary care NP's best course of action?
    1. Mix the medications as requested and stay with her while she consumes the preparation.

2. Consult with the attending physician to warn them about the patient's proposed course of action.
3. Seek an immediate order for an antidepressant.
4. Sit down with the patient and conduct a physical and psychological assessment.

11. The Patient Self-Determination Act (PSDA), passed by the U.S. Congress in 1990, resulted in which of the following policy changes?
    1. Hospitals are mandated to assist every patient to create a "living will."
    2. Federally funded managed care organizations (MCOs) are required to inform subscribers about their rights under state law to create "advance directives."
    3. Home health agencies are required to have "do not resuscitate" (DNR) orders on file for all terminally ill patients.
    4. Hospitalized patients are obligated to select a surrogate decision maker to make health care decisions for them if they become incapacitated.

12. Both the U.S. Food and Drug Administration (FDA) and Department of Health and Human Services (DHHS) have regulations governing research activities on human subjects. The principal investigator is responsible for:
    1. Securing a signed special research consent form.
    2. Reporting back to the Institutional Review Board if a subject is injured during the course of the study.
    3. Appearing before the Institutional Review Board to present the study and secure approval to proceed with subject recruitment at the facility.
    4. All the above.

13. If served with a summons and complaint (lawsuit documents), the adult-gerontology primary care NP should take which of the following actions as the first step?
    1. Call the patient to determine the basis for the action and nature of the alleged wrongdoing.
    2. Call the patient's lawyer (listed on first page of lawsuit) to obtain more information.
    3. Call the insurance company for instructions on how to proceed.
    4. Confer with colleagues and review the chart to determine if notes need to be clarified.

14. An adult-gerontology primary care NP in an impoverished rural area frequently encounters a female patient in a situation of domestic violence with few community options for referral. To address the situation, the adult-gerontology primary care NP participates in community education forums and fundraising for a safe house. The adult-gerontology primary care NP's participation is an example of applying what ethical principle?
    1. Autonomy.
    2. Nonmaleficence.
    3. Justice.
    4. Veracity.

15. Nurses practicing in expanded roles should carry professional liability insurance for which of the following reasons?
    1. Premiums are often modest and are a tax-deductible business expense.
    2. Even if the employer insures the adult-gerontology primary care NP, situations of conflict between employer and nurse may necessitate separate legal counsel.
    3. As roles expand, so do the liability potential.
    4. All the above.

16. The confidentiality of medical records is always a valid concern, especially with widespread computerization and fax machines. Release of medical information to third parties is:
    1. A "creature of state law," meaning that state statutes control the processing of such requests.
    2. Prohibited without the informed consent of the patient.
    3. Automatic when the requesting party is a third-party payer or insurer.
    4. Disallowed if the records contain proof of a diagnosis of acquired immunodeficiency syndrome (AIDS).

17. Which population is not included in the definition of disability under the Americans with Disabilities Act (ADA)?
    1. Profoundly deaf employees.
    2. Persons who are wheelchair bound.
    3. Current users of illegal drugs.
    4. Persons with mental retardation.

18. If a patient is having a problem with a managed care plan, the adult-gerontology primary care NP can offer to assist in which of the following ways?
    1. Suggest that the patient contact the customer service department (or "member services") for the care plan to resolve the issue; a formal grievance filing may be necessary.
    2. Remind the patient, who is a member of the "senior" plan for Medicare recipients, that the patient may complain to the federal Office of Personnel Management (OPM).
    3. Remind the patient that the state's insurance department also investigates complaints against health plans.
    4. All the above.

19. If a piece of equipment malfunctions while being used on a hospitalized patient, the risk manager would probably recommend which of the following courses of action?
    1. Return the item to the manufacturer with a description of the problem and a request for analysis.
    2. Tag and sequester the item at the facility and defer analysis pending risk management review of the litigation potential.
    3. Send the item to the biomedical engineering department with a request for immediate equipment breakdown and troubleshooting.
    4. Repair the item, either in house or by an outside contracted firm, and return it to service as soon as possible.

20. Nurse expert witnesses are essential in the adjudication of most professional negligence claims against nurses. Which of the following criteria do attorneys use in selecting adult-gerontology primary care NP experts?
    1. Appropriate professional education, preferably at the technical level.
    2. Relevant and recent professional work experience.
    3. Ability to understand and articulate the legal issues involved in the claim.
    4. Published authors of medical texts in the clinical subject areas.

21. Which federal law mandates the tracking of implantable medical devices?
    1. Administrative Procedures Act (APA).
    2. Patient Self-Determination Act (PSDA).
    3. Safe Medical Devices Act (SMDA).
    4. Omnibus Budget Reconciliation Act (OBRA) of 1987.

22. Which of the following are elements of a broad-based risk management program?
    1. Hazardous materials compliance program as part of a comprehensive safety and security system.
    2. Early-warning/incident reporting program to identify elements of risk.
    3. System of contract review to avoid assuming liabilities that should be borne by others.
    4. All the above.

23. What type of insurance coverage is purchased (or self-insured) by an organization to address employee job-related injuries?
    1. Professional liability insurance.
    2. Business interruption insurance.
    3. Directors and officers insurance.
    4. Workers' compensation insurance.

24. While driving your personal vehicle on a job-related errand, you are struck by a semitrailer on the interstate. The car is totaled and you are severely injured. Which insurance policies will respond to these losses?
    1. Your personal auto policy and your employer's workers' compensation policy.
    2. The employer's business auto policy and workers' compensation policy.
    3. Your homeowner's policy.
    4. The semitrailer driver's personal auto policy.

25. Adult-gerontology primary care NPs with hospital privileges may be impacted by the part of the Health Care Quality Improvement Act known as the National Practitioner Data Bank (NPDB). Which of the following statements about the Data Bank is not true?
    1. Professional liability insurance claims payments made on behalf of adult-gerontology primary care NPs are reported to the NPDB.
    2. The facility granting medical staff privileges must query the NPDB before approving a practitioner's privileges.
    3. The purpose of the NPDB is a nationwide flagging system that provides information about malpractice claims, licensure actions, and restrictions on privileges so that practitioners may not easily move from one jurisdiction to another to escape quality review.
    4. Insurance companies report all malpractice payments made on behalf of affected adult-gerontology primary care NPs within 30 days of the date the payment was made, if the amount of the claim is in excess of $11,000 and no matter how it was settled.

26. In 1985, the U.S. Congress took action against a phenomenon known as "patient dumping" by enacting what was known at the time as the COBRA law, now referred to the Emergency Medical Treatment and Active Labor Act (EMTALA). Which three statements about EMTALA are true?
    1. The original purpose of the statute was to prohibit the transfer of uninsured and untreated patients from the emergency department of one hospital to another (usually the county hospital).
    2. Subsequent rules and case law have expanded the statute so that almost any unauthorized transfer of a patient from one facility to another is potentially problematic.
    3. To effect a proper transfer, the forwarding facility need not notify or secure the acquiescence of the receiving facility.
    4. The transferring facility must utilize appropriate transport methods and send copies of patients' medical records.
    5. The patient can be transferred by family members to another facility awaiting the patient's arrival.

27. A adult-gerontology primary care NP who wants to effect change in the state's laws regarding the dispensing of prescription medications by adult-gerontology primary care NPs would take this case to the:
    1. State legislature.
    2. State board of nursing.
    3. State board of pharmacy.
    4. Nursing specialty organization.

28. What is the common meaning of "gag clauses" or "gag orders" in managed care?
    1. The managed care organization (MCO) declines to publish, in its subscriber contracts, the treatments that are excluded from coverage under the plan.
    2. The MCO refuses to allow its member services personnel to answer certain subscriber questions about covered benefits.
    3. The MCO contracts with providers to disallow providers from offering treatment alternatives that the providers know are not covered by patient plans.
    4. Providers are prohibited from offering experimental treatment to patients.

29. Under the Safe Medical Devices Act of 1990, which of the following health care providers or organizations are required to report the death of a patient to the Food and Drug Administration (FDA) if the death is related to the use of a medical device?
    1. Physician office staff.
    2. Hospitals, home health agencies, and ambulance companies.
    3. Nurse family members treating patients without compensation.
    4. Physicians making home visits.

30. A patient receives a medication that was intended for another person. Which is an appropriate way for the adult-gerontology primary care NP to document this event in the medical record?
    1. "Patient was given X mg of Y drug in error."
    2. "X mg of Y drug administered to patient. No adverse effects noted. Physician notified."
    3. "Patient received wrong medication. Incident report filed. Practitioner disciplined."
    4. "Practitioner inadvertently administered Y drug to wrong patient. Supervisor notified. Family threatening litigation."

31. What is the primary reason that patients give for suing adult-gerontology primary care NPs for medical negligence?
    1. The care they received was substandard.
    2. The provider made an honest mistake.
    3. The patient was not "heard" when attempting to communicate with the provider.
    4. The patient participated fully in all aspects of medical decision making, but the results were disappointing.

32. Informed consent is based on the ethical principle of:
    1. Beneficence.
    2. Respect for persons.
    3. Nonmaleficence.
    4. Autonomy.

33. The four elements of a professional negligence claim are:
    1. Duty, fulfillment of duty, professional relationship, and wrongful act.
    2. Professional responsibility, fault, harm to patient, and wrongful act.

3. Duty, breach of duty, causal connection between act and harm, and harm to patient.
4. Professional relationship, intentional wrongful act, proximate cause, and damage to patient.

34. An adult-gerontology primary care NP is making an initial home health care visit to an older adult woman. Her spouse states that she is often confused; he answers all the questions and dominates the discussion. On the initial assessment, the patient does seem to be oriented to time, place, and person. Who is the proper party to sign the written form to request consent for services?
    1. Spouse.
    2. Patient.
    3. Attending physician.
    4. Home health aide who will be providing continuing care.

35. Why is an expert witness usually required in a nursing negligence case?
    1. Knowledge of medical or nursing facts is not considered intuitive to a lay jury.
    2. Jurors are allowed to use their "sixth sense" regarding the facts presented to them.
    3. Fact witnesses are not able to present an unbiased account of the circumstances in dispute.
    4. Appropriately credentialed experts have more credibility in the eyes of lay jurors.

36. The standard of care for a adult-gerontology primary care NP will be established by an expert witness(es) in a trial. The expert opinion will be based on which three items?
    1. National norms for the specialty.
    2. Facility policies and procedures.
    3. Professional literature.
    4. Opinions of other NPs.
    5. Current events.

37. Alternative dispute resolution (ADR) is a process in which the parties to a dispute resolve their differences outside of a court trial. Advantages to this system of problem solving include three of the following:
    1. The parties usually prefer the process because they have their opportunity to be heard in a less formal and less intimidating environment.
    2. The process is often less time-consuming and less costly than traditional litigation.
    3. Damage awards are less likely to include nonfinancial compensation.
    4. Insurers are amenable to working with mediators with a track record of fairness and successful case resolution.
    5. The losing party may appeal the ADR decision to the court system.

38. The statute of limitations is:
    1. The state law that prescribes the time frames within which a nursing negligence action may be filed.
    2. The law that states that minors have no legal authority to sue nurses for malpractice.
    3. The law that limits the right of patients to sue adult-gerontology primary care NPs for negligent acts.
    4. The federal law that limits an adult-gerontology primary care NP's right to countersue a patient for malicious prosecution.

39. An adult-gerontology primary care NP is driving to a nursing seminar on an interstate highway. The NP observes a head-on collision and decides to stop to render aid. Which three statements are accurate with respect to the adult-gerontology primary care NP's potential liability for malpractice?
    1. There is no legal obligation to stop to render assistance; if the adult-gerontology primary care NP had driven by the accident, there would be no liability on the nurse's part.
    2. If appropriate nursing care is provided, gratuitously, the adult-gerontology primary care NP will be protected from liability under that state's Good Samaritan Law.
    3. Even if the adult-gerontology primary care NP acts in a grossly negligent manner, the Good Samaritan Law will shield the nurse from liability.
    4. The protections afforded by the Good Samaritan Law may differ from state to state; the adult-gerontology primary care NP should research the state's law on the subject.
    5. The adult-gerontology primary care NP must stop and render aid.

40. If an adult-gerontology primary care NP is subpoenaed to appear for a deposition in a nursing negligence case, appropriate preparation is prudent. Which advice from the attorney is appropriate? Select three responses.
    1. "Discreetly chew gum to calm your nerves, and dress for dinner because depositions usually take all day and you won't have time to change."
    2. "Review the patient's medical record and other pertinent material before appearing for questioning."
    3. "Take as much time as needed to think about your responses before answering; don't let the other lawyer put words in your mouth."
    4. "Be straightforward and truthful; remember that 'I don't know' and 'I don't remember' are acceptable responses."
    5. "Try to confuse the other attorney by displaying sophisticated medical knowledge and information."

41. Which four of the following suggestions for documentation are recommended?
    1. "Carefully document your criticism of a fellow provider's clinical decision in the patient's medical record. This will protect you if your treatment decisions need to be defended later."
    2. "Use standard abbreviations in the medical record so that subsequent readers will have no doubt as to your meaning and intent."
    3. "Document telephone conversations with the patient and adult-gerontology primary care NP in the medical record. Be particularly vigilant about recording changes in the patient's medications."
    4. "Document noncompliant patient behaviors in the medical record; be thorough, yet factual."
    5. "Always make notation of errors in the medical record according to agency policy."

42. If a patient is under the "age of majority" for the state, what three factors would be considered to determine whether the patient is "emancipated" and able to consent to medical treatment?
    1. The patient is married.
    2. The patient is in the military.
    3. The patient is living outside the "care, custody, and control" of a parent or guardian.
    4. A personal friend of the patient's tells you that the patient has been emancipated by an order of the court.

43. In 1987 and 1994, the U.S. Congress updated many of the regulations that govern the provision of long-term care services. What is important for an employer or nurse manager working in the long-term care environment to know?
    1. Nursing assistants working in long-term care facilities must be formally trained and certified.
    2. Patients or residents have specific rights, such as information about their physical condition, medical benefits, and associated costs.
    3. New and swifter sanctions are available to reviewers to impose on facilities with deficiencies.
    4. All the above.

44. An adult-gerontology primary care NP is employed in a private medical office. There is constant activity at the front desk, with patients checking in for appointments, staff scheduling tests, and telephone advice triage in progress. To preserve patient confidentiality, what changes should be implemented?
    1. Orient the computer monitor and printer, so that persons other than staff cannot read incoming reports and other data.
    2. Do all telephone scheduling from a more secure location, such as a conference room in the back office.
    3. Create a more private space to confer with patients who need follow-up information or explanations of tests or treatments.
    4. All the above.

45. Which activity could be considered grounds for a sexual harassment claim?
    1. A male employee tells an off-color joke to another man. The joke is overheard by a female co-worker who seems to appreciate the humor in it. The joke telling is an isolated incident.
    2. A nurse supervisor conducts an employee performance review. The supervisor does not mention a prior social relationship with the employee. The ratings are appropriate for the level of performance, and the employee receives a salary increase.
    3. A co-ed locker room is decorated with multiple centerfold photos from a popular men's magazine. The female employees find this offensive and have filed several complaints.
    4. A nurse is complimented on her appearance and asked on a date by her boss. She informs the boss that she is married and not seeking another relationship. The incident is forgotten.

46. A comatose female patient requires a feeding tube inserted for long-term nutritional needs. Her husband presents the adult-gerontology primary care NP with a document that he says is his wife's living will. It is signed by him, and he says that it sets out the wishes of his wife with respect to the feeding tube. Why is this living will not a legally binding document?
    1. The wife did not sign the document.
    2. The husband is not authorized to execute a living will on behalf of his wife.
    3. This type of advance directive must be signed by the individual (wife/patient) while this person is legally competent to execute the documents.
    4. All the above.

47. An adult-gerontology primary care NP is helping out at a clinic for homeless women. A diabetic patient in her third trimester of pregnancy has been reasonably compliant with respect to insulin therapy. Now, however, she has announced her intent to abandon her insulin regimen because she has heard "on the streets" that some drugs are harmful to fetuses. Which option is *not* legally appropriate for the adult-gerontology primary care NP, as this patient's health care provider, to consider?
    1. Seek the support of the clinic's attorney to file a petition for court-ordered treatment for the patient.
    2. Attempt to engage the patient in dialogue to provide her with accurate medical information.
    3. Detain the patient in the homeless shelter and administer the insulin, with or without her consent.

4. Confer with social services to find an appropriate interim placement for the patient until her medical and legal issues can be addressed.

48. What is the purpose of the Americans with Disabilities Act (ADA)?
    1. "Level the playing field" with respect to employment and other opportunities for disabled persons.
    2. Create a federal entitlement program for AIDS patients.
    3. Guarantee wheelchair access to every residential and commercial building.
    4. Authorize interpreters for deaf employees at all private businesses.

49. As a result of the U.S. Supreme Court's ruling on assisted suicide, which of the following is the current state of the law on this topic?
    1. Assisted suicide is still a criminal offense in most jurisdictions.
    2. A physician may prescribe a fatal dose of medication with the concurrence of the ethics committee.
    3. An adult-gerontology primary care NP may prescribe a fatal dose of medication with the concurrence of the supervising physician.
    4. A pharmacist may instruct a patient on how to mix and ingest a fatal dose of prescription medication.

50. A professional negligence or medical malpractice case is a civil action. What is the difference between a civil lawsuit and a criminal lawsuit?
    1. The damages sought in a civil suit are monetary; one private party sues another for money.
    2. If convicted in a criminal case, you are still covered by your professional liability insurer.
    3. In a criminal case, your state sues you for money; other penalties do not apply.
    4. In a civil suit, if you do not prevail, you could be incarcerated.

51. Which of the following are three forms of alternative dispute resolution (ADR)?
    1. Court or bench trial (judge's decision).
    2. Binding and nonbinding arbitration.
    3. Settlement conference.
    4. Jury trial.
    5. Mediation.

52. Why is it especially important for adult-gerontology primary care NPs caring for children to have adequate professional liability insurance coverage?
    1. Damages are always higher when a child is the injured party.
    2. Juries tend to award fewer dollars to injured children because the children are eligible for a variety of social programs that cover their medical expenses.

3. The statute of limitations is often tolled (put on hold) until the minor reaches majority, so the time frame within which the child can file a lawsuit is extended.
    4. Insurers are sensitive to the increased risk posed by minor claimants, so the coverage is difficult to obtain.

53. A health care provider has a duty to disclose certain information to the patient as part of the informed consent process. Exceptions to this duty would include all the following *except*:
    1. The patient has waived the right to receive the data.
    2. It is a bona fide emergency situation.
    3. The provider believes that the information would be harmful to the patient and invokes the therapeutic privilege.
    4. The patient is 80 years old, and older adult persons are unable to comprehend complex medical facts.

54. Before deciding to provide a detailed reference on a former employee, it would be important for the adult-gerontology primary care NP to consider which of the following?
    1. The requirements of the human resources department should be determined.
    2. If the comments are perceived as negative and the former employee becomes aware of them, the adult-gerontology primary care NP could be subjected to suit for defamation.
    3. If the employee exhibits unsafe patient care practices, it may be wiser to risk legal action from the employee than to subject future patients to this unsafe employee.
    4. All the above.

55. What is the primary purpose of a preemployment physical exam?
    1. Identify existing health problems that might adversely affect the company's insurance rates.
    2. Determine the mental status of the applicant.
    3. Determine if the applicant is physically capable of doing the job.
    4. Document any existing disabilities and recommend accommodations.

56. An adult-gerontology primary care NP involved in work-related surveillance knows all employers must report, according to Occupational Safety and Health Administration (OSHA), the following: (Select two responses.)
    1. Keep all OSHA records for 5 years.
    2. Report all work-related fatalities within 8 hours.
    3. Report all work-related inpatient hospitalizations, amputations, and losses of an eye within 24 hours.
    4. Report hospital-employee fatalities occurring 90 days following a work-related incident.

57. When treating a work-related injury, what is the adult-gerontology primary care NP required to do?
    1. Document thoroughly because of the high probability of legal action.
    2. Communicate directly with the patient's employer.
    3. File a report with the industrial commission documenting the injury and treatment.
    4. Notify the Occupational Safety and Health Administration (OSHA).

58. Which of the following situations would be considered reportable under the Occupational Safety and Health Administration (OSHA)?
    1. 3-cm abrasion of forearm.
    2. Warehouse worker with back strain reassigned to office work for a week.
    3. Twisted ankle that responded to ice and Ace wrap.
    4. Minor closed-head injury with no loss of consciousness.

59. The purpose of an Occupational Health and Safety Administration (OSHA) 300 log is to record:
    1. Occupational injuries and illnesses.
    2. Only work-related deaths.
    3. Dangerous workplace situations.
    4. Lost work days.

60. The American Disabilities Act (ADA) regulates how employers treat disabled persons. Under the ADA, disability is defined as a physical or mental impairment that substantially limits one or more major life activities of an individual, or a record of a situation in which an individual is regarded as having such an impairment. What would be included under this definition?
    1. History of addiction.
    2. Paralysis.
    3. Bipolar disorder.
    4. All the above.

61. The adult-gerontology primary care NP understands which of the following about the Health Insurance Portability and Accountability Act (HIPAA) of 1996?
    1. The HIPAA allows health insurance providers to deny insurance to patients because of preexisting medical conditions.
    2. The HIPAA provides easier access to all providers to obtain secure and private health information.
    3. A National Provider Identifier and Employer Identifier facilitates enrolment, eligibility, and claims processing and provides a mechanism to identify a specific provider, insurer, or patient.
    4. Healthcare organizations, insurers, and payers using electronic storage of patient data and performing claims submission must comply with the Final Rule for National Standards for Electronic Transactions.

62. Bioethical practice dilemmas are best described as situations in which proposed treatment alternatives are:
    1. Ranked from most acceptable to least acceptable.
    2. Not appealing to involved parties.
    3. Lacking acceptance by anyone.
    4. Less-than-perfect approaches to the situation.

Issues and Trends

63. Considering the four advanced practice roles of the clinical nurse specialist, nurse practitioner, certified nurse midwife, and nurse anesthetist, which role became accepted by and included into the practice arena without significant controversy?
    1. Clinical nurse specialist.
    2. Nurse practitioner.
    3. Certified nurse midwife.
    4. Nurse anesthetist.

64. In order to facilitate exchange of information in the clinical practice setting the adult-gerontology NP should provide educational materials that:
    1. Contain evidenced-based practice recommendations.
    2. Provide auditory as well as written instruction.
    3. Determine patient readiness to learn.
    4. Meet established health literacy standards.

65. What would be considered to be an expectation of the professional role of an adult-gerontology primary care NP based on practitioner competencies established by the American Association of Colleges of Nursing (AACN) 2010 standards?
    1. Teaching classes related to health promotion and disease prevention.
    2. Observing and maintaining professional boundaries.
    3. Providing mentorship to other practitioners.
    4. Prescribing medications within legally defined practice regulations.

66. Which three patients could be seen by an adult-gerontology primary care NP?
    1. A 16-year-old who is noted to be an emancipated minor.
    2. A 24-year-old female who needs prenatal care as she is 12 weeks pregnant.
    3. An 11-year-old male patient who has an ear infection.
    4. A 28-year-old male patient who needs a yearly physical exam.
    5. A 78-year-old male patient who suspects he has a urinary tract infection.

67. Historically, who was one of the most outspoken opponents of the adult-gerontology primary care NP role?
    1. Loretta Ford.
    2. Hildegard Peplau.
    3. Martha Rogers.
    4. Dorothea Orem.

68. Who started the first adult-gerontology primary care NP program?
    1. Hildegard Peplau.
    2. Mary Breckenridge.
    3. Agnes McGee.
    4. Loretta Ford.

69. Which is the most important action in developing health policy skills in the adult-gerontology primary care NP?
    1. Develop political allies in the U.S. Congress.
    2. Work on a campaign.
    3. Support causes (e.g., teen pregnancy; AIDS).
    4. Write letters and editorials.

70. Which is the least important barrier to collaborative advanced nursing practice?
    1. Prescriptive authority.
    2. Reimbursement privileges.
    3. Legal scope of practice.
    4. Political activism.

71. According to the APRN consensus model, the adult-gerontology primary care NP is categorized as which of the following?
    1. An APRN role.
    2. Representing a specialty.
    3. Specifying a practice population focus.
    4. Nurse practitioner.

72. To obtain reimbursement, the adult-gerontology primary care NP must understand which of the following?
    1. MNDS.
    2. ICD-10, CPT, and HCPC codes.
    3. HCPC codes and NANDA diagnoses.
    4. Medicare and Medicaid numbers.

73. Which four items that are part of a consensus model should be included in the curriculum for an individual who wants to become an adult-gerontology primary care NP?
    1. Completion of graduate studies.
    2. Meeting accreditation standards.
    3. Maintaining compliance with core competencies.
    4. Maintaining licensure.
    5. Nurse Residency Program.

74. According to Kurt Lewin, steps in the change process are as follows:
    1. Unsolving, mobilizing, recruiting, and finalizing.
    2. Building relationships, acquiring resources, choosing solution, and stabilizing.
    3. Unfreezing, moving, and refreezing.
    4. Forming, storming, and norming.

75. What was the major impetus for adult-gerontology primary care NP development?
    1. Need for an expert nurse clinician.
    2. Shortage of primary care physicians.
    3. Trend for specialized nurses to diagnose and manage unstable acute and chronic patients.
    4. Movement of graduate nursing education to diagnosis and treatment of major illness.

76. The adult-gerontology primary care NP understands that Medicare B provides:
    1. Hospitalization costs for insured patients.
    2. Health insurance benefits for low-income families.
    3. Benefits that cover physicians, adult-gerontology primary care NPs, medical equipment, and outpatient services.
    4. Outpatient laboratory services, radiography services, and skilled nursing care in appropriate facilities.

77. What was the impact of the Balanced Budget Act of 1997 on adult-gerontology primary care NP practice?
    1. Authorized all states to provide adult-gerontology primary care NPs prescriptive authority.
    2. Provided for only well visits and primary care services.
    3. Prevented a physician from billing 100% for an adult-gerontology primary care NP's services.
    4. Allowed direct Medicare payments to adult-gerontology primary care NPs in both rural and urban settings.

78. In the clinic, the adult-gerontology primary care NP must resolve a conflict between two medical assistants. The nurse has observed that one assistant is usually pleasant and helpful and the other is often abrasive and angry. What is the most important guideline that the adult-gerontology primary care NP must observe in resolving such a conflict?
    1. Require the medical assistants to reach a compromise.
    2. Weigh the consequences of each possible solution.
    3. Encourage ventilation of anger and use humor to minimize the conflict.
    4. Deal with issues, not personalities.

79. Which of the following is the name of an initiative that is part of the Affordable Care Act of 2009, which affects all health providers who practice in or admit patients to a hospital setting?
    1. APRN Compact Licensure Act.
    2. Interprofessional Education Collaborative (IPEC).
    3. Accountable Care Organization.
    4. Value-based Purchasing.

80. An adult-gerontology primary care NP approaches his friend, another adult-gerontology primary care NP, and tells him that a female physician at the clinic often follows him into the supplies room and tells him how "good looking" he is. Yesterday she patted his hand and said, "I wish we would get to know each other better. I would make it worth your while; better benefits at the clinic, more money." The staff nurse asks his friend, "What do I do? I don't want to date her, but I don't want to lose my job. I just want her to leave me alone." What would be the friend's best reply?
    1. "Tell her that her behavior makes you feel uncomfortable and that you want her to stop."
    2. "Go for it; date her and see if you get what she promises."
    3. "Go to the human relations office at the agency right away and relate to them the entire situation."
    4. "Contact your lawyer and get advice as soon as possible, in case she decides to turn the tables and accuse you of advances."

81. The adult-gerontology primary care NP understands that "incident to" services are reimbursed at which percentage?
    1. 75%.
    2. 80%.
    3. 85%.
    4. 100%.

82. What is the purpose of the Agency for Healthcare Research and Quality (AHRQ)?
    1. Develop cost-cutting strategies for healthcare.
    2. Provide assessment and treatment protocols and algorithms.
    3. Promote health care policy by lobbying efforts.
    4. Produce evidence to make a safer health care that is equitable and affordable.

19 Professional Issues Answers & Rationales

Legal and Ethical

1. Answer: 1, 2, 5

Rationale: Established adult-gerontology primary care NP competencies by the American Association of Colleges of Nursing (AACN) 2010 standards indicate that the NP should be prepared to provide patient care across the adult-older lifespan, provide direct care to the patient, inclusive of adults (young adults, adults, and older adults). Disease management is not limited to commonly occurring clinical diagnoses as practitioners are expected to manage both health and illness states. Practice management focuses on not only health promotion, but assessment, therapeutic management, health protection, and disease prevention.

2. Answer: 3

Rationale: Adult-gerontology primary care NPs' scope of practice is regulated by individual state law. Federal law does not address scope of practice. Academic institutions provide the necessary training for individuals to obtain an academic degree and assist in preparation for required certification in the specialty area. Scope of practice is not regulated by individual practice settings.

3. Answer: 2

Rationale: A clinical diagnosis of dementia for a patient indicates that in order to provide and obtain informed consent, an individual who has been designated as a health care surrogate and/or is acting as a power of attorney (POA) should be contacted to provide informed consent. The adult-gerontology primary care NP should not allow the individual patient to sign the form as informed consent process cannot be verified. Having a witness present when signing the form does not convey informed consent has taken place. Delaying medical treatment would not represent prudent practice.

4. Answer: 3

Rationale: If the adult-gerontology primary care NP suspects that physical abuse has occurred, then he or she is legally obligated to report the case to the appropriate agency based on state law. Admitting the patient to the hospital is not indicated unless confirmation of injury or trauma is justified. Reviewing the patient's chart for past history of abuse may be warranted but it is not the priority action. Arranging for home health to asses and monitor the patient does not preclude the legal responsibility of taking action to report the incident.

5. Answer: 2

Rationale: The most important advantage of an occurrence policy is that the coverage is available regardless of how long it takes to become aware of a claim (the long "tail" of a medical malpractice claim). The limits do not automatically increase. The carrier need not be notified during the policy period as is required with claims-made coverage. The coverage under each policy may be as broad as the carrier allows.

6. Answer: 2

Rationale: Fact witnesses and necessary paperwork are always easier to discover the sooner they are sought after a medical misadventure. Memories are fresh, and documents are less likely to be misplaced or destroyed. No rigid reporting window is required by insurance carriers, although they do want to be notified in a timely manner. Insurance premiums may be reduced if the insured's track record is clean (i.e., no claims), but not by mere compliance with policy requirements. Risk management employees prefer early notification so that damage-control efforts may be implemented promptly, not for regulatory reasons.

7. Answer: 2

Rationale: Assessment skills are presumed to be within the purview of the professional nurse, not those with fewer years of nursing education. Also, in this option, the LPN is an unknown entity to the delegator. Delegating to the LPN should be done cautiously after determining that person's skill level. The adult-gerontology primary care NP's license is not in jeopardy as they delegated appropriately to the RN, but an error was made and is attributed to the delegatee (RN). Activities such as providing nursing services and intervening when medical assistant personnel exceed their authority are appropriate for the role.

8. Answer: 3

Rationale: The patient's capacity to consent is questionable, so alternatives must be sought. If the patient has a court-appointed guardian, that person is the decision maker. The court has already made a determination of the patient's legal incapacity and appointed the person to whom the nurse will look for consent. If there were no guardian, the adult-gerontology primary care NP would analyze whether the patient himself may be able to consent or whether to look to his mother as the most appropriate surrogate decision maker. The group home employee has no automatic legal authority to consent to treatment for any resident.

9. Answer: 2

Rationale: Release of medical information by a patient to others requires documentation of intent and approval within the patient's chart. As the patient has left the office and there is no documentation related to medical release of information, the adult-gerontology primary care NP is bound by patient confidentiality and privacy laws (HIPAA [Health care Insurance Portability and Accountability Act]) to not answer any questions. Calling the patient to obtain verbal approval for release of medical information and/or having the patient come in to fill out a medical release form for release of information is not an expectation at this time.

10. Answer: 4

Rationale: Assisted suicide is still a criminal activity in most states (and in legal limbo in others). Circumventing the patient may seem to be an appealing option, but it substitutes paternalism for the autonomy we all claim as our due. A diagnosis of depression cannot be made with inadequate data; the necessary information can be determined only by conferring with the patient herself.

11. Answer: 2

Rationale: Managed care organizations (MCOs) are one group of health care organizations impacted by this law. All subscribers must be provided with the stated information at the time of enrollment. Advance directive documents, although extremely helpful in the health care setting, are never mandatory.

12. Answer: 4

Rationale: These are the basic requirements for conducting research at health care facilities.

13. Answer: 3

Rationale: Insurance carriers are thoroughly familiar with the processes of handling a claim. They will assist with every step, first by meeting their obligation to put the adult-gerontology primary care NP in contact with a lawyer. Conferring with the patient or the patient's lawyer is never a wise move. Colleagues can only offer moral support at this stage; the lawyer is the professional of choice at this time. The adult-gerontology primary care NP must never consider altering a record; it can turn a defensible case into a nondefensible one.

14. Answer: 3

Rationale: Lobbying for underserved patients is an example of justice, which is the duty to treat all patients fairly, without regard to age, socioeconomic status, or other variables. Autonomy is the patient's right to self-determination without outside control. Nonmaleficence is the duty to prevent or avoid doing harm, whether intentional or unintentional. Veracity is the duty to tell the truth.

15. Answer: 4

Rationale: These are all valid reasons to protect assets in the event of litigation. In an opposing view regarding the need for professional liability insurance, some professionals think that, if there are few assets to protect, insurance is an unnecessary expense. Adult-gerontology primary care NPs with professional liability coverage ("deep pockets") could be retained as defendants in a case for a longer time.

16. Answer: 1

Rationale: State law must be examined to define the circumstances under which confidential medical information may be disclosed. There may be additional requirements imposed by federal regulations (e.g., the handling of certain psychiatric records), but the bulk of the rule making on this issue is accomplished at the state level. Exceptions to the requirement of patient consent include communicable disease reporting to public health authorities and court-ordered record production. Third-party payers, although powerful with their fiscal controls, must produce some proof of patient consent to acquire records. An AIDS diagnosis does not shield a record from production, although many states have enacted extra levels of protection for this information. Again, knowledge of state laws is crucial.

17. Answer: 3

Rationale: Americans with Disabilities Act (ADA) does not protect this population. In fact, employers may test for illegal drug use; this is not considered a medical exam, which ordinarily is subject to specific requirements under the law.

18. Answer: 4

Rationale: These are all ways to achieve satisfaction from a health plan. The adult-gerontology primary care NP could also offer to help explain clinical issues to personnel who may not be clinically oriented.

19. Answer: 2

Rationale: The best immediate solution is to identify the item and remove it from service to avoid further patient injury. Then the risk manager, in consultation with the facility's attorneys and insurers, will determine how to proceed with equipment analysis. Returning the item to the manufacturer removes it from the nurse's control and diminishes the opportunity to defend against a charge of user error. Immediate repair may fail to uncover the real cause of the patient injury and impair a successful defense of a claim. If the litigation potential is high, the parties may want to pool their efforts (and costs) to conduct a third-party review of the equipment. If litigation is likely, it is also likely that the manufacturer and others in the distribution chain will be codefendants with the facility and staff.

20. Answer: 2

Rationale: The level of education preferred is that of a master's or doctoral of nursing practice (DNP) degree with adult-gerontology primary care NP specialization, not an associate's degree conferred on the technical nurse. The legal issues are the province of the attorneys and the judge; the nurse is expected to be the expert in the clinical issues. Published authorship on nursing issues does add an aura of credibility; specific work experience coupled with the educational credentials are more desirable.

21. Answer: 3

Rationale: The Safe Medical Devices Act (SMDA) of 1990 mandates the regulation and tracking of medical devices. The Administrative Procedures Act (APA) describes the workings of federal agencies. The Patient Self-Determination Act (PSDA) deals with advance directives, and the Omnibus Budget Reconciliation Act (OBRA) of 1987 changed the rule dealing with long-term care.

22. Answer: 4

Rationale: These and other elements combine to produce a program of systematic risk identification, analysis, treatment, and evaluation, with the overall goal of loss prevention.

23. Answer: 4

Rationale: Liability insurance is acquired to protect the organization from suits by patients arising from negligent acts of employees. Business interruption coverage is usually purchased in tandem with fire insurance. It reimburses an organization for losses sustained while the business is partially or completely shut down after a catastrophic event. The organization's management team (CEO and senior staff) is insured against losses based on business judgment errors through directors and officers coverage. Workers' compensation is the line of coverage that protects employees after on-the-job injuries. It is a no-fault system (negligence is not a factor) that covers employee medical bills and pays a percentage of wages while an employee is unable to work.

24. Answer: 1

Rationale: You were driving your personal vehicle, so your own auto insurer is "primary" (i.e., responds first to a loss). Because you were on company business, your injuries were sustained "within the course and scope of your employment," so there is coverage under the employer's workers' compensation policy for your medical bills and wage replacement. Depending on the circumstances and policy definitions, there could be some "excess" or additional coverage available under the employer's auto policy, but in no event would that carrier be primarily responsible for your losses. This is not the type of incident that homeowner's insurance is intended to cover. The semitrailer, presumably in use as a business vehicle, would not be insured under a driver's personal auto policy.

25. Answer: 4

Rationale: The intent of the National Practitioner Data Bank (NPDB) is to improve the quality of health care by encouraging state licensing boards, hospitals, and other health care entities and professional societies to identify and discipline those who engage in unprofessional behavior and to restrict the ability of incompetent physicians, dentists, and other health care practitioners to move from state to state without disclosure or discovery of previous medical malpractice payment and adverse action history. Adverse actions can involve licensure, clinical privileges, professional society membership, and exclusions from Medicare and Medicaid.

26. Answer: 1, 2, 4

Rationale: The forwarding facility needs to know whether the receiving facility has space for the new arrival and, more importantly, the ability to treat the particular illness for which the patient needs therapy. The receiving agency needs to be contacted and agree on the transfer. The transferring agency must send the patient's medical records. The transfer must be with qualified personnel and transportation equipment. A familiar example of a patient transfer is that of the burn victim, for whom specialty care is mandatory, and the locations of that specialty care are usually limited.

27. Answer: 1

Rationale: Health care policy within the states is codified or enacted into law by the respective state legislature. The state boards of nursing and pharmacy should have significant input in the process, providing the research data and expert "testimony" that the legislature needs to make informed decisions. Nursing organizations should also be willing to provide background information and nurse experts to educate the lawmakers.

28. Answer: 3

Rationale: The managed care organization's (MCO) cost-containment strategy is enhanced if providers practice within the treatment guidelines suggested by the plans. Providers who inform patients that a certain treatment regimen is the preferred alternative create difficulties if that alternative is excluded from coverage. MCOs usually clearly set out the exclusions in the plan documents, and member services personnel are expected to be able to explain the coverage to subscribers. Experimental treatment, if excluded, would be listed as such in the plan documents.

29. Answer: 2

Rationale: These are three of the agencies required to report. Events occurring in the other settings are exempt from reporting requirements under this federal law.

30. Answer: 2

Rationale: This is the most factual note; the writer does not apportion blame or assume liability. The other notes would be "red flags" for a chart reviewer. The mention of an incident report makes it virtually impossible to protect these documents from disclosure, especially in those jurisdictions still affording protection to these internal early warning documents that seek to alert risk management personnel to a potential claim.

31. Answer: 3

Rationale: Patients are often unable to evaluate the quality of the care they receive, but they do react to the way in which the care is delivered. Patient perceptions of rudeness or "uncaring" actions by the provider often spur patients to pursue legal action. Patients tend to be more forgiving of less-than-optimal outcomes if they have been involved in the process and are treated with respect.

32. Answer: 4

Rationale: Making one's own decisions is the basis for informed consent and the ethical underpinning of the Patient Self-Determination Act. "Doing good" (beneficence) and its corollary, "avoiding harm" (nonmaleficence), are ethic principles that are usually cited as the basis for other health care activities, such as maintaining professional competency. Respect for persons is a more global ethical principle supporting much of a nurse's personal philosophy of caring.

33. Answer: 3

Rationale: Usually phrased as duty, breach, proximate cause, and damages, these are the four elements of proof required to prevail in a medical negligence action. Intentional acts are not synonymous with negligent acts. Duty presumes a professional relationship and obligation to provide services. The breach is the error or mistake ascribed to the provider that results in the harm to the patient.

34. Answer: 2

Rationale: A competent adult patient is the person to whom the adult-gerontology primary care NP looks for consent to treat. A surrogate decision maker is sought only when the patient is unable to consent. Individual state laws must be checked for selection and priority of surrogate decision makers.

35. Answer: 1

Rationale: Lay jurors are not expected to know the clinical facts and circumstances involved in a professional negligence claim. The expert witness is necessary to educate the jurors about the medical facts and to testify to the standard of care to be applied. Witnesses with direct involvement in the case are no less credible because of their involvement; their testimony and personal bias, if any, will be evaluated by the jurors in the context of their roles.

36. Answer: 1, 2, 3

Rationale: With respect to nursing specialties, the standard of care is usually a national one. Facility policies, books, and journals are important to review, and physician input may be sought. In some cases, physicians may even be allowed to testify about the standard of care. Opinions of other NPs and current events are not considered a component of expert opinion.

37. Answer: 1, 2, 4

Rationale: One particular advantage of alternative dispute resolution (ADR) is the flexibility of the system. In mediation, for example, the mediator can assist with crafting a solution package that meets all the needs of a party, including such an apology from the health care provider. Money is not always the only answer. Insurers' goals, however, usually do focus on cash, avoiding huge damage awards to plaintiffs. If a mediator is successful in facilitating case settlements, the costs are usually significantly lower than the costs of a court trial. Insurers focusing on the bottom line are not averse to these advantages. Damage awards in the ADR process are generally financial awards. The parties may invest substantial time and money in the ADR process. The arbiter's decision can then be appealed to the district court, which is a disadvantage.

38. Answer: 1

Rationale: Statutes of limitations set out each state's rules for the timing of the filing of lawsuits, including malpractice actions. These statutes are procedural laws in that they describe the "how-to" parameters within which legal rights may be exercised. Minority is considered a legal disability; other state laws usually define it and describe its effects. Rights to sue are not governed by statutes of limitations.

39. Answer: 1, 2, 4

Rationale: Statutes may indeed differ from state to state with respect to the breadth of the protection but most will protect an adult-gerontology primary care NP who renders aid, without expectation of compensation and in a competent manner. Gross negligence will usually void the statutory protections. The adult-gerontology primary care NP is not required to stop and render aid.

40. Answer: 2, 3, 4

Rationale: A professional appearance boosts credibility as a witness. Inappropriate attire and gum chewing detract from the nurse's professional demeanor. Preparation is critical before the practitioner's words are recorded and transcribed as part of the official litigation transcript. The nurse should review documents but should refrain from bringing any materials to the deposition without the attorney's approval. The nurse should always ask for clarification of ambiguous questions. Speculation is not appropriate, as is trying to use sophisticated language and knowledge to confuse the other attorney. Questions about professional work history are always asked, so a copy of the adult-gerontology primary care NP's curriculum vitae (CV) is a useful tool to bring to a deposition.

41. Answer: 2, 3, 4, 5

Rationale: Jousting in the patient's medical record is never a good approach; it provides fodder for plaintiffs' lawyers and does not contribute to quality nursing care. The adult-gerontology primary care NP who has a conflict with another provider should deal with the provider directly, preferably in person. Another arena for resolving such disputes is the quality review process. The remaining options are good practice for documentation.

42. Answer: 1, 2, 3

Rationale: All these factors enter into an analysis of whether it is appropriate to accept a minor's consent to treatment. Another factor to consider is the type of treatment sought. Some states have statutes allowing minors to consent to specific therapies, such as treatment for venereal disease. A statement from a third party without supporting documentation to show that the patient is emancipated is not a factor.

43. Answer: 4

Rationale: Long-term care is a specialized area with layers of regulatory requirements, most stemming from the federal government. Nurses who work in this environment need to be vigilant about learning the rules and maintaining compliance. Ongoing, effective communication with regulators is essential.

44. Answer: 4

Rationale: Adult-gerontology primary care NPs tend to become careless with information management and the way they interact with patients and their personal data. The often wide-open and frantic front desk atmosphere of an office does little to calm patient fears that their information will be too easily accessible to those without a need to know.

45. Answer: 3

Rationale: The co-ed locker room with centerfold photos seems to fit the criteria for a hostile environment, a form of sexual harassment. The harassment seems to be pervasive and longstanding; the women have complained, and apparently no action has been taken. The isolated incident and single date request do not rise to the level of harassment. The participants did not find the actions objectionable, and job performance was not affected. Although the potential was there for the nurse to use the prior relationship either to downgrade the employee or to deny a benefit during the employee performance review, this result did not occur.

46. Answer: 4

Rationale: Advance directives are documents crafted by individuals who personally decide how they wish their future health care decisions to be handled. The documents must be prepared while the signer is fully capable of understanding their content and importance. Because the wife in this scenario is already comatose, she has missed her opportunity to prepare advance directives. This does not mean that the spouse is unable to decide on her medical treatment, only that a different consent process needs to be employed.

47. Answer: 3

Rationale: The option of detaining the patient would create liability potential for the adult-gerontology primary care NP under at least two legal theories: battery and false imprisonment. Talking with the patient would be the first prong of a planned approach to convince this patient that she needs the prescribed medical therapy. Conferring with social services would be the next choice. Court-ordered treatment is a consideration with a viable fetus.

48. Answer: 1

Rationale: This is the overall goal of Americans with Disabilities Act (ADA). It is not another entitlement program, and it cannot impose wheelchair ramp requirements on every building owner in America. Access ramps and interpreters may be required as a "reasonable accommodation" to qualified people in certain defined circumstances. No across-the-board mandate exists for these types of aid to the handicapped population.

49. Answer: 1

Rationale: The U.S. Supreme Court essentially deferred to the states to legislate on this topic. In most states, the activity is not permitted. In one of the states involved in the high court's case, a statute permitting assisted suicide is being challenged. Adult-gerontology primary care NPs need to look at their state laws on this topic for guidance. The providers referenced in the other options would act at their peril if their state laws followed the current majority view.

50. Answer: 1

Rationale: The purpose of a medical malpractice action is to make the claimant whole by the awarding of money damages. The award compensates the claimant or plaintiff for the wrong (or tort) he or she has suffered at the hands of the defendant. On the criminal side, the state sues on behalf of society for violations of society's criminal laws. The punishments are fines, imprisonment, or both. Professional liability insurance usually excludes criminal and intentional acts, so coverage for these types of activities is unlikely.

51. Answer: 2, 3, 5

Rationale: The full-blown jury trial and a bench or court trial is what alternative dispute resolution (ADR) seeks to avoid. Mediation and arbitration are the most well-known forms of ADR. Some jurisdictions use the settlement conference as a technique to attempt settlement after a lawsuit has been filed but before a trial begins. ADR hybrids include "med-arb," in which a proceeding starts out as a mediation, but if the case does not settle, it is referred to an arbitrator for resolution.

52. Answer: 3

Rationale: This is the so-called "long tail" of professional liability; there is always a time lag from the date of injury to the date a claimant files a malpractice action. In the case of an infant, the time lag may be many years because of the statute of limitations. This extends the period of potential risk to the nurse who cares for children. Although a sympathy factor may be involved when jurors decide damages awards, the judgment is usually proportional to the injury and not the age of the claimant. Insurance coverage for pediatric providers is no less available than for other specialties; insurers adjust premiums to account for the level of risk.

53. Answer: 4

Rationale: All patients are entitled to medical information to make an informed decision about treatment. Age, in and of itself, is not an exclusionary criterion. Providers may treat in the other circumstances.

54. Answer: 4

Rationale: If the human resources department has established guidelines for the handling of references, it would be wise to follow them. It is also an effective mechanism to deflect potentially problematic queries by passing requests to the department most equipped to handle them. Most employers will be very circumspect about the information released, often limiting the data to dates of employment only. Without protective state legislation, employers should be prudent about sharing comments on former employees' work histories.

55. Answer: 3

Rationale: The purpose is to determine the appropriateness of the applicant for the job. Identifying health problems to prevent hiring an individual is discriminatory. The mental status and disabilities may also be a part of the preemployment physical but are not the primary purpose.

56. Answer: 2, 3

Rationale: As of January 1, 2015, Occupational Safety and Health Administration (OSHA) requires that all employers must report all work-related fatalities within 8 hours and all work-related inpatient hospitalizations, all amputations, and all losses of an eye within 24 hours. Fatalities occurring within 30 days of a work-related incident must be reported to OSHA.

57. Answer: 3

Rationale: It is required by law that a report of any work-related injury be filed with the industrial commission of the state in which the injury occurred.

58. Answer: 2

Rationale: Occupational Safety and Health Administration (OSHA) requires the report of any injury or illness that requires more than first-aid treatment and/or involves loss of work time, limited work status, loss of consciousness, or death.

59. Answer: 1

Rationale: The purpose is to record occupational injuries and illnesses, including mortality reports and lost workdays, which could also reveal dangerous working conditions.

60. Answer: 4

Rationale: All the conditions listed would qualify under the American Disabilities Act (ADA) and may require accommodation in the workplace.

61. Answer: 4

Rationale: The four major goals of Health Insurance Portability and Accountability Act (HIPAA) of 1996 are to ensure health insurance portability by eliminating "job-lock" because of preexisting medical conditions, reduce health care fraud and abuse, enforce standards for health information, and guarantee security and privacy of health information. Because of protests from civil libertarians and others concerned about privacy issues, the National Individual Identifier has been put on hold until some compromise can ensure that no abuses of such an identifier system will occur. The first compliance HIPAA rule relates to national standards for electronic transactions.

62. Answer: 4

Rationale: The crux of a bioethical dilemma is that the proposed solutions are not perfect and, therefore, create some aspect of moral conflict.

Issues and Trends

63. Answer: 1

Rationale: According to the National Commission on Nursing (1983) and the Task Force on Nursing Practice in Hospitals (1983), the clinical nurse specialist (CNS) role was accepted quite rapidly. The psychiatric CNS role is considered the oldest and most highly developed of the CNS specialties and helped initiate the growth of other CNS specialties.

64. Answer: 4

Rationale: Educational materials given to patients should be based on meeting established health literacy standards in order to facilitate exchange of information. Although evidenced-based practice recommendations provide credible information, the reading level at which information is provided enables understanding. Providing auditory as well as written instruction address learning styles but does not specifically indicate that the information provided as written or discussed meets health literacy standards. Determination of a patient's readiness to learn helps to identify increased likelihood of interest but it does not address how the content of the information is provided in terms of meeting health literacy standards.

65. Answer: 3

Rationale: The adult-gerontology primary care NP should act as a mentor while acting within the professional role competency as identified by the American Association of Colleges and Nursing (AACN) 2010 standards. Teaching classes is part of the teaching competency. Observing and maintain professional bounda-

ries is part of the NP patient relationship. Prescribing medications is part of the management of patient health/illness status.

66. Answer: 1, 4, 5

Rationale: An adult-gerontology primary care NP can see adults (adolescents, late adolescents, as well as emancipated minors) and adults across the life expectancy ranging from young adults to older adults and the frail elderly. Providing prenatal care is not within the scope of practice for an adult-gerontology primary care NP. The patient who is 11 years old should be seen by a pediatric or family NP.

67. Answer: 3

Rationale: Martha Rogers argued that the development of the adult-gerontology primary care NP role was a ploy to lure nurses out of nursing and into medicine, thus weakening and undermining nursing's unique role in health care. This led to a major division within nursing, hindering the establishment of adult-gerontology primary care NP educational programs within the mainstream of graduate nursing education.

68. Answer: 4

Rationale: Loretta Ford, RN, PhD, and Henry Silver, MD, established the first pediatric NP program at the University of Colorado. Hildegard Peplau started the first psychiatric clinical nurse specialist (CNS) program at Rutgers University. Mary Breckenridge established the Frontier Nursing Service in the depressed, rural mountain area of Kentucky, which led to training nurse midwives. Agnes McGee is credited with offering the first postgraduate program for the nurse anesthetist role at St. Vincent's Hospital in Portland, Oregon.

69. Answer: 1

Rationale: Although all these answers are important for the adult-gerontology primary care NP in developing policy skills, the most important is developing political allies. Having political allies in decision-making places (legislature) will enable the adult-gerontology primary care NP to be active and informed regarding issues of regulation, limitations on admitting privileges and prescriptive authority, and managed care.

70. Answer: 4

Rationale: Three major issues are central to the expansion of the adult-gerontology primary care NP role: prescriptive authority, reimbursement privileges, and legal scope of practice. Although political activism is important, it is not specific to collaborative practice.

71. Answer: 3

Rationale: According to the APRN consensus model, there are four APRN roles: nurse anesthetist, nurse-midwife, clinical nurse specialist, and a nurse practitioner. Specialty areas include but are not limited to clinical areas of practice/health care needs rather than patient populations. The adult-gerontology primary care NP represents one of the six practice population foci that addresses specific populations across the lifespan.

72. Answer: 2

Rationale: The International Classification of Diseases (ICD-10) diagnostic codes identify the condition, illness, or injury to be treated and are used for billing insurance carriers. Physicians' Current Procedural Terminology (CPT) codes specify the procedure or medical service given. Medicare and state Medicaid carriers are required by law to use CPT codes. The Health Care Financing Administration Common Procedure Coding System (HCPC) is used for reporting supplies and medical equipment. Minimum Nursing Data Set (MNDS) is classification system of a set of items of essential nursing data with specific definitions and categories related to nursing and nursing care. Having a Medicare and Medicaid number is important, but additional information is required for reimbursement.

73. Answer: 1, 2, 3, 4

Rationale: Requirements for building an APRN curriculum reflecting a consensus model include: completion of graduate studies, meeting accreditation standards, maintaining compliance with core competencies, and maintaining licensure. Nurse Residency Programs are utilized in reference to new graduates who have just obtained licensure.

74. Answer: 3

Rationale: Lewin described three processes of change. Unfreezing involves "breaking the habit" or "disturbing the equilibrium." Moving involves development of new responses based on new information, with a change in attitudes, feelings, behaviors, or values. Refreezing involves reaching a new status quo by stabilizing and integrating new behaviors, with appropriate support to maintain the change. Forming, storming, and norming refer to the stages of group process development. Building relationships, acquiring resources, choosing a solution, and stabilizing lists steps in Havelock's change theory.

75. Answer: 2

Rationale: According to most sources, the adult-gerontology primary care NP role developed as a result of a shortage of primary care physicians in the 1960s and 1970s, when medical specialization was the trend.

76. Answer: 3

Rationale: Medicare is regulated by the federal government and includes the services described, plus outpatient laboratory and radiography. Hospitalization costs are covered under Medicare A.

77. Answer: 4

Rationale: The Balanced Budget Act is a crucial piece of legislation that allows direct payments to adult-gerontology primary care NPs at "80% of the lesser of either the actual charge or 85% of the fee schedule amount of the same service if provided by a physician." This does not change the "incident to" rule, which allows a physician to bill for 100% of an adult-gerontology primary care NP's services, provided the physician is in the suite at the time of the service and readily available to provide assistance.

78. Answer: 4

Rationale: Conflict must be addressed directly by the adult-gerontology primary care NP. The personal characteristics of the medical assistants must not enter into the conflict resolution process. The adult-gerontology primary care NP should determine the issue of conflict, and then work on possible solutions to resolve the issue. Compromise, in which both parties must be willing to give up something, is only one method of conflict resolution.

79. Answer: 4

Rationale: Value-based purchasing (VBP) is an initiative that affects all providers who practice in or admit patients to a hospital setting. VBP is part of the Affordable Care Act of 2009 with the goal to improve quality of patient care by linking payment from the Centers for Medicare and Medicaid Services for inpatient services to successful outcome measures. Essentially, the VBP program adjusts payments to hospitals based on the quality of care they deliver using hospital quality metrics. Accountable care organizations are groups of health care providers who come together voluntarily to give coordinated high quality care to their Medicare patients based on performance measures. The APRN Compact from the National Council of State Boards of Nursing and allows advanced practice registered nurses (APRNs) within the compact states who meet the compact requirements to obtain a multistate license, thereby expanding advanced nursing practice and mobility for APRNs. The Interprofessional Education Collaborative (IPEC) purpose is to connect various health professions to advance interprofessional learning.

80. Answer: 1

Rationale: There are two ways to deal with sexual harassment at work: informally and formally through a grievance procedure. The harassed person should always start with the direct approach and ask the person to stop. The male adult-gerontology primary care NP should tell the female physician in clear terms that her behavior makes him uncomfortable and that he wants it to stop immediately.

81. Answer: 4

Rationale: The adult-gerontology primary care NP is reimbursed at 100% of "incident to" services. Medicare services provided entirely by the adult-gerontology primary care NP are reimbursed at 80% of the lesser of the actual charge or 85% of the fee schedule amount of physicians.

82. Answer: 4

Rationale: The Agency for Healthcare Research and Quality's (AHRQ) purpose or mission statement is to produce evidence-based practice and research to make health care safer for all individuals that is of higher quality, more accessible, equitable, and affordable. The AHRQ works within the U.S. Department of Health and Human Services (USDHHS) and with other agencies to make sure that the evidence-based research is understood and used.

Bibliography

Adams, M., Holland, N., & Urban, C. (2014). *Pharmacology for nurses: A pathophysiologic Approach* (4th ed.). Boston: Pearson.

Administration for Community Living. (2015). The older American's act nutrition program. *Did you know?*. Retrieved from https://aoa.acl.gov/AoA_Programs/hpw/Nutrition_Services/DOCS/OAA-Nutrition-Program-FAQ.pdf.

Agrawal, P., Zane, R. D., & Kosowsky, J. M. (2011). *Pocket emergency medicine*. Philadelphia, PA: Wolters Kluwer Health/Lippincott Williams & Wilkins.

Aljarallah, K. M. (2017). Conventional and alternative treatment approaches for *Clostridium difficile* infection. *International Journal of Health Sciences, 11*, 50–59.

Alligood, M. R. (2014). *Nursing theorists and their work* (8th ed.). St. Louis, MO: Elsevier.

American Geriatrics Society. (2015). AGS updated Beers Criteria for potentially inappropriate medication use in older adults. *Journal of the American Geriatrics Society, 63*(11), 2227–2246.

Ball, J., Dains, J., Flynn, J., Solomon, B., & Stewart, R. (2015). *Seidel's guide to physical examination* (8th ed.). St. Louis: Elsevier/Mosby.

Balsells, E., Filipescu, T., Kyaw, M. H., Wiuff, C., Campbell, H., & Nair, H. (2016). Infection prevention and control of *Clostridium difficile*: a global review of guidelines, strategies, and recommendations. *Journal of Global Health, 6*, 1–18. http://dx.doi.org/10.7189/jogh.06.020410.

Banasikowska, A. K. (2017). Rosacea medication. *Medication summary*. Retrieved from http://emedicine.medscape.com/article/1071429-medication.

Bartlett, J. (2014, November 13). *Diagnostic approach to community-acquired pneumonia in adults*. Retrieved from UpToDate http://www.uptodate.com.contentproxy.phoenix.edu/contents/diagnostic-approach-to-community-acquired-pneumonia-in-adults?source=search_result&search=community+acquired+pneumonia&selectedTitle=2~150#H24.

Barzi, A., Lenz, H. J., Quinn, D. I., & Sadeghi, S. (24 Jan, 2017). Comparative effectiveness of screening strategies for colorectal cancer. *Cancer*. http://dx.doi.org/10.1002/cncr.30518.

Bigley, L. S., & Szilagyi, P. S. (2013). In *Bates' guide to physical examination and history taking*. Philadelphia, PA: Wolters Kluwer.

Browne, K. L., & Merrill, E. (2015). Musculoskeletal management matters: principles of assessment and triage for the nurse practitioner. *The Journal for Nurse Practitioners, 11*(10), 929–939.

Bodhidatta, L., Vithayasai, N., Eimpokalarp, B., Pitarangsi, C., Serichantalergs, O., & Isenbarger, D. W. (2002). Bacterial enteric pathogens in children with acute dysentery in Thailand: increasing importance of quinolone-resistant *Campylobacter*. *The Southeast Asian journal of tropical medicine and public health, 33*, 752–757.

Burns, N., Grove, S. K., & Gray, J. R. (2013). *The Practice of nursing research: appraisal, synthesis, and generation of evidence* (7th ed.). St. Louis, MO: Elsevier.

Buttaravoli, P. M., & Leffler, S. M. (2012). *Minor emergencies*. Philadelphia, PA: Elsevier/Saunders.

Buttaro, T. M., Trybulski, J., Bailey, P. P., & Sandberg-Cook, J. (2013). *Primary care: a collaborative practice* (4th ed.). St. Louis: Elsevier.

Camerota, A., Mastroiacovo, D., Bocale, R., & Desideri, G. (2014). Therapeutic challenges in management of chronic hyperuricemia and gout in the elderly. *Annals of Gerontology and Geriatric Research, 1*(3), 1–6. Retrieved from https://www.jscimedcentral.com/Gerontology/gerontology-1-1012.pdf.

Carey, M., & Lyder, C. H. (2011). Geriatric assessment: essential skills for nurses. *American Nurse Today, 6*(7). Retrieved from https://www.americannursetoday.com/geriatric-assessment-essential-skills-for-nurses/.

Centers for Disease Control (CDC). (1 September, 2012). *Tuberculosis fact sheet*. Retrieved from http://www.cdc.gov/tb/publications/factsheets/testing/skintesting.htm.

Centers for Disease Control (CDC). (26 November, 2014). *Latent tuberculosis infection: A Guide for Primary Health Care Providers*. Retrieved from http://www.cdc.gov/tb/publications/ltbi/diagnosis.htm#3.

Centers for Disease Control (CDC). (2015). *Algorithm for fall risk assessment & interventions*. Retrieved from https://www.cdc.gov/steadi/pdf/algorithm_2015-04-a.pdf.

Centers for Disease Control and Prevention. (2017). *Frequency measures*. Retrieved from https://www.cdc.gov/ophss/csels/dsepd/ss1978/lesson3/section1.html.

Centers for Disease Control (CDC). (2017). *Information for adult patients: 2017 Recommended immunizations for adults: by age and health condition*. Retrieved from https://www.cdc.gov/vaccines/schedules/downloads/adult/adult-schedule-easy-read.pdf.

Centers for Disease Control and Prevention. (2017). *Mortality frequency measures*. Retrieved from https://www.cdc.gov/ophss/csels/dsepd/ss1978/lesson3/section3.html.

Chalasani, N., Younossi, Z., Lavine, J. E., Diehl, A. M., Brunt, E. M., Cusi, K., & Sanyal, A. J. (2012). The diagnosis and management of non-alcoholic fatty liver disease: practice guideline by the American Gastroenterological Association, American Association for the Study of Liver Diseases, and American College of Gastroenterology. *Gastroenterology, 142*, 1592–1609.

Chey, W. D., Leontiadis, G. I., Howden, C. W., & Moss, S. F. (2017). ACG Clinical Guideline: treatment of *Helicobacter pylori* infection. *American Journal of Gastroenterology, 112*, 212–238. http://dx.doi.org/10.1038/ajg.2016.563.

Chowalloor, P. V., Keen, H. I., & Inderjeeth, C. A. (2013). Gout in the elderly. *OA Elderly Medicine, 1*(1), 2. Retrieved from http://www.oapublishinglondon.com/article/776.

Chinniah, N., & Gupta, M. (2014). Pruritus in the elderly: a guide to assessment and management. *Australian Family Physician*, *43*(10), 710–713. Retrieved from http://www.racgp.org.au/afp/2014/october/pruritus-in-the-elderly-%E2%80%93-a-guide-to-assessment-and-management/.

Chism, L. A. (2014). Guiding your patients through menopause. *American Nurse Today*, *9*(1). Retrieved from https://www.americannursetoday.com/guiding-your-patients-through-menopause/.

Clothier, A. (2014). Assessing and managing skin tears in older people. *Independent Nurse for Primary Care and Community Nurses*. Retrieved from http://www.independentnurse.co.uk/clinical-article/assessing-and-managing-skin-tears-in-older-people/63411/.

Curl, K. (2014). Hypothyroidism: clinical challenges in diagnosis and treatment. *Clinician Reviews*, *24*(7), 40–46.

Dains, J. E., Baumann, L. C., & Scheibel, P. (2016). *Advanced health assessment and clinical diagnosis in primary care* (5th ed.). St. Louis: Elsevier.

deLeon-Demare, K., MacDonald, J., Gregory, D. M., Katz, A., & Halas, G. (2015). Articulating nurse practitioner practice using King's theory of goal attainment. *Journal of the American Association of Nurse Practitioners*, *27*, 631–636.

Dellon, E. S., Gonsalves, N., Hirano, I., Furuta, G. T., Liacouras, C. A., & Katzka, D. A. (2013). ACG clinical guideline: evidence based approach to the diagnosis and management of esophageal eosinophilia and eosinophilic esophagitis (EoE). *American Journal of Gastroenterology*, *108*, 679–692.

Dickinson, B. T., Kisiel, J., Alhquist, D. A., & Grady, W. M. (2015). Molecular markers for colorectal cancer screening. *Gut*, *64*, 1485–1494. http://dx.doi.org/10.1136/gutjnl-2014-308075.

Dietrich, E. (2016). Choosing an SGLT-2 Inhibitor for a patient with type 2 diabetes: which agent (if any) is best? *Consultant*, *56*(11), 1008–1009.

DiPrio, J. T., Talvert, R. L., Yee, G., Matzke, G., Wells, B., & Posey, L. M. (2016). *Pharmacotherapy: a pathophysiologic approach* (10th ed.). New York: McGraw Hill Medical.

Domino, F. J. (Ed.). (2016). *The 5-minute clinical consult standard 2016* (24th ed.). Philadelphia: Wolters Kluwer Health.

Dougherty, T., Jr., Stephen, S., Borum, M., L., & Doman, D., B. (2014). Emerging therapeutic options for eosinophilic esophagitis. *Gastroenterology & Hepatology*, *10*, 106–116.

Dunphy, L. M., Winland-Brown, J. E., Porter, B. O., & Thomas, D. J. (2015). *Primary care: the art and science of advanced practice nursing* (4th ed.). Philadelphia: F.A. Davis Company.

Edmunds, M. W., & Mayhew, M. S. (2014). *Pharmacology for the primary care provider* (4th ed.). St. Louis: Elsevier.

Farrell, T. C., & Keeping-Burke, L. (2014). The primary prevention of cardiovascular disease: nurse practitioners using behavior modification strategies. *Canadian Journal of Cardiovascular Nursing*, *24*(1), 8–15.

Fenstermacher, K., & Hudson, B. T. (2016). *Practice guidelines for family nurse practitioners* (4th ed.). St. Louis, MO: Elsevier.

Ferri, F. F. (2015). *Ferri's Clinical Advisor 2015: 5 books in 1*.

Fischbach, F., & Dunning, M. (Eds.). (2015). *A manual of laboratory and diagnostic tests* (9th ed.) Philadelphia, PA: Wolters Kluwer.

Fitzpatrick, J. J. (2016). The peer review process revisited [Editorial]. *Applied Nursing Research*, *33*, 186.

Global Initiative for Asthma. (2016, April). *Pocket guide for asthma management and prevention*. Retrieved from http://www.ginasthma.org/.

Global Initiative for Chronic Obstructive Lung Disease. (2017, January). *Global strategy for the diagnosis, management, and prevention of chronic obstructive pulmonary disease*. Retrieved from http://goldcopd.com/guidelines-global-strategy-for-diagnosis-management.html.

Guidelines for advanced practice nursing. Role self-assessment using Benner's Novice to Expert Model. (n.d.). Retrieved from http://www.napnapcareerguide.com/wp-content/uploads/2013/02/Benners-Self-Assessment-Tool.pdf.

Habif, T. P., Campbell, J. L., Chapman, M. S., Dinulos, J. G., & Zug, K. A. (2011). *Skin disease: diagnosis and treatment* (3rd ed.). St. Louis, MO: Elsevier/Saunders.

Hain, D., & Fleck, L. M. (2014). Barriers to NP practice that impact healthcare design. *OJIN. The Online Journal of Issues in Nursing*, *19*(2). Manuscript 2. Retrieved from http://www.nursingworld.org/MainMenuCategories/ANAMarketplace/ANAPeriodicals/OJIN/TableofContents/Vol-19-2014/No2-May-2014/Barriers-to-NP-Practice.html.

Hamric, A. B., Hanson, C. M., Tracy, M. F., & O'Grady, E. T. (2014). *Advanced practice nursing: an integrative approach* (5th ed.). St. Louis: Elsevier/Saunders.

Han, J., & Han, S. (2014). Primary prevention of Alzheimer's disease: is it an attainable goal? *Journal of Korean Medical Science*, *29*(7), 886–892. Retrieved from https://www.ncbi.nlm.nih.gov/pmc/articles/PMC4101775/.

Hartnett, P. D., & O'Keefe, C. (2016). Improving skin care knowledge among nurse practitioners. *Journal of the Dermatology Nurses' Association*, *8*(2), 123–128.

Hossain, N., Kanwar, P., & Mohanty, S. M. (2016). A comprehensive updated review of pharmaceutical and non-pharmaceutical treatment for NAFLD. *Gastroenterology Research and Practice*, *2016*, 1–16. http://dx.doi.org/10.1155/2016/7109270.

Janz, T., Lu, K., Povlow, M. R., & Urso, B. (2016). A review of colorectal cancer detection modalities, stool dna, and fecal immunochemistry testing in adults over the age of 50. *Cureus*, *8*(12), e931. http://dx.doi.org/10.7759/cureus.931.

Jarvis, C. (2016). *Physical examination & health assessment* (7th ed.). St Louis, MO: Elsevier.

Jones, G. (2016). *Epocrates plus version*. BMJ Publishing.

Kashani, M., Eliasson, A., Vernalis, M., Bailey, K., & Terhaar, M. (2015). A systematic approach incorporating family history improves identification of cardiovascular disease risk. *Journal of Cardiovascular Nursing*, *30*(4), 292–297.

Katz, P. O., Gerson, L. B., & Vela, M. F. (2013). Guidelines for the diagnosis and management of gastroesophageal reflux disease. *American Journal of Gastroenterology*, *108*, 308–328.

King, S. (2012). Chronic pain management in the elderly: an update on safe, effective options. *Consultant*, *52*(5). Retrieved from http://www.consultant360.com/article/chronic-pain-management-elderly-update-safe-effective-options.

LoBiondo-Wood, G., & Haber, J. (2014). *Nursing research: methods and critical appraisal for evidence-based practice* (8th ed.). St. Louis, MO: Elsevier.

Lanza, F. L., Chan, F. K. L., Quigley, E. M. M., & the practice parameters committee of the American College of Gastroenterology. (2009). Guidelines for prevention of NSAID-related ulcer complications. *American Journal of Gastroenterology*, *104*, 728–738.

Levin, B., Lieberman, D. A., McFarland, B., Andrews, K. S., Brooks, D., Bond, J., & Winawer, S. J. (2008). Screening and surveillance for the early detection of colorectal cancer and adenomatous polyps, 2008: a joint guideline from the American Cancer Society, the US Multi-Task Force on Colorectal Cancer, and the American College of Radiology. *Gastroenterology, 134*, 1570–1595.

Lexicomp drug reference handbook for advance practice nursing. (2015). (16th ed.). Philadelphia: Wolters Kluwer.

Libman, D., & Cheung, A. (2015). A practical approach to osteoporosis management in the geriatric population. *Canadian Geriatrics Journal, 18*(1). Retrieved from http://www.cgjonline.ca/index.php/cgj/article/view/129/232.

LoBiondo-Wood, G., & Haber, J. (2014). *Nursing research: methods and critical appraisal for evidence-based practice* (8th ed.). St. Louis, MO: Elsevier.

Kern, B., & Rosh, A. J. (2014, September 4). *Hyperventilation syndrome treatment & management.* Retrieved from http://emedicine.medscape.com/article/807277-treatment#d10.

Kececi, A., & Bulduk, S. (2012). Health education for the elderly, Geriatrics. In C. Atwood (Ed.), *InTech* Retrieved from http://cdn.intechopen.com/pdfs/29304.pdf.

Kenny, K. A. (2016). Potential complications of herpes zoster. Early symptom recognition and vaccination is the key. *Advance for NPs & Pas.* Retrieved from http://nurse-practitioners-and-physician-assistants.advanceweb.com/Features/Articles/Potential-Complications-of-Herpes-Zoster.aspx.

Kiefer, M., & Chong, C. (2014). *Pocket primary care.* Philadelphia: Wolters Kluwer/Lippincott Williams & Wilkins Health.

Mackey, P. A., & Whitaker, M. D. (2015). Osteoporosis: a therapeutic update. *The Journal for Nurse Practitioners, 11*(10), 1011–1017.

Mandell, L. A., Wunderink, R. G., Anzueto, A., Bartlett, J. G., Campbell, G. D., Dean, N. C., & Whitney, C. G. (2007). Infectious Diseases Society of America/American Thoracic Society consensus guidelines on the management of community-acquired pneumonia in adults. *Clinical Infectious Diseases*, S27–S72.

McCance, K. L., & Huether, S. E. (2014). *The biologic basis for disease in adults and children* (7th ed.). St. Louis, MO: Elsevier.

Naganuma, T., Kuriyama, S., Kakizaki, M., Sone, T., Nakaya, N., Ohmori-Matsuda, K., & Tsuji, I. (2008). Coffee consumption and the risk of oral, pharyngeal, and esophageal cancers in Japan: The Miyagi cohort study. *American Journal of Epidemiology, 168*, 1425–1432.

Nickatis, D. M., & Frederickson, K. (2015). [Editorial]. Nursing knowledge and theory: where is the economic value? *Nursing Economic$, 33*(4), 3238–3239.

Pagana, K., Pagana, T. J., & Pagana, T. N. (2015). *Mosby's diagnostic and laboratory test reference* (12th ed.). St. Louis, MO: Elsevier.

Palmer, C. (2013). Dyslipidemia in adults: how recent research and recommendations affect nurse practitioner practice. *Journal of Nurse Practitioners, 9*(10), 669–678.

Pfenninger, J. L., & Fowler, G. C. (2011). *Procedures for primary care* (3rd ed.). St. Louis, MO: Elsevier.

Rajput, R., Chatterjee, S., & Rajput, M. (2011). Can levothyroxine be taken as an evening dose? *Journal of Thyroid Research.* http://dx.doi.org/10.4061/2011/505239. 505239.

Resnick, L. A., & Shufeldt, J. (2014). *Textbook of urgent care medicine.* Scottsdale: Urgent Care Textbooks.

Rice, P., Mehan, U., Hamilton, C., & Kim, S. (2014). Screening, assessment, and treatment of osteoporosis for the nurse practitioner: key questions and answers for clinical practice – A Canadian perspective. *Journal of the American Academy of Nurse Practitioners, 26*(7), 378–385.

Riddle, M. S., DuPont, H. L., & Connor, B. A. (2016). ACG clinical guideline: diagnosis, treatment, and prevention of acute diarrheal infections in adults. *American Journal of Gastroenterology, 111*, 602–622.

Roberts, M. E., & Davis, L. L. (2013). Cardiovascular disease in women: a nurse practitioner's guide to prevention. *Journal of Nurse Practitioners, 9*(10), 679–687.

Roebuck, H., Moran, K., MacDonald, D., Shumer, S., & McCune, R. L. (2015). Assessing skin cancer prevention and detection educational needs: an anagogical approach. *The Journal for Nurse Practitioners, 11*(4), 409–416.

Rubio-Tapia, A., Hill, I. D., Kelly, C. P., Calderwood, A. H., & Murray, J. A. (2013). ACG guidelines: diagnosis and management of celiac disease. *American Journal of Gastroenterology, 108*, 656–676.

Samadder, J., Valentine, J. F., Guthery, S., Singh, H., Bernstein, C. N., Yan, Y., & Smith, K. R. (2017). Colorectal cancer inflammatory bowel diseases: a population-based study in Utah. *Digestive Diseases and Science.* http://dx.doi.org/10.1007/s10620-016-4435-4. Jan 3.

Schaefer, P. (2011). Urticaria: evaluation and treatment. *American Family Physician, 83*(9) 1078–1074.

Song, S.-G., & Kim, S.-H. (2011). Pruritus Ani. *Journal of Korean Society of Colproctology, 27*, 54–57. http://dx.doi.org/10.3393/jksc.2011.27.2.54.

Stevens, K. (2013). The impact of evidenced-based practice in nursing and the next big ideas. *OJIN The Online Journal of Issues in Nursing, 18*(2). http://dx.doi.org/10.3912/OJIN.Vol18No02Man04.

Stollman, N., Smalley, W., & Hirano, I. (2015). AGA Institute Clinical Guidelines Committee. *Gastroenterology, 149*, 1944–1949.

Swartz, M. (2014). *Textbook of physical diagnosis: history and examination* (7th ed.). St. Louis, MO: Elsevier/Saunders.

Tack, J., & Drossman, D. A. (2017). What's new in Rome IV? *Journal of Neurogastroenterology Motililty.* http://dx.doi.org/10.1111/nmo.13053.

Tabibian, N., Swehli, E., Boyd, A., Umbreen, A., & Tabibian, J. H. (2017). Review Abdominal adhesions: a practical review of an often-overlooked entity. *Annals of Medicine and Surgery, 15*, 9e13.

Tenner, S., Baillie, J. M., DeWitt, J., & Swaroop, S. (2013). American College of Gastroenterology Guideline: Management of Acute Pancreatitis. *American Journal of Gastroenterology.* http://dx.doi.org/10.1038/ajg.2013.218.

Tse, Y., Armstrong, D., Andrews, C. N., Bitton, A., Bressler, B., Marshall, J., & LiuCan, L. W. C. (2017). Treatment Algorithm for Chronic Idiopathic Constipation and Constipation-Predominant Irritable Bowel Syndrome Derived from a Canadian National Survey and Needs Assessment on Choices of Therapeutic Agents. *Canadian Journal of Gastroenterology & Hepatology.* http://dx.doi.org/10.1155/2017/8612189.

Tintinalli, J. E., & Cline, D. (2012). *Tintinalli's emergency medicine manual.* New York: McGraw-Hill Medical.

Tomek-Roksandic, S., Mrcela, N. T., Narancic, N. S., Sostar, Z., Lukic, M., Durakovic, Z., Ljubicic, M., & Vucevac, V. (2013). Program of primary, secondary and tertiary prevention for the elderly. *Periodicum Biologorium, 115*(4), 475–481.

Touhy, T. A., & Jett, K. (2016). *Ebersole & Hess' toward healthy aging: Human Needs and Nursing Response* (9th ed.). St. Louis, MO: Elsevier.

Toy, E. C., Briscoe, D. A., & Britton, B. (2012). *Case files*. New York: McGraw-Hill Medical.

Toy, E. C. (2013). *Case files*. New York: McGraw-Hill Medical.

Velez, R., Donnelly-Strozzo, M., & Stanik-Hutt, J. (2016). Simplifying the complexity of primary hyperparathyroidism. *The Journal for Nurse Practitioners, 12*(5), 346–352.

United States Preventive Task Force Services. (2013, December). *Final recommendation statement lung cancer screening.* Retrieved from http://www.uspreventiveservicestaskforce.org/Page/Document/RecommendationStatementFinal/lung-cancer-screening.

United States Preventive Task Force Services. (2016). *Final recommendation statement osteoporosis screening.* Retrieved from https://www.uspreventiveservicestaskforce.org/Page/Document/RecommendationStatementFinal/osteoporosis-screening#clinical-considerations.

US Food & Drug. (May 12, 2016). *FDA Drug Safety Communication: FDA advises restricting fluoroquinolone antibiotic use for certain uncomplicated infections; warns about disabling side effects that can occur together.* Retrieved from https://www.fda.gov/Drugs/DrugSafety/ucm500143.htm.

Van Den Wijngaart, L. S., Sieben, A., Van Der Vlugt, M., de Leeuw, F. E., & Bredie, S. J. H. (2015). A nurse-led multidisciplinary intervention to improve cardiovascular disease profile of patients. *Western Journal of Nursing Research, 37*(6), 705–723.

Woo, T., & Robinson, M. (2016). *Pharmacotherapeutics for advance practice nurse prescribers* (4th ed.). Philadelphia: FA Davis.

Wood, J. W., & Gordon, P. (2012). Preventing CVD in women: The NP's role. *The Nurse Practitioner, 37*(2), 26–33.